The Complete Guide to

Women's Health

BRUCE D. SHEPHARD, M.D., F.A.C.O.G., is an obstetrician/gynecologist in private practice in Tampa, where he is also on the faculty of the University of South Florida College of Medicine. He serves on a statewide advisory committee on midwifery and has studied legislative issues affecting women's health care nationwide under a fellowship awarded by the American College of Obstetricians and Gynecologists.

CARROLL A. SHEPHARD, R.N., Ph.D., is a psychologist affiliated with the Counseling Center for Human Development at the University of South Florida. She is active in consumer health education and has taught childbirth preparation and parenting classes.

The Complete Guide to

Women's Health

Bruce D. Shephard, M.D., F.A.C.O.G.

Carroll A. Shephard, R.N., Ph.D.

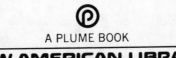

A PLUME BOOK

NEW AMERICAN LIBRARY

NEW YORK AND SCARBOROUGH, ONTARIO

Note to the Reader

The ideas, procedures, and suggestions contained in this book are not intended as a substitute for consulting with your physician. All matters regarding your health require medical supervision.

NAL BOOKS ARE AVAILABLE AT QUANTITY DISCOUNTS WHEN USED TO PROMOTE PRODUCTS OR SERVICES. FOR INFORMATION PLEASE WRITE TO PREMIUM MARKETING DIVISION, NEW AMERICAN LIBRARY, 1633 BROADWAY, NEW YORK, NEW YORK 10019.

Published by Arrangement with Mariner Publishing Company, Inc.

℗ PLUME TRADEMARK REG. U.S. PAT. OFF. AND FOREIGN COUNTRIES REGISTERED TRADEMARK—MARCA REGISTRADA HECHO EN FORGE VILLAGE, MASS., U.S.A.

SIGNET, SIGNET CLASSIC, MENTOR, PLUME, MERIDIAN and NAL BOOKS are published *in the United States* by New American Library, 1633 Broadway, New York, New York 10019, *in Canada* by The New American Library of Canada Limited, 81 Mack Avenue, Scarborough, Ontario M1L 1M8

Library of Congress Cataloging in Publication Data
Shephard, Bruce D., 1944–
    The complete guide to women's health.
    Includes index.
    1. Gynecology—Popular works.   2. Obstetrics—Popular works.   3. Women—Health and hygiene.   I. Shephard, Carroll A., 1944–   . II. Title.   [DNLM: 1. Gynecology —popular works.   2. Obstetrics—popular works. WP 120 S548c]
RG121.S533   1985   618   84-29501
ISBN 0-452-25673-9 (pbk.)

First Plume Printing, June, 1985

2 3 4 5 6 7 8 9

PRINTED IN THE UNITED STATES OF AMERICA

Dedicated to our parents

Madelyn R. Shephard, 1914–1979
Richard G. Shephard
Georgianna C. Swanson
Eldon C. Swanson, M.D.

Contents

Tables

Preface

This book was written for you and for all women who wish to participate more actively and more knowledgeably in their own health care.

Until fairly recently, health care meant, for most women, a visit to the doctor when there was a medical problem. Health care meant finding a "good" doctor who would make the right medical decisions for his or her patient. Today this concept is being challenged as more and more women are discovering that, even without a medical background, they can learn to use a vast amount of information about their own health care. The intention is not to replace medical care but to shift some emphasis for maintaining good health from the medical professional to the individual.

The problem has been: What resources does today's woman have at her disposal to gain this needed knowledge? The result, during this trend toward self-education and self-responsibility, has been health care books by the score.

So why another women's health book?

We prepared this book because we felt it would fill a special need, in the following two ways:

(1) *By serving as a single, comprehensive resource on women's health.* We think it is important to provide information in many significant areas of women's health in addition to those related strictly to gynecology and childbirth. (A glance at the table of contents and the list of tables will give a good idea of the book's wide coverage.)

(2) *By providing specific strategies for health care problems.* Forty chapters of the book provide step-by-step diagrams to help the reader determine when she should seek medical treatment and when she can successfully care for her own health problems. Elsewhere in the book we have encouraged decision-making approaches in matters like birth control, birthing alternatives, estrogen replacement therapy, and surgery, as well as in many other areas.

To add to the reader's knowledge and understanding, we have included in the appendices a *glossary* of common medical terms used throughout the book, a suggested *further reading* list, and a list of *resource groups* that may provide supplementary information on specific subjects.

Our goal in writing this book was to help women to better understand their body functioning, to become aware of the alternatives open to them in the many areas of health concerns, and to learn about the various parts of our complex health care system that might have seemed a mystery before. We hope you will be able to use this information to realize your own potential for medical self care and to be able to make informed decisions about many of your own health problems.

Bruce D. Shephard, M.D., F.A.C.O.G.
Carroll A. Shephard, R.N., Ph.D.

July, 1982

Foreword

Women seeking a complete and up-to-date health guide for the 1980s will find this thoughtful, professional volume a most valuable resource. The Shephards, a husband-wife, doctor-nurse team, have taken a humanistic perspective that is oriented to women as informed users of health care services. The authors talk as people talking with other people about medical issues that are important to all women concerned about their health.

The Complete Guide to Women's Health offers an extraordinary amount of practical information about such subjects as pregnancy, birth control, sexually transmitted disease, menopause, sterilization, and hysterectomy. In fact, the Shephards might have titled their book *Everything You Need to Know about Obstetrics and Gynecology*, except that they cover other issues as well. In the book specialists assist women in choosing and using services within the often-confusing health care system. Other parts of the book deal with preventive health concerns. Nutrition, exercise, and drug problems are well covered with separate discussions for both the pregnant and nonpregnant woman.

The Complete Guide to Women's Health is a leader among "consumer-oriented" health books for women which have been published in recent years. Like the field of medicine, such books have become more and more specialized and technical. It is increasingly difficult to find an up-to-date single volume overview on the subject of women's health simply because of the amount of material involved. The Shephards have combined their mutual professional expertise and relied upon sixteen consultants to produce a work which is both exhaustive and meticulously researched.

What makes *The Complete Guide to Women's Health* different from other books is its emphasis upon the reader's active involvement in decision making as opposed to merely passive understanding of medical facts. This problem-oriented approach is most obvious in Section Eleven, where forty common health problems, covered in chapters alphabetically from *acne* to *weight gain and weight loss*, are discussed. In each of these forty chapters, step-by-step diagrams are used to indicate whether home treatment or medical care represents the best choice. The reader will find outlined elsewhere in the book strategies for dealing with other problems, such as finding the right doctor (Section One), selecting a method of birth control (Section Two), deciding whether to take estrogen hormones (Section Six), and determining whether or not to have female surgery (Section Nine).

The wide range of symptoms and problems covered in *The Complete Guide to Women's Health* will enable readers to identify warning signs and take appropriate measures when health problems are in their early stages. Use of this book will go a long way toward helping a woman better understand her body, her health, and her options when she needs medical care.

Louise B. Tyrer, M.D., F.A.C.O.G.
Vice-President for Medical Affairs
Planned Parenthood Federation of America, Inc.
New York, New York

Acknowledgments

A book of this type would not be possible without the generous cooperation and support of many people. We are especially indebted to our editor, Shirley M. Miller, for her constructive guidance, enthusiasm, and painstaking attention to detail throughout an intensely busy four-month period of reorganizing, revising, and editing. We also owe a very special thanks to Carole Cheeley, R.N., for her creative suggestions toward the book's organization and for her able, sensitive assistance in editing the manuscript's preliminary draft.

We want to thank the nurses and office staff of Tampa Obstetrics and Gynecology Associates, and the physicians of this association: Ralph M. Stephan, Cyrus L. Gray, and Nicholas G. Fallieras. To all of these individuals we are most grateful for their patience and support during the past three years. We are no less indebted to the many patients who shared their enthusiasm with us and made suggestions about the book and who were most understanding during office interruptions and scheduling delays related to the book's publication.

We want to add a special note of appreciation to Priscilla Adkins for the skill, patience, and cheerfulness with which she accomplished the voluminous typing of a much revised and difficult manuscript. In addition we are grateful to Margaret B. Horacek, Associate University Librarian at the University of South Florida, who assisted us throughout our research. We also want to thank several other people who helped with research or manuscript preparation, including Marion Reid, Carol Guerriere, Doris Fletcher, June Owrey, Melinda Gray, Susan Fallieras, Linda Gentry, Etta Breit, Nancy Major, Suzan Pagano, and Steven Lieber, D.M.D.

We likewise extend our thanks to the administration, nursing staff, operating room technicians, and anesthesia department of Women's Hospital, Tampa, for their cooperation and assistance in setting up many of the photographs used in this book. We appreciate the creative work of Joseph Traina in producing the photographs and drawings for the book. We want to acknowledge the help of G. D. Searle & Co. and Parke-Davis, division of Warner-Lambert Company, for permission to reproduce several illustrations appearing in the book. A special thanks is extended to Terry Peterson for her capable assistance in preparing the initial drawings for the book.

We wish to thank the following people for their counsel, friendship, and warm support during many difficult and challenging stages of the book's development: Doritha Poole, Minnie Dennard, Angela and Sonja Ossorio, Fredric Mendes, Joanne Swanson, Lori Del Rossi, Nancy Segall, Richard and Bonnie Hoffman, Maria Vega, Richard Swanson, Lee Minton,

Carol Lieber, and Nancy Bruemmer. We are especially grateful to Hugh Rawson for his encouragement during the manuscript's early stages which later turned out to be so valuable.

We want to thank our children, Christopher and Carleton, for the patience they showed their parents during the seemingly endless time of "working on the book."

Finally, we wish to thank M. N. Manougian, President of Mariner Publishing Company, and his staff. It was he who recognized the timeliness and need for this work and provided the patience and support so essential to the development of a high-quality book.

Bruce D. Shephard, M.D., F.A.C.O.G.
Carroll A. Shephard, R.N., Ph.D.

Consultants

We very much appreciate the kindness of our various colleagues (listed alphabetically below) who reviewed selected portions of the manuscript dealing with their particular areas of expertise. Their comments and suggestions were an invaluable contribution toward making the book accurate, complete, and up-to-date.

John S. Breen, M.D.
  Assistant Professor, Department of
    Internal Medicine
  University of South Florida College of
    Medicine
  Chief, Section of Infectious Diseases
  VA Hospital
  Tampa, Florida

Sexually transmitted diseases

Denis Cavanagh, M.D., F.A.C.O.G.
  American Cancer Society, Ed C. Wright
    Professor of Clinical Oncology
  University of South Florida College of
    Medicine
  Tampa, Florida

Cancer of the female reproductive system

Carole Cornell, R.N., B.S.
  Operating Room Supervisor
  Women's Hospital
  Tampa, Florida

Hospital care before and after surgery

Kathleen J. Dolan, R.N., M.S.
  Assistant Director of Nursing Service
  University of California
  San Francisco Medical Center
  San Francisco, California

Pregnancy and childbirth

Charles R. Engle, R.Ph.
  Eckerd Drugs
  Tampa, Florida

Drugs

Nicholas G. Fallieras, M.D.
  Fellow, American College of Obstetrics
    and Gynecology
  Tampa, Florida

Pregnancy and childbirth

Dianne Swanson Gaines, M.S.
  Registered Physical Therapist
  Palatka, Florida

Joint and back problems and physical fitness

Susan Howard, M.S., M.P.H. 　Registered Dietician 　Tampa, Florida	Nutrition
Lorraine Kushner 　Childbirth Educator 　Certified by the American Society for 　　Psychoprophylaxis in Obstetrics 　Supervisor, Lamaze Childbirth Preparation 　　Program 　Hillsborough Community College 　Tampa, Florida	Pregnancy and 　childbirth
Norman R. Miller, Ph.D. 　Executive Director 　Guidance Center of Hernando County 　Brooksville, Florida	Depression; nervousness 　and anxiety
Marilyn Myerson, Ph.D. 　Assistant Professor, Women's Studies 　　Program 　University of South Florida 　Tampa, Florida	Female sexuality
Frank C. Riggall, M.D. 　Fellow, American College of Obstetrics 　　and Gynecology 　Assistant Professor of Obstetrics and 　　Gynecology 　University of Florida College of Medicine 　Gainesville, Florida	Pregnancy and 　childbirth
John R. Tagler, R.Ph. 　Eckerd Drugs 　Tampa, Florida	Drugs
Susan H. Tagler, R.Ph. 　Eckerd Drugs 　Tampa, Florida	Drugs
Kathleen E. Toomy, M.D. 　Assistant Professor of Pediatrics 　Division of Genetics 　Children's Hospital 　National Medical Center 　Washington, D.C.	Genetics
Barry S. Verkauf, M.D. 　Fellow, American College of Obstetrics 　　and Gynecology 　Associate Professor of Obstetrics and 　　Gynecology 　University of South Florida College of 　　Medicine 　Tampa, Florida	Infertility; hormone 　problems

one

Health Strategies for Women

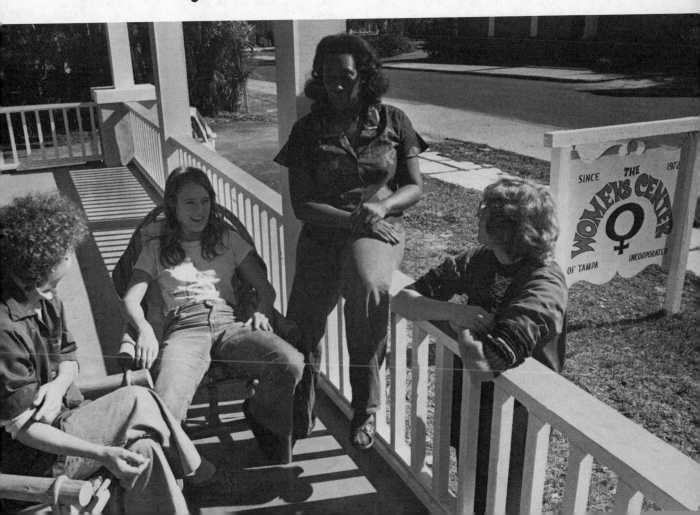

1

Choosing the Right Doctor or Other Health Professional

The best time to choose a physician is when you don't especially need one. Common sense tells us that if you wait until an emergency arises, then you must accept whatever care, good or grim, is available. Your health is too precious to settle for this hit-or-miss course of action. This chapter aims to ease the way for you to leisurely research and find the best doctor for your needs and your money. Although in many parts of the country there are reliable cost-saving alternatives to the doctor—nurse-midwives and nurse practitioners —(and we'll talk about them before this chapter ends), we'll concentrate first on demystifying the M.D.

Four Types of Physician

Most women who want a doctor as their primary health care provider choose from four types of physician: the general practitioner (often called a G.P.), the family practitioner, the internist, or the obstetrician-gynecologist (referred to by some people as an OB-GYN, pronouncing each letter separately). Each of these doctors attended medical school for four years and each must pass an exam in order to be licensed to practice in his or her State. The educational differences among these doctors lie in their postgraduate training.

A general practitioner (the G.P.) is either an M.D. (Doctor of Medicine) or a D.O. (Doctor of Osteopathy) whose knowledge of obstetrics (which deals with women during pregnancy and childbirth) and gynecology (the study of the functions and diseases of the female organs) may be limited, because these areas of study are now electives in most medical schools. The first postgraduate year, formerly called "internship," may or may not include a period of study in obstetrics and gynecology. In fact, in some States, this postgraduate training has been abolished as a requirement for State licensure.

The family practitioner is a new form of specialist who is replacing the G.P. in many parts of the country. The three years of training following medical school includes a minimum of three months of obstetrics and gynecology. Both the G.P. and the family practitioner are oriented as primary care physicians to treat the entire family. They generally do not perform surgery but will refer patients to surgeons or other specialists if special problems arise. These generalists may also make referrals for obstetrical and gynecological care.

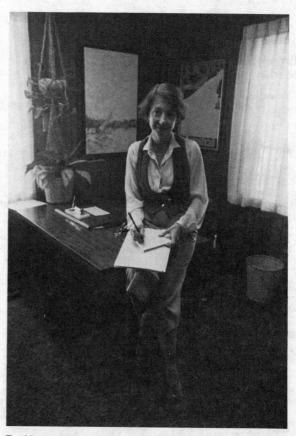

Dr. Nancy C. Bruemmer, gynecologist.

The internist, a specialist in internal medicine, has three or more years in postgraduate training with possibly three months in obstetrics and gynecology. In addition, the internist may have a subspecialty in one of many areas of study: the heart (cardiology), the joints (rheumatology), the digestive system (gastroenterology), and so on. Again, if a medical condition outside the expertise of the internist occurs, he or she will refer patients to a qualified specialist. The internist may or may not perform routine gynecology checkups; that's something you'll need to ask.

The obstetrician-gynecologist takes three to four years of specialty training after medical school, including a minimum of eighteen months of obstetrics and eighteen months of gynecology. Similar to the internist, the OB-GYN may take subspecialty training in areas such as high-risk pregnancy or gynecological cancer. Obstetrician-gynecologists, who often provide primary care for women because of the declining numbers of general practitioners, also guide patients to the right health professional when serious medical problems occur.

Alternative Health Professionals

As health care costs continue to rise in the 1980s, *physician extenders*—especially nurse-midwives and nurse practitioners—will become more visible providers of women's health care because they can save you money without your having to sacrifice quality of care. These alternative health care providers, who usually work under the supervision of a physician, may be the right choice for the woman who is in general good health. Both perform routine breast and pelvic exams and provide excellent contraceptive counseling. And both are usually trained to send you to the appropriate physician if unusual medical problems develop. Be aware, however, that their educational backgrounds vary.

A certified nurse-midwife (CNM) is a registered nurse who has taken at least one year of additional specialized training in a program approved by the American College of Nurse-Midwives. The CNM usually works closely with an obstetrician and is trained to provide complete obstetrical care including delivery in uncomplicated pregnancies.

Registered nurses in many States can train to become family or gynecology nurse practitioners through specialized training programs ranging from a few months up to nearly two years. The programs consist of a formal curriculum leading to either a certificate or Master's degree in nursing. Nurse practitioners can order diagnostic procedures under the supervision of a physician. There is also emphasis on social, psychological, and preventive health in their training.

Another type of health provider, the lay midwife, is sometimes confused with the certified nurse-midwife. Lay midwives include at least two groups—"granny midwives" who traditionally have assisted at childbirth in areas where medical care has been unavailable and a younger, more radical group who have been staunch proponents of home birth. Historically the lay midwife has depended upon hand-to-hand passage of information and experience to get her training and has tended to have little formal education. However, some states are beginning to license lay midwives and have established training programs.

Questions to Consider When Selecting a Health Professional

In addition to educational differences, health professionals vary in personality, ability, and style as much as professionals do in every field. In the beginning stages of choosing among them, you should consider these basic questions:

1. Do you want everyone in your family to see the same physician? If so, a family practitioner or general practice physician can provide you and your family with preventive health services.

2. Would you feel more comfortable with a male or female health professional? Some women believe that only another woman will fully grasp their problems. Ninety percent of gynecologists are males, so the availability of female doctors, while increasing, is somewhat limited. Most physician extenders, however, are women.

3. Is age an important factor to you? Some young women prefer a younger physician since he or she is more likely to share their views, particularly of contemporary life

styles. Older women may prefer more mature physicians for the same reason.

4. Do you have a diagnosed medical problem (say, heart disease)? If so, then the applicable specialist (in this case, a cardiologist) may be the wisest choice as your health professional.
5. Are you planning to become pregnant in the future? You might want to choose the obstetrician-gynecologist who can ultimately provide maternity services as well as fill your current gynecological needs.
6. Do you have definite ideas about the type of birthing experience you want? It is a good idea to ask about any special desires you may have, such as Leboyer delivery, at the initial phone call or visit. Sometimes nurse-midwives, nurse practitioners, and/or physicians organize as a group to offer special services, such as delivery at an alternative birth center.
7. Do you prefer to see primarily one physician or would you rather have the services of several who are part of a group? There are both advantages and drawbacks in choosing solo-practice doctors as well as group-practice doctors. This area of decision making requires further discussion.

Group Practice Vs. Solo Practice

The solo practitioner, who may be a G.P. or specialist, has no partners or organizational affiliation. He or she may be your sole source of medical help if you live in a rural area. Some women prefer the solo physician because they feel strongly about seeing the same physician with each office visit and establishing an intimate doctor/patient relationship. In most cases, even if you choose a group practice, you can usually elect to schedule your planned office visits with one specific member of the group. In emergencies, however, whether you are seen by the group or the solo practitioner, you may be seen by a doctor who is a stranger to you if your own physician is sick or on vacation or otherwise not available.

There are two types of group practice. One is simply a group of the same kind of specialist—an OB-GYN group, for example. The other is a group composed of several major specialties, perhaps including one or more obstetrician-gynecologists.

The idea behind these groups is pooling office expenses and sharing coverage for weekends and nights so that the individual physician can have more free time. The multispecialty group offers the additional advantage of more comprehensive care because the several specialists can offer various perspectives on medical problems. If you do select a group practice, remember that the larger the group, the less likely your own doctor in the group will be on call on any given night or weekend when you might need him or her.

Making a Smart Choice

There are three basic viewpoints from which to select a health care provider: availability, amiability, ability. Although we'll be talking about the "Three A's" as they apply to physicians, these principles can be adapted to your choice of any health professional.

Availability

Access to a doctor depends partly on the size, organization, and type of practice the doctor has. Be sure you understand the scope of a doctor's practice in terms of your own needs or possible future needs. Some doctors, for example, limit their practices to gynecology and infertility; it would be stressful, for example, to develop a sound relationship with such a physician only to have to change doctors when you become pregnant. Sometimes, however, such a change is happily necessary when your earlier visits were made for infertility problems that have been solved.

If you are considering a group practice, you'll need to ask how the "on call" schedule operates, as it varies widely. Obviously, a doctor in a solo or small group practice will be more readily available to you than one in a large group practice. Whether you choose a solo or a group practice, it is often easier to get an appointment with a young doctor just out of training. He may have more flexible office hours, such as evenings or Saturdays, and have more time to spend with patients.

Amiability

Amiability means an attitude that leads to a comfortable doctor/patient relationship. Your psychological and emotional needs determine what you seek in a doctor/patient relationship. If you have strong beliefs about certain issues, such as contraception, abortion, rooming-in, or breast-feeding, it is essential to find a physician who shares at least some of these beliefs. You should be completely comfortable in being yourself with your physician without worrying that his or her personal value judgments will influence how he or she provides for your care. Amiability is a factor that is difficult to evaluate prior to meeting the physician. However, a friend who has attitudes and values similar to yours may be able to advise you on a doctor with whom she has developed a satisfying relationship.

Ability

The most difficult quality to judge—ability—is also the most important. As in any profession, there is a spectrum of skill and judgment. Most doctors specialize—that is, they limit their practice to one area of medicine. However, specialization does not automatically mean the doctor has had additional supervised training in that area unless he is board-certified. This additional attainment, board-certification, based on written and oral exams, is one measure that a doctor is qualified to practice his or her specialty. You can determine if a physician is board-certified by looking at his or her wall diplomas or stationery, by calling your local county medical society, or by looking in the *Directory of Medical Specialists* available at your public library. Another diploma worthy of note is the American Medical Association's Physician Recognition Award, which is given for continuing education and teaching during a three-year period. This certificate, issued only in recent years, indicates that a physician is likely to be medically up-to-date. Usually, a diploma signifying completion of a residency program is also readily visible. Residency programs in hospitals associated with medical schools are often superior in depth of preparation to programs that are not university-affiliated. Occasionally board-certified specialists will take further training in the form of a fellowship: the internist in cardiology or gastroenterology, the obstetrician in high-risk pregnancy or gynecological cancer, to name a few. Certificates indicating fellowships of one or two years in one of these subspecialties do indicate a significantly greater level of skill and knowledge in that area.

Some consumers feel safe in judging a doctor's ability according to the hospitals in which he or she has staff privileges. The presence of staff privileges means little since controls placed on physicians are minimal. The total absence of staff privileges, however, is not a good sign, especially if a large hospital is close to the doctor's office. Most doctors limit their practice to one or two hospitals for convenience.

Many people choose a doctor who is recommended by their friends. Be cautious; while it may be possible to assess amiability and attentiveness on the basis of another's experience, assessing medical ability is another matter. A fine cosmetic scar, for instance, says nothing about the judgment required in determining the need for surgery. The advice of a labor-and-delivery or operating room nurse would be a more reliable referral source for an obstetrician or surgeon. These nurses observe their doctors daily and can offer a valuable perspective for you. Or, if you know or utilize other doctors, ask them where their wives go for health care.

Shopping for the right health professional for your needs is not easy. The highest quality in this marketplace is found only if you take the time and energy to seek it out. Your body and peace of mind deserve your best efforts.

Saving Money in Our Health Care System

The Hospital

Hospitalization is the costliest part of medical care in terms of your wallet and probably your psyche as well, so you should avoid it when possible. If you can have minor surgery or a series of tests on an outpatient basis, then make every effort to do so.

Of course, there are times when admission to a hospital cannot be avoided. If you are pregnant or you need surgery and you do not have health insurance or a prepaid health plan, consider using a county or university hospital where a sliding-scale fee may be used rather than a flat fee-for-service. When a medical school is affiliated with a hospital, the technical side of care—the lab tests and procedures—is likely to be superior, though the human warmth element may suffer at times. More tests than you actually need may be ordered by a zealous doctor in training. However, you will have close supervision by resident physicians trained with the latest available knowledge. The level of obstetrical care afforded by supervised OB-GYN residents at hospitals affiliated with medical schools is generally very good.

Whenever you obtain obstetrical care, investigate the possibility of an early hospital discharge.

You cannot use our health care system wisely or economically if you are unaware of alternative health care services available to you. The last chapter told you about your choices in health care professionals. This chapter will point out your options in health care facilities. Again, it is smart to familiarize yourself with the existing facilities in your area. This knowledge can save you money and heartache.

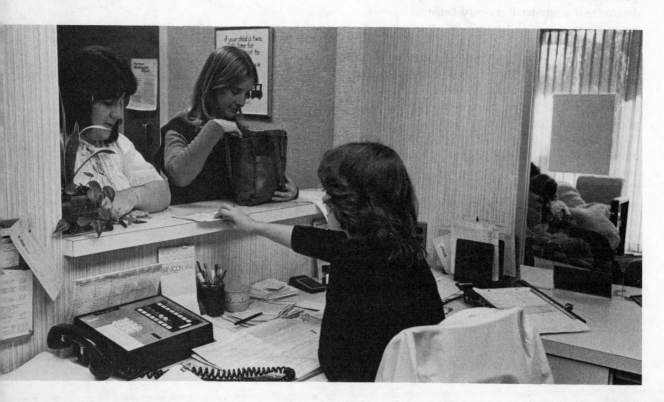

Many hospitals are adopting cost-saving so-called family-centered policies including discharge within twenty-four hours of normal delivery.

The Emergency Room

The emergency room at your local hospital is a valuable resource for urgently needed medical help. The care is given by general or family practitioners, internists, or physicians with specialized training in emergency room medicine. However, keep in mind that emergency room costs, based on fee-for-service policies, are typically higher than those of a private physician. Among other disadvantages of using the emergency room for routine health problems are the following: long waits (the true emergency must be handled first), impersonal attention, and minimal or no follow-up care. Unless your situation is life-threatening, the last place to go for health care is the emergency room.

Prepaid Health Care Groups

This rapidly growing form of health care consists largely of Health Maintenance Organizations (HMOs). The consumer or her family joins the HMO by making regular monthly payments. Comprehensive health care including hospitalization, surgery, and referral to medical specialists is provided when the need arises. Freedom to select your health care provider may be limited as is your choice of hospitals, depending on the institutions participating in the HMO. (See Table 1 to find out how to obtain more information on possible HMOs in your area.)

Free Clinics

The Public Health Department's Free Clinics provide general primary care as well as contraceptive counseling and prenatal care. Financial eligibility may be required and a small fee asked for the service. Pregnancy screening and VD (venereal disease) detection and treatment is usually free of charge. Staffing may be by a physician or nurse practitioner. Continuity of care varies, depending on the physician/nurse turnover and continued State and local funding. Referral for specific health problems is provided.

Birth Centers

A birth center may be an alternative available in your area. The popularity of these centers derives from their warm, homelike atmosphere as well as from their cost savings. Patients go home within twenty-four hours of delivery and pay a single fee to the center and its staff. The staff may consist of nurse practitioners, certified-nurse or lay midwives, and/or obstetrician-gynecologists. Transportation capability on the part of the center is important for those times when an emergency arises during a delivery. Local arrangements are usually established beforehand with nearby hospitals. A helpful rule of thumb is that the time from diagnosis of an emergency to arrival at the hospital should be less than fifteen minutes.

Planned Parenthood

Excellent contraceptive counseling, especially for women with an uncomplicated health history, can be obtained at a reasonable fee at Planned Parenthood centers. This organization also offers pregnancy counseling, abortion and sterilization services, or referral for such services on an outpatient basis. Some branches of Planned Parenthood give special educational programs for marriage, sex education, prenatal care, and a variety of health-related topics. Staffing is variable, consisting of nurse practitioners, physicians, and lay persons.

Women's Clinics for Pregnancy Termination

Pregnancy termination is simply another way of saying abortion. These clinics, which offer free pelvic exams and pregnancy tests as an introductory feature, usually present a single-fee package that includes first-trimester abortion (up to 12 weeks) with pre- and post-abortion counseling, pertinent laboratory tests, and contraceptive counseling. Special problems, such as RH sensitization due to pregnancy, can be treated at the clinic for an extra fee. Local anesthesia as opposed to general anesthesia is usually given, and the procedure is done on an outpatient, short-stay basis usually requiring less than three hours. Some clinics will perform second-trimester abortions (between 12 and 24 weeks) usually in a nearby hospital. Staffing is typically provided by board-certified OB-GYNs, nurse practitioners, and trained counselors. If you are researching this service, inquire not only as to costs but also as to what follow-up care exists. Many physicians are now doing pregnancy terminations in their own offices at fees competitive with these clinics and sometimes with better follow-up care.

Women's Crisis Centers

These centers provide immediate counseling to women in crisis situations, such as rape, divorce, and physical abuse. Frequently free of charge, they depend largely on volunteer services, and as such the quality and experience of counselors varies greatly. Referral services for health problems are usually available.

It bears repeating that the time to look into and even visit the health care facilities in your locale is before you desperately need them. Table 1 lists various resources to help you in your search.

Table 1   RESOURCES FOR FINDING HEALTH CARE ALTERNATIVES

1. Local branch of American Nurses Association

2. Local women's organizations, e.g., National Organization for Women

3. Local university, Department of Women's Studies or College of Nursing

4. Local medical school, Department of Internal Medicine, Family Practice, or Obstetrics and Gynecology

5. Local hospital, Department of Nursing Service or In-service Education

6. Local county medical association

7. Local public library

8. Classified section of newspaper or phone book

9. Local branch, Planned Parenthood association

10. Local Public Health Department

11. Group Health Association of America, Inc. Communication and Information Department 624 Ninth Street, N.W., 7th Floor Washington, D.C. 20001
    (This organization will provide information about HMOs in your area.)

12. Health Maintenance Organization Room 3-10, Parklawn Bldg. 12420 Parklawn Drive Rockville, Maryland 20857
    (This office within the Department of Health and Human Services (HHS) will provide information about government-certified HMOs in your area.)

13. American College of Nurse-Midwives 1522 K Street, N.W., Suite 1120 Washington, D.C. 20005

14. The Nurses Association of the American College of Obstetricians and Gynecologists 600 Maryland Avenue S.W. Suite 200 East Washington, D.C. 20024

3

Understanding Female Anatomy and Its Functioning

The women's movement has encouraged greater individual responsibility for health and body awareness. In the past (and still in the present for some) the natural urge for self-exploration in childhood was inhibited, and women often learned to ignore their sexual organs. Not so much anymore. Many women openly discuss, among friends or in women's groups, their concerns about their body functioning. They can choose from among a great many books that explain female anatomy and sexuality. Self-examination, too, is a way many women are learning. We hope this chapter will increase your knowledge of basic female anatomy and physiology and will make you more comfortable with the terms used by your clinician.

The easiest way to examine yourself is with a mirror, which should be at least four or five inches wide. Plan for a few private moments to look at yourself and identify your external genitalia, or sexual organs. You can squat, or lie on your back with your head and knees elevated, or sit on the edge of a chair. If you have a full-length mirror, you might be able to position yourself in front of it. In any case, find a position that is comfortable and relaxing to you.

The External Female Anatomy

This is the area you can see in your mirror (see Figure 1). As you read about each organ, remember that individual differences in size, shape, and coloration are normal and may be due to racial factors, childbirth, or genetic factors. If you have any doubts or questions, consult your clinician.

The *mons veneris* is the triangular area of fatty tissue that covers the pubic bone. Pubic hair, usually coarse and curly, covers the mons and may continue up to your navel. The thickness and amount of pelvic hair varies greatly. Pubic hair makes its appearance during adolescence as the result of an increased output of sex hormones.

The *vulva* is the name of the entire outer area of a woman's genital-urethral organs. The vulva includes the labia majora (large lips), labia minora (small lips), the clitoris, the urethral opening, and the vaginal opening.

The *labia majora* are two soft folds of outer skin that cushion and protect the vaginal opening. Like skin elsewhere in the body, they are covered with hair and sebaceous (oil) glands. As a woman becomes older, these lips become more flaccid, or looser; after childbirth they may no longer completely cover the labia minora.

Figure 1
External female anatomy.

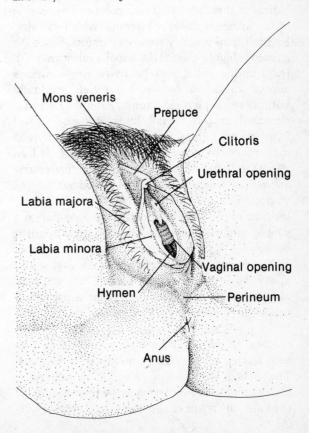

Mons veneris

Prepuce

Clitoris

Urethral opening

Labia majora

Labia minora

Vaginal opening

Hymen

Perineum

Anus

The *labia minora* are small, sensitive lips just inside the labia majora. They play an important role in sexual activity, becoming engorged during excitation, thus providing a tighter grip around the penis.

As you separate the labia majora, you will see the *clitoris* at the top of the folds where the larger and smaller lips come together. The *prepuce*, or clitoral foreskin, sits on top of the smaller lips and looks like a small triangle. When you feel the small rounded clitoris with your finger, you will find it to be very sensitive. With manipulation, it becomes stiff and enlarged, filling with blood during sexual activity, similar to the engorgement of the male penis.

Directly below the clitoris is a small dark "dimple" called the *urethral opening*, which is the opening through which you urinate. The *urethra* is the canal through which urine is passed from the bladder.

Below the urethral opening is the *hymen* or its remnants. The hymen is the thin fibrous tissue that partially covers the vagina, leaving a small opening for vaginal or menstrual discharge. This opening can be stretched or torn through such athletic activities as horseback riding or bicycle riding or through initial intercourse. The tearing of the hymen may cause bleeding, which will stop by itself, and possibly some discomfort. Since the hymen is highly elastic, the use of a lubricant (K-Y jelly) during initial sexual activity almost always allows an intact hymen to stretch gradually without much physical trauma. After the hymen is stretched or torn, small folds of tissue, called *hymenal tags*, may remain. Rarely, the hymen may cover the entire vaginal opening (called an *imperforate hymen*), blocking normal intercourse as well as trapping menstrual blood within the vagina. This condition requires correction about the time of the onset of puberty; the procedure is a simple surgical one easily done on an outpatient basis.

The *perineum* is the area below the vagina and above the anus. If you have given birth, you may observe small thin scars here from a procedure called an *episiotomy*. This procedure involves making a small cut (and then repairing it with stitches) in the perineum during delivery to prevent tearing of the vaginal muscles into the anus. The *anus* is the opening into the rectum. After childbirth, small skin tags may be present around the anus, the result of stretching and pressure during pregnancy and the delivery process. These skin tags are remnants of previous hemorrhoids and are quite common.

The Internal Female Anatomy

The internal female organs are normally "felt" by the clinician during the pelvic examination, which will be discussed in Chapter 4. Figure 2 shows you the location of each of these organs, which include the vagina, cervix, uterus, Fallopian tubes, and ovaries.

The *vagina*, an elastic organ similar to a tiny tunnel, connects the cervix (opening of the uterus) to the outside of your body. The vagina varies in length from three to five inches. Sometimes called the *birth canal*, the vagina can expand during childbirth to five inches in width. The length of the vagina does not affect the ease of delivery or sexual enjoyment. Unless the hymen is intact, inserting one or two fingers into the vagina will not cause discomfort. The vagina should feel soft, moist, and pliable. The vagina lies between the bladder (above) and the rectum (below) (see Figure 7). Using a flashlight and a plastic speculum, available from your gynecologist or local women's self-help group, you may better visualize the vagina in your mirror. As you insert your fingers into the vagina, you may touch something hard and dimpled which feels similar to the tip of your nose. This is the *cervix*, or mouth of the uterus. If you have an intrauterine device (IUD), the string may be felt in the vagina, but the IUD itself should be located above the cervix. The cervical opening is very small; thus tampons are prevented from being pushed up into the uterus. Two glands, called *Bartholin's glands*, open into the vagina, one gland on either side, near the hymen and produce a thin mucus that helps to lubricate the vagina. These glands are not visible on the outside unless blockage of the gland opening occurs, producing a cyst or infection.

The *uterus*, a shiny, pink, pear-shaped, muscular organ, is designed to nourish and support the developing fetus. It is normally about the size of a fist. An amazingly versatile organ, the uterus stretches to many times its size during pregnancy and contracts its powerful muscles to begin the birth process. The inner lining of the uterus, called the *endometrium*, is composed of soft, blood-enriched tissue that sloughs (drops off

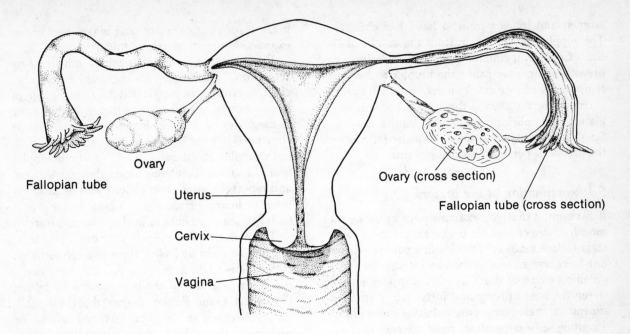

Figure 2   *Internal female anatomy.*

or sheds) each month during your menstrual period. The uterus has three openings: two upper openings into the Fallopian tubes and one lower opening (cervix) into the vagina. The top portion of the uterus, called the *fundus*, is what nurses and doctors are feeling when they push on your stomach following childbirth. The only time you can normally feel your uterus is at this time, too. For the first few days after delivery you can push on your abdomen with your hand and feel a hard, round ball about the size of a grapefruit.

Women often think of the *Fallopian tubes* as the pathway of the egg into the uterus. It is sometimes forgotten that it is here, in one of the two Fallopian tubes, where embryonic life begins. The sperm, after successfully negotiating its trip up the vagina, cervix, and uterus, meets the egg (called an *ovum*) in the upper portion of one Fallopian tube, and fertilization takes place. During the six-day journey it takes for the fertilized egg to migrate down the tube, specialized cells along the passageway maintain and protect the egg, as they wave it on its way to the uterus.

The two *ovaries*, one located on either side of the uterus adjacent to the opening of each Fallopian tube, produce the sex hormones estrogen and progesterone. These are the major female hormones that stimulate the development of female characteristics during puberty and make reproduction possible. The eggs (ova) are also housed here and

number about 400,000 at the time of puberty, although only one out of every thousand ova will be used in a woman's lifetime. The process of *ovulation*, the release of a matured egg from the ovary, will be discussed later in this chapter.

The Breasts

Probably no other part of a woman's anatomy is as obvious as the breasts, yet many women know very little about them. The breasts function both as milk producers following childbirth and as organs of sexual stimulation. Breast tissue contains essentially fat cells and a network of milk-producing glands (see Figure 3). The fat cells, unlike the general fat elsewhere in the body, are a specific type which grow in response to the increase in sex hormones during adolescence. Breast development starts in a girl anywhere from one to two years before she begins to menstruate. The size of one's breasts is determined largely by genetic factors and depends on the amount of fatty tissue present. Breasts respond to normal cyclic hormonal changes and may swell or feel tender just before a menstrual period. A slight difference in the size of the two breasts is also normal.

The pinkish-red or brownish portion around the nipple of each breast is called the *areola*. The color of the areola is usually darker in pregnant women and in women who have had children. The nipple may protrude from the areola or lie flat. Cold temperature, sexual stimulation, or breast-feeding may cause the nipples to become temporarily more erect. You may see small bumps surrounding the areola; these are sebaceous (oil) glands that lubricate the nipple during nursing. Small hairs sometimes arise from the follicles in the areola, a perfectly normal situation.

Self-examination of the breasts

It is essential that you examine your breasts each month to detect possible breast cancer in its early stages. Breast cancer is the leading cause of death due to cancer among women and is also the most common cause of death in American women between the ages of forty and forty-five. With rare exception, these tumors are painless; and without a routine self-examination, their presence may go undetected. (See Appendix E.)

The best time to examine your breasts is right after your menstrual cycle. Sometimes just before or during your period, your breasts may feel more tender or thickened. For this reason, breast examination, either by you or your clinician, is most reliable when performed just after a period rather than the week before. If you are past menopause, pick a particular day of the month, say the first,

Figure 3
Normal breast anatomy.

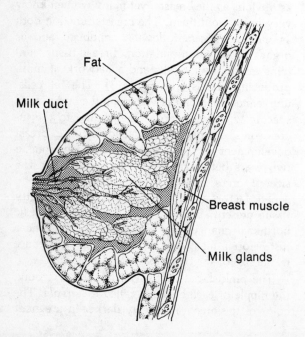

Fat

Milk duct

Breast muscle

Milk glands

mark it on your calendar, and make your breast examination each month on this day.

First, look at your breasts in a mirror. Any retraction, discharge, scaling, or other skin changes around the nipple may be an early sign of breast cancer. Any breast bulging, dimpling, or redness should be noted and reported to your clinician. Do your breasts seem symmetrical, with both nipples at the same level? Do both nipples look the same? Raise your hands above your head and repeat the same observation. This helps to expose the lower surface of the breasts and makes it easier to see any changes in shape or contour.

The next step is to palpate your breasts, that is, to examine them by feeling them in a certain way. Here is how to do it. Because you can more easily detect irregularities of the breast tissue by letting the breast tissue flatten against the chest wall, simply lie down on the floor, on a bed or sofa, or perhaps in the bathtub. As you examine, for example, your left breast, raise your left arm above your head, resting your left hand behind your head. Placing a small pillow or towel under your shoulders may help you in this examination of the breast tissue. Gently feel your left breast with the fingers of your right hand, beginning around the nipple, pressing lightly with your fingers. Move your fingers in widening circles or slightly back and forth so that you systematically cover the entire breast. What you are feeling for is a lump or thickness. Repeat this examination with your left arm lying down by your side. Pay special attention to the area between the nipple and the armpit as this is one of the most common locations of tumors. To examine your right breast, simply reverse the procedure, with your right hand behind your head, and so on. Check each nipple for possible discharge by gently squeezing it between your thumb and forefinger. Ask your clinician or the nurse to demonstrate this technique to you. They may have special teaching materials, such as videotapes or pamphlets, for your use.

Regular self-examinations help you to know what your breasts feel like normally. With practice you will be able to detect any lump, thickness, or irregularity that may appear.

Hormonal Changes During a Woman's Life Cycle

The word *menses*, which means the same as menstrual period, comes from the Latin word "mensis," meaning month. The menstrual cycle averages 28 days in length, with normal variation ranging from 21 to 35 days. Menstrual bleeding is traditionally considered the beginning of the menstrual cycle. Times of emotional and physical stress can delay or speed up the start of the menstrual cycle. Breast-feeding may delay the resumption of menstruation, perhaps for several months after delivery, even after you have stopped breast-feeding.

What causes menstruation?

Menstruation is a complicated hormonal process initiated by the brain hormones LH (luteinizing hormone) and FSH (follicle-stimulating hormone), both of which come from the pituitary gland, at the base of the brain. LH and FSH start the process by stimulating the ovaries to produce their own hormones, estrogen and progesterone. The hypothalamus, also located in the brain, regulates the release of FSH and LH from the pituitary gland. This helps explain the effect of psychological stress on the menstrual cycle since the hypothalamus is considered a principal emotional center in the brain. If you are overly upset, the message gets to the hypothalamus; the hypothalamus contacts the pituitary gland, and your menstrual cycle may arrive early or be delayed.

The first half of the menstrual cycle is dominated by the production of FSH by the pituitary. This hormone is responsible for the maturation of the egg in one of the ovaries prior to ovulation. The maturing egg is located in a special part of the ovary called the follicle; this follicle secretes estrogen. Each month estrogen stimulates the growth of a whole new uterine lining (endometrium) in which a fertilized egg can implant itself. Approximately halfway through the menstrual cycle, LH causes the release of the egg from its follicle. This release is called *ovulation* and it may be accompanied by a brief, sharp pain on one side of the abdomen. An increase in vaginal mucus discharge or slight spotting may also occur near the time of ovulation.

The second, or postovulatory, half of the menstrual cycle is characterized by increasing levels of both estrogen and progesterone which some authorities believe are responsible for many of the symptoms of premenstrual tension. After releasing its egg, the ovarian follicle is called the *corpus luteum*, which continues to secrete hormones. The released egg enters one of the Fallopian tubes, usually on the same side that ovulation occurred, and begins its six-day journey to the uterus. Fertilization must take place during this time period. Rarely, a fertilized egg may implant in the tube, causing a *tubal*, or *ectopic*, *pregnancy*. If the egg isn't fertilized, it disintegrates and is released in the menstrual blood.

The corpus luteum stops producing estrogen and progesterone at the end of the cycle if conception has not occurred. As the hormone levels drop, the blood supply ceases to nourish the uterine lining and menstrual bleeding begins. The low production of estrogen eventually acts as a stimulus for pituitary production of FSH to begin the next menstrual cycle. In the absence of fertilization, the corpus luteum normally recedes, leaving only a small scar on the surface of the ovary. Occasionally it may persist as a small cyst for several weeks or months, accounting for one of the most common causes of mild pelvic pain in women.

How does fertilization occur?

Fertilization, or conception, occurs with the union of one egg and one sperm in the Fallopian tube. The male testes continuously produce sperm, and millions of sperm leave the penis upon ejaculation during intercourse. The sperm quickly "swim" up through the cervix and the uterus to the tiny entrance into the tubes. Pregnancy begins when the sperm and the egg unite (see Figure 4).

What happens if fertilization occurs?

When conception takes place, the hormone production of the last half of the menstrual cycle is changed. With implantation of the fertilized egg about one week after ovulation, the *placenta*, which is the organ for receiving oxygen and nutrients and discharging waste products, begins to develop. The developing placenta soon produces HCG (human chorionic gonadotropin), sometimes known as the pregnancy hormone, which prevents the cyclic hormonal changes of menstruation from taking place. It acts as a stimulus to the corpus luteum to continue its production of estrogen and progesterone for the first three months of pregnancy, after which production is taken over by the placenta. HCG is the hormone measured in all pregnancy tests.

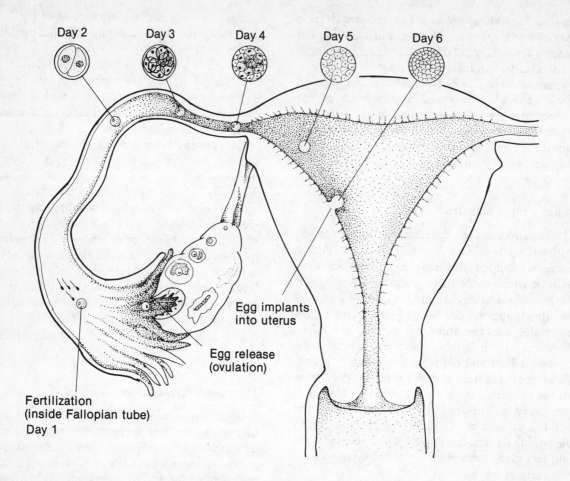

Day 2   Day 3   Day 4   Day 5   Day 6

Egg implants
into uterus

Egg release
(ovulation)

Fertilization
(inside Fallopian tube)
Day 1

Figure 4   *The first six days of life. Fertilization results when a sperm from the male unites with an egg from the female. If fertilization occurs, division of the egg begins. It then takes about six days for the fertilized ovum to travel through the tube and reach the uterus where the mass of cells implants into the uterine lining. Modified with permission of Parke-Davis, division of Warner-Lambert Company (Female Reproductive Organs—in Health and Illness, 1978).*

During this time twinning may occur in one of two ways. Fraternal twins will result if the woman produces two eggs within the same month and they are fertilized by two different sperm. Identical twins result from the splitting of a single fertilized egg in the first few weeks of development. The chance of having twins is about one in ninety. Fraternal twins are more common than identical twins by a ratio of about two to one. It is not clear which factors make a woman susceptible to having identical twins; however, a slight increase in the frequency of fraternal twins has been linked with increasing maternal age, large family size, and a family history of twins, especially involving the maternal side of the family.

The ovaries rest during pregnancy, with no stimulation of follicles or ovulation taking place. Menstruation resumes within the first three months following delivery in about 85% of women. The remaining 15% usually begin menstruating again in the next four to six months.

At what age does menstruation begin?

A girl experiences her first period, called the *menarche*, usually at about the age that her mother did. The average age of menarche today is about twelve years, although it is common to find menarche beginning anywhere between the ages of ten to fourteen. If a woman has not started to menstruate by the age of sixteen, she should consult a physician for evaluation.

The menstrual cycle is usually irregular for the first two years or so. Many initial periods may be *anovulatory* (no ovulation) while the adolescent body matures and hormone production becomes more regular. The anovulatory cycles prevent pregnancy from occurring in a young girl until her body and bone structure are sufficiently mature. If she is engaging in sexual activity, however, and if pregnancy is not desired, a method of birth control should be considered because there is no certainty that each successive period will be anovulatory.

How do you know when you are ovulating?

The basal body temperature (BBT) chart is a way commonly used to determine the time of ovulation. The basal body temperature refers to the temperature of your body at rest. To determine your BBT, take your temperature *immediately* upon awakening every day. This means *before* you get out of bed. Record your temperature from a special thermometer used for this purpose on a chart supplied by your physician or pharmacist. (This procedure is discussed in more detail in Chapter 6.) There is a slight but definite elevation of your BBT at the time of ovulation. The rise is caused by the production of progesterone at ovulation and usually measures no more than 0.4 to 1.0 degree Fahrenheit. This rise in temperature persists until the progesterone production stops prior to menstruation. If you become pregnant, your temperature will stay at the higher level. Infertility caused by failure to ovulate can be determined by use of the BBT. Figure 9 shows examples of different temperature chart patterns. Cervical mucus charting, as discussed in Chapter 6, is another method used for determining ovulation.

Some women experience "middle pain" (*mittelschmerz*) each month around the time of ovulation. This brief, sharp pain felt on one side (or the other) of the lower abdomen occurs just as the egg is released from the surface of the ovary (ovulation).

How does menopause occur?

Anovulatory cycles, similar to those in adolescents, usually start around forty-five years of age

Parents greeting their newborn twins.

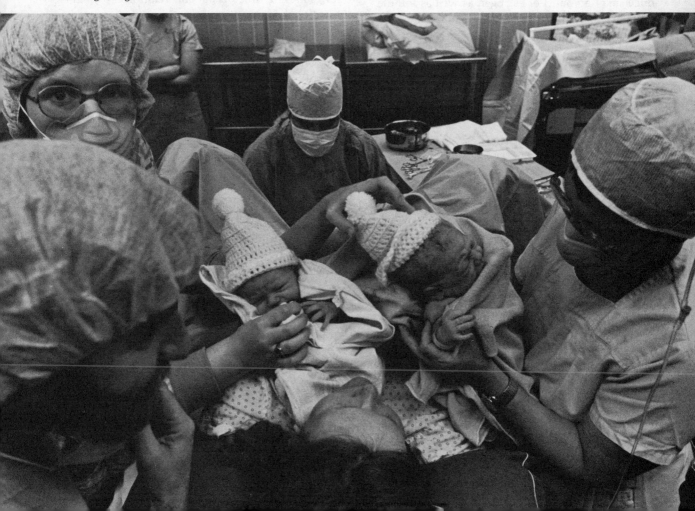

and are due to declining production of hormones by the ovaries. The premenopausal years, called the *climacteric*, usually span a four- to six-year period; it takes this long for the ovaries to stop producing hormones. The age a woman experiences menopause, while bearing no relationship to the woman's age of menarche, is closely correlated with the age that her mother stopped having periods.

The first indication that the ovaries are slowing down is menstrual irregularity. Periods usually become lighter and less frequent with some variation from month to month. A woman is considered to have reached menopause when she has not had a period for twelve consecutive months.

As the ovaries gradually stop production of estrogen, the pituitary produces increasing amounts of FSH and LH in a futile attempt to stimulate estrogen production by the ovary. Some authorities believe these high levels of FSH and LH account for certain menopausal symptoms, such as hot flashes and night sweats. For many years following menopause, the ovaries continue to produce small amounts of estrogen as well as minute amounts of male sex hormones (androgens), accounting for the slight hair growth noticed by some women at this time.

4

Getting the Most Out of Your Office Visit

Most women feel reluctant and a little fearful about their initial visit to a gynecologist or other health professional. The pelvic examination is often an unnerving intrusion of privacy even in longstanding doctor/patient relationships. This emotional and physical discomfort can be diminished if you know what to expect. This chapter provides a step-by-step guide to the exam and offers specific suggestions to help you get the most out of your office visit.

Making Your Appointment

Evaluate your needs before making an appointment. If your problem is not urgent, schedule your appointment between menstrual periods. If you unexpectedly start your period prior to a scheduled exam, check with your doctor to see if you need to reschedule. Otherwise you may spend your time and money on two visits, one for a checkup and the other for a Pap smear. Do not douche or use a vaginal cream for at least twenty-four hours before your appointment; you may be washing away important clues to diagnosing some vaginal conditions. Having intercourse prior to your visit does not in any way affect the doctor's exam. If your reason to see the doctor will not require an exam, try to handle the problem with a phone call.

Medical Records

You have a legal right to see your medical records at any time. Hospital records are usually more detailed than office records and are thus more useful to a physician unfamiliar with your health history. Three aspects of hospital charts are usually well documented. These are the nurses' progress notes, the operative note (what was found and what was done), and the pathology report which reflects the findings at surgery. For obstetrical patients, the labor-and-delivery record contains the essential information about previous childbirths. In requesting your records from other doctors' offices, it is particularly important to obtain these portions of the hospital record.

Patients often assume that medical records are detailed and complete. Unfortunately this is not so. You can keep a record of any symptoms or findings you have with much more accuracy than is usually documented in the records. Your keeping your own record is a good idea especially if pelvic abnormalities are found. From the examination, your doctor should be able to provide you with information about abnormal cysts, swellings, or tumors to the centimeter. Because written infor-

mation about your medical history may be sketchy, it is important to verbally recount your history to your doctor in addition to requesting that records be sent to your doctor.

The Pre-Exam Interview

Physicians and other health care providers are taught to take a medical history according to a prescribed format. In practice this format is considerably shortened depending on the time allotted and the severity of the problem. Physician extenders may take a more thorough history than do physicians. More often than not, a diagnosis is made from a careful history rather than from the physical exam. In preparing for an initial office visit, it is helpful if you have a written record of your health history. At the back of this book a Health History Profile checklist is provided (see Appendix A). The checklist emphasizes women's health problems and is designed to cover most of

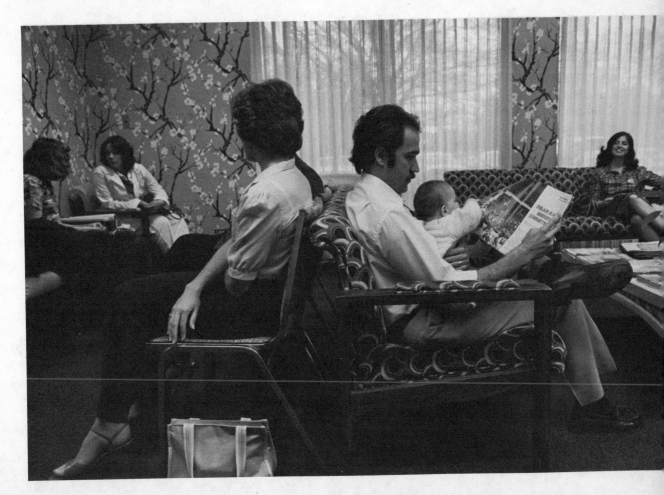

Table 2   AREAS OF INFORMATION COVERED BY THE HEALTH HISTORY PROFILE*

Area of Information	Comment
1. Current problems	1. Are there specific concerns or problems that you want to discuss with your clinician?
2. Menstrual history	2. Are your periods regular? Any unusual bleeding or pain?
3. Contraceptive history	3. What birth control method(s) have you used? Any problems or side effects?
4. Pregnancy history	4. Be sure to mention any complications of pregnancy or childbirth you have experienced.
5. Previous conditions	5. Include any past illnesses requiring medical treatment.
6. Previous hospitalizations	6. Include any previous surgery.
7. Family history	7. It is especially important to include any family history of breast cancer, high blood pressure, or diabetes.
8. Medication history	8. Include your drug allergies and side effects you have experienced.

* The complete Health History Profile checklist appears in the back of this book (Appendix A).

the questions you are likely to be asked. Table 2 shows what general areas of information the Health History Profile covers.

You can either make photocopies of the blank Health History Profile checklist directly from the one at the back of this book; or you can tear it out of the book and perhaps make some blank copies of it, to use one for each different doctor you visit who asks for this information. You can thus take more time before your appointment to prepare this information carefully for your doctor, and you will also be able to check out things that may not come to mind immediately in the doctor's office, like family history. The more accurate the information is that you give your doctor, the better able he or she is to evaluate your health problem. After you have completed the Health History Profile, you may want to make a copy of the completed form and keep it for your own records to use in the future. You can bring the completed form with you at the time of your office visit.

Before, rather than after, your pelvic exam, make clear your reason for coming so that your doctor will be alert for your specific concern. If your problem has been a chronic one, be certain to explain why it concerned you enough to make the appointment at this particular time. If the reason for your visit is a second opinion about a problem, you may wish to keep this to yourself until after

the examination to see if your second doctor's diagnosis confirms the first doctor's opinion. Your doctor should know that you are selective about your care. If the problem is something you feel is not directly related to the gynecological area, mention it. Gynecologists are the principal physicians for many women and can readily treat simple nongynecological problems. For more serious or chronic ailments, inquire about a referral to a specialist.

The Gynecological Exam

Most gynecologists do a modified form of the complete physical examination. This includes determination of weight and blood pressure, a urinalysis, and a blood count as well as examination of the skin, throat, neck, chest, heart, breasts, abdomen, and pelvis. There is some controversy about the benefits of the complete physical exam, especially in individuals under forty. The American Cancer Society now recommends that women without any symptoms should have breast and pelvic exams every three years between age twenty and forty and annually after age forty (see Table 3). Pap smears are recommended at least every three years after two negative Pap smears one year apart. Some controversy surrounds these new Pap smear guidelines—refer to Chapter 36 for more information. Most gynecologists recommend continuing the yearly checkup regardless of age to examine for other medical conditions, especially if the gynecologist is the woman's primary physician. Table 3 also suggests a time schedule for other recommended medical procedures, based on your age and medical history. Discuss with your doctor those areas mentioned in Table 3 that apply to you.

The breast exam

More than 90% of palpable breast cancers are detected through self-examination. In Chapter 3 we described how you can do this simple, quick exam yourself. You should learn how to do this procedure and perform it on a regular basis. When the clinician examines your breasts, point out any areas that concern you. You may want to ask for a demonstration of the breast self-exam at this time also. Fortunately, the vast majority of breast masses detected are benign. (See Appendix E.)

The pelvic exam

The self-pelvic and self-Pap exams are not as convenient or as easy to do compared to the breast self-exam. For this reason, it can be done more reliably by a doctor or nurse who has the experience to differentiate normal from abnormal. Because of normal changes throughout the menstrual cycle, changes brought about by childbirth, and individual variation, there is a wide spectrum of what is considered normal pelvic findings. The nurse or family practitioner will often refer a questionable normal finding to an OB-GYN specialist for clarification. A nurse or female assistant is almost always present to assist during the pelvic exam for medical-legal reasons and to provide you with empathetic support.

It is important to urinate just prior to the pelvic exam, both for your own comfort and so that your doctor won't misdiagnose a full bladder as a cyst. (You may have just given a urine specimen to the nurse or a lab assistant, but after a long waiting-room wait you may have the urge to urinate again. Don't hesitate to do so.) Before the exam, you are usually given a drape sheet or examining gown. The purpose of the drape sheet is to cover your lower abdomen and thighs to help preserve your remaining modesty—not to cover

up what the physician is doing. If you prefer, the drape can be arranged to permit eye contact with the doctor. However, if the gown is objectionable to you and you are wearing a slip, ask if you can wear your own slip instead of the gown.

Pelvic examining tables have metal stirrups (sometimes plastic covered) for resting your heels while you slide your hips down to the edge of the table. Let your knees spread apart comfortably and relax as much as possible. The more relaxed your abdominal and vaginal muscles, the more comfortable and thorough will be the exam. To facilitate relaxation, ask your doctor to let you know what he or she is doing during each step of the exam.

The pelvic exam consists of four steps which should take no more than a few minutes to complete. In the first step, the external genitalia, or vulva, is inspected, including the labia majora, labia minora, clitoris, urethral opening, and outer vagina. You may want to request that your examiner clarify any questions you have concerning your anatomy by use of a mirror. Point out areas of irritation or lesions you have noticed. Because of the rich supply of nerve endings of the vulva, a very small area may be the source of a lot of discomfort to you but may go unnoticed by the physician. The pelvic support provided by your vaginal muscles is tested next; childbirth may have caused some normal stretching and loss of support, especially in women who have had large babies or more than three children. The clinician inserts one or two fingers into the vagina and presses down while you are asked to strain or cough to bring out any bulge or muscle weakness in the upper or lower vagina (*cystocele* or *rectocele*). Be sure to mention if you have noticed any vaginal protrusion, loosening of the vaginal muscles during sex, or some loss of bladder control.

The second step in the exam involves insertion of a plastic or metal speculum and is called the *speculum exam*. If a metal speculum is used, don't hesitate to request that it first be warmed. This insertion is done by slowly introducing the closed speculum into the vagina. After insertion, the speculum is opened just wide enough to permit the doctor to see the cervix and upper vagina (see Figure 5). Aside from pressure or mild discomfort, any pain or pinching you may experience indicates either inflammation or an impatient examiner. Let your doctor know if his or her technique is not a gentle one.

Table 3 AMERICAN CANCER SOCIETY GUIDELINES FOR CANCER-RELATED CHECKUPS*

Exam and/or Procedure	Age 20 to 40	Age 40 and Over	Exceptions (Higher-Risk Women Who May Need More Frequent Testing)
General checkup including breast and pelvic exam as well as exam of skin, mouth, thyroid, and lymph nodes	Every three years	Every year	See exceptions below; women at risk for uterine (endometrial) cancer (see Table 61) should have an endometrial tissue sample (biopsy) at menopause
Breast self-exam	Every month	Every month	
Pap test	At least every three years** (includes women under 20 if sexually active)	At least every three years**	Higher risk for cervical cancer (see Table 58)
Breast X-ray (mammogram)	One base line X-ray between 35 and 40	Every one to two years after age 40	Higher risk for breast cancer (see Table 53)
Guaiac slide test (to check for blood in stool)	Not applicable	Every year after age 50	Higher risk for colon or rectal cancer (personal or family history of polyps in the rectum or colon or of cancer in the rectum or colon; personal history of ulcerative colitis)
Sigmoidoscopy (procto exam—see glossary)	Not applicable	Every three to five years after age 50	Higher risk for colon or rectal cancer (personal or family history of polyps in the rectum or colon or of cancer in the rectum or colon; personal history of ulcerative colitis)

* Guidelines set forth by the American Cancer Society for women without symptoms. The A.C.S. recommends that you talk with your doctor to see how these guidelines relate to you.

** After two initial negative tests one year apart. Some doctors believe Pap smear testing should be more frequent—see Chapter 36.

The primary purpose of the speculum part of the exam is to do the Pap test (see Figure 6). This painless test, named for its inventor, Dr. George Papanicolaou, involves gently scraping the cervix with a small wooden or plastic spatula to collect cells, which are smeared on a glass slide and then sprayed with a fixative. The slides are then sent to a cytology laboratory for microscopic examination of the cell characteristics. A few days later, the doctor receives a report indicating whether the cells are normal, atypical, or malignant (see Chapter 36 for a fuller explanation of Pap test results). Fortunately, abnormalities detected by this test are usually due to inflammation (vaginitis) and not to cancer. Usually, precancerous changes in the cells show up several years before actual invasive cancer develops in the tissues. Regular checkups, therefore, practically insure against development of a life-threatening cervical cancer. Most authorities recommend that an initial exam, including a Pap smear, be done on a woman by the age of eighteen or at the beginning of sexual activity, whichever is earlier.

Another purpose of the speculum exam is to diagnose various vaginal and cervical inflammatory conditions, some of which are infectious and most of which produce more discharge than usual. If your problem concerns a vaginal infection, a *wet prep* may be done. This is a slide preparation obtained from secretions of the

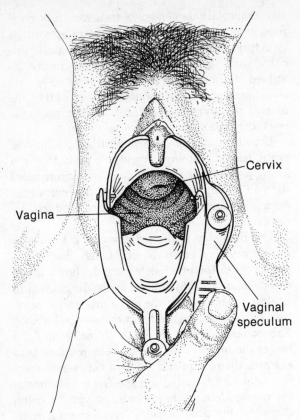

Figure 5

*View of cervix and vagina
during the pelvic examination.*

vagina for microscopic examination. If you are concerned about the possibility of a venereal infection, a *transgrow* culture, a standard test for gonorrhea, may be done. You have to ask for this test specifically in most doctors' offices. The test is accomplished by swabbing a sample of cervical secretions with a cotton-tipped applicator onto a culture plate, which is then sent to a bacteriology lab. It takes up to seventy-two hours for the results of the test because it takes that long for the bacteria to grow on the culture medium. In general, other types of vaginal cultures for monilia (yeast) or nonspecific bacteria have little practical value in the diagnosis and treatment of most vaginal infections.

The speculum exam provides other information, too. The diagnosis of miscarriage is made exclusively from the speculum exam. If miscarriage has occurred, the cervical opening will be dilated and there will be evidence that tissue has been passed. Also, if ovulation has occurred within the last day or two, it is theoretically possible to detect this occurrence from the speculum exam. At

ovulation there will be clear, copious mucus present and the mouth of the cervix will be widened. Previous pregnancy affects the appearance of the cervix; the cervical opening will be widened and the amount of glands on the surface will be increased. This normal increase in glands accounts for the slightly greater amount of vaginal secretions in women who have been pregnant. The pill may produce this effect as well. IUD placement, if an IUD is present, is also checked at the time of the speculum exam.

The third step of the woman's pelvic exam involves evaluation of the uterus, tubes, and ovaries and is called the *bimanual exam*. The physician removes the speculum and inserts two fingers into the vagina alongside the cervix while the other hand presses the lower abdomen and directs the pelvic organs toward the examining fingers (see Figure 7). Using this method, the examiner first attempts to outline the uterus to determine its size, contour, position, and consistency. The interior of the uterus, that is, the uterine cavity, cannot be evaluated by this exam. Uterine size varies with age and childbirth. Adolescents and women beyond the menopause will normally have a smaller uterus than women in the childbearing years. With succeeding pregnancies the uterus enlarges. Physicians sometimes refer to the size of a uterus by using the equivalent size during pregnancy as a reference point. For example, a "six-weeks size uterus" would be about two cubic inches in size. After several pregnancies, the uterus may become

Figure 6

Obtaining a Pap smear.

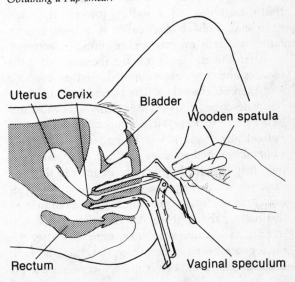

as large as six-weeks size as a result of the hyper-trophy, or stretching process, after childbirth. A uterus larger than six-weeks size would be considered enlarged. Even if no periods have been missed, pregnancy is considered a possibility since the apparent last menstrual period may actually have been due to bleeding resulting from the implantation of the fertilized egg.

If your doctor feels that you have a significantly enlarged uterus, you may be able to feel it with your hand by the following procedure. While the doctor is examining you through the vagina, have him or her elevate the uterus with the examining fingers and ask him or her to place your hand over the lower abdomen where he or she is feeling the uterus. If you can easily feel the uterus in this manner, this usually confirms that the uterus is indeed enlarged. This procedure may be difficult in some individuals because of pain, immobility of the uterus, or "backward tilting" of the uterus.

Abnormalities in uterine contour or shape are unusual. They most often represent either a growth, such as a small fibroid, or a variation in the embryonic formation of the uterus. These variations are completely harmless except that they may occasionally give rise to problems in pregnancy and childbirth.

Because the uterus is mobile, its position can change according to your activity. In the past, it was mistakenly thought that a tilted, or retroverted, uterus (see Figure 8) could cause a miscarriage or infertility; however, this position is now known to be a normal variation. The uterus has various muscular and fibrous supports. During childbirth these supports may be weakened or stretched so that the uterus sits just slightly lower in the vaginal canal. This change, called *descensus* or *prolapse*, is usually minimal and requires no treatment.

After the uterus is felt by the examiner, the ovaries and tubes are examined, first on one side and then on the other. The same bimanual technique described above is used. This is the most difficult part of the pelvic exam for the doctor and patient alike, and it will be helpful if you relax your abdominal muscles as much as possible. It may help to take deep breaths in and out through your mouth to help you relax. In many individuals it is not really possible for the examiner to distinctly palpate (feel) the Fallopian tubes and ovaries as separate structures, especially after the menopause because then these structures become smaller. The examiner is mainly concerned with

any abnormal enlargement of the ovary-tube complex, which is normally felt on exam as a single structure measuring up to approximately one cubic inch. The Fallopian tubes are rarely involved in cancer and more commonly are associated with infectious diseases. Like the uterus, the ovaries and tubes do not normally swell during a normal menstrual cycle.

If you feel any tenderness during the bimanual exam, tell the examiner. It will help your doctor to know if you have more discomfort than is usual for you. Compared to the uterus, the ovaries are normally more sensitive to pressure produced by the exam.

The final step in the pelvic exam is known as the *rectovaginal exam*. Most women, during this step of the exam, experience some discomfort; you can decrease this discomfort by bearing down or straining. This part of the exam involves a variation of the bimanual techniques described above. The examiner places one finger in the rectum and leaves the other in the vagina. The purpose is to examine the rectum and the area between the rectum and vagina called the *cul-de-sac*. The rectal exam may detect hemorrhoids, polyps, or colon cancer (a rare occurrence). A rectal exam is sufficient in examining adolescents or others where only a small hymenal opening is present. Because the doctor can reach higher than through the vaginal route alone, greater palpation of the ovaries is possible. If you have hemorrhoids, ask your doctor to omit the rectovaginal exam.

You may wonder about what your doctor can actually determine about you from the pelvic exam and what conditions cannot be determined from the exam. Table 4 outlines and answers some of the questions you may be thinking about in this respect.

The Post-Exam Interview

If no abnormalities are found, you may be told "everything is fine." However, if you came to the office with specific symptoms unexplained by the exam, you should not leave without a clear understanding of your condition and plans for follow-up care. It is not always possible for doctors to be completely sure that the exam is normal. Unless a definite problem can be determined, the doctor may recommend a follow-up exam rather than starting treatment without a definite diagnosis.

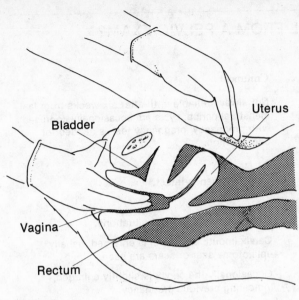

Figure 7
Side view of the pelvic examination.

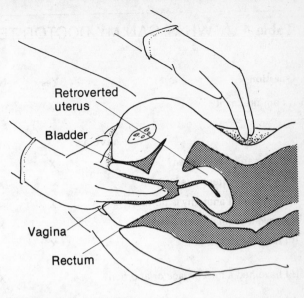

Figure 8
Side view showing the pelvic examination with a retroverted uterus. A rectal examination will allow a more complete evaluation of the uterus.

For example, stool may be confused with a pelvic tumor; in this case, your doctor may suggest an enema before your next visit. If some doubts exist in your mind about your exam, questions you may want to ask are:

1. Is my uterus enlarged?
2. Is there a question of pregnancy?
3. Is an ovary enlarged?
4. Is there any inflammation of the cervix?
5. Is anything abnormal?

You should know before leaving the office:

1. Are any tests to be scheduled and, if so, what are they for?
2. Could follow-up be handled without an office visit?

If any treatment is planned, ask these questions:

1. Is any printed literature available? If not, ask your physician to make a simple drawing to facilitate your understanding of the problem. Some physicians have audio-visual cassettes for their patients on various subjects such as surgical procedures.
2. If medication is prescribed: What are the actions and side effects? How will the prescribed medication react with any other

medication I may be taking? When should I or should I not take the medication, for example, on an empty stomach, with food, or not with certain foods? Is free sample medication available? All physicians are visited regularly by pharmaceutical representatives who leave samples of all the commonly used drugs, including birth control pills.
3. Specifically what is the program of treatment? Are alternate treatments possible? If necessary, get a second opinion, especially if surgery is proposed following an initial visit.

The post-exam interview offers an additional opportunity to evaluate your physician's approach to the doctor/patient relationship and to influence to some extent the course it will take in subsequent visits. Classically doctors have been taught they should have much more authority than is actually necessary. This approach encourages women to become very dependent upon their physicians. Many health professionals now follow more of a patient-participation type model, in which patients actively share in the process of determining their own health needs and alternatives. You are probably best off with a doctor

Table 4   WHAT CAN MY DOCTOR TELL FROM A PELVIC EXAM?

Question	Yes	No	Comment
If I am pregnant?	X		Not always reliable until after six weeks from last menstrual period; cysts are occasionally confused with pregnancy; pregnancy test is needed for confirmation.
If I have an intact hymen?	X		
If I have had intercourse?		X	Unless hymen is intact.
If my external anatomy is normal?	X		
If I have a vaginal odor?		X	Rarely apparent in most situations.
If I have had a baby?	X		Cervix (mouth of uterus) is enlarged; usually episiotomy scar or scars are seen.
If I have had a miscarriage or abortion?		X	Occasionally the cervix is slightly enlarged, indicating previous pregnancy.
If I masturbate?		X	
If I have gonorrhea?		X	A laboratory test (culture) is the only way to confirm the diagnosis.
If I have a vaginal infection?	X		
If I have venereal warts?	X		
If I have had sex recently?	X		If a slide test of vaginal secretions is done, sperm are often seen.
If I can have an orgasm?		X	
If I can get pregnant?		X	The majority of causes of infertility cannot be detected by exam alone; several tests are usually required.
If I can deliver a baby normally?		X	Most women have normal vaginal deliveries. Little can be accurately predicted about whether you will need a cesarean section.
If I get pregnant, am I likely to have premature labor, a miscarriage, or a breech birth?		X	This cannot be predicted by examination alone except in rare instances.
If my uterus, or womb, is enlarged?	X		
If my cervix is inflamed?	X		
If my vaginal muscles are loose?	X		
If my bladder is "dropped"?	X		
If there is weakness or decreased support of vaginal muscles?	X		
If my uterus is "dropped," or prolapsed?	X		
If I need hormones?	X		This is recognized when the vagina is very dry and the vaginal wall tissues appear extremely thin.
If I have a pregnancy in my tube?		X	This requires surgery to confirm.
If my tubes are blocked or scarred?		X	This diagnosis is presumptive; only by certain tests or surgery can this condition be confirmed.
If I have a spastic colon?		X	Diagnosis is made by X-ray and history.

table continues

Table 4   Continued

Question	Yes	No	Comment
If I have endometriosis?		X	Confirmation by surgery is required.
If I have cancer?		X	Diagnosis can be suspected but biopsy is required to prove.
If my periods are heavy?		X	
If I have fibroids?		X	This common diagnosis is always a presumptive one.

whose approach allows you to participate in decisions involving your health care.

At the close of a patient's visit, doctors often expect pressing, last-minute questions. Even if you don't have such a question, ask one just so you can determine your doctor's willingness to give you the explanations and answers you need.

Leaving the Office

Sometimes you may feel depressed or frustrated when leaving the office. If you do, try to figure out why. Did you ask all the questions you wanted to? Sometimes a patient is too tense to ask all her questions or to understand what the physician has said. Only when the patient is home rethinking the interview or is trying to explain to someone else what the doctor has said does she realize that she is confused. If this happens to you, don't hesitate to call the physician to clarify your information, especially if something new or unexpected is discovered. Sometimes the nurse can simply help you over the phone by looking over your record. Don't be afraid to inquire, repeatedly if necessary, about anything pertaining to your office visit—it is your right and your responsibility to be well-informed.

References for Section One

Lewis, C. E., and Lewis, M. A. The potential impact of sexual equality on health. *New England Journal of Medicine* 297(16):863-869, 1977.

Gibson, R. M., and Mueller, M. S. National health expenditures, fiscal year 1976. *Social Security Bulletin* 40:3-22, 1977.

American Cancer Society report on the cancer-related health checkup. *Ca-A Cancer Journal for Clinicians* 30(4):194-232, 1980.

Weiss, L., and Meadow, R. Women's attitudes toward gynecologic practices. *Obstetrics and Gynecology* 54:110-114, 1979.

Foster, R. S., Jr., et al. Breast self-examination practices and breast cancer stage. *New England Journal of Medicine* 299:265-270, Aug 10, 1978.

Greenwald, P., et al. Estimated effect of breast self-examination on breast cancer mortality. *New England Journal of Medicine* 299:271-273, Aug 10, 1978.

Martin, L. L. *Health Care of Women.* Philadelphia: Lippincott, 1978.

Rakel, R. E. The changing role of the family physician. *The Female Patient* 6(1):8-10, 1981.

Jonas, S. *Health Care Delivery in the United States.* New York: Springer Publishing Co., 1977.

Huguley, C. M., and Brown, R. L. The value of breast self-examination. *Cancer* 47(5):989-995, 1981.

Two.

A Woman's Guide to Birth Control

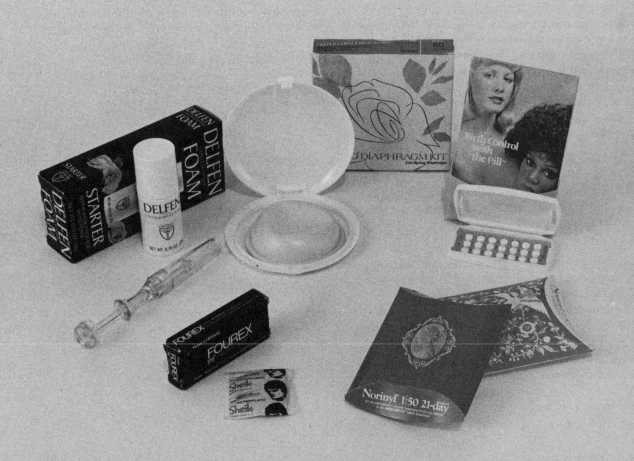

5

An Overall Look at Birth Control

Contraception is a continuing concern for many women. Despite recent medical advances, a *completely* safe, effective, and reversible method of birth control has yet to be developed for men or women. No major contraceptive breakthroughs occurred in the 1970s, a decade in which women became aware of serious side effects associated with popular contraceptives and turned to more traditional forms of birth control such as the diaphragm and the rhythm method. The 1980s promise to continue this trend while research focuses on more acceptable methods of contraception for men as well as for women. Vaginal rings containing hormones, cervical caps, and long-term injectable contraceptives are among the types currently being studied but not yet approved for general use.

There are four major types of birth control methods in use today, as follows:

1. Natural family planning methods.
2. Barrier methods.
3. Intrauterine devices (IUD).
4. Birth control pills (also called oral contraceptives).

In each of the next four chapters of this section we will discuss in some depth each of these major types. In the last chapter of this section we will give you information designed to help you select the contraceptive method which is best for you.

Birth control pills continue to be the most popular method, used by 30% of married couples using contraception in the United States. The barrier methods, such as the diaphragm and condom, are used by 18% of women, especially those who plan to get pregnant within a year or who cannot use birth control pills or an IUD for medical

reasons. The IUD, although it is selected by only 8% of women, has the most prolonged use of any method, partly because active steps must be taken in order for the woman to stop using it. The rhythm method, now expanded and known as natural family planning, is the least frequently used birth control method (about 3%) although it is probably the one gaining fastest in popularity at this time. These four methods add up to much less than 100% since nearly 50% of married couples now choose a permanent method of birth control (voluntary sterilization). Coitus interruptus, or "withdrawal," in which the man withdraws his penis just prior to ejaculation was used as a contraceptive method much more in past times. Today, coitus interruptus cannot be considered an effective birth control method for a woman who chooses not to conceive.

With the number of new and sometimes conflicting reports in the media about health risks, decreased fertility, or cancer-causing effects of various contraceptive methods, it is often hard for a woman to decide which method is best for her. To help you make this decision, we have divided the process of contraceptive selection into three simple steps, outlined in Table 17 at the end of this section. This chart, along with the information presented throughout this section, will guide you in your choice of the most appropriate method of birth control for your personal needs.

6

Natural Family Planning

The traditional *rhythm methods* have increased in popularity recently and have acquired new emphasis as a "natural" means of family planning, requiring no artificial devices or medication. Its growing popularity is probably related to women's concern about medical hazards of birth control pills and the IUD as well as the high cost of medical care. It is estimated that natural family planning will overtake the IUD in the 1980s as the third most popular method of birth control. All methods of natural family planning depend upon abstaining from intercourse (or using other forms of contraception) during the fertile days of the menstrual cycle. This fertile period includes the days just prior to and after ovulation, which occurs approximately midway between menstrual periods. Ovulation can be determined by the *temperature method*, the *calendar method*, or the *cervical mucus method*, all of which are considered rhythm methods.

Keep in mind that any penile-vaginal contact without protection at any time during your fertile days, even though you don't actually have intercourse, allows the possibility, however small, of your becoming pregnant.

The Temperature Method

The temperature method is based on the fact that a woman's basal (resting) temperature (known as basal body temperature (BBT)) drops briefly and then rises half a degree following ovulation. The temperature remains elevated until just before menses begins. Normal resting temperature usually ranges from 96 to 98 degrees before and 97 to 98 degrees after ovulation. A rise in temperature that

persists for at least three days indicates that ovulation has occurred. Safe days are from the fourth day of a sustained temperature rise through the last day of your next period. You should avoid intercourse between the last day of your next period until the temperature again rises for three days in the next cycle (see Figure 9). The temperature method requires a long abstinence period since this method, while accurately detecting ovulation, cannot predict its onset. If you use a temperature rise as the indication to abstain, you may already be too late to prevent conception. Here is the reason. Sperm may survive for two to three days following ejaculation. If you have had intercourse (without contraceptive protection) at some time during the two to three days before ovulation, the sperm may still be alive to fertilize the egg when you do ovulate.

Your temperature should be taken and recorded daily, preferably on a special chart, immediately upon your awakening, before you get out of bed. You can purchase a basal body thermometer and temperature charts at a drugstore, to make this method more convenient.

The Calendar Method

Before you can actually use the calendar method as your sole method of birth control, you will need to keep a written record of when each menstrual period begins. You will need to keep a record of the *length* of each cycle, that is, how many days from the start of one period to the start of the next period, for about eight months before beginning to use this method, unless your cycles are perfectly regular. This requirement may be an initial disadvantage because another form of contraception, but not the pill, should also be used during these first eight months. The pill cannot be used because the pill influences your normal pattern of ovulation. Each month, update your record so you are always using your most recent eight months in the calculations you will be using for the calendar method.

The calculations are based on the fact that the interval from ovulation until the beginning of your next period is always 14 days, regardless of cycle lengths. In other words, if you have a short cycle for one month, say 21 days, ovulation should occur on or about day 7 (21 minus 14 days). Day number 1 is always the first day of

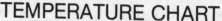

TEMPERATURE CHART

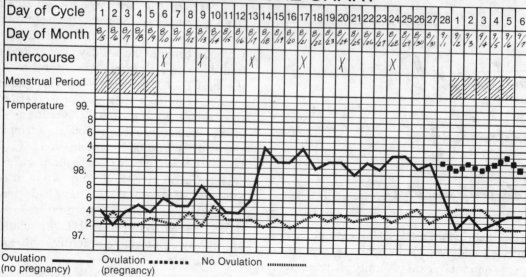

Ovulation —— (no pregnancy)　Ovulation ▪▪▪▪▪▪▪ (pregnancy)　No Ovulation ·············

Figure 9 *The solid line represents a typical temperature chart pattern for ovulation. The temperature rises after ovulation and remains elevated if pregnancy occurs (thick broken line). The thin broken line represents the pattern you would see if no ovulation occurred. The temperature chart can be used for birth control as a part of "natural family planning" or as a guide to help time intercourse in couples who wish to conceive.*

your period. In a longer cycle, for example 34 days, ovulation occurs on day 20 (34 minus 14 days). Since it is the time before ovulation that can vary in length—postovulation time (that is, from the day of ovulation to the first day of your next period) is always 14 days—you cannot predict ovulation without a knowledge of previous cycle lengths. Less variation in cycle length means you have a smaller range of possible fertile days and, therefore, fewer days of abstinence. In other words, the more regular your cycle, the better this method will work. If your cycles vary by a week or more in length, this method of birth control may be too risky for you.

Here's how to calculate the fertile days, remembering that day number 1 is always the first day of your period:

1. To determine your *first fertile day*: select the shortest cycle from the previous eight months and subtract 18. The number 18 is derived by using the 14-day interval to pinpoint ovulation and then adding four days to cover sperm survival. For example, if your shortest cycle was 27 days, your first fertile day is day number 9 (27 minus 18). This means that the first day you should abstain from intercourse during this month is the 9th day of your cycle.

2. To determine your *last fertile day*: select the longest cycle from the previous eight months and subtract 11. The number 11 is derived by using the 14-day interval to pinpoint ovulation and then subtracting three days to allow for egg survival. For example, if your longest cycle was 32 days, your last fertile day is day number 21 (32 minus 11). This means that the last day you should abstain from intercourse during this month is the 21st day of your cycle. In this example, fertile days would be from the 9th to the 21st day, a total of 13 days.

If you had an unusually long cycle during the preceding eight months, the number of calculated fertile days would increase accordingly. But if your cycles are always about the same length, the number of abstaining days are less and decrease to an absolute minimum of eight days a month for a woman whose cycles are always exactly the same length.

The Cervical Mucus Method (Billings Method)

The cervical mucus method is the latest, least studied, and most controversial method of natural

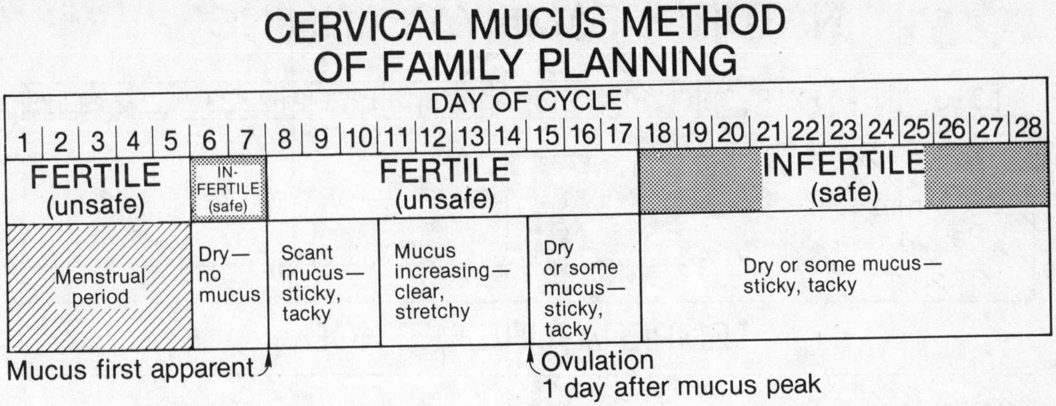

CERVICAL MUCUS METHOD
OF FAMILY PLANNING

DAY OF CYCLE																											
1	2	3	4	5	6	7	8	9	10	11	12	13	14	15	16	17	18	19	20	21	22	23	24	25	26	27	28
FERTILE (unsafe)					IN-FERTILE (safe)		**FERTILE** (unsafe)										**INFERTILE** (safe)										
Menstrual period					Dry— no mucus		Scant mucus— sticky, tacky			Mucus increasing— clear, stretchy				Dry or some mucus— sticky, tacky			Dry or some mucus— sticky, tacky										

Mucus first apparent ⌐

Ovulation
1 day after mucus peak

Figure 10 *Intercourse is "safe" during infertile days. During "unsafe," or fertile, days another method of birth control must be used if you have intercourse.*

family planning. It depends on a thorough understanding of your anatomy and menstrual cycle because you predict ovulation by observing and recording daily changes in the amount, consistency, and color of the cervical mucus. To obtain the mucus sample, you can touch the cervix directly, reach inside the vagina, or simply wipe the vulva.

Figure 10 summarizes the cervical mucus changes in a typical cycle. Usually no mucus is present for a few days after your period ends. During these "early dry days," intercourse is safe although there is a small chance of pregnancy due to sperm survival into the first "wet" (fertile) day which follows. A mucous discharge is present within the vaginal opening about six days before ovulation. This is the start of the "wet" days. As ovulation approaches, the mucus changes from cloudy and thick to clear and thin (like raw egg white) and suddenly increases in amount for one or two days. Intercourse should be avoided from the start of your "wet" days until at least three days after the amount of mucus "peaks." Ovulation occurs about twenty-four hours after this mucus peak. After ovulation the mucus decreases in quantity, becomes cloudy and thick again, and may be absent altogether for a few "late dry days" before your next period starts. Strict proponents of the mucus method also recommend abstinence during the menstrual period since mucus cannot be evaluated at this time.

The mucus method is not appropriate or feasible for everyone. Women using foam or other vaginal contraceptives may find it difficult to "read" their cervical mucus. Mucus evaluation is also less reliable in the presence of a vaginal infection, following childbirth, and in women ap-

proaching menopause when glandular secretions are less likely to occur according to a cycle.

Combining Rhythm Methods

Various combinations of rhythm methods are possible to increase effectiveness or decrease abstinence days, or both. For example, your first fertile day may be determined by the calendar method (subtract 18 from your shortest cycle) and your last fertile day by the temperature or cervical mucus method. This combination decreases the number of days requiring abstinence but may be slightly less effective than the temperature method alone, which permits intercourse only after ovulation. When combining methods, rely on the calendar prediction for your last fertile day whenever you have doubts about interpreting your temperature or mucus pattern, or if you have a cold or vaginal infection which could alter these signs. If you don't use the calendar method, the safest approach when in doubt is to abstain or to use other birth control until you have a clear indication that ovulation has occurred.

Another approach is to combine all three methods (see Figure 11). High rates of effectiveness approaching 91% have been reported in recent studies of this combination, known as the *Sympto-Thermal Method.* Many couples combine barrier contraception with natural family planning on the fertile days of the cycle to allow greater sexual freedom and spontaneity. Although medical checkups are not required for this method of contraception, some instruction from a professional or a woman familiar with the techniques involved is often helpful, especially in the beginning.

NATURAL FAMILY PLANNING

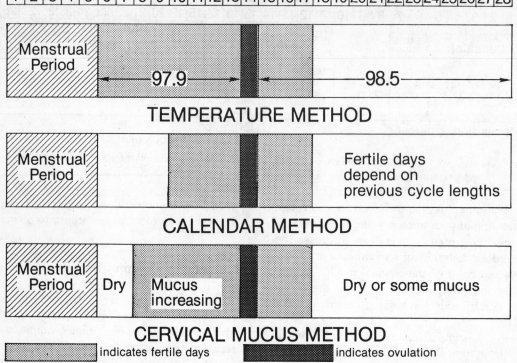

DAY OF CYCLE

| 1 | 2 | 3 | 4 | 5 | 6 | 7 | 8 | 9 | 10 | 11 | 12 | 13 | 14 | 15 | 16 | 17 | 18 | 19 | 20 | 21 | 22 | 23 | 24 | 25 | 26 | 27 | 28 |

Menstrual Period — 97.9 — 98.5

TEMPERATURE METHOD

Menstrual Period — Fertile days depend on previous cycle lengths

CALENDAR METHOD

Menstrual Period — Dry — Mucus increasing — Dry or some mucus

CERVICAL MUCUS METHOD

indicates fertile days   indicates ovulation

Figure 11   *This illustration indicates fertile days in a typical month for each method of natural family planning. By combining the temperature method with either the calendar or cervical mucus method you can reduce the number of abstinence days.*

Advantages and Disadvantages

Although the rhythm method is economical, free of medical side effects, and successfully practiced by many women, physicians are often reluctant to recommend this method, perhaps partly because of the time required to explain its use. Physicians also point to studies which show rhythm to be one of the least effective methods of birth control, averaging less than 80% effectiveness. This high

---

Table 5   COMPARISON OF THE THREE RHYTHM METHODS OF BIRTH CONTROL

	Temperature	Calendar	Cervical Mucus
Effectiveness*	over 90%	70—85%	over 90%
Number of fertile days (28-day cycle)	12	8	15
Affected by vaginal infection	no	no	yes
Requires regular cycles	no	yes	no
Requires daily record keeping	yes	no**	yes

---

* Based on a limited number of studies, these rates assume abstinence or use of a barrier method during fertile days.

** Only first day of each cycle.

failure rate is due in part to the fact that many women who use natural family planning do not have regular menstrual cycles with clear-cut temperature and cervical mucus discharge patterns. Women who do have regular cycles may use this method with a much higher degree of effectiveness.

Another disadvantage to rhythm is the need for time-consuming, almost compulsive, record keeping, which demands a high-level commitment to a method that requires abstinence nearly half of the time. There is one unnatural aspect to natural family planning: if pregnancy does occur, there is a greater chance of fertilizing an overmature egg, one that was released from the ovary several days before fertilization. If this occurs, the chance of a fetal abnormality may be slightly increased.

Table 5 shows a comparison, according to certain factors, of the three rhythm methods discussed here.

7

The Diaphragm and Other Barrier Methods

The barrier methods of birth control act in one of two ways: the sperm is either immobilized by a

Contraceptive decision making—for some women, the diaphragm has become an increasingly popular alternative.

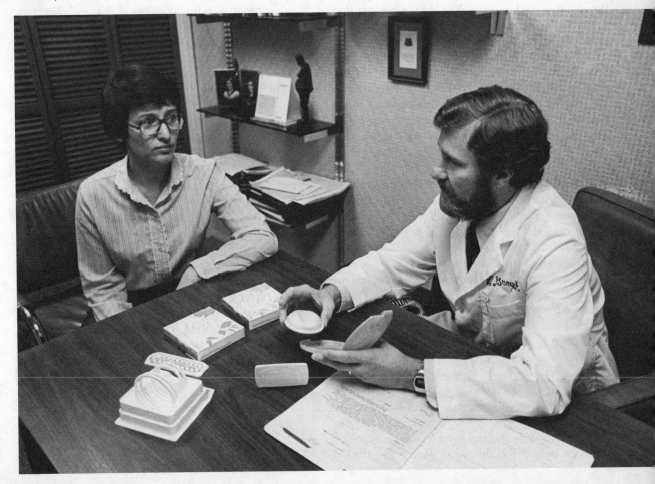

chemical (cream, foam, jelly, or suppository) or mechanically blocked from entering the uterus (diaphragm, condom). In actual practice, the effectiveness of barrier methods varies from 64% to 97% depending on how carefully the method is used. Remember that the barrier method needs to be applied before there is any penile-vaginal contact. Most studies show lower pregnancy rates with the diaphragm and condom methods than with either foam or suppositories. Contraceptive effectiveness increases tremendously if you combine two barrier methods.

The Diaphragm

The diaphragm is the oldest consistently reliable method of contraception; it was used by women for generations before the introduction of the IUD and the pill. The diaphragm is a soft rubber cuplike device (with a flexible, spring rim) that is used with a sperm-killing (spermicidal) cream or jelly and is inserted into the vagina by the woman or her partner so that it covers the cervix, that is, the entrance to the uterus. You need a prescription to obtain a diaphragm since it must be fitted to your exact size. There are about seven sizes ranging from 60 to 90 millimeters in diameter. A snug fit is important: since your vagina will expand slightly during sexual activity, a diaphragm that is too small could become dislodged during intercourse; one that is too large may be uncomfortable. Be sure to have the size of your diaphragm checked every two years and replaced at that time, even if the size has not changed. You are also likely to need a change in size after childbirth, miscarriage, or abortion, or if you have gained or lost over twenty pounds.

Learning the technique of diaphragm insertion takes time and patience (see Figure 12). Try it in the clinician's office and make sure he or she checks your proper placement of the diaphragm when it is initially fitted. You might feel more comfortable having the nurse help insert the diaphragm. During insertion, make sure the diaphragm is directed toward your tailbone, not toward the midback. This prevents positioning the diaphragm in front of (above) your cervix. In most women, the diaphragm slips naturally over the cervix regardless of the direction of insertion. As you finish inserting the diaphragm and you tuck the front of the rim up behind your pelvic bone, proceed to feel the cervix (it feels like the tip

of the nose) through the soft, cuplike dome of the diaphragm to confirm that it is positioned correctly.

Instead of using manual insertion (accompanied by pinching the rim of the diaphragm between thumb and forefinger), you may find it helps to use a plastic introducer, which can be included in the prescription for the diaphragm. This method will also make the insertion less messy because the introducer easily guides the diaphragm into the vagina. If any doubt about placement remains (and it often does), come back into the clinician's office with your diaphragm in place to have the position rechecked.

Here are some tips to maximize the effectiveness of diaphragm use:

1. Always use your diaphragm when you have intercourse, even during your period. Be sure to insert the diaphragm before any penile-vaginal contact.
2. You might find it convenient to insert the diaphragm routinely at bedtime. Although the manufacturer's instructions may indicate protection for six hours after the diaphragm, with jelly or cream, is inserted, it is a good idea to use additional cream, jelly, or foam if you have intercourse after an hour or more from the time of insertion.
3. Do not douche or remove the diaphragm for at least six hours after intercourse, or after the last intercourse.
4. Apply additional cream or jelly before each time you have intercourse while the diaphragm is still in place. A plastic applicator for this purpose may be provided along with the diaphragm, if you ask for it, or it may be bought separately at the drugstore. It may be more convenient for you to purchase prepackaged foam with an applicator and use that instead of the vaginal cream or jelly if you have intercourse more than once while the diaphragm is still in place.
5. Keep in mind that during intercourse the position most likely to dislodge the diaphragm is that of the woman on top.
6. After use, wash your diaphragm with mild soap and water, rinse and dry it well, and powder it with cornstarch (not talcum powder) to reduce moisture, which may weaken the rubber.
7. Check the diaphragm frequently for tiny,

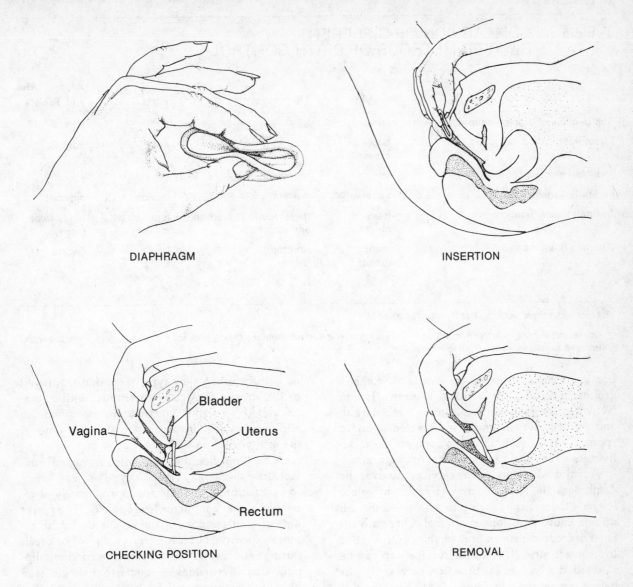

DIAPHRAGM

INSERTION

CHECKING POSITION

Vagina

Bladder

Uterus

Rectum

REMOVAL

Figure 12 *Using a diaphragm.*

pinpoint holes by holding it up to the light
or filling it with water. It is a good idea to
have a spare available in case you need it.

8. The diaphragm may be left in place for
twenty-four hours. If left for longer periods
of time, there is a small chance of developing
a vaginal discharge or uterine infection.

The Cervical Cap

This small, thimble-shaped rubber or plastic
(formerly metal) device covers the cervix like a

mini-diaphragm and is inserted and removed by
the woman. Like the diaphragm, you need a prescription since it must be fitted to your size. But
the cervical cap has run into barriers of its own,
according to some gynecologists in women's
clinics. The cervical cap is classified by the FDA as
experimental—and thus cannot be marketed in the
U.S.—since no modern studies have proved its effectiveness and safety as a contraceptive. Although
used widely in Europe, the cervical cap remains
largely unavailable in this country except through
a few physicians and an estimated 150 clinics
which obtain the device from a distributor in

Table 6   COMPARISON OF DIFFERENT BARRIER METHODS OF BIRTH CONTROL

	Condom	Diaphragm	Foam	Suppositories and Tablets
Approximate effectiveness in actual use	90%	85%	80%	80%
Effect upon sensation during sex	some decrease*	little or none**	none**	none**
Available over-the-counter	yes	no; cream or jelly is	yes	yes
Protection against VD	substantial	moderate	minimal	minimal
Aesthetic considerations	least messy	messy during insertion and removal	tends to be messy	tends to be messy
Common brand names	many brands	Koromex Ortho	Delfin Emko Koromex	Encare

* Least with animal skin products (Fourex, Naturalamb).

** Occasional burning or irritation affecting you or your partner may occur from the cream, jelly, foam, or suppository. If the burning or irritation continues, switch to another brand.

London. Primarily due to the efforts of women's groups, including the National Women's Health Network, the National Institute of Child Health and Human Development is expected soon to sponsor a research program to compare the effectiveness of cervical caps with that of diaphragms.

A major advantage of the cervical cap over the diaphragm is that it may remain in place longer—theoretically for up to a week—although no one knows how long is optimal. Other advantages include disassociation of the contraceptive from intercourse (that is, the cervical cap can be inserted at a convenient time, not necessarily just before intercourse), low price, lack of serious side effects, and possible venereal disease prevention. The main disadvantage with the cervical cap appears to be its sometimes difficult insertion and removal, which require more skill on the woman's part than with the diaphragm. Also, because of limited sizes currently available, some women cannot be fitted without a significant risk of dislodgment during intercourse.

The Condom

The condom is a rubber sheath that fits over a man's erect penis, preventing the sperm from entering the uterus. Of all methods of birth control, the condom offers the best protection against ve-

nereal disease. A new type of condom approved in 1982 by the FDA comes lubricated with a spermicide. This spermicidal condom may provide an additional safeguard against pregnancy should the semen spill on withdrawal.

A condom should be used prior to vaginal contact since sperm may be discharged or "leak" prior to ejaculation. Condoms are approximately as effective as the diaphragm (see Table 6). The newer animal skin condoms (Fourex, Naturalamb) are more expensive but less likely to slip off or break during intercourse. To prevent the condom slipping after lovemaking, your partner should take hold of the condom with his hand after ejaculation and withdraw before his erection is lost. For the woman who wants her partner to use this method, condoms can be carried conveniently in a purse so that one is immediately available.

Contraceptive Foam, Cream, Jelly, and Suppositories

These preparations contain spermicides. (Don't confuse them with feminine hygiene products, which are often on the same shelf in your local drugstore.) Cream and jelly products are used with a diaphragm. Foam is often used by itself partly because of its easy application. However, contraceptive effectiveness is greatly enhanced when the condom is used in addition to foam. Foam is packaged in a pressurized container which comes with either a plastic applicator or a nozzle for direct release of foam into the vagina. If you use an applicator, buy only a refill the next time since the applicator is reusable.

Insert the applicator deep into the vagina to be sure the foam will be ejected close to the cervix. You can do this while you are lying down or squatting or with one leg up on a chair. Foam, unlike vaginal suppositories or tablets (Encare) which take ten to fifteen minutes to melt or dissolve, is immediately effective. Remember to shake the container before use to enhance foam effectiveness.

The Vaginal Sponge

This relatively new over-the-counter contraceptive was approved for use by the FDA in 1983. The vaginal sponge is a soft, donut-shaped device measuring two inches in diameter. It consists of a spongy material containing spermicide which is activated by wetting the sponge with water just before use. The vaginal sponge works both by deactivating sperm and by blocking sperm passage into the cervix. The vaginal sponge has some advantage over other barrier methods by permitting twenty-four hours of continuous contraception. No additional spermicide need be added during this time. Initial studies indicate that the sponge's safety and effectiveness is similar to that of the diaphragm. Rare cases of toxic shock syndrome have been reported in users of the vaginal sponge (see Chapter 32). As a precaution this contraceptive is not recommended during menstruation.

Advantages and Disadvantages

An advantage of the barrier methods is their complete lack of serious side effects. The only possible adverse reaction is minor irritation or burning from the spermicide or the rubber used in the contraceptive material itself. No fetal abnormalities or cancer have been associated with any barrier method of contraception. Probably the greatest criticism of barrier contraception is inconvenience—the need to apply the method close to or just before the time of lovemaking.

Table 6 compares the various barrier methods of contraception.

8

Intrauterine Devices

The intrauterine device (IUD), a relatively new method of contraception, involves the insertion by a clinician of a small object into the uterus (see Figure 13). No one knows exactly how these devices work, but we do know they prevent the fertilized egg from implanting in the uterus and thus prevent pregnancy. The traditional IUDs include the Saf-T-Coil and Lippes Loop. Some of the more recent IUDs have the addition of metal (Copper 7 and Tatum-T models) or a hormone, progesterone (Progestasert model) in an attempt to decrease certain side effects. These newer IUDs are associated with less bleeding and fewer expulsions of the devices compared to the traditional models. The major disadvantage of the newer IUDs is their limited period of effectiveness—three years for the copper models and one year for the Progestasert. One of the older IUDs, the Dalkon Shield, has been banned by the FDA because of a high incidence of side effects, including rare instances of fatal infections. If you are still wearing a Dalkon Shield, you should have it removed.

Effectiveness of IUDs varies from 94% to 99% depending on which study you read. Although IUDs are indeed highly effective, they have several serious side effects which you should consider before choosing this method of birth control.

Side Effects to Consider Before You Choose the IUD

There are a number of common problems you should discuss with your clinician before choosing to use an IUD (see Table 7). Occasionally an IUD causes an infection within the uterus (*endometritis*). This infection may spread from the uterus to the tubes and ovaries, resulting in chronic pain or abscess formation. Sterility may

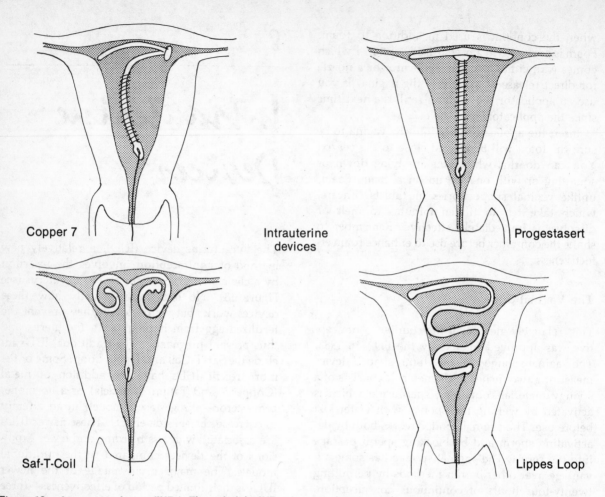

Copper 7

Intrauterine
devices

Progestasert

Saf-T-Coil

Lippes Loop

Figure 13 *Intrauterine devices (IUDs). The end of the IUD string extends just past the cervical opening.*
Modified with permission of G. D. Searle and Co. (The Female Reproductive System. *San Juan, Puerto Rico, 1976*).

result when repeated infections cause scarring and blockage of the tubes. For this reason, a history of previous tube, ovary, or venereal infection is probably a good reason to avoid the IUD. Women with chronic vaginal discharges, especially when due to bacteria or trichomonas (as opposed to yeast), also may be at higher risk for developing tube infections if they use this method of contraception. If you have severe menstrual cramps or heavy periods, you should also mention this to your clinician because these symptoms are a common side effect encountered with the IUD. Since placement of an IUD into the uterus of a pregnant woman may cause miscarriage, be sure to mention any symptoms of pregnancy, especially if your period is unusually light or delayed.

IUD Insertion

The IUD is inserted during your menstrual period for two reasons: 1) you will feel less discomfort at

that time because the cervix is slightly dilated, and 2) menses is presumed evidence that you are not pregnant.

Mild *cramping* is common during and following insertion of the IUD. A transitory fainting reflex occasionally accompanies IUD insertion and may require IUD removal if this symptom is associated with nausea and severe cramping. Such symptoms are more likely to occur in women who have never been pregnant.

Expulsion of the IUD may occur at any time; but if it is going to occur, it usually occurs within the first month after insertion. During this first month, you might want to use a second method of contraception, such as foam or condoms. Expulsion occurs in fewer than 5% of women using the IUD, most commonly during or after a menstrual period, and occurs more frequently in women who have never been pregnant.

You will be told to check for expulsion by examining your cervix to feel for the IUD string. If

Table 7 POSSIBLE CONTRAINDICATIONS TO THE IUD

Before selecting the IUD as your method of birth control, tell your clinician if you have a history of any of the following conditions, which may make the IUD unsuitable for you:

1. Allergy to copper
2. Anemia
3. Bleeding between periods
4. Fainting attacks
5. Heart disease
6. Heavy menstrual flow
7. Infection of the uterus, cervix, or tubes
8. Pelvic infection, including venereal disease
9. Recent abortion or miscarriage
10. Severe menstrual cramps
11. Suspected or possible pregnancy
12. Suspicious or abnormal Pap smear
13. Vaginal discharge or infection

you cannot feel it, keep in mind the string often curls up within the uterus, but call your doctor for an appointment just in case. If you can feel the string (but not the IUD itself), the IUD is likely to be in place. The most important reason to check yourself periodically is to make sure the IUD itself is not protruding from the cervix since this increases the risk of pregnancy.

Have your doctor or nurse practitioner check the position of the IUD a few weeks after it is fitted and at subsequent checkups. If the string cannot be seen or felt by the examiner, he or she will try to locate the IUD by inserting a small probe within the uterus. An alternate and costlier approach is to obtain an X-ray or sonogram.

Advantages and Disadvantages

The main advantages of IUDs are their high rate of effectiveness and their convenience (no need for abstinence or for diaphragm insertions). The major disadvantages are serious side effects. The overall serious risks associated with the IUD are about the same for women under the age of thirty-five as the risks for the pill. There are fewer fatal complications but more hospitalizations related to birth control side effects with IUD users as compared to pill users. Problems with IUD use are discussed below, and warning signals requiring a call to your clinician are listed in Table 8.

Increased *bleeding* is one of the most common side effects of the IUD. Periods may increase in duration or flow; or, less commonly, bleeding may occur between periods. Excessive bleeding may lead to anemia. These side effects usually subside after the first few months of IUD use.

Increased *menstrual cramping* is a common side effect of IUD use, especially among women who have never been pregnant.[1] Pelvic pain, including painful intercourse, may be a sign of uterine *infection* particularly when associated with fever, bad-smelling discharge, or spotting between periods. There is a definite increased risk of such infection among IUD users. Women who have never been pregnant are at highest risk especially where there are multiple sexual relationships or a history of previous tube infections. Treatment of IUD-related infections which most commonly involve the uterus (*endometritis*) consists of antibiotics and usually does not require removal of the device. More severe infections causing low abdominal cramping pain involve the tube or ovary and may require hospitalization and sometimes surgery. A primary consideration with IUD-related infections is the question of irreversible tubal scarring which may result in sterility. Only since 1977 have the potentially damaging effects upon the tubes from IUD use become clear, indicating a small but definite reduction in fertility among IUD users. This problem is of special concern to and a possible contraindication for many young women who have not yet started their families.

Table 8 WARNING SIGNALS FOR IUD USERS

Call your clinician if any of the following conditions occur:

1. Unusually heavy or prolonged menstrual bleeding
2. Pelvic pain, unusually severe menstrual cramps, or painful intercourse
3. Exposure to venereal disease
4. Missed period

Table 9   QUESTIONS COMMONLY ASKED ABOUT THE IUD

Can I use the IUD if . . .	Yes	No	Comment
I have had a cesarean section?	X		
I have a heart murmur?	X		Use may be contraindicated if murmur is due to rheumatic heart disease or congenital heart disease.
I delivered six weeks ago?	X		Expulsion and perforation rates are slightly higher until at least 8 weeks postpartum.
I had a therapeutic abortion two to three weeks ago?	X		If you were more than 12 weeks pregnant, wait until 6 to 8 weeks after your abortion.
I have an infection of the cervix or an abnormal Pap smear?		X	Wait until after diagnosis and/or treatment is completed for IUD insertion.
I have had a tubal (ectopic) pregnancy?		X	The risk of subsequent tubal pregnancy is much higher compared to other women using the IUD.
I douche or use tampons?	X		
I have never been pregnant?	X		Chances of IUD expulsion, painful menstrual cramps, and infection are somewhat greater compared to women who have given birth.
I am allergic to copper?		X	Applies only to the copper-containing IUDs.

Severe, persistent pain immediately after insertion of the IUD, accompanied by the fact that you are unable to feel your IUD string, may indicate perforation of the device through the wall of the uterus. Perforation occurs less than one percent of the time and is usually treated by removal of the IUD by laparoscopy (see glossary).[2]

Pregnancy may occur after an unnoticed expulsion or with the device still in place. In the latter case, miscarriage occurs approximately half of the time if the IUD is not removed and significantly less often when it is removed. Sometimes when the string is not visible and pregnancy is suspected, a sonogram is done to determine if the IUD is within the uterus, outside the uterus (perforated), or not present at all (expelled). Certain complications to both mother and fetus are more frequent if the IUD is retained within the uterus. These complications include delayed miscarriage (up to 20 weeks), premature delivery, stillbirth, and various infections either before or after childbirth. No increase in birth defects is known to occur in women who become pregnant while wearing an IUD. The effects on the fetus of progesterone-medicated IUDs are unknown. Tubal (ectopic) pregnancy has recently been found to be more frequent among IUD users, occurring in one pregnancy out of twenty, as compared to the usual rate of one in eighty.

Table 9 answers some questions you may have about the IUD.

[1] If menstrual cramping occurs you may want to ask your clinician to prescribe one of the "antiprostaglandin" drugs such as Anaprox, Motrin, or Ponstel (see Chapter 77). These drugs have been recently approved by the FDA for relief of menstrual cramps. Antiprostaglandin drugs work by blocking the action of prostaglandin, a hormone that plays a major role in causing uterine contractions and cramping and is found in excessive amounts in IUD wearers.

[2] Recently, a government-sponsored research project, the Women's Health Study, reported finding an unusual frequency of uterine perforation among IUD users who were breast-feeding. The timing of insertion did not change the perforation risk—those who had IUDs inserted at the time of the six-weeks postpartum checkup were not more likely to experience perforation during lactation than those with later insertions. The increased perforation risk for breast-feeding women may be because the walls of the uterus remain thin during lactation due to lower estrogen levels at this time.

9

Birth Control Pills (Oral Contraceptives)

About twelve million American women use oral contraceptives, the most effective and most popular method of birth control presently available. Despite controversial and often adverse reports, it is estimated that 85% of women do not have medical contraindications to the pill and can safely use this form of contraception. Since the mid-1970s, researchers have more precisely identified women at risk to develop serious side effects from the pill. This has led to lower-dose pills and a subsequent wider margin of safety for pill users.

If your doctor recently prescribed birth control pills for you, you may have received a lengthy government pamphlet called a Patient Package Insert (PPI). We will cover the major points covered in the PPI in terms that will help clarify the benefits and risks of these pills.

Considerations Before You Choose the Pill

There are five conditions under which you *must not take the pill* (oral contraceptives) *under any circumstances*; these conditions are listed in Table 10. There are also many relative, or less serious, contraindications to the pill; these are summarized in Table 11. You should think very carefully before choosing the pill if any one of the factors in Table 11 applies to you. If any two or more factors apply, you should strongly consider finding another method of contraception.

Side Effects of the Pill

Most side effects of the pill are not serious and some are beneficial (see Table 12). Common side effects usually subside after a few menstrual cycles. It usually takes that long for the body to adjust, so it is better not to switch pills during the initial two to three months of use. Adverse reactions to the pill are also usually mild, and these, as well as serious effects, are also noted in Table 12.

Blood clots are the most serious side effects of oral contraceptives and require immediate medical attention. Most large studies indicate that users of birth control pills are several times more likely than nonusers to develop blood clots, which can cause heart attacks and strokes. Each year approximately one woman in two thousand who take birth control pills is hospitalized for treatment of blood clots; although these conditions may be fatal, 98% are not. The great majority of women who develop blood clots have various risk factors associated with pill use. Before you decide to take birth control pills, you should consider these three important risk factors that increase your chances of serious side effects:

1. Your age—if over age thirty-five, especially if over age forty.
2. Whether you smoke—especially more than fifteen cigarettes per day.
3. If you plan to take pills containing more than 50 micrograms of estrogen—see below under *The combination pill*.

How Birth Control Pills Differ

There are two basic types of pills: the *combination pill* and the *mini-pill*. Ninety-nine percent of the

---

Table 10   ABSOLUTE CONTRAINDICATIONS TO BIRTH CONTROL PILLS

1. Present or previous blood clots including clots in the leg (thrombophlebitis), in the lung (pulmonary embolus), in the brain (stroke or cerebrovascular accident), or in the heart (heart attack or coronary thrombosis). History of angina or chest pain due to heart disease.
2. Present active liver disease such as hepatitis or cirrhosis.
3. Present or previous cancer of the breast or uterus.
4. Pregnancy—known or suspected.
5. Abnormal or unexplained vaginal bleeding.

Table 11 RELATIVE CONTRAINDICATIONS TO BIRTH CONTROL PILLS

If this risk factor applies to you . . .	You should have . . .	You should probably stop taking the pill if . . .
uterine fibroids	a pelvic exam every six months	fibroid growth occurs
migraine headaches	checkups* at least every six months; consider neurologist evaluation if headaches persist after stopping pill	headaches increase in frequency or severity
epilepsy	checkups* every six months and periodically by internist	seizures increase in frequency
diabetes (requiring insulin)	checkups* every six months and periodically by internist	insulin control is difficult
high blood pressure	your blood pressure checked within three months initially and then every six months	blood pressure increases
infrequent periods, every three to six months (possible relative infertility)	(see Chapter 76, Menstrual Periods—Infrequent, Short, or Absent)	pregnancy is planned within one to two years
depression	(see Chapter 60, Depression)	severe anxiety or depression develops
vaginitis	a wet smear (office test); glucose tolerance test if repeated yeast infections	yeast infections do not respond to treatment
gallbladder disease	liver function tests annually	tests are abnormal or gallbladder attacks increase in frequency or severity
liver disease	liver function tests annually	tests are abnormal
sickle-cell anemia (see glossary)	a sickle-cell test if unsure whether you have sickle-cell anemia	any worsening of disease, such as bone pain, occurs
cystic breast disease	a breast exam every six months; base line mammogram (see Chapter 33)	you have a family history of breast cancer or previous breast biopsy showing atypical cells
family history of heart attacks before age 50	blood cholesterol and triglycerides annually	either of these is abnormally elevated
family history of uterine cancer	a Pap smear semiannually	you have frequent abnormal bleeding on the pill and are over age 35
family history of breast cancer	periodic mammograms after age 35 (see Chapter 33)	you have an abnormal mammogram, severe cystic breast disease, or a breast biopsy showing atypical cells
jaundice (see glossary) during pregnancy	liver function tests annually	tests are abnormal
diabetes during pregnancy	a glucose tolerance test annually	tests are abnormal
high blood pressure during pregnancy	your blood pressure checked every one to three months initially	blood pressure increases
over age 35	checkups* every six months	you are over age 40, or over 35 and have been on the pill more than five years
history of cigarette smoking	or consider having a cardiac treadmill test (stress test) after age 30	you are over age 30 and presently smoke

* by your gynecologist or other primary care clinician.

Table 12 POSSIBLE SIDE EFFECTS OF BIRTH CONTROL PILLS

Mild Side Effects

(usually subside in three months):

Nausea (most common)
Weight gain (usually less than five pounds)
Fluid retention
Spotting between periods
Breast tenderness

Moderately Serious Side Effects

(advise clinician if any of these symptoms develop; consider switching pills or stopping altogether):

Breast pain, discharge, or engorgement
Rash, itching, or jaundice (see glossary)
Reduced tolerance to contact lenses
Lack of periods
Headaches (may be migraine or related to high blood pressure)
Nervousness
Depression

Serious Side Effects—Danger Signals

(stop pill and contact clinician immediately if any of these symptoms occur):

Symptom	Possible Cause
Leg tenderness or swelling	Thrombophlebitis (inflammation of leg vein with possible formation of blood clot)
Sudden chest pain, shortness of breath, coughing up blood	Pulmonary embolus (blood clot in lung sometimes originating in legs) or coronary thrombosis (heart attack—blood clot in heart)
Sudden, partial or complete loss of vision in an eye	Retinal thrombosis (blood clot in eye)
Sudden weakness, numbness, or inability to move a part of the body; impaired speech, blurred vision, blackouts	Stroke (blood clot in brain)

Possible Beneficial Effects

Decreased menstrual pain, bleeding, and premenstrual tension
Predictable control of menstrual cycle
Fewer ovary and breast cysts
Decreased endometriosis
Improved complexion
Decreased rheumatoid arthritis (slight effect)
Less ovarian and uterine cancer
Less pelvic inflammatory disease

time, doctors prescribe the combination pill. There are presently nearly thirty brands of combination pills on the market, each of which contains estrogen and progesterone. In general, the dosages of estrogen and progesterone vary in each pill. The most important component in the combination pill is estrogen. Effectiveness and most of the serious side effects have been related to the dosage of estrogen. However, researchers are now showing concern about the dosage and type of progesterone as well, since this hormone recently has been linked to such effects as high blood pressure, elevated cholesterol, and heart disease.

The combination pill

The combination pills can be categorized into three groups based on the amount of estrogen (see Table 13). Pills with 50 micrograms of estrogen or more have the same effectiveness; that is, Norinyl 1/80 with 80 micrograms and Norinyl 1/50 with 50 micrograms each have an effectiveness of 99.7% when taken properly. However, serious side effects are likely to be more frequent when a pill containing *more* than 50 micrograms is taken.

Pills with less than 50 micrograms of estrogen are called low-dose pills. No one knows for sure that they are safer as to side effects than 50-microgram pills, but many authorities believe they are. However, the *sub-50s*, as the low-dose pills are called, do have more minor side effects such as spotting or irregular, infrequent periods.

So the optimal dosage of estrogen seems to be 50 micrograms or less. Above 50 micrograms of estrogen the risks of *major* side effects increase, and below it, *minor* side effects are more likely to occur. These differences are summarized in Table 13. For most women starting on the pill, the safest one with the fewest side effects will be a pill containing 35 to 50 micrograms of estrogen.

All combination oral contraceptives come in packages of 21 or 28 pills. Both packages contain 21 hormone pills. The 28-day pack also contains 7 "blanks," which have no active ingredients. These are reminder pills so that you avoid a break in the pill-taking schedule. You can select whichever type you prefer. Some women find it easier to take 28-day pills because the pills are taken without interruption, presumably with less chance of missing taking a pill on the first day of the next cycle.

Some 28-day pills (e.g., Norlestrin Fe 1/50) contain small amounts of iron in the last seven pills. This offers no particular advantage. Women with iron deficiency anemia should be on daily supplemental iron.

The mini-pill

The second type of birth control pill, sometimes called the *mini-pill*, contains only progesterone in each tablet. The advantage of the mini-pill is that it has no estrogen, the hormone believed to be responsible for most serious combination pill side effects. Certain serious side effects, such as blood clots, have not been associated with the use of the mini-pill. However, the mini-pill does have significant disadvantages: a higher pregnancy rate (3% compared to less than 1% for the combination pill) and a rather high frequency of minor side effects (irregular spotting or lack of periods). The three mini-pills currently on the market are Ovrette, Micronor, and Nor-Q-D.

The "Morning-After" Pill

The "morning-after" pill refers to high-dose estrogen tablets, taken usually for only five days. This form of contraception is an emergency measure only and must be used within three days of unprotected intercourse. The brand called Premarin has fewer side effects, such as nausea and breast tenderness, than other pills, some of which contain DES (see Chapter 37).

How to Take Birth Control Pills

Complete this checklist before starting to take the combination pill for the first time:

1. You have no *absolute* contraindications to the pill (see Table 10).
2. You have no or only one *relative* contraindication to the pill (see Table 11).
3. You have had a recent breast and pelvic examination as well as a blood pressure check—preferably the exam should take place within a month before starting the pill.

Table 13   COMPARISON OF BIRTH CONTROL PILLS* BY DOSAGE

	Brand Name	Estrogen Dose (Micrograms)	Serious Side Effects	Minor Side Effects	Theoretical Effectiveness
Group I, High Dose (greater than 50 micrograms of estrogen)	Enovid E	100			
	Enovid 5	75			
	Norinyl 1/80	80	More frequent than Group II or III	Few	99.7%
	Norinyl 2	100			
	Ortho-Novum 1/80	80			
	Ortho-Novum 2	100			
	Ovulen	100			
Group II, Average Dose (50 micrograms of estrogen)	Demulen 1/50	50			
	Norinyl 1/50	50			
	Norlestrin 1/50	50			
	Norlestrin 2.5	50	Very few	Few	99.7%
	Ortho-Novum 1/50	50			
	Ovcon 50	50			
	Ovral	50			
Group III, Low Dose (less than 50 micrograms of estrogen)	Brevicon	35			
	Demulen 1/35	35			
	Loestrin 1/20	20	Similar to or possibly less frequent than Group II	More frequent than Group I or II	99%
	Loestrin 1.5/30	30			
	LoOvral	30			
	Modicon	35			
	Nordette	30			
	Norinyl 1/35	35			
	Ortho-Novum 1/35	35			
	Ortho-Novum 10/11	35			
	Ortho-Novum 7/7/7	35			
	Ovcon 35	35			
	Tri-Norinyl	35			
	Triphasil	30/40			

Recommendations for pill selection:

1. For maximum safety, select a pill in Group II or III. (A pill with less than 50 micrograms of estrogen may be slightly safer than one containing 50 micrograms, but this is not yet proven.)
2. The most recent pills (Ortho-Novum 7/7/7, Tri-Norinyl, and Triphasil) are known as triphasics because their formulations contain three phases in which the hormone dosage is varied to simulate changes in a normal menstrual cycle. In each triphasic pill the progesterone dosage varies and in Triphasil the estrogen dosage varies as well.
3. Women who have a tendency toward high blood pressure or premenstrual weight gain should consider starting with a pill in Group III.
4. Women desiring to avoid spotting or breakthrough bleeding (see glossary) should select a pill from Group II rather than Group III as an initial choice.

* Mini-pill not included.

4. The pill you will use contains 50 micrograms or less of estrogen (discuss this with your clinician at the time of the office visit).

The suggestions below may help you to use the combination pill as effectively as possible.

If you have not had prior intercourse, you can start taking the pill any time, although starting just after a period is usually most convenient. If you are sexually active, begin your cycle of pills only after a normal period. Take your first pill on the fifth day of your period whether or not the bleeding has stopped. Take the pill at the same time each day for a total of 21 days. Then for the next 7 days take no pills (if you have the 21-pill packet) or take pills 22 through 28, which are a different color (if you have the 28-pill packet). During these 7 days a menstrual period usually occurs. After these 7 pill-free days (or days when a different colored pill is taken in the 28-pill packet), take the first pill of your next packet and begin the sequence again.

If you start the pill following pregnancy, follow these guidelines:

1. *After a normal pregnancy:* It's a good idea to ask your clinician to prescribe the pill for use two to three weeks after the baby is born; this way you will be protected prior to your six-week checkup in case you have intercourse before this time. The pills are contraindicated if you are breast-feeding.

2. *After a miscarriage or therapeutic abortion (up to 12 weeks):* Use of birth control pills should begin immediately since ovulation resumes much more quickly following miscarriage or abortion than after a full-term pregnancy.

3. *After a late therapeutic abortion or late miscarriage (after 12 weeks):* Start one week after the procedure. Ovulation occurs sooner than after a normal pregnancy but not as soon as following early miscarriage or early therapeutic abortion.

If you forget to take a pill, take two pills the next day. The chance of getting pregnant is unlikely. If you lose a pill (for example, if it falls down the sink), you have two alternatives. You could take a pill from another pill package, which you then would not be able to use (except as replacements for future lost pills, until the expiration date for that package); or you could simply take the next pill from your current pack. In the latter case, you will finish your pill cycle one day early and subsequent cycles will start a day earlier (for example, Saturday instead of Sunday).

If you miss two days in a row, take two pills a day for the next two days. For example, if you miss taking your pills on Monday and Tuesday, take two pills on Wednesday and two pills on Thursday. Use a back-up method of birth control for the rest of that cycle.

If you miss more than two days of taking the pill, don't take any more pills from that pack. Use an alternative method of birth control for the rest of that cycle.

When to Stop the Pill

If you develop any serious side effects of the pill (see Table 12), you should consult your physician about stopping the pill. If you develop other side effects listed in this table, you may want to switch pills or stay with the same pill for two or three months since many of these symptoms subside on their own. Consult your doctor.

Go off the pills two to three months prior to attempting pregnancy and use another method of birth control such as foam or condoms during this time.

Go off the pills one to two months prior to elective surgery. This will decrease the risk of blood clot complications after surgery as well as blood loss. Use another method of birth control during this time.

Most authorities advise going off the pill at about age forty, if not by the age of thirty-five because of the increasing risk of serious side effects that occur with age. Whether certain risks increase with duration of pill use (say, five years or more) remains uncertain. So some clinicians recommend that all women on the pill have screening tests (for example, for glucose tolerance and cholesterol level) every few years or more often if you have risk factors for diabetes or heart disease (see Table 11). If abnormalities in these tests develop, you probably should stop the pill. Talk with your doctor.

When to Switch Pills—Common Pill Problems

Fortunately, most pill problems are not serious and subside on their own in two or three months and do not require changing to a different pill. Much has been written about the relationship of the hormonal dosages in the combination pill to specific side effects. However, the particular hormone ratios in each pill have a combined action that is not the same in each woman. Clinicians often use trial and error in switching pills to lessen troublesome side effects. Nevertheless, there are a few useful guidelines to follow when dealing with certain side effects:

Light bleeding or spotting may occur on days when you take the pill especially during the first three cycles while your body adjusts to the pill. This is known as *breakthrough bleeding.* If the bleeding is heavy, take two pills a day (one in the morning and one before you go to bed) on pill days when spotting occurs. Take the second pill from a separate packet used for this purpose. If breakthrough bleeding persists after the first few cycles, then try a pill with more estrogen. If you have been using a sub-50 pill, try one with 50 micrograms. If you have been using a 50-microgram pill, remember that in going up to, say, an 80- or

100-microgram pill, your chances of serious side effects increase slightly because of the increase in estrogen. With some 50-microgram pills, such as Norlestrin 1/50, it may be possible to control breakthrough bleeding by increasing the amount of progesterone component (switching to Norlestrin 2.5 in this case) while keeping the same dose of estrogen.

An absent period is not the same as minimal spotting. Even a single brown spot each month is normal for some women on the pill. Complete absence of a period is more common with the mini-pill and with the sub-50s. This may be corrected by increasing the estrogen dosage in the case of combination pills. Get a pregnancy test if you miss two periods on the pill, even if you have not missed any pills.

Nausea, breast tenderness, or breast swelling are characteristic estrogen side effects which may subside or lessen by reducing the amount of estrogen in the pill. These symptoms are a good indication for stepping down to the sub-50s if you currently take a pill with 50 micrograms or more of estrogen. Premenstrual fluid retention is sometimes reduced by using a pill with less estrogen, but the response to switching pills is less consistent than with the other estrogen-dependent side effects.

Acne or oily skin can be dealt with in two possible ways: first, avoid pills which contain certain progesterones, which tend to promote acne and hair growth in some women. These progesterones are found in Ovral, LoOvral, Norlestrin, and Loestrin. If you are not taking one of these pills, the second way to reduce these side effects is by switching to a pill with more estrogen: use Demulen 1/50, instead of Demulen 1/35, for instance.

Depression, fatigue, and noncyclic weight gain are due mainly to progesterone, found in the mini-pill or with progesterone-dominant combination pills, such as Ovral, LoOvral, or Loestrin. By switching to other 50 or sub-50 combination pills, you can reduce these side effects.

The Pill and Pregnancy

Although the risk is very low, several studies have suggested the risk of fetal malformations in women taking hormones, including the pill, *during* the first three months of pregnancy. The risk appears to be somewhat greater for women who took hormones as a diagnostic test for pregnancy, or for treatment of threatened miscarriage, than for those taking birth control pills in early pregnancy. No definite evidence links birth defects or miscarriages to pregnancies conceived immediately *after* going off the pill. A 1978 report by the Harvard School of Public Health found no increased risk of fetal malformation in women who became pregnant one month or more after stopping the pill. Some newer evidence indicates a higher frequency of twins when conception occurs within two months of going off the pill.

Previously women were urged to wait six months after going off the pill before attempting pregnancy. This long wait now appears to be unwarranted. A wait of two to three months is sufficient since after that time there appears to be no increased risk of twins or fetal abnormalities. Furthermore, if you become pregnant without menstruating subsequent to your last pill period, it is difficult to determine when you became pregnant because the timing of the first ovulation following your last cycle of pills is often variable. Once your regular menstrual cycle becomes established after you stop the pill, calculation of your due date if pregnancy should occur becomes much more reliable. The due date is especially important for the high-risk mother-to-be.

Does the Pill Cause Infertility?

The overall fertility of pill users and nonusers is identical, regardless of how long a woman is on oral contraceptives. In the first cycle after the pill is stopped, ovulation is sometimes delayed a few weeks, but overall capacity for becoming pregnant is unchanged. In women who have very infrequent periods, the pill may be associated with some difficulty in their becoming pregnant because of their failure to ovulate. It isn't clear whether such delay of ovulation is pill-related or would have occurred anyway. Women who have had infrequent periods prior to pill use are more likely to experience a prolonged delay (six months or more) in the onset of their first period subsequent to stopping the pill. Usually ovulation can be restored, if pregnancy is desired, by taking a so-called fertility drug such as Clomid (see Chapter 13). These ovulation problems affect fewer than 1% of women using the pill.

The Pill and Cancer

There is presently no convincing evidence that oral contraceptives cause any type of cancer in

Table 14   QUESTIONS COMMONLY ASKED ABOUT BIRTH CONTROL PILLS

Question	Yes	No	Comment
Are all birth control pills equally effective?		X	The mini-pill has a failure rate of about 3% compared to less than 1% for combination pills.
Can the pill stunt growth in a young woman?		X	Not if taken after menstrual periods have begun.
Should I wait two to three months after stopping the pill before planning to get pregnant?	X		The chances of fetal malformations and of twins may be slightly increased if you get pregnant during the first month after stopping the pill.
Can I take the pill if I have varicose veins?	X		Unless they are quite severe, not considered a contra-indication.
Should the pill be taken during the months I am breast-feeding?		X	Although the risks to the newborn are not clearly defined, taking the pill during breast-feeding is not recommended.
Do I need to take iron while on the pill?		X	Unless you are already anemic.
Are periodic "rest periods" desirable (that is, going off the pill for a length of time)?		X	There are no benefits to "rest periods" and you are exposed to a greater risk of unplanned pregnancy at this time.
Does the pill usually decrease sex drive?		X	There is no clear pattern toward increasing or decreasing sexual feelings or responsiveness.
If my mother took DES during her pregnancy with me, can I take the pill?*	X		While no adverse effects have been reported, routine check-ups are advisable approximately every six months.
Is spotting during the first cycle on the pill normal?	X		This light bleeding usually subsides after the first few cycles on pills.
Is facial skin pigmentation which develops while a woman is on the pill improved by switching pills?		X	This pigmentation may occur with different pills regardless of dosage and is made worse by exposure to sunlight.
Should I use a second method of birth control during the first cycle on the pill?	X		Until after the first seven pills are taken; after that you are safe.
Is my fertility increased or decreased after going off the pill?		X	Wait two to three months before attempting pregnancy.

* For more information on DES see chapter 37.

women, although the long-term effects of the pill are not completely known. However, three types of malignancy—breast cancer, uterine cancer, and malignant melanoma (a form of skin cancer)—are associated with increased tumor growth when estrogen is taken. Because the pill contains estrogen, you should not take the pill if you have had any of these types of cancer.

With respect to breast cancer, a number of conflicting reports previously suggested that a few women with severe cystic breast disease may harbor precancerous cells which could be stimulated to grow by estrogen in the pill. For this reason, many authorities have considered cystic breast disease a relative contraindication to the pill. Actually many women with breast cysts and breast tenderness notice an improvement of symptoms while on oral contraceptives.

In March 1983, the Journal of the American Medical Association published reassuring findings from the Cancer and Steroid Hormone Study, a large government project examining long-term effects of the pill. Early results from this study show that long-term pill use (eleven years or more) does not increase a woman's chances of developing breast cancer. The study also found that women who have taken the pill have a 50% reduction in risk for developing cancer of the endometrium or ovary. The relationship between long-term pill use and the development of cancer of the cervix is less certain. Most recent studies have failed to confirm an overall increase in the risk of cervical cancer with pill use. However, women who have taken the pill for five years or more do have nearly twice the risk of developing cancer of the cervix or precancerous changes (see Chapter 36). Whether this finding represents cause and effect or merely the association of other cancer risk factors among the population of pill users is unclear.

10

Selecting Your Method

We hope you have a good working knowledge about contraception after reading the previous chapters. Now comes the difficult part: selecting the contraceptive method best for you. Your doctor is a good source of specific information. It would be easy to let him or her decide for you, but we think you are the one to make the most appropriate choice. Table 15 summarizes the advantages and disadvantages of the major birth control methods.

Table 15 ADVANTAGES AND DISADVANTAGES OF BIRTH CONTROL METHODS

Method	Advantages	Disadvantages
Pill	almost complete effectiveness; convenient and does not interfere with sexual spontaneity; decreased menstrual blood loss and cramping	not safe for all women; rare serious and numerous minor side effects
IUD	very effective; does not interfere with sexual spontaneity; most convenient method	frequent side effects, especially in women who have not had children; if pregnancy occurs, serious infection or other complications may develop; perforation or expulsion may occur and be unnoticed
Barrier (*diaphragm, condom, foam*)	very effective if properly used; no major medical complications; possible prevention against venereal disease	may interfere with sexual spontaneity; may be inconvenient or messy; chance of pregnancy higher than for pill or for IUD
Rhythm (*natural family planning*)	no physical side effects; accepted by all religions	high chance of pregnancy; abstinence or back-up method required nearly half of the time; requires diligent record keeping; may be difficult to use if periods are irregular

Table 16   EFFECTIVENESS RATES* FOR VARIOUS BIRTH CONTROL METHODS

Method	Theoretical Effectiveness Rate	Use Effectiveness Rate
Combination pill	99.9%	96% to 99% (98% average)
IUD	98%	94% to 99% (98% average)
Diaphragm (with spermicide)	97%	80% to 97% (85% average)
Condom	97%	64% to 97% (90% average)
Condom and spermicide	99%	94%
Foam	97%	71% to 97% (80% average)
Rhythm (natural family Planning)	95% to 99%	53% to 99% (70% average)

* Based on rates reported from various studies.

Three Steps to Selecting Your Method

There are three essential steps to follow in selecting your birth control method:

1. How *effective* does your chosen method need to be?
2. How *safe* will the method be for you?
3. How *acceptable* is the method for you?

The three-step decision-making process is outlined in Table 17.

Step 1—Effectiveness

Effectiveness here means how well the method keeps you from becoming pregnant. Begin by selecting from Table 16 the method which offers the highest effectiveness required for your needs. Remember that effectiveness is directly related not only to the inherent efficiency of the method (known as *theoretical* effectiveness) but also to how carefully the method is going to be used (known as *use* effectiveness). The theoretical effectiveness and use effectiveness rates are very close for the various IUDs and the pill. Note that the widest difference between the theoretical effectiveness rate and the use effectiveness rate is found with the barrier methods (diaphragm, condom, and foam) and the rhythm methods. To know which end of the effectiveness range for a specific method applies to you, you should add a fudge factor based on your own motivation to consistently use these methods properly. With proper use, the barrier methods or rhythm methods may be nearly as effective as the pill or IUD. The question you need to answer is: How careful and painstaking am I likely to be in using the method I choose? Be honest with yourself. Remember also that effectiveness increases considerably when you use two methods at the same time.

Step 2—Safety

Safety here refers to the health risks involved with the use of each method. The risk for each method has two components:

1. the risk of side effects and death associated with the method itself (higher for the pill and the IUD); and
2. the risk (medical and death) associated with unexpected pregnancy (or therapeutic abortion) if the method fails (higher for barrier and rhythm methods).

When these two risk components are combined, the overall risk of any one of the four methods (pill, IUD, barrier, and rhythm) in nonsmoking women under age thirty is essentially the same—namely, 1 to 2 deaths per 100,000 women per year. In other words, based on the experience of hundreds of thousands of nonsmoking women, *up to age thirty* your overall risk calculated statistically is similar, regardless of which birth control method you choose. After age thirty, the picture changes in four ways:

Table 17 THREE-STEP APPROACH FOR SELECTING YOUR BIRTH CONTROL METHOD

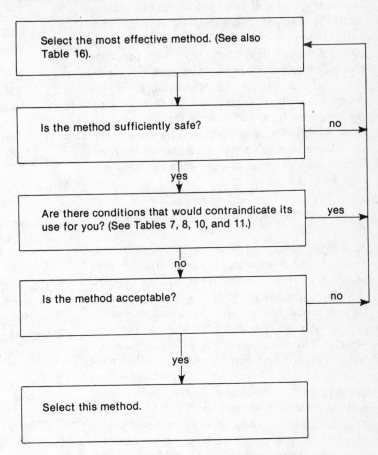

Step 1: Effectiveness — Select the most effective method. (See also Table 16).

Step 2: Safety — Is the method sufficiently safe? → no

yes

Are there conditions that would contraindicate its use for you? (See Tables 7, 8, 10, and 11.) → yes

no

Step 3: Acceptability — Is the method acceptable? → no

yes

Select this method.

---

1. The risk of death (mortality) in pill users who smoke rises disproportionately with increasing age. This risk is four to seven times the risk compared to that for non-smoking pill users and from seven to over twenty-five times more risky than for users of other birth control methods (IUD, barrier, rhythm).

2. The method of birth control with the lowest overall mortality regardless of age is the IUD (1 to 2 deaths per 100,000 women per year even in women over forty). These risks are due to a combination of risks inherent in the method itself and to pregnancy risks associated with method failure.

3. The mortality risk among pill users who do not smoke increases only slightly between age thirty and age thirty-five at which point it goes up to about 5 to 7 deaths per 100,000

women per year. These risks are due largely to risks associated with the method itself.

4. The mortality risk among users of traditional contraception (barrier method and rhythm method) increases somewhat after age thirty to 2 to 4 deaths per 100,000 women per year. These risks are due largely to pregnancy risks from failure of the method.

Step 3—Acceptability

Acceptability is a subjective determination; that is, every person has a different idea of what is acceptable, and this determination is one you must make for yourself. The method selected in the first two steps of this process must now conform to your personal needs for convenience and sexual spontaneity, as well as your tolerance for side effects. For example, if you are planning to get pregnant in the next year, the IUD or the pill is probably not for you. If you have never been pregnant, the IUD may be unacceptable because of a clearly increased risk of side effects, including possible decreased fertility. For some women the barrier method may be unsatisfactory for aesthetic reasons, while for other women who have infrequent intercourse or who want possible increased protection against venereal disease, such methods may may be better suited.

Hormonal Birth Control—Future Methods

Enormous costs and years of research are involved in the development of new drugs, including contraceptives. Unfortunately the Federal government has not made research into new birth control methods a priority and annually spends about ten cents per capita on contraceptive research. FDA drug testing regulations require extensive animal and human testing, so that most drugs take five to ten years or more before they are approved. Some drugs which are widely used in other countries do not meet the FDA's strict requirements for safety or effectiveness. An example is Depo-Provera, a long-acting injectable hormonal contraceptive used worldwide, especially in many Third World nations.

Probably the most promising development in hormonal contraception besides an improved birth control pill is the use of a contraceptive implant. The implant consists of several tiny pellets that are injected subcutaneously into the skin of the upper arm using local anesthesia. The pellets continuously release progesterone (at concentrations much less than in the pill), providing highly effective contraception for up to five years. The pellets are then removed in the doctor's office—a potentially cumbersome disadvantage. To eliminate this problem biodegradable pellets are being developed that will not have to be removed. The hormonal implant system should become available by the late 1980s.

Resources

For further information on birth control and fami-

ly planning clinics, contact your local women's center or write to the following:

Planned Parenthood Federation
of America, Inc.
810 Seventh Avenue
New York, New York 10019

Zero Population Growth, Inc.
1346 Connecticut Avenue, N.W.
Washington, D.C. 20036

References for Section Two

Chapter 6—Natural Family Planning

Lanctot, C. A. Natural family planning. *Clinics in Obstetrics and Gynecology* 6(1):109-128, 1979.

Hilgers, T. W., and Prebil, A. M. The ovulation method—vulvar observations as an index of fertility/infertility. *Obstetrics and Gynecology* 53(1):12-22, 1979.

Hilgers, T. W., Abraham, G. E., et al. Natural family planning. *Obstetrics and Gynecology* 52(5):575-582, 1978.

Wade, M. E., McCarthy, P., et al. A randomized prospective study of the use-effectiveness of two methods of natural family planning. *American Journal of Obstetrics and Gynecology* 141(4):368-376, 1981.

Chapter 7—The Diaphragm and Other Barrier Methods

Family Planning Perspectives Digest: Seven-year prospective study of 17,000 women using the pill, IUD, and diaphragm show benefits of each outweigh risks. *Family Planning Perspectives* 8(5):241-245, 1976.

Maine, D. Barrier methods—renewed interest but more research is needed. *Family Planning Perspectives* 11(4):237-240, 1979.

Dent, T., and Brueschke, E. E. Barrier contraceptives. *The Female Patient* 57-66, Oct 1981.

Chapter 8—Intrauterine Devices

The Medical Device and Drug Advisory Committees on Obstetrics and Gynecology: *Second Report on Intrauterine Contraceptive Devices*, 1978, U.S. Dept. of HEW, Food and Drug Administration, Washington, D.C. (Stock #017-012-00276-5).

Kaufman, D. W., et al. The effect of different types of intrauterine devices on the risk of pelvic inflammatory disease. *Journal of the American Medical Association* 250:759–762, 1983.

Segal, S. J. What's the latest on IUDs? *Contemporary OB/GYN* 16(special issue):115-118, 1980.

Dept. of HEW. Intrauterine contraceptive devices: Professional and patient labelling published in Federal Register, 1977.

Eschenbach, D. A. Do IUDs increase relative risk of infection? *Contemporary OB/GYN* 14:93-97, Oct 1979.

Burkman, R. T., and The Women's Health Study. Association between intrauterine device and pelvic inflammatory disease. *Obstetrics and Gynecology* 57(3):269-276, 1981.

Chaudhury, R. R. Current status of research on intrauterine devices. *Obstetrical and Gynecological Survey* 35(6):333-338, 1980.

Chapter 9—Birth Control Pills (Oral Contraceptives)

Lincoln, R. The pill, breast and cervical cancer, and the role of progestogens in arterial disease. *Family Planning Perspectives* 16(2):55–62, Mar/Apr 1984.

Wahl, P., et al. Effect of estrogen/progestin potency on lipid/lipoprotein cholesterol. *New England Journal of Medicine* 308:862–867, 1983.

Connell, K. B. Update on oral contraceptives. *Current Problems in Obstetrics and Gynecology* 2(8):3-30, 1979.

Huggins, G. R. Contraceptive use and subsequent fertility. *Fertility and Sterility* 28:603-610, 1977.

Ory, H. W. Association between oral contraceptives and myocardial infarction. *Journal of the American Medical Association* 237:2619-2622, 1977.

Fisch, I. R., and Frank, J. Oral contraceptives and blood pressure. *Journal of the American Medical Association* 237:2499-2503, 1977.

Rothman, K. J., and Louik, C. Oral contraceptives and birth defects. *New England Journal of Medicine* 299:522-524, Sept 7, 1978.

Kretzschmar, R. M. Oral contraceptives and cancer. *Ca-A Cancer Journal for Clinicians* 28(2):118-123, 1978.

Speroff, L. A brief for low-dose pills. *Contemporary OB/GYN* 17(5):27-32, 1981.

Ory, H. W., Rosenfield, A., et al. The pill at 20: an assessment. *International Family Planning Perspectives* 6(4):125-129, 1980.

The Walnut Creek contraceptive drug study. a supplement to *The Journal of Reproductive Medicine* 25(6), 1980.

Swan, S. H., and Brown, W. L. Oral contraceptive use, sexual activity, and cervical carcinoma. *American Journal of Obstetrics and Gynecology* 139(1):52-57, Jan 1981.

Chapter 10—Selecting Your Method

Darney, P. D. What's new in contraception? *Contemporary OB/GYN* 23(6): 117–138, June 1984.

Zatuchni, G. I. Advances in fertility control. *The Female Patient* 9:17–26, May 1984.

Ory, H. W. *Making choices: Evaluating the Health Risks and Benefits of Birth Control Methods.* Washington, D.C.: The Alan Guttmacher Institute, 1983.

Garcia, C. R. Contraception at the crossroads. *Contemporary OB/GYN* 13:81-87, Jan 1979.

Flowers, C. E. Psychological aspects of contraception. supplement to the *Journal of Continuing Education in Obstetrics and Gynecology* 21(7), 1979.

Brenner, P. F. Contraceptive counselling. *The Female Patient* 60-62, Feb 1979.

Ford, C. V. Psychological factors influencing the choice of a contraceptive method. *Medical Aspects of Human Sexuality* 98-106, Jan 1978.

Hatcher, R. A., et al. *Contraceptive Technology 1984–1985,* ed. 12. New York: John Wiley and Sons, 1984.

Mishell, D. R., Jr., and Davajan, V. *Reproductive Endocrinology, Infertility and Contraception.* Philadelphia: F. A. Davis, 1979.

three

Planning Pregnancy

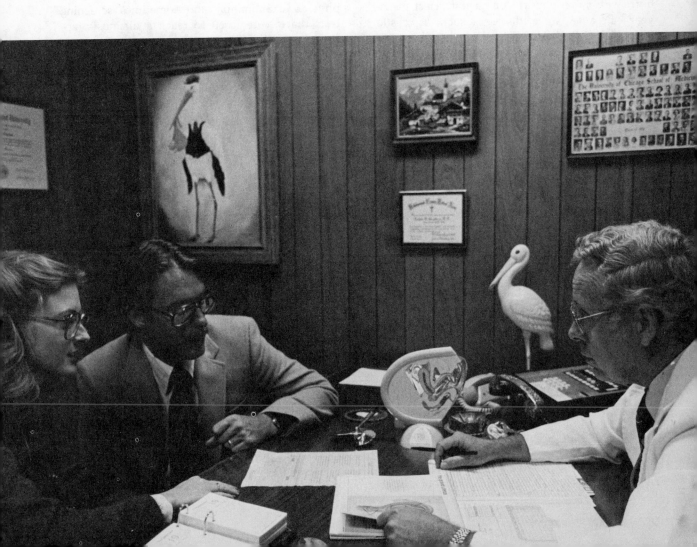

11

Identifying Birth Defects

Concern with preventing genetic birth defects has grown steadily in the past decade among the general population and health professionals alike. Genetic disease or genetically influenced conditions now account for nearly one-third of infant deaths, and major defects affect about 2.5% of all live-born infants. In all, about 250,000 babies are born with some physical or mental defect every year. Because some diseases, such as cystic fibrosis, Tay-Sachs disease, and sickle-cell anemia (see glossary), may not show up for several months, the real chance of a birth defect is about 5%. Looking at it another way, 95% of infants appear healthy at birth and will not develop major birth defects in later life.

The causes of birth defects range from genetic roots that result in, say, Down's syndrome, to underlying environmental influences, like drugs, exposure to radiation, or maternal infection (German measles). Few birth defects have a single, major environmental or genetic cause. Most are believed to result from the interaction of several genes, possibly in combination with subtle environmental influences. As a result, birth defects usually occur irregularly and unpredictably. However, couples with known risk factors, such as a family history of an inherited genetic disease, previous birth of a defective child, or advanced maternal age, often want to know their chance of having a healthy baby. Genetic counseling deals with these and other factors in helping such couples plan their families.

What is Genetic Counseling?

Genetic counseling is the process of educating couples who want to have children about how some birth defects happen, what the couple's chances are of having a normal baby, and what alternatives are open to them if they are at risk of having a baby with a birth defect. Genetic counseling uses the science of genetics to help prevent birth defects. If you have a child with a birth defect and/or mental retardation, you would be wise to seek genetic counseling before attempting another pregnancy. Primary care physicians, such as family practitioners or obstetricians, often provide initial counseling since they are the ones who see the patients first. At times, the medical geneticist and his or her specialized laboratory may be needed as well.

Counseling explains the risks of having a child with a certain disorder and what that disorder means. It also offers the couple alternatives for dealing with the risk. Valuable clues from your medical and family health history can often determine the pattern of inheritance or expected frequency of a certain genetic disorder. After a physical examination and sometimes screening tests that are required to reach a diagnosis, appropriate alternatives can be considered: for example, prenatal testing, adoption, artificial insemination, sterilization. The option selected depends on the severity of a given defect and the risks involved. Fortunately, 95% of the time, couples seeking genetic counseling about a particular disorder can expect reassurance that their baby will not be affected by the disorder in question.

Genes and Chromosomes

You can understand how different disorders may be inherited by looking at the basic body unit—the cell. Every human cell except the sperm cell and egg cell contains 46 chromosomes, each filled with thousands of genes arranged in pairs. Half of each gene pair comes from the egg cell of the mother and half from the sperm cell of the father. Genes contain the genetic material that controls all of our physical features from eye color and ear shape to critical parts of the heart and nervous system. The genetic information carried in genes directs the growth, development, and function of our bodies throughout life. Considering the vast information contained in our genes, it is amazing that mistakes resulting in genetic disorders occur as infrequently as they do. Most people are carriers of a few genes for inherited diseases. However, normal genes most often outweigh the effects of faulty genes. Unless both parents carry the same abnormal genes, the offspring is usually unaffected.

Genetic disorders can be classified into three basic types: *chromosomal disorders*, *single-gene disorders*, and *multifactorial inheritance*.

Chromosomal disorders result from an abnormality in the number or structure of the chromosomes in each cell. These disorders occur during an isolated accident (such as acquiring an extra chromosome) in the development of the fertilized egg. Such chromosomal errors are then transmitted to all other cells from the moment of fertilization. It should be stressed that parents of offspring with a chromosomal defect are almost never the carriers of that defect because chromosomal abnormalities are rarely inherited. The risk of bearing a child with this defect, however, does increase with maternal age.

Most chromosomal errors have serious medical consequences and many result in miscarriage. This is nature's way of handling severely defective embryos. Less often, chromosomal problems result in stillbirth or multiple birth defects. Chromosomal abnormalities of varying severity occur in about one out of two hundred newborns.

In Down's syndrome (which used to be called Mongolism), the most common chromosomal defect, the affected child has 47 chromosomes in each cell, rather than the normal 46. The disorder causes mental retardation and a typical so-called mongoloid appearance: small head, slanting eyes, and other physical abnormalities. Down's syndrome and other chromosomal disorders can be diagnosed prenatally.

Single-gene disorders, hereditary conditions caused by a single defective gene, affect approximately 1% of newborns. According to the laws of genetics, there are three ways in which these defects may be transmitted from generation to generation: *dominant inheritance*, *recessive inheritance*, and *X-linked inheritance*.

With *dominant inheritance* (see Table 18) it takes just one defective gene from either parent to cause a disorder in the offspring. If that faulty gene is passed to the offspring, the faulty gene always dominates the normal counterpart gene from the other parent and causes the child to inherit the defect. Since the child will inherit from the affected parent *either* the normal gene *or* the

defective gene, then each child has a 50% chance of inheriting the defect. To understand this percentage, you need to picture the genes of each parent in pairs. Let's say one gene of one parent's pair is faulty; the other gene of that same pair is normal. Only one of the gene twosome is passed to the offspring. If the normal gene is passed, the child will be normal. If the faulty (dominant) gene is passed, the child will have a birth defect. This is one of the *laws of inheritance*. Examples of dominantly inherited disorders include hypercholesterolemia (high blood cholesterol), Huntington's disease (progressive nervous system degeneration), and certain forms of dwarfism. At present, very few dominantly inherited disorders can be diagnosed during pregnancy.

Recessive inheritance (see Table 19) requires one defective gene from each of *both* the parents to cause the disorder in the offspring. In the case of *recessive* inheritance, if a person has one normal gene and one defective gene, the normal gene takes precedence over its defective recessive counterpart. This means that this person is not *affected* by the disease but can be a *carrier*, that is, can pass the defect on to offspring. Each child has a 25% chance of inheriting the defect when both

---

Table 18 HOW DOMINANT INHERITANCE WORKS (SINGLE-GENE DISORDERS)

(Only one parent is affected whose single faulty gene (D) dominates its normal counterpart (A).)

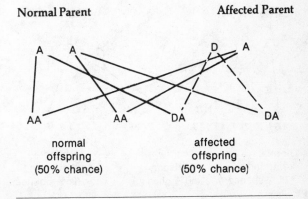

Normal Parent   Affected Parent

| normal offspring (50% chance) | affected offspring (50% chance) |

parents are carriers. If only one parent is a carrier, the offspring cannot inherit the defect but each child has a 50% chance of being a carrier of the defect. Single-gene defects include many inborn errors of metabolism, so called because they don't allow normal chemical reactions in body cells. Many of these metabolic conditions cause mental retardation or death in early childhood. Examples of recessively inherited disorders include cystic fibrosis (disorder of the mucous and sweat glands), galactosemia (inability to digest milk sugar), phenylketonuria (a biochemical disorder causing mental retardation), sickle-cell disease (severe form of anemia), and Tay-Sachs disease (fatal brain damage). Since this form of inheritance occurs when neither parent seems to be affected (but both are carriers), diagnosis is usually made only after the birth of an affected child. If a child has been diagnosed with one of these disorders, the child's parents may be advised to have an amniocentesis in subsequent pregnancies, because this test can detect about seventy of the four hundred known recessively inherited disorders.

X-linked, or sex-linked, *inheritance* disorders occur when a genetic condition is transmitted through the X chromosome. Normal females have two X chromosomes in each cell. Normal males have one X chromosome and one Y chromosome. In X-linked inheritance, the mother usually carries an abnormal gene on one of the X chromosomes but is usually not affected herself. Each son has a 50% chance of inheriting this disorder. Each daughter has a 50% chance of being a carrier, like her mother. Examples of X-linked disorders are hemophilia (defect in blood-clotting mechanisms), some forms of muscular dystrophy (progressive muscle wasting), and color blindness. Most X-linked disorders cannot be diagnosed during pregnancy, but amniocentesis does establish the sex of the fetus and consequently whether or not the child could be affected.

Table 20 summarizes the chances of an offspring being a carrier or being affected, according to certain existent conditions, in the three ways that single-gene disorders may be inherited.

Multifactorial inheritance refers to defects resulting from the interaction of faulty genes and possibly a negative environment. The risks for these defects are based on their statistical frequency in the population rather than on laws of inheritance. If you have one affected child, the risk of having another with the same defect is approximately 5%. Certain malformations in this group, including spina bifida (open spine) and anencephaly (failure of brain development), can be diagnosed during pregnancy by amniocentesis. Nearly all other genetic diseases in this category, although they include 90% of all birth defects, cannot be diagnosed by prenatal testing.

Preventing Genetic Disease

Carriers of genetic diseases are not affected themselves but may be at risk for passing a defect to their children. Couples who carry (but are not themselves affected by) harmful traits may thus not be aware of their risk status unless there is an affected relative in the family or they themselves have an affected child. Medical screening tests can presently detect about seventy separate genetic diseases. These tests detect the parents who are the carriers of faulty genes that may lead to a birth defect. Carrier detection has been most widely applied to screening for sickle-cell disease and Tay-Sachs disease because each of these diseases occurs so frequently within a specific population. Ten percent of U.S. blacks are carriers of sickle-cell

Table 19   HOW RECESSIVE INHERITANCE WORKS (SINGLE-GENE DISORDERS)

(Both parents are usually unaffected and have a normal gene (A) which takes precedence over its faulty recessive counterpart (r).)

Carrier Mother   **Carrier Father**

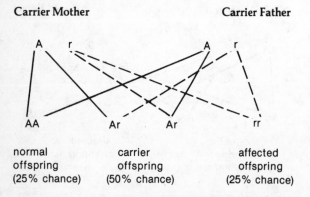

| AA | Ar | Ar | rr |

| normal offspring (25% chance) | carrier offspring (50% chance) | affected offspring (25% chance) |

Table 20 CHANCES OF INHERITING SINGLE-GENE DISORDERS

Type of Inheritance	Parent Affected?	Parent Carrier?	Chance of Offspring Being a Carrier	Chance of Offspring Being Affected
Dominant inheritance (1 parent carries faulty gene, 1 parent genetically normal)	yes	no	0%	50%
Recessive inheritance (1 parent carries faulty gene, 1 parent genetically normal)	no	yes	50%	0%
Recessive inheritance (both parents carry same faulty gene)	no (neither)	yes (both)	50%	25%
Sex-linked inheritance (mother carries faulty gene, father genetically normal)	no	yes (mother)	25% (50% of all females, 0% of males)	25% (50% of all males, 0% of females)

disease and 3% of Jewish persons of eastern European ancestry are carriers of Tay-Sachs disease. Both of these diseases are transmitted by recessive inheritance and affect 25% of the offspring when both parents are carriers.

Another form of genetic screening involves chromosomal analysis called *karyotyping* to search for abnormalities in parental chromosomes. This blood test presently costs about $200 and takes a technician several days to perform, making it impractical for mass screening. As stated previously, most chromosomal defects result from isolated accidents rather than from inheritance. In rare cases, however, parents who are carriers of chromosomal abnormalities may transmit the defect to their offspring. Often the only clue to the person carrying a chromosomal abnormality is a history of reproduction problems. Therefore, couples with a history of any of the following pregnancy-related difficulties should consider chromosomal testing to see if either partner carries abnormal chromosomes:

1. Three or more miscarriages.
2. Two miscarriages plus a child born with a birth defect.
3. Two miscarriages and a stillbirth.
4. Stillbirth where birth defects are present.
5. Infertility if routine tests prove negative.
6. Previous child with a birth defect (some instances).

Some couples who feel they may be at risk undergo these screening tests to detect single-gene

or chromosomal defects so they can make informed decisions about pregnancy. If affected, some partners elect to remain childless; others take the risk of having their own child, or they adopt children. Artificial insemination is another option when only the husband is a carrier. The affected couples who do attempt pregnancy often undergo prenatal testing to determine if a given genetic defect is present in the fetus.

Prenatal testing for birth defects

Nearly 90% of birth defects are *not* subject to prenatal diagnosis; that is, it is not possible with 90% of birth defects to determine through a prenatal test whether a birth defect exists. Of the 10% remaining, those most suitable for prenatal diagnosis include:

1. Chromosomal abnormalities (such as Down's syndrome).
2. Metabolic disorders (rare).
3. Sex-linked disorders (rare).
4. Specific disorders of the central nervous system (anencephaly, spina bifida).

With rare exception, all these conditions require a relatively new procedure called *amniocentesis*, which is performed between the fourteenth and sixteenth week of pregnancy. The procedure involves removal of a small amount of amniotic fluid (the "waters" surrounding the baby) through a hollow needle inserted through the mother's abdomen into the uterine cavity (see

Figure 22 in Chapter 20). The use of local anesthesia makes the procedure no more uncomfortable for most women than a blood test. Amniotic fluid cells shed from the fetus are then sent to a laboratory and tested for chromosomal defects or for specific biochemical abnormalities, such as Tay-Sachs disease. Chromosomal analysis also reveals the sex of the child.

Amniocentesis takes about five minutes to perform. Although the risk of fetal injury is practically zero, the chance of spontaneous miscarriage as a direct result of this procedure is approximately one out of two hundred. Other complications, such as infection and bleeding, are rare. Sonography (see Chapter 16), a procedure using sound waves, is usually performed prior to amniocentesis to help guide the needle to a "pocket" of fluid away from the placenta. Passing the needle through the placenta is likely to cause leakage of fetal blood cells into the maternal circulation, possibly resulting in complications for Rh negative women. For this reason, even if sonography is used, Rh negative women now receive a small dose of RhoGAM, a drug to prevent complications, after amniocentesis. In addition to its uses for amniocentesis, sonography confirms the gestational age of the fetus and identifies the presence of twins.

Table 21 lists the possible reasons for genetic amniocentesis. A couple should seriously consider having the procedure performed if any of the conditions apply. The most common reason for prenatal amniocentesis is advanced maternal age. As women grow older, they have increased chances for bearing children with chromosomal problems, such as Down's syndrome. Advanced paternal age is not nearly as important. The reason for this may be that a man continuously produces sperm throughout his life, whereas a woman is born with the number of eggs she will have throughout life. As the eggs age, chromosomal accidents during ovulation or fertilization may occur with increased frequency. After the age of thirty-five, the risk of Down's syndrome and other chromosomal abnormalities increases significantly. There is some debate as to whether the risk in women between the ages of thirty-five and thirty-nine justifies the procedure; however, taking into account the increased risk of *all* chromosomal abnormalities in this age group—approximately 2%—many authorities believe that amniocentesis is indicated. After age forty, amniocentesis is definitely recommended.

Another common reason for genetic amniocentesis is the previous birth of a child with a chromosomal defect, including Down's syndrome. A woman with this history has a 1% to 2% risk for recurrence, regardless of her age. A much higher risk for recurrence—25%—exists for couples who have children with inherited metabolic disorders where both parents are carriers. Prior to the use of amniocentesis, such carrier parents had two options: to go with the throw of the genetic dice or to remain childless. Now, some of these disorders can be identified by amniocentesis. At this time, practical methods are not available to screen a given individual for all of the known metabolic abnormalities. A person is tested only for the abnormality at risk. In couples who have had children with certain abnormalities of the brain (anencephaly) and spinal column (spina bifida), the woman should undergo amniocentesis, because the recurrence risk for these defects is approximately 5%.

Among all the new procedures for prenatal diagnosis of genetic disorders, amniocentesis is the most accurate and safest.

A new technique called chorion biopsy may replace amniocentesis by the late 1980s as the procedure of choice for diagnosing genetic disorders in early pregnancy. Chorion biopsy or chorionic villus sampling (CVS) allows doctors to screen for genetic defects as early as the eighth week of pregnancy and gives results within forty-eight hours. CVS involves insertion of a small tube through the cervix into the uterus to take a sample of the chorion, a membrane surrounding the fetus. Cells from the chorion have the same genetic makeup as the fetus. The earlier detection and more rapid diagnosis of birth defects by this method would be a major advantage over amniocentesis, which is performed near the sixteenth week of pregnancy and takes two to four weeks for results. At this time, however, CVS remains an experimental procedure which may turn out to have a higher rate of miscarriage and other complications compared to amniocentesis.

Sonography can detect very gross abnormalities such as anencephaly (where the fetal skull is not formed) but needs far more research before it can be relied upon as a tool for diagnosing other physical defects. Fetoscopy is a technique that diagnoses blood diseases, such as sickle-cell anemia, thalassemia, and hemophilia. The procedure permits direct sampling of fetal blood by means of a pencil-sized instrument inserted through the ab-

Table 21   POSSIBLE REASONS FOR AMNIOCENTESIS TO IDENTIFY BIRTH DEFECTS

Possible Reason	Incidence of Birth Defect
Age over 35, especially if over 37	1% to 2%
Three or more miscarriages	less than 1%
Either parent has a known chromosomal abnormality	1% to 100% (average 10%)
The mother has had a chromosomally abnormal child in the past, such as Down's syndrome	variable* (average 1% to 2%)
There is a history of Down's syndrome (or other chromosomal abnormality) in either parent's family	variable (average less than 1%)
The mother has male relatives with muscular dystrophy, hemophilia, or other sex-linked disorder	25%
Both parents are carriers for or have had a child with a hereditary metabolic disorder (e.g., Tay-Sachs disease)	25%
The mother has had a child with spina bifida (open spine) or anencephaly; or the disorder is present in a close family member (parent or sibling)	3% to 5%

* The recurrence risk in 95% of women who have given birth to a child with Down's syndrome is 1% to 2%. In the other 5% of women, either parent may carry an abnormal chromosome which has a recurrence risk of approximately 5% to 10%.

domen of the mother. Although presently an experimental and potentially hazardous technique, fetoscopy may be justified for couples carrying certain diseases for which no other means of diagnosis is currently available.

Limitations of amniocentesis

The relative rarity of genetic abnormalities even in high-risk populations is a major factor limiting the wider use of amniocentesis for detection of genetic disease. Even if amniocentesis were done on all women over thirty-five, the frequency of Down's syndrome, for instance, would be decreased by less than 50% since the *average* maternal age for this condition is less than thirty-four years. For the genetic diseases that can be diagnosed, the options are presently limited by the inability to treat the vast majority of diseases either in utero (in the uterus) or following childbirth. Consequently, for those few women who have a positive prenatal diagnosis, there are really only two alternatives: abortion or risking the birth of a deformed child. Couples who select abortion often experience depression following termination of the pregnancy. Despite the emotional trauma involved, couples selecting therapeutic abortion may consider this option preferable to the birth of a severely defective child.

Sex Determination

Choice of a girl or a boy may become a parental option by the end of the 1980s. As of 1984, however, techniques enabling sex selection are far from perfected. Scientists have long known that the sex of a child depends on whether a "male" or "female" sperm fertilizes the egg; the sperm carrying the Y chromosome will produce a boy and one bearing the X chromosome is responsible for producing a girl.

Numerous methods of sex determination have been proposed. Popular but unsubstantiated theories in the 1960s emphasized the use of coital timing and baking soda or vinegar douches to enhance the survival of male or female sperm, respectively. The most promising method of sex selection today involves separation of male and female sperm. A technique for sperm separation was originally developed by a reproductive physiologist, Dr. Ronald Ericsson, in 1973. Ericsson's patented method takes advantage of the fact that male and female sperm "swim" at different rates. A sperm race is set up by suspending a drop of semen onto a solution of albumin, a dense fluid found in blood. The technique allows collection of the faster-moving male sperm which swim to the bottom of the albumin-filled glass

Table 22   INFORMATION ABOUT COMMON BIRTH DEFECTS

Name	Frequency of Occurrence	Risk of Recurrence	Detectable in Pregnancy	Genetic Classification
Anencephaly (failure of brain development)	1:1000	1:20	yes (amniocentesis; sonography)	multifactorial
Cleft lip and/or palate	1:1000	1:20	no	multifactorial
Clubfoot	1:1000	1:30	no	multifactorial
Congenital heart disease	1:1000	1:50	no	multifactorial
Congenital hip dislocation	1:1000	1:25	no	multifactorial
Cystic fibrosis	1:2500	1:4	no	single gene
Down's syndrome	1:650 (age-dependent)	1:50	yes (amniocentesis)	chromosomal
Hemophilia	1:3000	1:4 (50% of all males)	yes (amniocentesis detects fetal sex; fetoscopy***)	single gene (sex-linked)
Pyloric stenosis (obstructed opening from stomach into intestine)	1:1000	1:30	no	multifactorial
Sickle-cell anemia	1:500*	1:4	yes (fetoscopy***)	single gene
Spina bifida	1:1000	1:20	usually (amniocentesis)	multifactorial
Tay-Sachs disease	1:3000**	1:4	yes (amniocentesis)	single gene

*   frequency among blacks
** frequency among Jews of eastern European ancestry
*** this procedure not generally available

tube. Using these sperm for artificial insemination would increase a woman's chances to conceive a boy to perhaps 75%. Still, many infertility experts remain skeptical of successful reports of sex determination since the number of successful cases reported is very small. Thus, for at least the present, a proven method of sex determination remains unavailable.

Where to Get Help

If you need more information about birth defects and genetics (see Table 22), start with your family physician or obstetrician, who may make the ap-

propriate local referral if he or she cannot do the counseling. There are counseling centers located in most major cities throughout the U.S.

For further information on genetic counseling, write to:

March of Dimes Birth Defects Foundation
1275 Mamaroneck Avenue
White Plains, N. Y. 10605

National Clearinghouse for Human Genetic
  Diseases
805 Fifteenth Street, N.W., Suite 500
Washington, D.C. 20005

12

Pregnancy After Thirty-Five

In the 1980s many women are choosing to wait, for one reason or another, until their thirties or even early forties to have babies. Other women may not have the opportunity to experience motherhood prior to this time. The trends toward first establishing one's career, having later marriages and smaller families, having children in second and third marriages, and spending fewer years at home as a full-time homemaker have all paralleled one another. The impetus of the women's movement, changing life styles, modern methods of birth control, and availability of child-care facilities have also contributed toward this shift in the timing of childbearing.

There is probably no "perfect" time to have a baby. There can be advantages and disadvantages at every age of childbearing when all the factors—social, financial, psychological, and medical—are considered. Your marital happiness, financial security, and, when you have the opportunity, the satisfaction that comes from planning a child when the time is right for you are important considerations which you must weigh against strictly medical factors.

Let's consider here first the medical concerns of pregnancy and childbirth after the age of thirty-five. Although no specific age separates "young" mothers from "old" mothers, many authorities use age thirty-five and older in discussing special pregnancy problems affecting the "older" woman. Actually the likelihood of medical complications increases gradually, without sudden escalation, starting at about the age of thirty. For example, the risk of pregnancy-related deaths per 100,000 births increases from 11 in the late twenties to 18 in the early thirties, rising to 46 in the late thirties, and so on; but keep in mind that this rate is still a very small percentage.

Although it is true that certain birth defects increase with maternal age, many of these abnormalities are detectable in early pregnancy and they affect a very small percentage of women over the age of thirty-five. The most well-known and frequent risk of pregnancy after age thirty-five is the birth of an infant with a chromosomal abnormality, such as Down's syndrome (see Chapter 11). The incidence of Down's syndrome rises from less than one per thousand before age thirty to one per hundred by age forty. Women over thirty-five have a 2% chance of having a child with a chromosomal birth defect.

Infertility increases with age and may become a concern for couples in their thirties. Human reproductive capacity peaks for both sexes in the midtwenties and then appears to decline steadily in women over thirty and in men over forty. Tubal infections, endometriosis, and fibroid tumors occur more often in older women and are among the common causes of infertility in this age group.

Other pregnancy complications which are at least twice as frequent in mothers over the age of thirty-five compared to those in their twenties include miscarriage, stillbirths, placenta previa, diabetes, and high blood pressure. (See index for more information.) Multiple births also occur more often with increasing age, so that women in their thirties have a 30% greater chance of having twins than they did in their twenties. The risk of premature births and infant deaths is only *slightly* greater in older mothers, even up to age forty-four; and it is not nearly so great as in pregnant teen-agers.

With adequate rest, diet, and prenatal care, some of these risks can be minimized. Amniocentesis (see Chapter 20) and sonography (see Chapter 16) identify possible pregnancies at risk and make early intervention—sometimes by cesarean section—possible.

Psychologically, there are special concerns and advantages for the woman who delays pregnancy until after age thirty-five. If a pregnancy complication, such as miscarriage, does occur, the disappointment may be much greater as she waited longer to have her family. Or she may be concerned about potential problems with sibling rivalry because of the need to have her children spaced closer together in age than she ideally would like. Keep in mind, however, that sibling rivalry occurs no matter what the age spacing of children, and planning for spending individual time with each child will help to minimize it. If you are a mother with older children, you may feel excited or depressed, or both, initially at the thought of giving birth to and rearing another child. When the baby arrives, depending on your circumstances, you may find you react either more or less enthusiastically toward caring for this newborn and observing his or her development compared to your initial feelings with your earlier children.

You may feel isolated from your friends who are close to your age and who are freer from child care responsibilities and involved with other things. In this case, getting more help with child care is important. You may decide to go back to work and spend less time at home with this child than you did with your previous children. Or you may feel more relaxed and want to spend more time to "enjoy" this child than you did with your others.

More and more today when both parents work, couples are electing to wait until their thirties to start a family. One advantage of this delay is often

that both parents are more mature and more likely to have had time to establish their marriage as well as to consider their desire for parenthood. Parenthood is an adjustment regardless of age; and a couple's past experience, separately and together, in coping with stress and change may help smooth their transition into parenthood.

Having a clear idea of career goals is particularly helpful to the older woman just starting a family. A woman who is comfortable and secure with her own career plans may find it easier to maintain her identity as an individual with her own needs as separate from those of her developing family.

Financial concerns connected with raising children are often a matter of major importance. Having a child today represents a substantial economic commitment, and a couple may feel more financially secure at this later point in their lives. If both parents work, it may be possible for either or both of them to arrange a leave of absence or to work part-time during the baby's first years.

In this chapter, we have dealt with some of the special concerns, medical and otherwise, you may

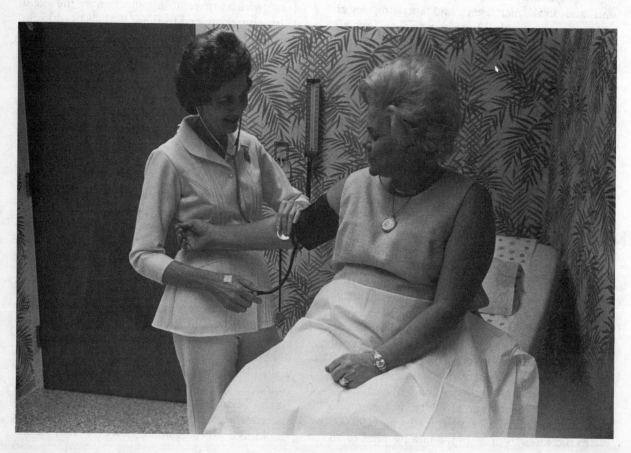

have if you are, or plan to be, pregnant and are over the age of thirty-five. As a result of later marriage, infertility problems, or other reasons, you may suddenly be faced with the fact that if you are to have children, you will be an older-than-average mother. But the dangers are not nearly so great as is often believed. What is "ideal" for your body biologically may not suit your personal, social, or emotional needs, and, on balance, the advantages to delaying pregnancy until later in life often outweigh the disadvantages. For the woman in good general health, the medical risks of childbearing after thirty-five are indeed relatively low. Although childbearing complications for mother and baby do increase with age, this factor cannot be isolated from other aspects of your life. The truth is that over 95% of women over thirty-five have healthy babies and little or no pregnancy complications. Good nutrition, early prenatal care, and genetic counseling can help maximize your chances for having a normal, enjoyable pregnancy and childbirth.

13

Infertility— Causes and Treatment

Despite apparent dwindling social pressures to have children, pregnancy and childbirth remain major milestones in the lives of many women. Psychiatrists report that even women who choose to remain childless often experience depression during their thirties related to unfulfilled motherhood. The psychological impact of an inability to bear children that are desired can be even more devastating.

A predictable and nearly universal sequence of feelings accompanies the infertility experience. The sequence resembles the pattern of coping that people go through during other crises, such as serious illness or the loss of a loved one. Couples entering infertility evaluation are already in a state of crisis. The evaluation itself produces further stress in the form of embarrassing questions, physical discomfort, costly tests, and the emotional anguish of having to wait several months for results. Even though a couple undergoes evaluation because they suspect they are infertile, a diagnosis suspecting or confirming infertility shocks them. They may even initially deny this diagnosis.

As the investigation proceeds, feelings of isolation and anger often develop. During this time, many couples experience marital discord or sexual difficulties, such as impotence or a decrease in sex drive. Sex, misguidedly planned around temperature charting, often becomes work instead of play. A cycle may develop with increasing emotional tension after ovulation, followed by depression when menses ensues. At this point, guilt feelings add to an already lowered sense of self-esteem. Many women may ask themselves why they have been singled out not to achieve what the rest of the world takes for granted. They may attribute infertility to some past deed, such as abortion or infrequent medical checkups. Such factors rarely account for infertility but may explain the severe depression and guilt that infertile couples so often experience.

Grief normally becomes a prominent emotional feature of an infertility evaluation. Since infertility is rarely absolute, the process of grieving may be prolonged by uncertainty surrounding the outcome of the evaluation and the potential treatment. Grieving involves acknowledging many losses in addition to the loss of potential children. There is also the loss of genetic continuity, the loss of all that fertility means to one's sexuality, and the loss of the pregnancy itself. When these feelings are dealt with openly, couples can begin to accept infertility. This acceptance allows couples to consider their remaining alternatives.

Counseling may be helpful at this point. Counseling is sometimes available through local support groups consisting of couples who have also experienced infertility problems. Many of these groups have been established through RESOLVE, Inc., a national organization offering infertile couples a variety of services, including telephone counseling and referrals for medical help. For further information, write to: RESOLVE, Inc., P.O. Box 474, Belmont, MA 02178.

What Is Infertility?

Infertility is the inability to become pregnant after one year of unprotected intercourse. Sixty percent of couples achieve conception after six months and 85% by one year. On this basis, an estimated 15% of all married couples are infertile. After the age of thirty, when a woman's fertility begins to decline somewhat, most authorities recommend an infertility evaluation if pregnancy is unsuccessfully attempted for more than six months. Infertility currently affects at least five million couples. An increasing trend to put off childbearing until after age thirty, or to stop having babies and not start again until after thirty, may increase the number of couples seeking infertility evaluation in the 1980s.

This infertility evaluation is usually done by a primary care physician such as an obstetrician-gynecologist. OB-GYNs can handle most infertili-

ty problems. Frequently gynecologists list themselves in the yellow pages of the phone book as infertility specialists. However, fewer than five percent of gynecologists have received additional subspecialty training required for treating the more uncommon infertility problems.

About half of all couples seeking infertility evaluation and treatment will ultimately be able to have children. Sometimes pregnancy occurs fortuitously during the evaluation, which takes several months or more to complete. Over 80% of the time a specific diagnosis is made. Among known causes of infertility, about one-third are attributed to a problem in the male, one-third to a problem in the female, and a final third to factors that involve both male and female partners.

Ideally the infertility evaluation is a mutually shared investigation that begins with a medical history and physical examination; the history taking includes some questions that could be directly related to the infertility (see Table 23). A sequence of laboratory tests follows the examination. In practice, this evaluation often starts with the woman who seeks advice from her gynecologist during a regular office visit. Most infertility experts recommend having both partners present at least initially to explain the upcoming tests and to lessen misplaced guilt that either one may experience by feeling responsible for the infertility. Since the initial evaluation of the man is usually simpler, basically consisting of a semen analysis, this test should be one of the first steps. If the semen analysis is normal, the woman can then be evaluated.

The Causes and Treatment of Infertility

Problems found in the four areas investigated in an infertility evaluation account for over 95% of known causes of infertility. The following part of this chapter covers these four areas in terms of causes, tests, and treatment.

Tubal factors

Tubal problems contribute to infertility nearly 30% of the time and are now the leading cause of female-related infertility. Tubal blockage often occurs as a result of scarring of the Fallopian tubes due to previous infection. Although such infection is usually transmitted sexually (venereal infection),

Table 23   QUESTIONS COMMONLY ASKED BY THE DOCTOR DURING THE INFERTILITY HISTORY

Question	Significance	Treatment
Are your periods regular?	infrequent periods often associated with faulty ovulation	fertility drug (e.g., Clomid) to stimulate ovulation
Do you have painful intercourse?	may be associated with certain causes of infertility affecting the tubes—infection, adhesions, or endometriosis	laparoscopy; possible tubal microsurgery
Do you have an irritating vaginal discharge?	may be associated with cervical infection	antibiotics or vaginal creams
Do you have very painful periods?	may be associated with cervical stenosis from previous surgery involving the cervix (cone biopsy) or with endometriosis	D & C (for cervical stenosis); laparoscopy (to evaluate for endometriosis)
How often do you have intercourse?	too frequently—decreases sperm count; too infrequently—decreases sperm activity	ideally, have intercourse every other day during midportion of the cycle
Have you had previous abdominal surgery?	may have caused adhesions	laparoscopy; release of adhesions if present
Have you had several miscarriages?	may be due to a uterine abnormality	diagnosis by hysterosalpingogram; may require uterine surgery
Have you noticed dry skin, sudden weight gain, and intolerance to cold?	may be due to low thyroid	thyroid pills

previous surgery or the prior use of an IUD could be responsible. Other tubal problems associated with infertility include endometriosis (see Chapter 35) and tubal (ectopic) pregnancy which may require surgical removal of the involved tube.

Common tests to evaluate the Fallopian tubes: There are three basic tests to evaluate whether the Fallopian tubes are open.

The *Rubin test*, an office procedure, involves injecting carbon dioxide gas through the cervix and into the uterus and tubes. When the tubes are open, the test produces slight shoulder pain. This is due to an irritating effect of the gas, which refers pain from the abdomen to the shoulder area.

A somewhat more elaborate test, a *hysterosalpingogram* (see Figure 14), is an X-ray performed in the radiology department. The radiologist injects a special dye into the uterus and tubes, allowing an outline of the inside of the uterus and tubes to be seen on the X-ray. Both the Rubin test and hysterosalpingogram (HSG) involve some discomfort, and both are subject to about a 25% error.

An apparently blocked tube, for example, may only be in spasm.

The Rubin test is not used widely today because the test results are often unclear or misleading. For example, a woman with damaged Fallopian tubes may have an apparently normal Rubin test (indicated by shoulder pain) unless her tubes are completely blocked. The HSG is a much more complete test, however, which identifies certain uterine abnormalities, pinpoints the location of tubal blockage, and provides a permanent record.

Laparoscopy, the third method of tubal evaluation, is the most definitive method. In an infertility evaluation, laparoscopy should be one of the last procedures since it is also the costliest and most hazardous. Laparoscopy, usually done on an outpatient basis under general anesthesia, involves inserting a long, thin, telescopelike instrument into the abdominal cavity through a small incision in the navel. This allows direct visualization of the pelvic organs. During this procedure, an assistant injects dye through the cervix while the clinician

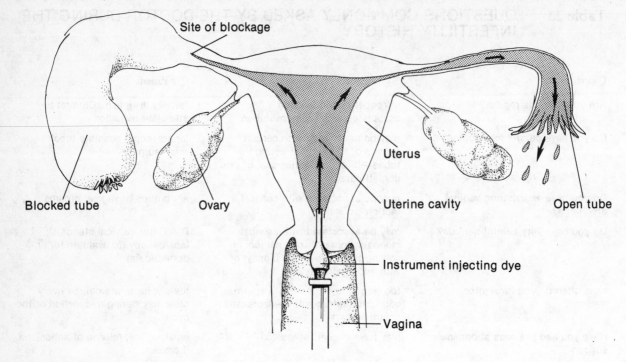

Site of blockage

Blocked tube   Ovary   Uterus   Open tube

Uterine cavity

Instrument injecting dye

Vagina

Figure 14   *Diagram of an X-ray of uterus and tubes (hysterosalpingogram).*

observes the dye as it comes out the tubes into the abdominal cavity. The location of any tubal blockage can be determined, and sometimes adhesions around the tubes can be cut apart by the clinician as a part of this procedure. Approximately 40% of women with infertility will have some unsuspected abnormality at the time of laparoscopy. The most common findings include infection of the tubes, endometriosis involving the ovaries or tubes, and pelvic adhesions.

The usual reasons in an infertility evaluation for having laparoscopy include:

1. Failure of preliminary tests to determine the cause of infertility.
2. An abnormal hysterosalpingogram or Rubin test.
3. Failure to become pregnant after taking a fertility drug for six months in the absence of other identifiable causes.
4. To determine whether a tubal ligation (a tying off of the tubes) that was done can be reversed.

If blocked tubes are discovered at the time of laparoscopy, you can arrange in advance to have your surgeon perform tubal surgery at the same time to prevent the need for a second operation. Because the extent of disease with blocked tubes

varies widely, many physicians recommend discussing the findings of the laparoscopy first and planning definite tubal surgery later. Another reason to wait is that following any of the diagnostic procedures—Rubin test, hysterosalpingogram, or laparoscopy—your chances of pregnancy increase slightly. This may be due to the procedure itself, which can open up small adhesions inside the tubes.

Treatment: Tubal infections are treated with antibiotics. As noted, minor adhesions can be cut apart at the time of laparoscopy without making a regular abdominal incision. (Tubal adhesions occur when tissue surfaces stick together during the healing process after surgery, from infections involving the internal pelvic organs, or from diseases such as endometriosis.) More serious adhesions, either surrounding or within the tube, require special surgery. Until a few years ago, less than 25% of women benefited from tubal surgery. Now, close to 50% of women with blocked tubes may be able to get pregnant through the use of the new technique of microsurgery.

A doctor experienced in microsurgical technique has had extensive training not included in many OB-GYN residency programs. So if you need this special surgery, it is best to have it done at a hospital affiliated with an infertility center or with a medical school that does include microsurgery in its program.

Tubal surgery requires special magnifying glasses or an operating microscope, along with special instruments. The success of this surgery depends partly on the location of the blockage. Obstructions at either end of the tube have less than a 50% pregnancy rate after surgery. When blockage is at the uterine end of the tube, the least common location, repair may be accomplished by implantation. That is, the blocked area of tube is removed and the healthy portion implanted back into the uterus. Blockage at the far end of the tube may result from venereal infection, causing the end of the tube to close off. The scar tissue must then be cut away and a new opening created. A higher success rate is achieved with reconstruction of the midportion of the tube. In this procedure, known as *anastomosis*, the blocked segment of the tube is cut out and the cut ends are sewn together. This procedure is most often done to reverse previous elective tubal sterilization. In this instance, the best results are obtained when the sterilizing technique involved a nonburning surgical procedure to mechanically block the tube, using a "clip" or "band." (See Chapter 42.)

The carbon dioxide laser (see Chapter 36) represents a new technical development in the field of tubal microsurgery. The laser allows relatively bloodless surgery and permits a clear field of view, which is an advantage in performing microsurgery. Although the laser seems promising, it's too early to tell whether the technique will improve the results of infertility surgery.

Candidates for any tubal microsurgery must be screened very carefully because the presence of severe tubal disease lessens the chances of good results. Restoring normal tubal anatomy, moreover, is not the same thing as restoring tubal function. Once severe damage occurs, no amount of plastic reconstruction can guarantee the tube's ability to maintain a fertilized egg during its journey from ovary to uterus.

Complications of tubal surgery include an increased rate of ectopic (tubal) pregnancy and pelvic infection. To prevent infection, antibiotics are usually prescribed before and after surgery.

Ovarian factors

Absent or infrequent ovulation accounts for 10% to 15% of infertility problems. Women who menstruate every two to four months ovulate infrequently. Among the causes of infrequent periods and ovulation are polycystic ovaries (see Chapter 76), serious illness, and emotional stress. Thyroid problems, especially hypothyroidism (see glossary), occasionally cause infrequent ovulation.

Common tests to evaluate the ovaries: The basal body temperature (BBT) chart is the simplest test to determine if you are ovulating. The sex hormone produced in the second half of the menstrual cycle causes a slight (half a degree) but abrupt rise in temperature twenty-four hours after ovulation. This rise can be documented on a chart by taking your temperature every morning. (The correct method for this procedure is described in Chapter 6, Natural Family Planning.) Failure to ovulate as noted by the pattern on the BBT chart implicates the ovaries as the source of infertility. If the results of the BBT test are unclear, the clinician may determine if ovulation has occurred by performing an endometrial biopsy or by obtaining a blood hormone (progesterone) level approximately ten days after ovulation. The biopsy, an office procedure, involves removal of a tiny amount of uterine tissue by means of a small instrument inserted into the uterine cavity. The appearance of the tissue under microscope indicates whether ovulation has occurred.

Additional tests measuring the level of various hormones are rarely necessary and add considerable cost to the infertility evaluation. However, women who have never had a period (see Chapter 76) or who have experienced other hormonal problems such as hair growth (see Chapter 64) or breast discharge (see Chapter 55) may need to have further diagnostic testing.

Treatment: Fertility drugs effectively induce ovulation within three months in more than 90% of women with infrequent or absent ovulation. Clomid, the principal fertility drug, acts on the brain, causing release of the hormones which stimulate ovulation. Clomid is indicated only in women who do not ovulate or ovulate infrequently. For the woman who produces an egg each month, fertility pills are of no value. Further, pregnancy rates average only about 40% with Clomid since not all women who ovulate as a result of taking this drug conceive. Eight percent of women who conceive while taking Clomid experience multiple births; this rate is ten times more often than multiple births in the general population.

Clomid is usually taken for five consecutive

days starting from the fifth day of your menstrual period. To increase chances of conception, you should have intercourse every other night starting five days after you take the last pill. More frequent intercourse may actually decrease the sperm count slightly. Women who do not have regular periods may need to have a period induced each month with a drug containing progesterone, such as Provera, before starting Clomid. Clinicians evaluate Clomid therapy by using the BBT chart to detect the presence of ovulation. If your temperature does not rise, ovulation has not occurred and subsequently the dose of Clomid may need to be increased.

Contraindications to the use of Clomid may include the presence of ovarian cysts, liver disease, or abnormal vaginal bleeding. Clomid is not known to cause congenital abnormalities, but, like any other drug, its use is best avoided in pregnancy. Relatively common side effects of Clomid include hot flashes, nausea, headaches, and breast tenderness. Blurred vision is an uncommon side effect and indicates that Clomid should be discontinued. Approximately 14% of women taking Clomid develop ovarian cysts. For this reason, you need a pelvic exam at least every two months when you are taking this drug, to check for ovarian enlargement. Such cysts shrink on their own after the drug is discontinued.

If ovulation does not occur after adjustments in Clomid dosage, the clinician may prescribe another fertility drug, called Pergonal. Compared to Clomid, Pergonal has more serious side effects, is more costly (presently $200+ per menstrual cycle), and requires constant monitoring by a fertility expert, preferably one with subspecialty training. Ovarian cyst formation and rupture occur far more frequently with this drug than with Clomid. Also, the chance of twins is two and a half times as likely with Pergonal. Pregnancy rates with Pergonal average between 50% and 70%.

Uterine factors

Approximately 20% of infertility results from a problem within the uterus, often involving the cervix. For a few days before ovulation, the cervical glands secrete a watery mucus that supports sperm migration from the vagina into the uterus. Most of the time no one knows what causes impairment of the quantity and quality of cervical mucus. Cervical stenosis, a narrowing of the cervical canal, may block the passage of sperm into the uterus or

diminish mucus quantity. The scarring associated with this condition can result from overzealous cautery (see glossary) of the cervix or from previous dilatation and curettage (D & C) or cone biopsy (see Chapter 36). One of the least frequent uterine factors responsible for infertility is the presence of sperm antibodies in the cervical mucus. Such antibodies prevent conception by destroying sperm just as other types of antibodies in the body destroy bacteria.

Common tests to evaluate the uterus: The postcoital, or *Sims-Huhner*, test involves microscopic examination of sperm and cervical mucus a few hours after intercourse. The clinician performs this painless test near the time of ovulation when the mucus is most copious. A normal test, showing copious clear mucus within the cervix and active sperm, would indicate that a tubal or an ovarian factor more likely accounts for the infertility.

Hysteroscopy, a new and increasingly used office procedure, allows visualization of the cervical canal and inside the uterus. Hysteroscopy requires the use of a thin, telescopelike instrument similar to the laparoscope. The clinician can utilize the hysteroscope to visualize and often release adhesions and remove cervical polyps and other growths inside the uterus. The tubes, ovaries, and outer side of the uterus cannot be seen.

Treatment: Antibiotics, vaginal creams, and occasionally cryosurgery (see glossary) are used to treat cervical infections that may contribute to abnormal cervical mucus. Women with inadequate cervical mucus production respond well to treatment with low doses of estrogen. Those with stenosis of the cervix may need a D & C to widen the canal or artificial insemination to bypass the narrowed cervix. Uterine suspension, once a common operation to straighten a so-called tipped uterus, is rarely done. It is now known that a tipped, or retroverted, uterus is rarely a cause of infertility.

Male factors

Approximately 40% of infertility problems are due to male factors, initially evaluated by sperm count or semen analysis. Normal counts range from 20 million to over 100 million sperm per cubic centimeter. Counts below 20 million are often associated with some degree of infertility. Azospermia, a very uncommon finding, refers to complete absence of sperm. A small and often temporary decrease in the sperm count may be due to a variety of factors such as fatigue, poor diet, excessive alcohol or other drug abuse, smoking, occupational exposure to chemicals, or prostate gland infection. A common and surgically correctable form of male infertility is due to varicose veins in the scrotum (varicocele). This condition raises the temperature near the sperm, thus impairing their development.

The *common test* to evaluate male infertility is called a semen analysis. In addition to measuring volume and acidity of the ejaculate, the semen analysis test involves microscopic evaluation of sperm activity, appearance, and number. For the semen analysis test, the man should abstain from sexual activity for three days before producing a sperm sample, and the sample should be collected by masturbation into a clean, dry container. To get the most accurate evaluation, he should bring the sample to the lab at once since sperm activity decreases with time.

Treatment: An abnormal semen analysis requires referral to a urologist or another infertility specialist. Men with low sperm counts occasionally respond to Clomid or other hormonal therapy. Alternatives to raising the count by medical means in order to achieve pregnancy include the use of a split-ejaculate technique and artificial insemination.

In the split-ejaculate method, the husband allows only the first portion of the semen to enter the vagina by withdrawing midway through ejaculation because the first portion usually contains more sperm. Artificial insemination may be conducted with sperm from the husband or from a donor. In either case, the technique involves introduction of semen into the upper vagina or cervix. To enhance the chances for pregnancy, several inseminations are performed during a single cycle near the time of ovulation as calculated by use of the BBT chart (see above under the paragraphs on *Ovarian factors*).

Results of artificial insemination using the husband's sperm (AIH) have been disappointing. The low pregnancy rate of 25% reflects the fact that the usual indication for AIH is low sperm count. When performed for reasons such as impotence, the success rate of AIH increases.

Artificial insemination from a donor (AID) may be indicated if the husband is sterile, is impotent, has a very low sperm count, or carries a genetic disease likely to be transmitted to the child. Donors are carefully selected by the physician, who searches the donor's background to rule out hereditary diseases, chronic conditions, or current infection. Pregnancy rates with AID run between 50% and 80%.

The legal status of AID is complicated. Most States do not have laws establishing legitimacy of children conceived by artificial insemination from donors.

The psychological implications of AID are enormous. Some couples or religious groups find AID immoral. Many couples experience guilt feelings resulting from the secrecy that often surrounds the procedure, owing to the anonymity of the donor. Men may feel left out when their wives conceive by AID, and women may feel there is something improper about being fertilized by another man's sperm. The long-term psychological effects of AID upon husband, wife, child, and donor remain unclear. Certainly artificial insemination, particularly by a donor, aggravates the emotional stress normally associated with infertility.

Information concerning physicians who perform artificial insemination may be obtained by contacting: The American Fertility Society, 1608 13th Avenue South, Suite 101, Birmingham, AL 35256.

Sperm Banks

Sperm banking was initially heralded as a possible method of so-called reproductive insurance for men who planned to have vasectomy. Recent interest has focused on the use of this technique in infertility. Sperm banks permit a man with a low sperm count to pool his own multiple ejaculates, allowing concentrated specimens for artificial insemination. Such attempts have been largely unsuccessful because of the inability of these sperm to withstand the freezing necessary for storage. Even sperm from males with normal counts often become damaged or lose their activity as a result of cold shock. How long sperm can survive freezing remains unclear although pregnancies have occurred after several years of sperm storage. No one knows how the freezing of semen affects the rate of mutations or other abnormalities since so few babies are conceived through the use of stored sperm. Fertility experts report somewhat lower conception rates with stored compared to fresh semen, so fresh semen is favored for artificial insemination. For more information on sperm banks, write to: Barren Foundation, 6 East Monroe Street, Room 1407, Chicago, Illinois 60603.

Table 24   HOW A DOCTOR EVALUATES INFERTILITY

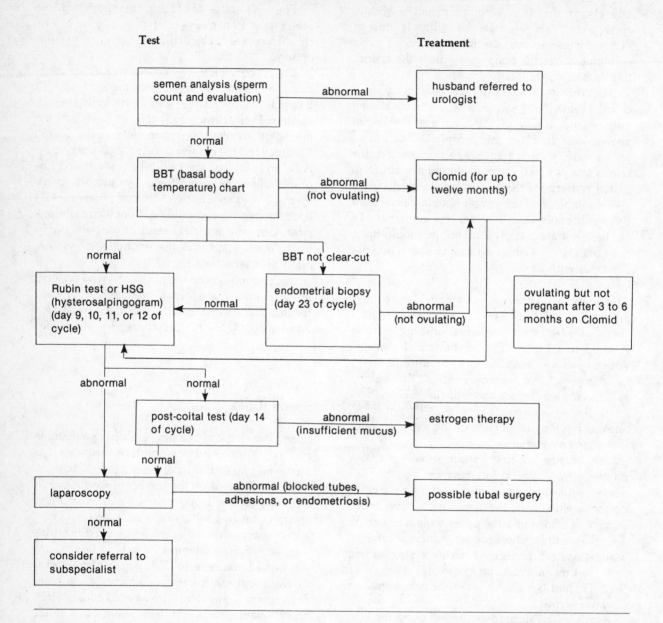

In Vitro Fertilization

The work of British researchers Patrick Steptoe and Robert Edwards culminated in 1978 with the birth of the first baby conceived by fertilization outside the body, a process known as "in vitro fertilization" (IVF).

The first "test-tube" baby successfully overcame a major cause of infertility: blocked Fallopian tubes. To accomplish this, the British team, using laparoscopy, removed an egg from the woman's ovary prior to ovulation and fertilized the egg, using the husband's sperm, in a laboratory dish. After fertilization, the embryo incubated in a culture dish whose environment was carefully controlled while the cells began to divide. About two days later, the embryo was "transferred" from the dish into the wife's uterus, where implantation occurred. From then on, pregnancy proceeded as it would have following normal ovulation and fertilization.

Although IVF offers hope to select childless

couples, the procedure is costly, time-consuming, and complicated. Fees range from $3,000 to $5,000 for each treatment cycle and two or three cycles may be needed. One to two weeks of preliminary testing, including daily sonograms and blood tests to measure hormone levels, are necessary to accurately establish when the egg is about to be released. Then follows an intricate series of steps coordinated by the IVF "team"—removal of an egg (or eggs) by laparoscopy, fertilization using the husband's sperm, and finally transfer of the embryo into the mother's uterus.

Despite only a 20% overall success rate, waiting lists of several months or more for IVF are not unusual. Couples must meet certain requirements. For example, most clinics list forty as their age limit. Most couples will need to travel some distance to reach one of the nearly fifty IVF centers in the U.S. For information about the IVF facility closest to you contact the American Fertility Society (see Appendix D).

Among the untested and ethically controversial uses of "test-tube" fertilization is the use of donor eggs in women who do not respond to ovulatory drugs or who are carriers for genetic disorders. Even more controversial is the use of a surrogate mother to incubate embryos conceived by "test-tube" fertilization. This option might be selected by the woman who had a hysterectomy early in life but retained her ovaries, which in this case would supply the egg. While the legal ramifications of such arrangements are mind boggling, these alternatives will likely become reality for some women in the 1980s.

References for Section Three

Chapter 11—Identifying Birth Defects

Nordenskjold, F., and Gustavii, B. Direct-vision chorion villi biopsy for prenatal diagnosis in the first trimester. *Journal of Reproductive Medicine* 29(8):572–574, Aug 1984.

Kaback, M. M. Genetic screening for better outcomes. *Contemporary OB/GYN* 13:123–129, Jan 1979.

Golbus, M. S. Analyzing genetic defects in the fetus. *Contemporary OB/GYN* 13:133–139, Feb 1979.

Luthy, D. A., Karp, L. E., et al. What part do chromosomes play in repeated reproductive failure? *Contemporary OB/GYN* 13:98–105, Apr 1979.

Simpson, J. L. Directions in diagnosing chromosomal disorders antenatally. *Contemporary OB/GYN* 13:135–143, Jan 1979.

Karp, L. E. *Genetic Engineering: Threat or Promise?* Chicago: Nelson-Hall, 1976.

Simpson, J. L. What causes chromosomal abnormalities and gene mutations? *Contemporary OB/GYN* 17(3):99–114, 1981.

Simpson, J. L., et al. Genetic counseling and genetic services in obstetrics and gynecology: implications for educational goals and clinical practice. *American Journal of Obstetrics and Gynecology* 140(1):70–77, May 1981.

Chapter 12—Pregnancy After Thirty-Five

Naeye, R. L. Maternal age, obstetric complications, and the outcome of pregnancy. *Obstetrics and Gynecology* 61(2):210–216, Feb 1983.

Daniels, P., and Weingarten, K. A new look at the medical risks in late childbearing. *Women and Health* 4(1):5–36, 1979.

Kajanoja, P., and Widholm, O. Pregnancy and delivery in women aged 40 and over. *Obstetrics and Gynecology* 51(1):47–51, 1978.

Benson, R. C., et al. *Current Obstetrics and Gynecologic Diagnosis and Treatment*, ed. 4. Los Altos, Calif.: Lange, 1982.

Chapter 13—Infertility—Causes and Treatment

Speroff, L., et al. *Clinical Gynecologic Endocrinology and Infertility*, ed. 3. Baltimore: Williams and Wilkins, 1983.

Grimes, E. M. For infertile couples—a holistic approach. *Contemporary OB/GYN* 23(2):179–196, Feb 1984.

Toth, A. The role of infection in infertility. *The Female Patient* 9(7):16–28, July 1984.

Menning, B. E. Counseling infertile couples. *Contemporary OB/GYN* 13:101–108, Feb 1979.

Kaufman, S. A. New solutions for infertility. *The Female Patient* 52–54, Jan 1979.

Curie-Cohen, M., et al. Current practice of artificial insemination by donor in the U.S. *New England Journal of Medicine* 300:585–590, Mar 15, 1979.

Wallach, E. E., et al. Helping the "normal" infertile couple. *Contemporary OB/GYN* 17(5):102–125, 1981.

Johnson, W. G., Schwartz, R. C., et al. Artificial insemination by donors: the need for genetic screening. *New England Journal of Medicine* 304(13):755–757, 1981.

four

Pregnancy and Childbirth

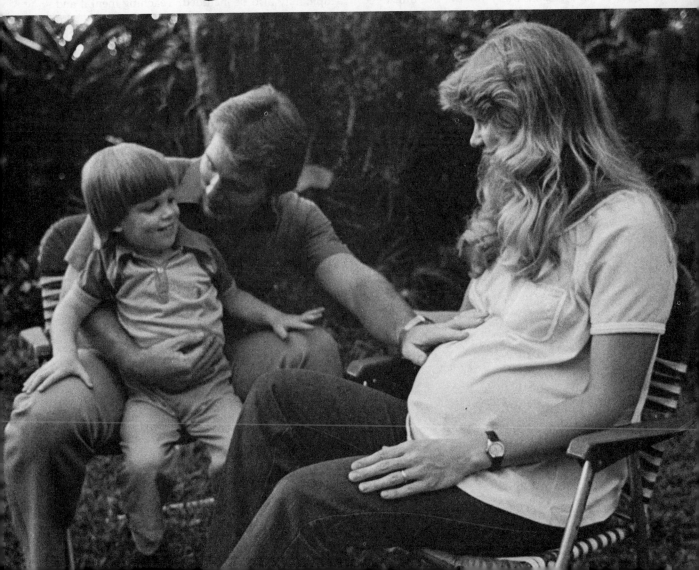

14

Childbirth Education

During the late nineteenth century, attempts to reduce maternal and infant infections and to provide relief from pain brought childbirth from the home setting into the hospital. As the hospital began to take responsibility for the birthing experience, childbirth education became limited to what one could hear about it from one's mother or among peers. But because many women of this era were put to sleep under general anesthesia during childbirth, even they were not sure what happened. Pregnant women thus found themselves unprepared for childbirth and dependent on their physicians to "deliver" them. Before long, women grew dissatisfied with their passive role in childbearing.

There's a lot to learn about childbirth.

Today's pregnant woman wants to be more fully informed and involved in decisions that affect her pregnancy and delivery. For this reason, you'll find classes for expectant parents in almost every community in the United States. Hospitals, community colleges, the American Red Cross, private organizations, and some physicians now provide courses to meet the increasing demand for childbirth preparation. Some goals of prepared childbirth are to minimize the discomfort of labor and delivery, to decrease potential risks to you and your newborn, and to help you and your family have the best experience possible for your unique situation.

Most childbirth preparation classes provide nutrition counseling and information about labor and delivery, as well as the opportunity for you to share experiences with other mothers-to-be. Because of the increased rate of cesarean deliveries, this topic may also be included. Teaching mental and physical relaxation techniques to deal with contraction discomfort is an important part of the classes. Childbirth education emphasizes minimal use of pain medication during labor and more active participation of the father. With such preparation, a mother is likely to be less anxious and fearful and she may feel greater satisfaction by actively participating in the birth process.

Choosing prepared childbirth, which requires

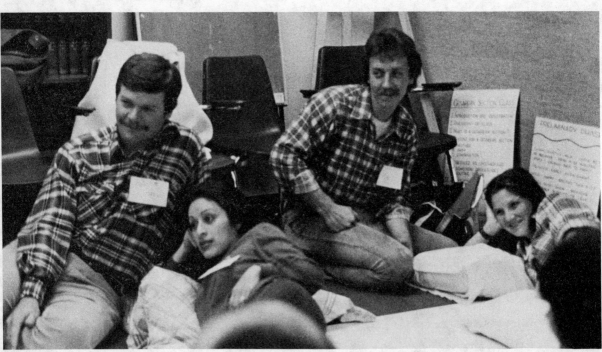

an active decision on the parents' part, means that you elect to become more aware of what will happen to you so that you can make informed choices throughout your labor, delivery, and postpartum period. *Choosing* to be prepared for childbirth is more important, we feel, than the particular method you select. The types of prepared childbirth classes are discussed below. Ask your clinician or a nurse which methods are available in your community, or write for more information to the organizations that interest you; you'll find a list of addresses at the end of this chapter, in Table 25.

The Dick-Read Method

About 1914, Dr. Grantly Dick-Read, a British obstetrician, pioneered the concept of childbirth as a normal, natural process, as opposed to a medical condition. Women, he believed, had been unnecessarily conditioned to fear the pain of labor. Dr. Dick-Read believed that this fear produced muscle tension that led to much of the experienced "pain of childbirth." The Dick-Read method attempts to break the fear-tension-pain cycle by making the woman more knowledgeable about childbirth and by teaching muscle relaxation exercises ("passive relaxation"). Some of the techniques used resemble yoga in that the mother

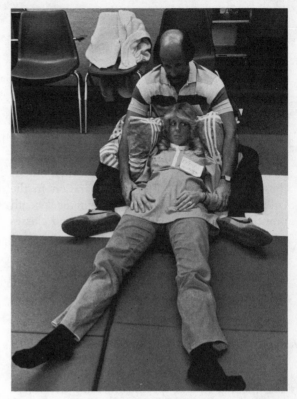

Practicing breathing techniques in preparation for labor and delivery.

Discussing the three stages of labor.

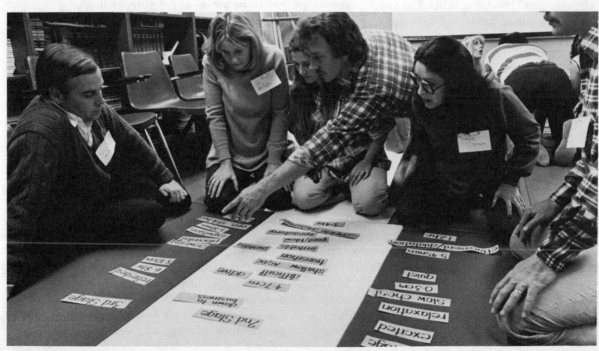

learns to develop an attitude of passivity and acceptance toward childbirth. She becomes conditioned to focus inward, concentrating on herself and meeting each contraction as it comes. This method relies heavily upon close communication between the laboring woman and the hospital staff, who help to reduce childbirth fears by answering questions about what to expect each step of the way.

Many other childbirth preparation techniques have been developed from the Dick-Read method, the oldest type of childbirth preparation in the United States. Classes, which begin in the seventh month, last eight weeks. Husbands attend classes with their wives to learn how to appropriately give their wives support during labor and delivery.

Lamaze (Psychoprophylaxis)

In the early 1950s, Dr. Fernand Lamaze developed a method of childbirth preparation to minimize the pain and discomfort of labor and delivery. This method teaches specific breathing techniques for dealing with painful contractions. Proper exercise and a thorough knowledge of the labor and delivery process are also stressed. Essential to the Lamaze technique is the use of a coach (usually but not necessarily the husband), who attends the classes and helps the mother-to-be practice her relaxation and breathing skills. The coach accompanies her during labor and delivery, to provide support, to time contractions, and to help her relax. Lamaze is currently the most popular method of childbirth preparation in the United States. Classes are usually six weeks in length and begin about the seventh month of pregnancy. Elisabeth Bing, R.P.T., a prominent authority on the Lamaze method, has written *Six Practical Lessons for an Easier Childbirth*, which has become the standard text for many Lamaze classes.

Bradley Husband-Coached Childbirth

In 1947, Dr. Robert A. Bradley developed the concept of husband-coached natural childbirth, a method heavily emphasizing the use of husband support and supervision during the childbearing process. Using a more rigid approach than other methods, Bradley strongly advocates the use of totally unmedicated births, breast-feeding immediately following birth, and early, frequent contact between mother and baby.

Bradley classes also differ from others in that the first class, which covers nutrition and exercise, is held early in the third month. Eight more classes follow, beginning during the sixth or seventh month of pregnancy, followed by review classes every two weeks in the final months. Breathing exercises and pushing techniques differ from the other methods. Because Bradley stresses nonmedicated participation during childbirth, this method has become popular for some home births.

Hypnosis

Although hypnosis can lessen childbirth pain in certain individuals, it has received limited use because this method requires more time and money than other types of childbirth preparedness. Hypnosis may produce total amnesia or may selectively abolish perception of pain. A form of self-hypnosis, called autosuggestion, can decrease the time needed for hypnosis. A woman conditions herself by silently repeating to herself a phrase that, with daily practice, triggers physical and mental relaxation. This phrase becomes a stimulus for the woman to go into a mild trance which mentally removes her from painful stimuli while allowing her to be aware of her surroundings.

Hypnosis offers the advantage of posthypnotic suggestion—for example, in some individuals episiotomy pain can be reduced at the suggestion of the hypnotist. There are no drug dangers or discomfort to being hypnotized; however, it requires considerable time and commitment from both the hypnotist and the patient.

Prenatal Yoga

Prenatal yoga classes, a helpful way to psychologically approach pregnancy through exercise and breathing techniques, can be used during your entire pregnancy. These classes focus on teaching relaxation techniques but they seldom include the physiology of labor and delivery and other practical aspects of childbirth. For this reason, if you use prenatal yoga, we recommend that you attend another form of prepared childbirth classes as well.

Early Parenting Classes

Some "prenatal" classes that are taught by private organizations last twelve months. After delivery, the classes cover the needs and activities of the infant during the first year of life as well as those of the parents. You'll be able to "practice" taking care of your baby because parents bring their babies to class where they can also observe normal variations in growth and development. These classes provide an opportunity to share ideas and support for those first difficult months of adjustment to parenthood.

Prenatal Classes For Repeat Parents

Pregnancy, birth, and parenting are not necessarily easier for experienced parents. Many repeat parents feel that they need more than a simple review of the labor-and-delivery breathing techniques. Some communities offer classes to meet the special needs of repeat parents. Subject matter usually includes preparation of siblings for the baby and new ideas on how to fit the proper rest and nutrition into a busy mother's schedule. Many women worry about differences in fetal movement between this pregnancy and their previous pregnancies. Some are concerned as to whether they can love another child as much as they loved their older child or children. Often mothers feel more uncomfortable or tired with a second or subsequent pregnancy than with the first pregnancy. Getting support from mothers in similar situations

Childbirth education class.

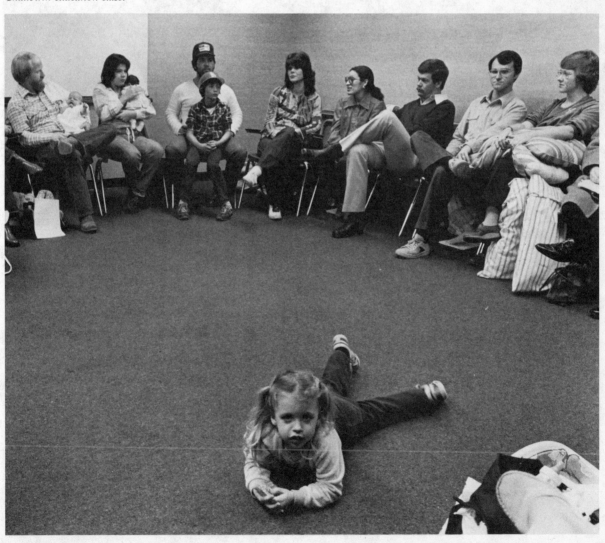

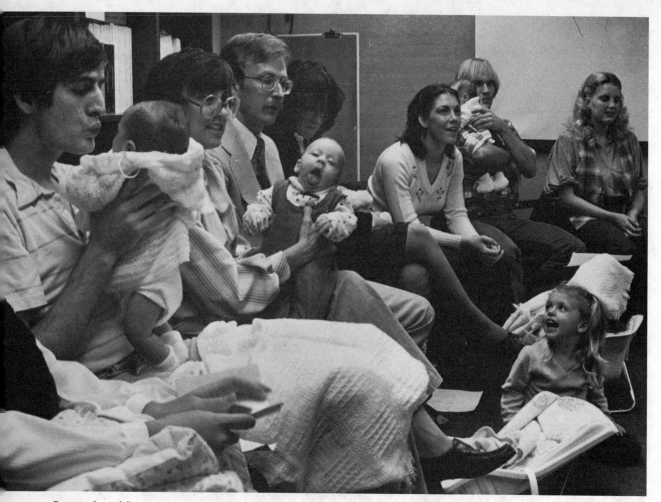

Parents share delivery experience and show off their newborns at a prenatal class reunion.

helps to make up for the usually less enthusiastic reactions of friends and relatives to a second pregnancy. A repeat mother knows what it is like to be responsible for a child's care twenty-four hours a day and is realistically concerned about the demands of this additional child. She is in some ways more aware of the realistic stresses that she will face with a new child than is the mother who is pregnant for the first time.

If no such classes exist in your community, you might approach your local chapter of the International Childbirth Education Association or childbirth educator. Or organize your own group of second- and third-time mothers to share ideas about adjusting to the second or third baby.

Table 25 CHILDBIRTH EDUCATION ORGANIZATIONS

Type of Childbirth Education	Where You Can Get Information
Dick-Read	Read Natural Childbirth Foundation, Inc. 1300 S. Eliseo Drive, Suite 102 Greenbrae, California 94904
Lamaze	American Society for Psychoprophylaxis in Obstetrics, Inc. (ASPO) 1411 K Street, N.W., Suite 200 Washington, D.C. 20005
Bradley Husband-Coached Childbirth	The American Academy of Husband-Coached Childbirth P.O. Box 5224 Sherman Oaks, California 91413
Hypnosis	To request information about a physician near you who practices hypnosis, write: The American Society of Clinical Hypnosis 2250 East Devon Avenue, Suite 336 Des Plaines, Illinois 60018
General information	International Childbirth Education Association P.O. Box 20048 Minneapolis, Minnesota 55420

15

Hospital Birth and Its Alternatives

More than in any other area of women's health, people have been urgently challenging the way care is provided during pregnancy, labor, and delivery. The feminist movement and consumer activism have much to do with new options that are now available for the pregnant mother and her family. Birthing alternatives vary greatly from community to community and often reflect the differing reference points from which physicians and pregnant women view pregnancy and childbirth. Physicians tend to think of potential *medical* risks to both mother and baby and how they can best anticipate and treat emergencies that might occur. The obstetrician clearly prefers to deliver the baby in the hospital, where equipment and personnel are available to meet any emergency. More and more women, on the other hand, view pregnancy as a natural biological process involving the whole family and needing minimal medical attention. They aren't sick—they're just pregnant! These women sometimes prefer to share the childbearing experience with their family in the warmer, more intimate surroundings of their home or a birth center. They reason that they can always go to a hospital should an emergency occur.

Because the birth rate has decreased and the number of home deliveries has increased in the last decade or so, hospitals now have an economic incentive to provide birthing alternatives in order to attract prospective parents to their institution. Many hospitals have therefore developed the concept of *family-centered maternity care*. The meaning of family-centered maternity care varies among

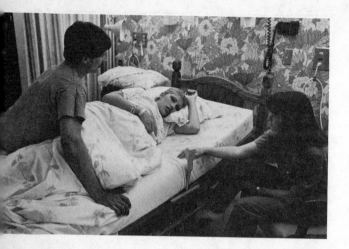

Labor and midwife-attended delivery in a birthing room.

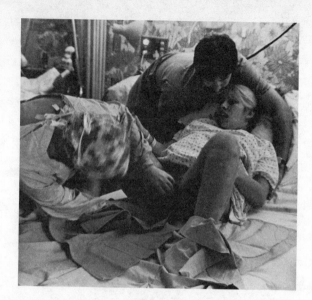

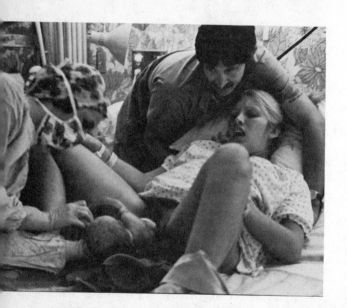

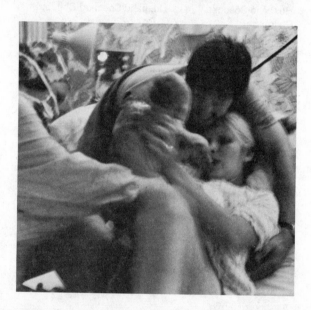

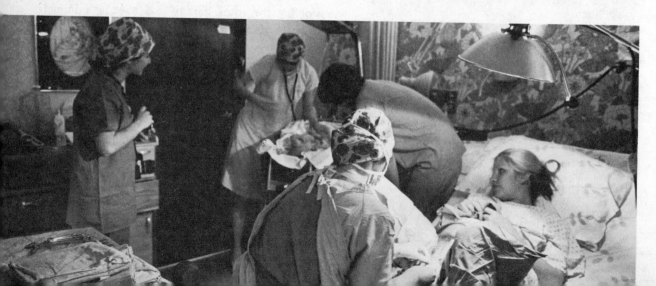

hospitals, but it may include classes for expectant parents, a tour of the hospital before delivery, and birthing alternatives such as fathers being present in the delivery room, rooming-in, bonding periods, and sibling visitation (see Chapter 19).

A recent trend in birth-setting alternatives is the designation of regional centers for high-risk mothers. These facilities, often located at university medical centers, employ special staff round-the-clock to care for mothers with complicated pregnancies. If your pregnancy is identified as being high risk (see Chapter 20), you may be referred to one of these centers.

Physicians, nurses, and other people who are concerned about the availability of alternative birth settings have formed their own organizations to which you can write for further information:

National Association of Parents and
  Professionals for Safe Alternatives in
  Childbirth (NAPSAC)
P.O. Box 267
Marble Hill, Missouri 63764

The Cybele Society
Suite 414, Peyton Bldg.
Spokane, Washington 99201

The Cybele Society provides information and consultative services to health professionals interested in promoting family-centered maternity care.

How Do I Choose Where To Have My Baby?

There is no *one* right way to have your baby. You won't be a better mother just by choosing a birthing center, for instance, over a traditional hospital setting. Some parents feel guilty about not selecting a new, trendy alternative. What may be most suitable for another couple may not be the best choice for you. It's a good idea to investigate the alternatives your community has to offer and to see what meets your personal goals. Here is a preview of the birth-setting alternatives you may find during your investigation.

Alternatives Within the Hospital

Traditional childbirth

Hospitals vary widely in their labor-and-delivery policies, but many hospitals do provide childbirth

preparation classes. If you are having your baby in the hospital, insist on a tour of the labor and delivery area beforehand. This will help you feel more comfortable when you enter the hospital for childbirth. Under traditional hospital care, the laboring woman is admitted into a small, so-called labor room, either private or shared, and is usually permitted a limited number of visitors. The physician usually orders an enema, some form of perineal shave, and an IV (intravenous solution). Electronic monitoring of the unborn fetus and pain medication or anesthesia may be prescribed routinely unless you specifically request otherwise at the time of hospital admission.

When completely dilated, the woman is transferred by stretcher to the sterile delivery room; her husband might accompany her, if the hospital permits. Following delivery, she may stay in the delivery room or go to a recovery room for several hours. Here, nurses evaluate uterine bleeding and then transfer the stable patient to a hospital room. The baby may stay with the mother during this period or may be immediately taken to a newborn nursery. The mother may see her baby only at feeding time, or the baby may be with her constantly if rooming-in is available.

The average length of stay in the hospital following delivery varies from two to four days. Some hospitals have an early-discharge program where you can leave within twenty-four hours of normal delivery. The program sometimes includes home visitation by a nurse. Most hospitals offer classes on breast-feeding and newborn care.

Birthing rooms

Birthing rooms offer an alternative to home births in providing a more intimate, personal experience within the hospital setting. A birthing room is cheerfully decorated and informal, with a couch, magazines, and often a television available to both the mother-to-be and her visitors. The labor bed easily transforms to a delivery bed as the mother stays in one room for both labor and delivery. Some of these beds allow a woman to deliver in any position she desires.

Birthing room practices vary in their flexibility of birthing experiences. Some hospitals limit visitors while others let the parents decide who may be present during labor and delivery. Medical care may not include certain standard procedures such as enemas, episiotomies, and fetal monitoring

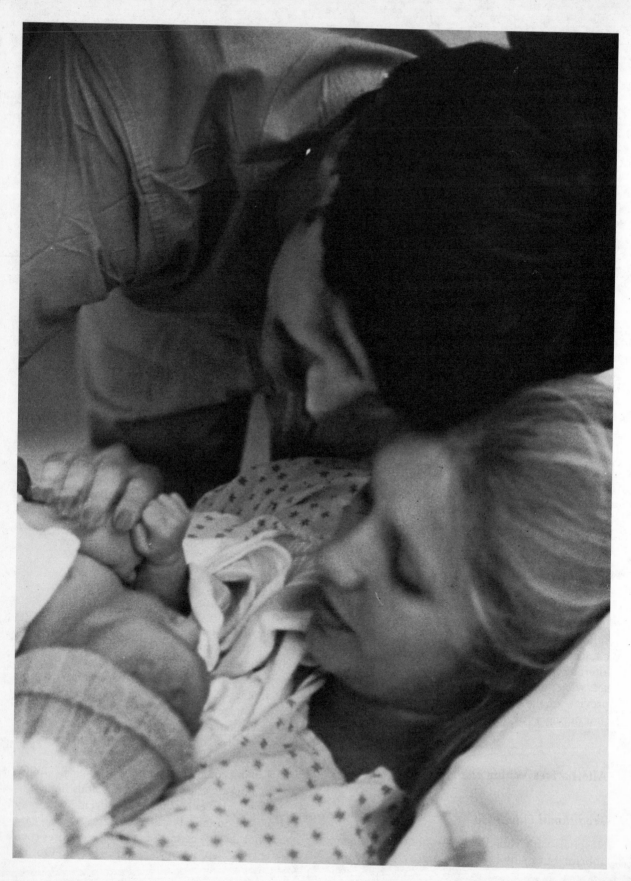

unless you want them. Sometimes fathers participate in the actual delivery. Some hospitals with birthing rooms offer complete maternity care for low-risk patients by midwives under physician supervision. In hospitals where early discharge is possible, mother and baby may stay in the birthing room for three to six hours after delivery and then leave for home if all has progressed normally. This markedly reduces hospital costs. So-called gentle birth (Leboyer delivery), bonding, immediate breast-feeding, and sibling participation are typical options in the birthing room setting (see Chapter 19).

Alternatives Outside the Hospital

Birth centers

These centers provide for a labor-and-delivery experience in a low-cost, homelike setting. Use of birthing centers is increasing as an economic and personal alternative to private-physician care and hospitalization. A mother-to-be and her family usually stay in one room for labor, delivery, and the immediate recovery period under the supervision of a nurse-midwife. Bonding, gentle birth, breast-feeding, sibling participation, and early discharge are readily available. Should an emergency occur, these centers usually have arrangements for immediate transfer to a hospital or back-up service by a physician. Extensive parent education classes are usually part of the center's prenatal program.

Because requirements for licensure differ from State to State, birth centers vary greatly both in the quality of professional care and emergency provisions. If you select this option, make sure the birth center has an arrangement with a nearby hospital to accept patients from the center should an emergency arise that requires hospitalization during labor.

Home births

In 1950, only half of all childbirths took place in the hospital; by 1975, that figure had climbed to 99%. Home births have become a controversial issue in the United States although they remain commonplace in other countries throughout the world. Even proponents of home birth do agree, however, that home birth should be considered only for mothers who have little risk of complications and that advance arrangements for immediate transfer to a hospital should be made for unpredictable, last-minute emergencies that might occur even in low-risk pregnancies.

Although a good deal has been written about the outcome of home births, little statistical data has actually been collected. This lack of data arises partly from the fact that in some States the birth setting may not be recorded on the birth certificate. One study done in northern California in 1977 showed a low maternal and newborn complication rate in a carefully selected low-risk population. However, these findings do not justify concluding that delivery at home is as safe as in the hospital. Other reports have reached opposite conclusions. The American College of Obstetricians and Gynecologists compiled statistics on out-of-hospital births from twelve States that showed a two- to five-times-higher stillbirth or newborn death rate for births outside hospitals. Although there is no consensus among the various reports available as to the safety of home birth, the response of physicians to home birth generally has been negative. Many physicians view home birth as an irresponsible risk to mother and child and hence refuse to support or attend home delivery.

The number of couples selecting home birth is increasing. A few studies indicate that such couples tend to be white, middle-class, and often college-educated. Women often choose to have their babies at home because the home is seen as the most natural place to have a baby, to celebrate the miracle of a new member of the family. Home birth is much less costly and gives the mother much greater control of her birth experience. For some women the experience of a previous hospital childbirth, including the subtle pressure to take drugs for pain relief, is their main reason for wanting a home birth. The parents' desire for early and unlimited contact with the newborn, photographing and recording the childbirth, and flexibility of delivery position are other reasons often given for the choice of home birth delivery, especially when these options are unavailable in a nearby hospital.

The types of home birth services that are available vary widely, and their number is increasing. The delivery may be done by a physician or by a certified or lay midwife with or without a back-up physician available. Home birth services usually include medical screening by a physician, nutrition counseling, preparation for childbirth,

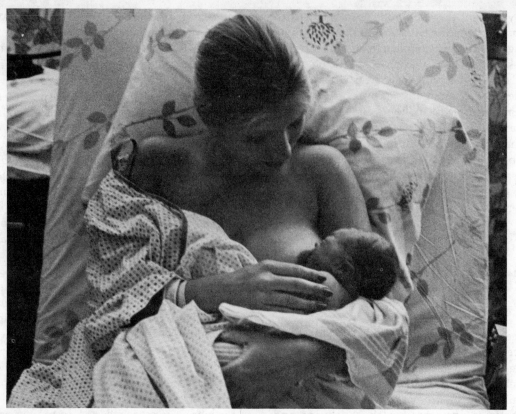

Bonding (below) and breast-feeding (above) immediately following delivery.

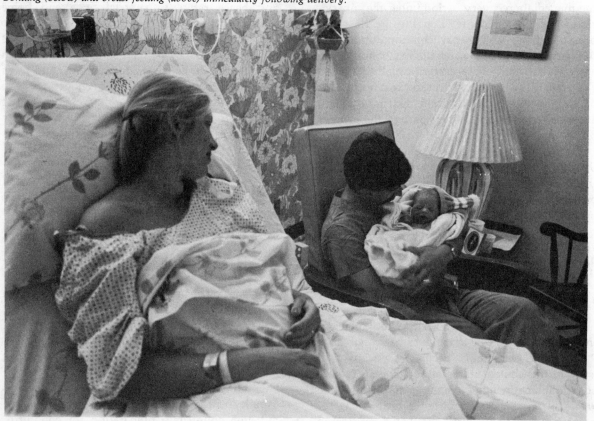

and a postpartum checkup. Enemas, IVs, and episiotomies are usually not performed at home. Some home birth services teach couples to recognize the signs of hemorrhage and to learn newborn resuscitation should it be needed. Self-birthing, where the parents actually do the delivery with supervision, is now part of some home birth classes. Comprehensive health insurance often pays for maternity hospitalization and prenatal care but may not pay for costs of a home delivery.

For information about home births, write to:

Home Oriented Maternity Experience (HOME)
511 New York Avenue
Tacoma Park, Maryland 20012

Midwives' Alliance of North America
30 S. Main Street
Concord, New Hampshire 03301

For information about birth centers, write to:

National Association of Childbearing Centers
R.D. 1, Box 1
Perkiomenville, Pennsylvania 18074

16

Pregnancy

When you decide to become pregnant, we hope you are already in good physical condition. Frequent exercise, proper nutrition, and plenty of rest are good habits for keeping healthy and are especially important in preparing for pregnancy (see Chapters 46 and 47). You can't expect to suddenly quit smoking (see Chapters 31 and 59), watch your weight (see Chapter 87), give up junk foods, and begin jogging at the moment you find out you are pregnant! Pregnancy is usually confirmed after the second month, so if you want your pregnancy to benefit from a new life style, make any changes that are beneficial early, well before conception takes place. Avoid taking any drugs (see Chapter 31) as soon as you begin trying to conceive. If at that time your clinician prescribes medication, alert him or her to the fact that you could be pregnant. Many pregnant women intend to give up alcohol and smoking "for the baby." It's better to make these changes as soon as you plan pregnancy, rather than after you conceive—and do it for *yourself*!

Today's alternative forms of birth control make it possible for women to become pregnant by choice. Still, unplanned pregnancies do occur. If you are uncertain about whether you want to continue your pregnancy, contact your clinician, Women's Center, or local Planned Parenthood chapter for counseling. It should be *your* decision, and early medical attention is beneficial and important whether you continue your pregnancy or seek abortion.

How Can I Tell If I'm Pregnant?

Some women say they know they are pregnant from the moment of conception. When asked how they can tell, they often reply that they "feel different" but can't explain in what way. Other women are pregnant for several months without

Table 26 EARLY SIGNS OF PREGNANCY

1. Missed period(s)
2. Breast changes (enlargement, tenderness)
3. Nausea, vomiting (morning sickness)
4. Increased frequency of urination
5. Fatigue
6. Slight weight gain
7. Abdominal enlargement

realizing it. You may have some or none of the early signs of pregnancy listed in Table 26. If you have been taking your basal body temperature (see Figure 9 in Chapter 6) and it stays elevated for sixteen days with no menstruation, you can be reasonably sure you are pregnant. If you haven't been taking your temperature, then confirmation of pregnancy requires a test and an examination.

Confirmation of pregnancy

Both a pregnancy test and a pelvic exam are necessary to confirm pregnancy because either procedure alone may be misleading. The test may be inaccurate, or uterine enlargement detected during pelvic examination may be due to some cause other than pregnancy. For most women, the simplest approach is to have a pregnancy test two weeks after a missed period—or earlier (see below)—followed by an appointment with her clinician if the test is positive. If the test is negative, you can repeat the test in one to two weeks and put off the examination until after the second test report. If you have unexpected pain or unusual vaginal bleeding, however, see your clinician immediately even if your pregnancy test is negative.

The main purpose of the pelvic exam in early pregnancy is to evaluate the size of the uterus. The clinician determines how many weeks you have been pregnant by evaluating uterine enlargement, initially detectable about four weeks after conception (that is, two weeks after your period was due). Besides uterine enlargement, the clinician looks for two other findings indicative of pregnancy: uterine softening and a slight bluish coloration of the cervix.

Urine pregnancy tests: All pregnancy tests are based upon the detection of pregnancy hormone (see Chapter 3) found in the urine or blood. There are two types of urine pregnancy tests. The *slide test,* which is done in most offices and clinics, takes the clinician two minutes to perform and is approximately 97% accurate when obtained two weeks or more after a missed period. The *tube test,* commonly used when the slide test is negative, requires one to two hours for results. The most widespread use of tube testing is in the form of simple-to-use home pregnancy tests, such as Daisy II, Acu-Test, and E.P.T., usually available at your local drugstore. Home pregnancy tests reliably detect pregnancy about nine days after a missed period. Home pregnancy tests are often as reliable as lab tests; that is, a positive test is 97% accurate, a negative test is 80% accurate, and a negative test repeated one week later is about 91% accurate. Since urine pregnancy tests depend upon the concentration of pregnancy hormone, always use your first urine specimen of the day because it is the most concentrated.

Recently, even more sensitive tube tests have become available for commercial use. These newer tube tests allow your clinician to diagnose most normal pregnancies at or before your expected menstrual period at a lower cost than the blood pregnancy tests described below.

Remember that urine pregnancy tests are normally positive for up to a week following a miscarriage or abortion, and they may be falsely positive because of "hormone interference" in women who are entering menopause. The greatest number of incorrect tests are false negatives, occurring in up to 20% of women using home tests and in a much smaller percentage when the tests are performed in the hospital lab or a doctor's office. Most false negatives occur because the test was performed too soon or with a dilute urine specimen. Very occasionally a false negative test may also result if an ectopic pregnancy (see glossary) has developed. For this reason a woman should consult her clinician if symptoms of pregnancy continue after a negative reading.

Blood pregnancy tests: Blood pregnancy tests are the costliest as well as the most sensitive and reliable of pregnancy tests. The basic type is called the *radioimmunoassay* (RIA) or beta-subunit HCG. This test is often reserved for pregnancy complications such as a suspected tubal pregnancy, but it can also be used to determine if a woman is pregnant *before* the missed period. Essentially 100% accurate, test results usually take one to three hours. This test can also establish approximately how far your pregnancy has progressed in weeks. The *radioreceptor assay* (RRA) is a somewhat less expensive form of the RIA and provides results within two hours with nearly 100% accuracy. Blood pregnancy tests, done at private laboratories or in hospitals, must be ordered by your clinician.

How Is My Due Date Determined?

The clinician calculates your due date from the first day of your last known period (since the date of conception is usually unknown) using Nägele's Rule: count back three months from the first day of your last menstrual period and add seven days. For example, if your last menstrual period began May 1, your due date would be February 8. Fewer than 10% of women deliver exactly on their due date, and it's normal to have your baby as much as two weeks early or two weeks late. Because of the inaccuracies of calendar calculations, a number of fetal maturity tests have been developed to determine the age of the fetus. *Sonography* is one type of fetal maturity test.

Uses of Sonography During Pregnancy

During pregnancy sonography may be used to evaluate the fetus, amniotic fluid, and placenta. It works like this: sound waves are sent out by an instrument called a *scanner*, and the reflected waves (the echo) are displayed on a screen, appearing as a black-and-white image that looks similar to an X-ray. The sonography procedure is painless except for the discomfort of lying on your back and temporarily having a full bladder. You will be asked to drink fluids and not urinate until after your sonogram, because the clinician can read the pattern better when your bladder is full. The clinician coats your abdomen with mineral oil or aqua gel to improve the quality of sound waves from the hand-held scanner. As you watch the screen, you can see the outline of the fetus (and see movement with some of the newer machines which use so-called real-time imaging). Your clinician can point out the head and other parts of the body.

Sonography is largely used to assess fetal growth and age. Abnormal growth may be suspected if the fetus seems small for the progression of pregnancy

or if your weight gain is very low. Using sonography, the clinician measures the head size, called the *biparietal diameter* (BPD). This measurement closely correlates with the precise age of the fetus, measured from the date of conception (called *gestational age*), especially when determined between the sixteenth and twenty-fifth week of pregnancy. At this time the BPD measurement can accurately determine fetal age to within ten days. After twenty-six weeks the BPD is less reliable because of the greater variability in fetal head growth during the latter part of pregnancy.

Other uses of sonography include assessment of the position of the fetus (head first or breech) and detection of twins. Localization of the placenta by sonography allows the physician to identify a "pocket" of amniotic fluid as well as the placenta and fetus, both of which must be avoided by the amniocentesis needle (see also Chapter 20). Sonography is also used to diagnose certain placental disorders causing bleeding in late pregnancy (see Chapter 53). Ectopic pregnancies (abnormally located outside the uterus) and ovarian cysts can also be identified as well using this technique.

Your body is exposed only for a fraction of a second to the sound waves and there are no known harmful effects. Despite its apparent safety, sonography is not recommended for routine use during pregnancy unless there is a reason for it. Table 27 summarizes some of the reasons for the use of sonography during pregnancy.

Progression of Pregnancy

Pregnancy lasts about nine months and averages 38 weeks from the date of conception, or about 40 weeks from the first day of your last menstrual period, depending on the usual length of your cycle. After your initial visit to your clinician, you will usually have a checkup once a month until your seventh or eighth month when visits become more frequent. During these visits, your clinician measures fetal growth by recording the expansion of your uterus (see Figure 15). Your weight and blood pressure are checked and urine samples are taken to check for albumin (indicator of toxemia) and sugar (indicator of diabetes). You and your clinician should use these visits to get to know and feel comfortable with each other. It is important to thoroughly discuss attitudes and decisions about your childbirth experience so your plans and expectations coincide.

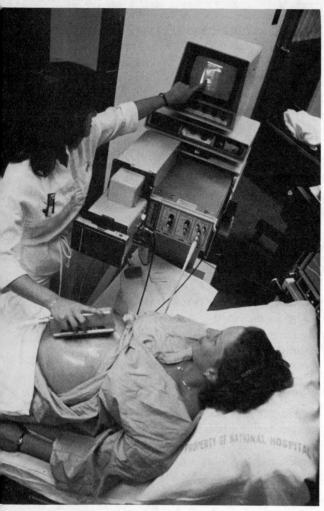

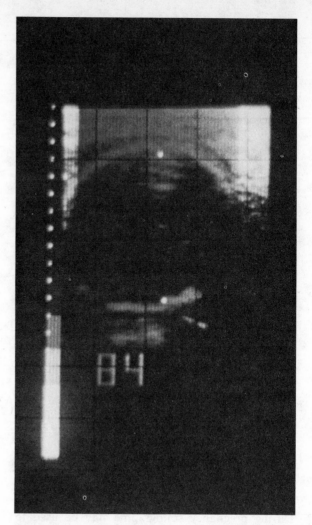

Obtaining a sonogram. The X-ray technician presses a sound-wave emitting device (scanner) lightly against the mother's abdomen. This procedure results in a sound-wave "picture," indicated by the technician.

The outline of the baby's head as viewed on a sonogram.

The events of pregnancy fall naturally into three equal time periods, called *trimesters* of pregnancy. The physical and emotional changes in the mother, which are discussed below, vary predictably within each trimester. It is important to remember, however, that each pregnancy is unique and that this discussion is only a general outline of what you might experience. If you notice symptoms that worry you, look them up in the symptoms section of this book (Section Eleven) for their possible causes and treatment. Diet and nutrition in pregnancy are discussed in Chapter 46.

Warning signs in pregnancy—that is, indica-tions that your pregnancy may be threatened—are shown in Table 28.

The first trimester (1 to 3 months)

During the first trimester (the first three months), the fetus makes its greatest developmental strides. The head, brain, heart, body, and limbs begin to form. Fingers and toes are recognizable. Sex organs begin to develop but cannot yet be observed. Except for the first week after conception, all drugs and chemicals to which you are exposed may cross the placenta and possibly influence the development of the fetus.

Table 27 POSSIBLE REASONS FOR A SONOGRAM (ULTRASOUND) DURING PREGNANCY

When Performed*	Reason or Indication	What Sonogram Shows
6—12 weeks	Bleeding in early pregnancy.	Fetal movement is detectable (using real-time scanner) by nine weeks: absence of movement indicates miscarriage; fetal movement is reassuring sign.
6—12 weeks	Pelvic pain in early pregnancy.	Can detect some causes of pain—e.g., ovarian cyst and ectopic pregnancy.
16—18 weeks	Amniocentesis is planned to screen for genetic defects.	Identifies "pocket" of amniotic fluid as well as placenta and fetus, both of which must be avoided by amniocentesis needle.
16—25 weeks	History of previous child with anencephaly, spina bifida, or hydrocephaly.	These abnormalities are detectable.
16—25 weeks	High-risk pregnancies in which labor may be induced (e.g., high blood pressure, diabetes) or repeat cesarean section planned.	Measurement of fetal head size allows calculation of gestational age and due date.
16—25 weeks	Maternal family history of twins or suspected twins because of apparent large size of fetus.	Shows presence of one fetus or more (may be detected as early as 10 weeks).

* Counting from the first day of your last menstrual period.

Your physical changes: You may experience some or none of the early signs of pregnancy listed in Table 26. The most common symptoms of early pregnancy are a missed period, morning sickness, breast tenderness, and frequent urination.

Your emotional changes: Most women have conflicting feelings about pregnancy throughout the first trimester. Even women who have had difficulty conceiving go through mood swings that pass from exuberance to despair. Both parents-to-be often worry about the financial and psychological responsibility of parenthood. You may wonder if you want to be a mother after all, or if you can be a good mother. Sometimes a father finds himself feeling just as worried and torn about the pregnancy as his wife is. It often helps to share your feelings with each other.

During the first trimester, many women are preoccupied with the changes in their bodies and what seems to be happening to them. They frequently feel at this time more dependent upon others. The need to share the frustrations and

Table 28 TEN WARNING SIGNS IN PREGNANCY

Report any of these symptoms to your clinician immediately:

1. Any vaginal bleeding or spotting
2 . Severe, persistent headaches
3. Prolonged vomiting (over one to two days, preventing adequate intake of liquids)
4. Blurring of vision; spots before the eyes
5. Fever (over 100° F.) and chills not accompanied by symptoms of a cold
6. Sudden intense or continual abdominal pains
7. Sudden gush of fluid from the vagina
8. Sudden swelling of hands, feet, and ankles
9. Frequent, burning urination
10. Pronounced decrease in fetal movement

pleasures of pregnancy is likely to continue through the entire nine months. It's best to depend on someone besides your clinician since he or she may not always be available. Ideally, the person you select should also be the one who will be with you in labor and delivery. If you have a close friend who is pregnant at the same time, you can offer each other mutual support and understanding.

The second trimester (4 to 6 months)

The heart and circulatory system of the fetus develops during this time; and by the fifth or sixth month the clinician, using an instrument called a *doptone* (see glossary), can hear the heartbeat. By the end of the sixth month, the fetus will have grown to about six inches in length. The clinician continues to measure uterine growth in centimeters during your monthly checkups. This is the time to start preparing for breast-feeding if that is what you wish to do. You may want to contact your local La Leche League office for group sup-

port and instruction. See Chapter 19 for more information about breast-feeding.

Your physical changes: If you felt some discomfort during the first trimester, you are likely to feel better the second trimester. If you felt well during the first trimester, you may feel even better during this time.

As the fetus increases in size, so does your waist. You gain weight more rapidly in the second trimester and find that your clothes become uncomfortably tight. By the twentieth week or so of your pregnancy, the fetus becomes large enough for *you* to feel its movements, called *quickening*. Repeat pregnant mothers usually notice it earlier in their second pregnancy since they are familiar with the fluttering movement. Be sure to tell your clinician the date on which you first felt fetal movement.

Indigestion problems such as heartburn, gas, and constipation may appear. Your heart is working harder because your blood volume has increased, and this circumstance may lead to greater fatigue and some fluid retention. You may find

Figure 15   *Curved marks indicate the location of the top of the uterus (fundus) at various weeks of pregnancy. The approximate weight of the fetus at each of these weeks is shown. Note that by 40 weeks, the fundus has become slightly lower than at 36 weeks because the fetus "drops" in the last month of pregnancy. Most of the fetal weight is gained in the last 12 weeks.*

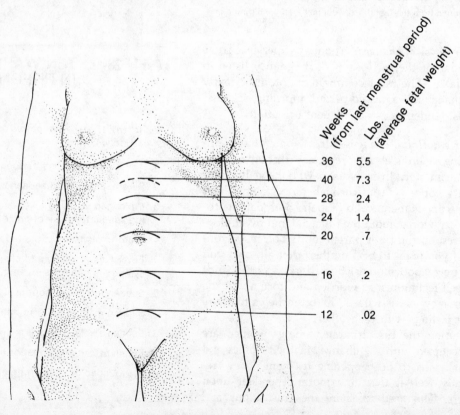

Weeks (from last menstrual period)	Lbs. (average fetal weight)
36	5.5
40	7.3
28	2.4
24	1.4
20	.7
16	.2
12	.02

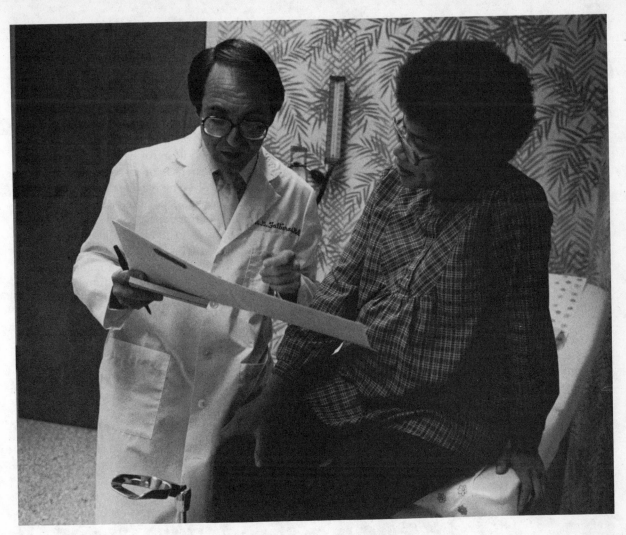

that some discomfort can be relieved by continued regular exercise (see Chapter 47). Other conditions which may begin to occur in midpregnancy include varicose veins, hemorrhoids, and skin changes, including the appearance of stretch marks, called *striae*.

Your emotional changes: Many women feel very well during this time, partly as a result of the disappearance of the unpleasant symptoms of early pregnancy. You are obviously pregnant yet not too big to move around comfortably. The reality of the pregnancy is obvious to everyone, and you will probably get more immediate support and recognition from others.

The feelings of the movements of the fetus can be thrilling. If you are upset about your pregnancy, however, the movements may seem to focus your anger and make you feel less in control of your body. Repeat mothers often compare their current pregnancy with their previous pregnancies and the amount of fetal movement, wondering how the differences between this pregnancy and earlier pregnancies will be reflected in this newborn's personality.

As you begin to wear maternity clothes and lose your figure, you may still experience conflicting feelings toward this pregnancy. A change in your image—in the way you see yourself physically—normally occurs by the second trimester. You may experience many different emotions as you watch the growth of your abdomen and realize you have been sharing your body with a growing fetus. You may feel protective and maternal toward what is inside your abdomen. It is common to continue to wonder if your newborn will be normal.

Even in the most wanted and planned pregnancies, feelings of confusion, anxiety, or depression may lurk below the surface. It is normal to turn your thoughts more to yourself, to look more into your own mind and feelings, and to spend time thinking about your own mother and your childhood. If you have a close relationship with your mother, and she is nearby, you may find her support comforting. If your mother is far away or you have conflicts in your relationship, you may use a great deal of energy in trying to develop your own separate, distinct style of maternal role and identity. Second and subsequent pregnancies may be harder at this point because of the demands of older children. Every pregnant woman needs some time to think about becoming a mother and to identify her feelings about it.

The third trimester (7 to 9 months)

The fetus grows rapidly during the last three months, multiplying its weight about three to four times. You may note the hands or feet of the fetus poking out in a lump in your abdomen or appearing as a wave when it changes position. You are constantly aware of its movements, from kicking

to hiccuping. The last trimester is usually the time to begin preparation classes for childbirth (see Chapter 14).

Your physical changes: Your abdomen is very large, and you can see the movements of the fetus clearly. Your abdomen feels very firm and big; your navel may be pushed out flat. The fetus moves into the position for delivery, usually head down. Your awareness of these movements may wake you, and sleeping may be difficult. Finding a comfortable sleeping position isn't easy. Sometimes slight contractions, called *Braxton-Hicks*, cause your uterus to tighten. These contractions seem like menstrual cramps and usually go away quickly. Shortness of breath is a common symptom during this period; this condition is due to the fact that the uterus is pushing up other abdominal organs and thus restricting movement of the diaphragm. At the end of the eighth month, the top of the uterus may be felt just below the lower edge of the ribs. This may cause an uncomfortable feeling of stretching below your lower ribs.

The fetal heartbeat can be heard through a special stethoscope called a fetoscope (below) or with an instrument called a doptone (opposite page).

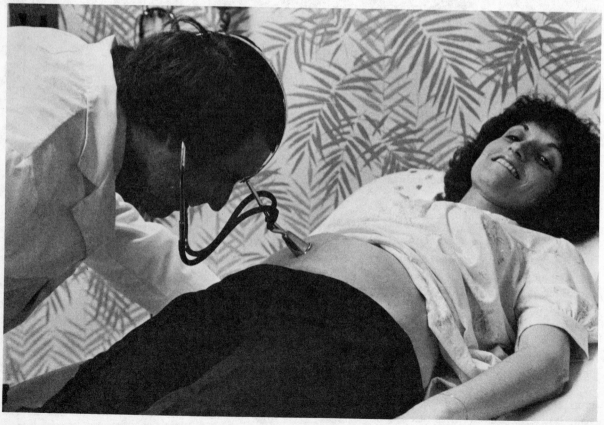

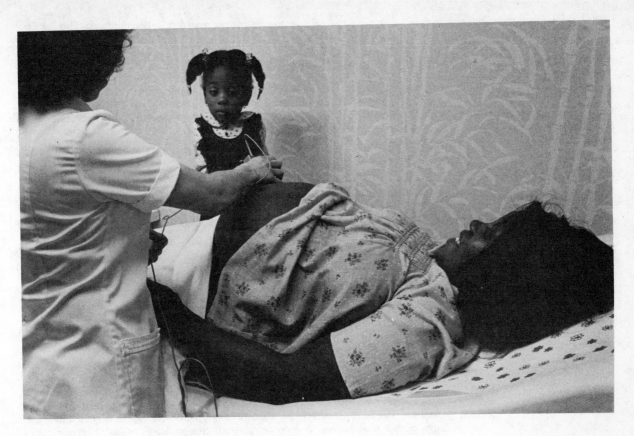

Pressure from the fetus may be felt in many ways: aches and pains in the legs, thighs, or perineum; frequent urinating; and occasional lightheadedness or dizziness. You may experience indigestion because the uterus presses against your stomach. Backache, too, is common because you tend to lean backward to compensate for your heavy abdomen. *Lightening* refers to the slight descent of the uterus that occurs when the head of the fetus drops into the birth canal; it usually occurs two to four weeks before delivery. This process is more pronounced in first-time mothers and may not occur until labor in repeat mothers. Lightening relieves the pressure on your stomach and diaphragm, making it easier to breathe. Lightening means that your body is getting ready for delivery.

Your emotional changes: Now is a time of expectancy, of waiting for labor to begin. Many women experience a feeling of wanting the delivery soon but at the same time fear the experience of labor and delivery. Taking childbirth preparation classes helps you to lessen your anxiety as well as to share your excitement with other pregnant women. Anxiety about birth defects may increase. You may feel a deep sense of oneness and at the same time be ready to give up this oneness in order to see and hear and touch what you have anticipated for nine months.

You begin to picture your newborn's appearance. You may dream or fantasize about what he or she looks like; these thoughts are quite normal. The baby's increasing activity won't let you forget him or her or the fact that you are soon to be a mother. The last month may drag by as you eagerly await the arrival of the baby. People constantly ask you how you feel and when you expect to have the baby. These comments can be upsetting as you have no answer for what you want to know most, and no one can tell when "labor day" will arrive. The last few weeks of pregnancy are a hard time during which to plan anything, and most women stay close to home. Each day you wonder if this will be "the day," though you know the waiting is well worth it.

Feelings of dependency on friends and relatives increase. This is the time, it is hoped, when you should be getting some extra help. Your husband or an older son or daughter can help with the heavier chores, and perhaps one of them can spend more time with your other children. If you are alone, stay close to a friend who will be available for help.

Table 29 COMMON CONCERNS DURING PREGNANCY

Trips by car . . .	Wear a seat belt and shoulder strap at all times, fitting the belt loosely over your thighs as opposed to tightly around your abdomen. Take frequent (hourly) breaks for exercise and nourishment. Stay close to home during your ninth month in case the baby decides to make an early appearance.
Air travel . . .	Fly only in a pressurized aircraft. It is recommended that you move about every 45 minutes to promote circulation.
Sex . . .	During a normal pregnancy, sexual intercourse is in no way harmful. Some women experience increased sexual desire during pregnancy. Avoid intercourse if you have vaginal bleeding or ruptured membranes, or in the last six weeks of pregnancy if you are pregnant with twins or have a history of premature labor. (See Chapter 23.)
Pets—like cats . . .	Cats may carry a rare microorganism that causes a disease called toxoplasmosis and that is excreted in their stools. An ample precaution is to have someone else change the kitty litter and to wash your hands after you have handled a cat.
Exercise . . .	A safe rule to follow is to continue whatever exercise you were doing before pregnancy as long as you feel comfortable. Jogging, horseback riding, swimming, and skiing have all been done safely by pregnant women. Use your common sense and if you find you are uncomfortable and tired, stop. Walking and prenatal exercises are particularly helpful. Check with your clinician about your exercise program. (See Chapter 47.)
Work . . .	In most uncomplicated pregnancies the woman can work throughout the pregnancy, including the ninth month. In general, avoid strenuous activity, extreme temperatures, smoking areas, and excessive stair climbing. Take frequent breaks, stop working when fatigued, elevate your legs periodically, and wear support hose. Prolonged standing (greater than four hours), repetitive heavy lifting (greater than twenty-five pounds), and frequent stooping and bending below knee level should be avoided in the last three months. Women with previous preterm babies or other high-risk factors such as high blood pressure, diabetes, or inadequate fetal growth should seriously consider only light duties throughout pregnancy. Exposure to environmental toxic substances (that is, chemicals) may be hazardous to the fetus, especially in early pregnancy.
Video display terminals . . .	VDT's have not been found to be a hazard to the fetus, but you may experience neck pains or headaches from sitting in a fixed position for prolonged periods.
Hot tubs . . .	Animal experiments suggest that high maternal temperatures result in a reduction of blood flow to the fetus. In uncomplicated pregnancies, short stretches in a sauna or hot tub are probably not harmful if the temperature is less than 102° F and exposure does not exceed ten minutes.

Common Concerns During Pregnancy

There are many concerns that women may have during pregnancy. Table 29 discusses some of the more common ones.

Further Information

For more information about what to expect during pregnancy, you can write to the American College of Obstetricians and Gynecologists, which provides free patient information booklets, including:

Pregnancy and Daily Living
Food, Pregnancy, and Health
Travel During Pregnancy

The address is:
Resource Center
American College of Obstetricians and
    Gynecologists
600 Maryland Ave., S.W.
Washington, DC 20024

You can also write to the following for more information:
Office of Maternal and Child Health
U.S. Dept. of Health and Human Services
5600 Fishers Lane, Room 7-39
Rockville, MD 20857

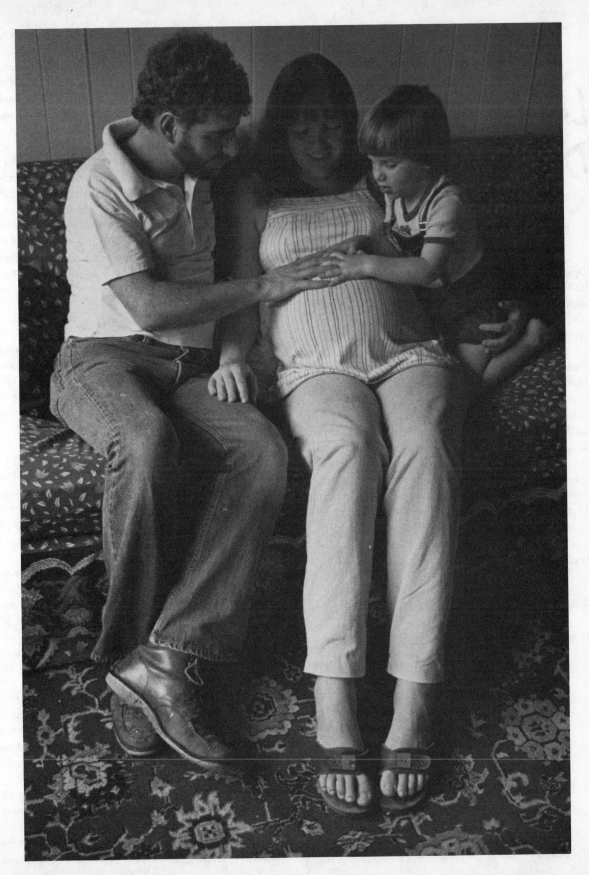

17

Labor and Delivery

Labor is the process by which uterine contractions cause the cervix to dilate (become widened), allowing delivery of the baby. No one knows what causes these involuntary contractions to begin. Prior to labor the cervix undergoes a process (sometimes called *ripening*) in which it becomes thinner (*effaced*), more pliable, and slightly dilated. Dilation refers to the size of the cervical *opening*. During the final two or three prenatal visits, the clinician estimates by pelvic examination how much dilation and effacement have occurred. Even if your cervix is closed, labor can begin within twenty-four hours. Once the cervical opening widens to two to three centimeters, however, labor often starts within one or two days. During labor, uterine contractions will complete the process of cervical dilation, which must reach ten centimeters (about four inches) for vaginal delivery to occur.

How Do I Know When Labor Begins?

There are three signs that labor may soon begin:

1. You may notice a blood-tinged mucous discharge known as *bloody show*. This discharge means that the mucus plug sealing the bottom of the uterus has been dislodged. Labor often begins within twenty-four hours following bloody show.
2. Leakage of fluid from the vagina, in a constant trickle or a sudden gush, usually indicates rupture of the bag of waters. ("Waters" means simply the amniotic fluid surrounding the fetus during pregnancy.) Spontaneous rupture of your membranes usually means that labor will begin sometime during the next twenty-four hours. If your membranes rupture, contact your clinician.
3. Frequently, backache or painless abdominal tightening (*false labor*) indicates that labor will soon begin. These Braxton-Hicks contractions help prepare your uterus for real labor, which is characterized by regular, often painful contractions which occur initially at ten- to fifteen-minute intervals. As a general rule you should contact your clinician and prepare to leave for the hospital (or other birth setting) once these contractions become regular, occurring at least every ten minutes and lasting thirty seconds or longer. Table 99 in Chapter 81 explains differences between real labor and false labor.

Stages of Labor

There are three stages in the labor and delivery process. The first stage of labor is the time it takes the cervix to dilate ten centimeters (see Figure 16). The first stage averages thirteen hours in a woman having her first baby; in subsequent childbirths, this period is shorter, averaging about eight hours. This stage is divided into three phases: *early, active,* and *transition*. Often the *early* phase (up to three to four centimeters dilation) will not be too uncomfortable. Walking, watching TV, and talking with your labor coach (if you have one) help the time pass. Your clinician or a nurse will record the length, strength, and frequency of contractions and listen to fetal heart tones. Decisions on enemas and type of perineal shave will be made. The *position* of your baby is determined, and you may have an X-ray if the baby is in a breech position (see Chapter 21). You may be reminded to empty your bladder frequently. This avoids bladder distention (stretching) which may require catheterization. Vaginal exams are done periodically between contractions.

During the *active* phase (four to seven centimeters), when contractions become more intense, you will rely more on breathing techniques to help relieve discomfort. At this time you may want to request pain medication or an epidural anesthetic (see Chapter 19).

The final phase, known as *transition* (eight to ten centimeters), is the time when most intense pressure and pain occur during contractions. This phase is the hardest but also the shortest part of labor. You may want to "push" or bear down

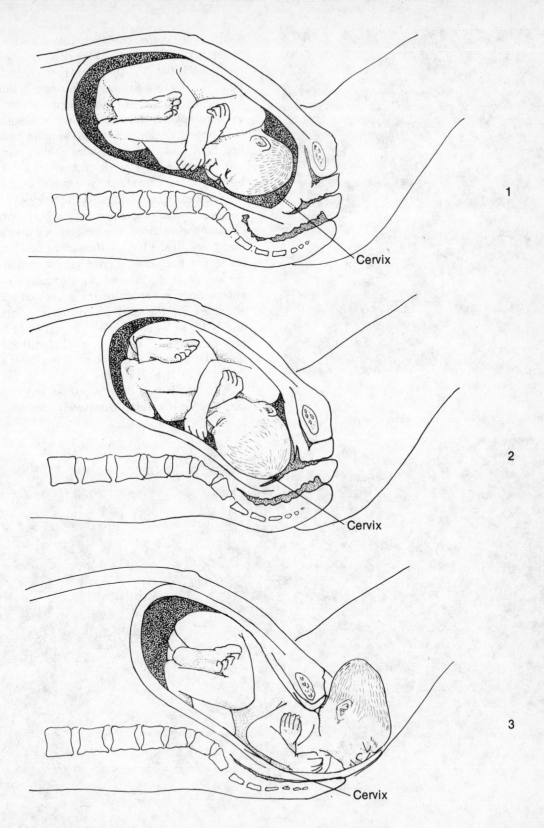

Figure 16 *Prior to labor the cervix is closed or slightly dilated (1). As labor begins, the cervix begins to dilate (2). For delivery to occur the cervix must be completely dilated (3).*

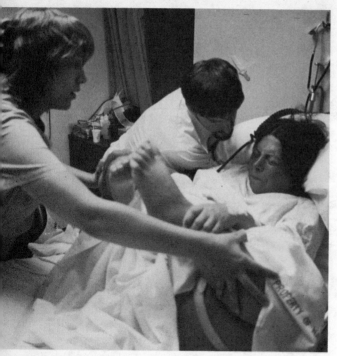

"Pushing" during the second stage of labor.

Footprinting the newborn in the delivery room.

before you reach complete dilation (ten centimeters). You need the most support and encouragement at this time to help you stay in control. Once you are fully dilated, the hardest part is finished.

The second stage of labor begins when the cervix is completely dilated. The second stage usually lasts no more than an hour in a woman having her first baby and averages less than thirty minutes in subsequent childbirths. It ends when the baby is born. During this stage, you feel a tremendous urge to bear down and push the baby out. It can be a very satisfying experience to push with each of your contractions. Pushing lessens the contraction pains. If the birth setting and situation allow for it, you can observe your baby's head in a mirror as you push. If you have a spinal or epidural anesthetic, your coach or the nurse can feel your abdomen for the start of your next contraction and tell you when to push. If you have had no other anesthesia, either a local anesthetic or a pudendal block (see Chapter 19) is almost always used just prior to delivery.

After the baby's head is pushed out, the baby may cry before being completely delivered. The

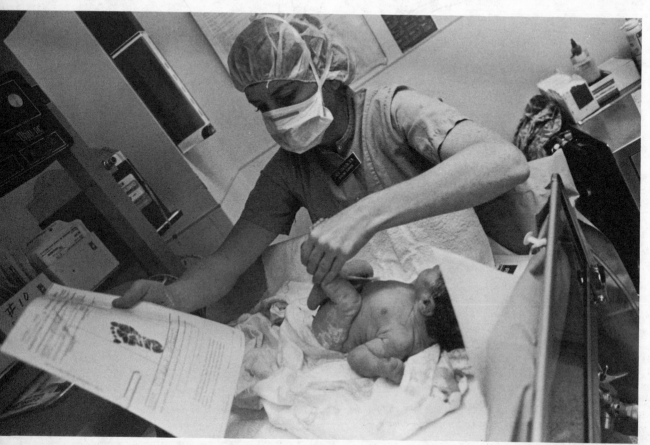

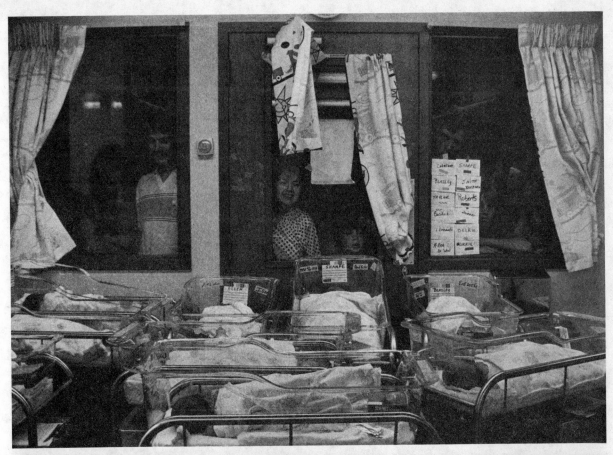

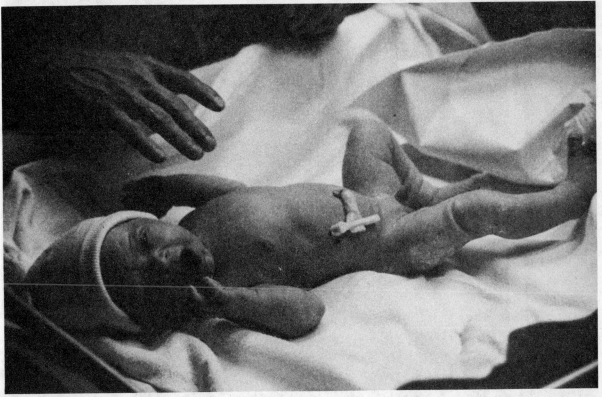

baby's shoulders come next followed quickly by the rest of the body. Your baby can be placed on your abdomen, where the cord is cut. Or the cord may be cut while the baby is still in the hands of the clinician. Mucus from the baby's mouth is quickly removed by a small suction bulb.

When you first see your newborn, don't be surprised if your baby doesn't look like the pictures you've seen in magazines. He or she may appear smaller and is usually wet looking and covered with a white, creamy substance called vernix. Normally a newborn's hands and feet may look blue. The baby's head may look strange—often swollen or elongated—a result of passing through the birth canal. This temporary condition is known as *molding*. Newborns seem so tiny and fragile; even the most experienced parents feel awkward in holding them. It's natural for you and your husband to want to hold and touch your

baby, to fully realize the reality of your having given birth. Childbirth is such an amazing process that it takes a while to absorb the experience.

The third stage of labor includes delivery of the placenta (afterbirth), which usually occurs within fifteen minutes after birth. The clinician examines the expelled placenta to make sure it is complete, because any part left in the uterus may cause subsequent bleeding or infection. After delivery of the placenta and repair of any tears and the episiotomy, if performed, you are usually taken to a recovery area. There the nurses observe you closely for bleeding and other complications and massage your uterus to minimize blood loss. Your baby is also closely observed in the recovery area or in the newborn nursery. When you and your baby appear to be progressing without complications, you will be transferred to a room or allowed to go home, depending on your birth setting.

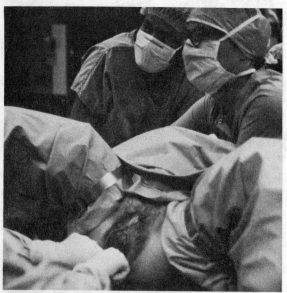

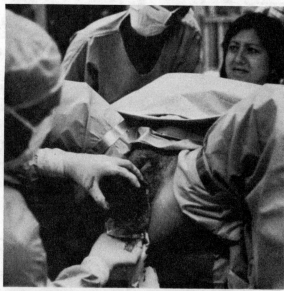

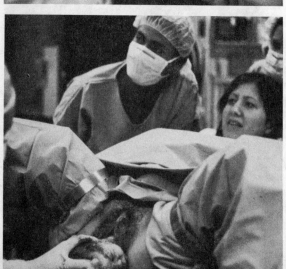

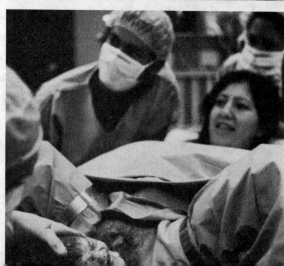

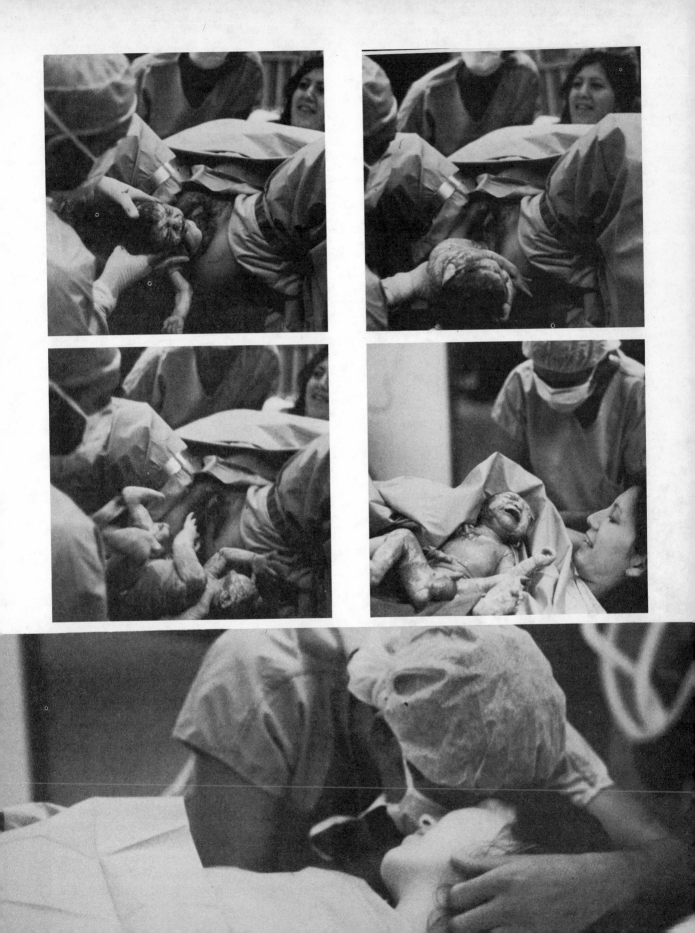

Your First Weeks as a Mother

Birth climaxes months of waiting. With the birth of a first child, it transforms spouses into parents and converts a marriage into a family. The new mother undergoes changes in her physical state, feelings, and style of living. These first few weeks after your baby's birth are known as the postpartum period. It may take several days after child-

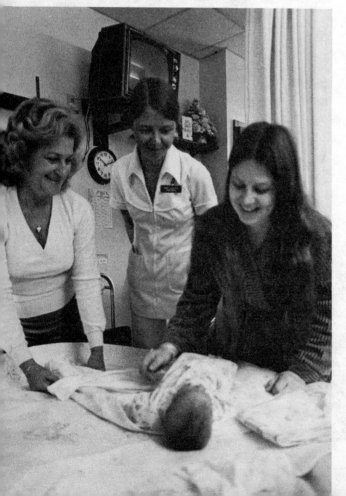

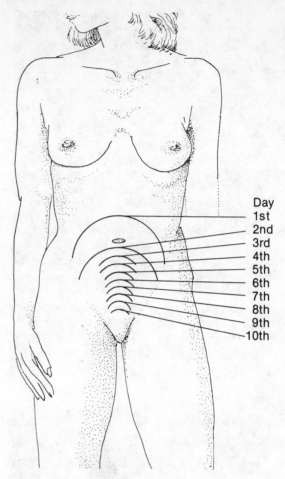

Figure 17
The location of the top of the uterus (fundus) during the first ten days after childbirth. After about a week the fundus can no longer be felt by pressing on the abdomen.

Day
1st
2nd
3rd
4th
5th
6th
7th
8th
9th
10th

birth for a woman to feel she has regained control over the physical changes affecting her body. This chapter talks about what to expect physically and emotionally in the postpartum period.

Physiologic Changes

The uterus gradually returns to its nonpregnant size in a process called *involution*, which takes about six weeks (see Figure 17). The uterus continues to mildly contract following delivery, thereby controlling possible bleeding. Immediately after delivery, you can feel the top of the uterus (fundus) above your umbilicus (bellybutton). The fundus feels round and solid, somewhat like a grapefruit, for the first few days after you deliver. The nurse will press on your abdomen to check for the firmness of your uterus, and she may massage it to keep it firm in the first few hours after childbirth. You may be encouraged to massage the fundus, as well, to help prevent bleeding. The periodic cramping some women experience for a few days after having a baby is called *afterpains.* These uterine contractions are less common in women having their first baby and thus may come as a surprise to a woman having a subsequent child. These contractions after childbirth may feel especially strong during breast-feeding, which stimulates them.

The abdominal wall muscles remain stretched following childbirth. When you first stand up after your delivery, the abdominal muscles will fall forward, pushed out somewhat by the uterus, giving you a slight still-pregnant appearance. This is very disappointing, especially if you had expected to be flat right away! In the next few days, your abdomen will begin to firm up; and with fre-

quent postpartum exercise (see Chapter 47), you can be zipping up and buttoning your pants in about six weeks. Most women require at least three months to return to their prepregnancy weight. You may want to wear a supporting girdle initially to hold these muscles in, although it really isn't necessary.

Some women worry that if they begin walking too soon after delivery "everything will fall out." This isn't true; nor is the belief that walking increases vaginal bleeding true. Vaginal bleeding continues for three to six weeks after delivery. All women experience vaginal drainage called *lochia* for the first few days after childbirth. Normally this vaginal discharge changes in a few days from red or pink to brown or yellow. It is important to wash the vaginal area with warm water (usually from a squeeze bottle or pitcher) when you change your sanitary napkin or urinate. This helps to keep the area clean and reduces the chance of infection.

Women who breast-feed may not menstruate while they are nursing. Menstruation usually

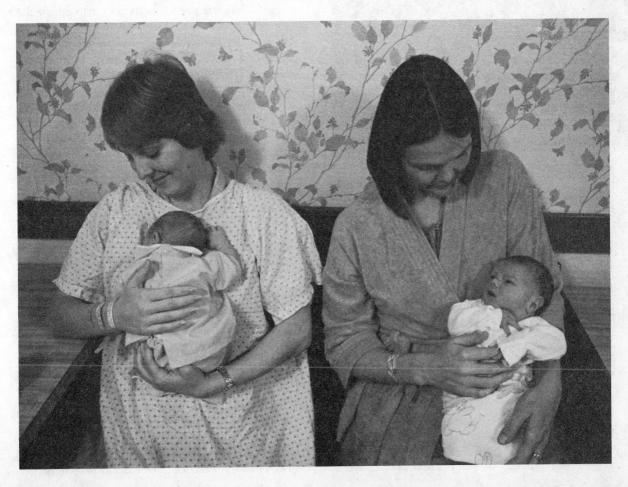

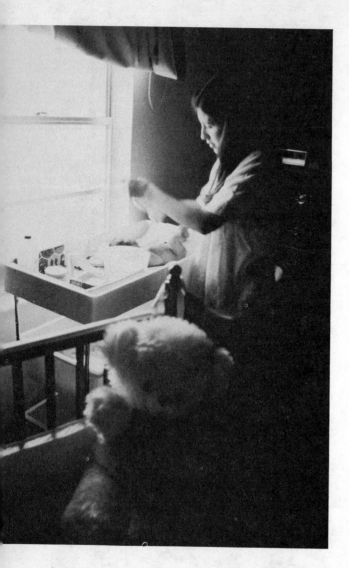

pre-moistened gauze pad (available in your drugstore), held in place by your sanitary napkin also help relieve the pain from stitches. When you go home, you may want to ask for pain medication; but remember, if you are breast-feeding, that the drug will pass into your milk (see Chapter 31). Ask your clinician for examples of postpartum exercises that will help to reduce your discomfort.

Adequate Rest and Sleep

A few hours after delivery, you will feel very tired, though excited from the delivery. It is important to continue to force yourself to rest so you won't become frustrated and irritated in taking care of your new baby. If you are breast-feeding but really exhausted, you might want to let the nurses feed the baby water through the night so that you can get some sleep. The baby mainly needs fluids at this time.

With the first baby it is easy to nap; but when older children are at home, it is very difficult. If possible, ask friends or relatives to help during the first few weeks so that you can rest. Involve the other family members in housekeeping chores by delegating some day-to-day tasks. Limit your visitors during the first few weeks. It is easy to overdo at first, and you may suddenly find yourself exhausted. Arrange for some time to be alone with your husband. Remember that chronic sleep loss will make you less able to enjoy your new baby, and *you* are more important than the chores to be done.

Postpartum Blues

Postpartum blues refers to the slight depression normally experienced by most women after childbirth. The blues may occur as a letdown following initial excitement of childbirth, or it may come three to six weeks later. These feelings may reflect changes in hormone levels after delivery or may be due to the realization of the reality of motherhood. Some women never acknowledge or experience any depression, while others find themselves crying frequently for several days.

A new mother is often unprepared for how the baby will upset her former life style. She often finds herself juggling baby's needs, possibly older children's needs, and husband's needs while her own needs go unmet—no wonder she may get

begins in two months in women who do not nurse and in four months or so in women who do. Remember, it is possible to get pregnant before you menstruate, so use contraception as soon as you resume sexual intercourse.

Many women worry about the discomfort of having their first bowel movement, which normally does not occur until a few days after delivery. This delay is usually a result of the lack of recent food intake or if you had an enema during labor. Stool softeners are frequently given after delivery; a laxative will also help. A nutritious diet of vegetables and fruit as well as plenty of fluids is also beneficial (see Chapter 46).

Your stitches may cause discomfort or itching for several weeks. Sitting on an inflatable cushion that is shaped like a doughnut or on a pillow helps to relieve direct pressure on your incision. Heat from a tub bath or heat lamp and a Tucks pad, a

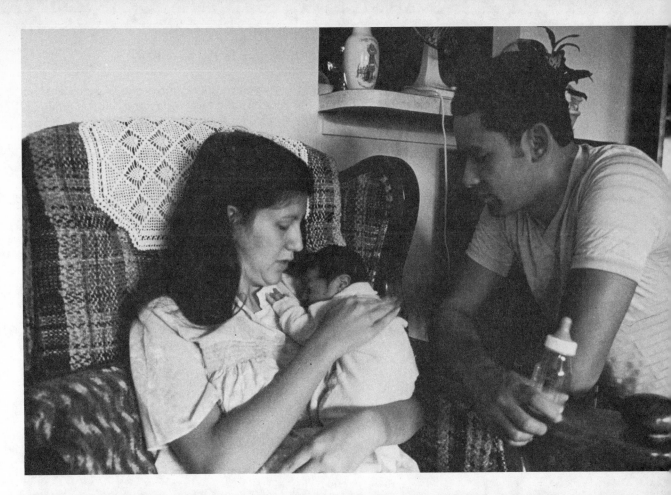
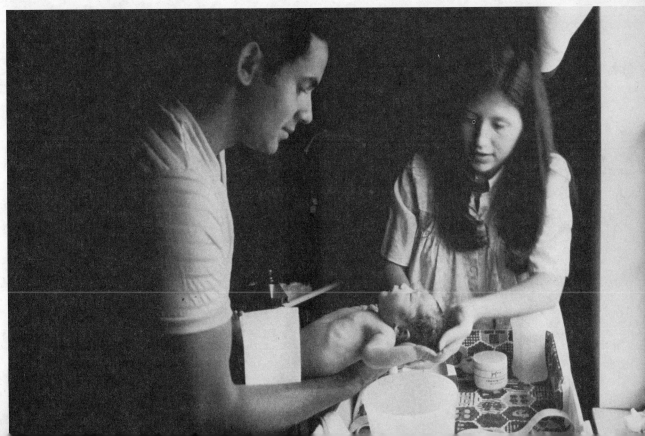

angry! It often helps to express your feelings to your husband and friends. Ask for emotional support from your family and close friends, especially if they have been helpful at stressful times in the past. If you find yourself overly tired and unmotivated to do necessary tasks, seek out professional help (see Chapter 60, Depression).

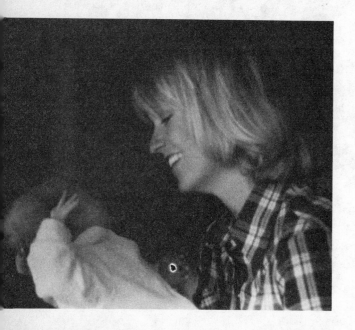

Adjusting to the New Baby

Most women have unrealistic expectations for themselves and their behavior as mothers. Parenting behavior is learned—not instinctive—and our society provides few personal opportunities to learn about infant care until parenthood. It may take as long as a year to "feel like a mother" and adjust to your new role in life. And it also takes time for you to understand your newborn's needs. Each baby is so different! Baby-care classes are offered at most hospitals with obstetrical services, and the hospital nurses can help you with specific questions about caring for your baby. The American Red Cross offers parenting classes for parents of newborns. When you are at home, call your clinician's office if you need help or have questions. Your physician can refer you to a public health nurse if you need one. You could also call the nursery nurses if you have a question and, of course, your pediatrician's office. Other young mothers or relatives with whom you are comfortable may be among your best resources.

Each family member has his or her own period of readjustment when the new baby arrives. New parenthood necessarily involves reduction of some nonfamily needs and interests, but don't let

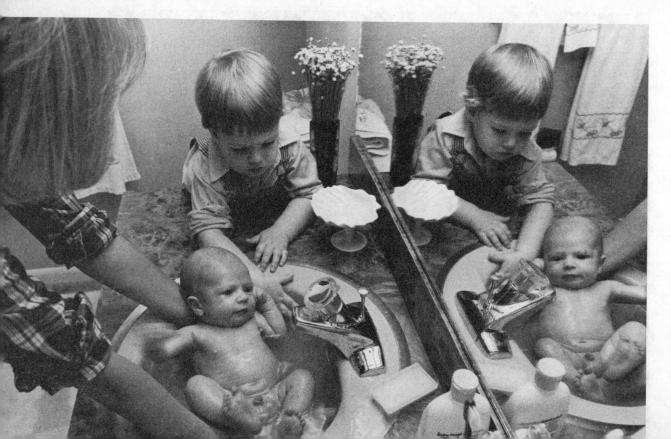

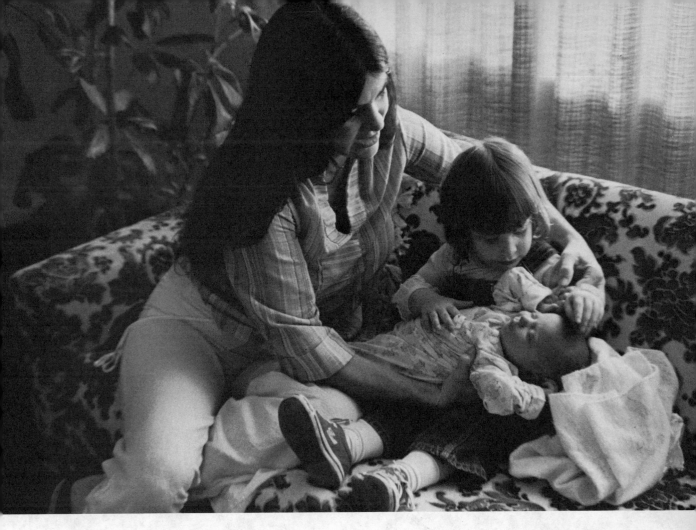

them all go. It is important to return after a few weeks to some outside activity that interests you. If you have stopped working, you may miss the loss of income as well as the social contacts involved in your job. The additional laundry and caretaking activities may seem overwhelming. You may find your husband or your other children, or both, more demanding, and this relationship may worry you. Your husband may feel an increased financial pressure now that he is a family man or now that there is an additional family member. Siblings, too, usually have mixed feelings about the attention paid to the new baby—although they may outwardly act otherwise. It is important to acknowledge these normal feelings in your other children. In time, with support and understanding, these stresses will resolve and your family will stabilize once again.

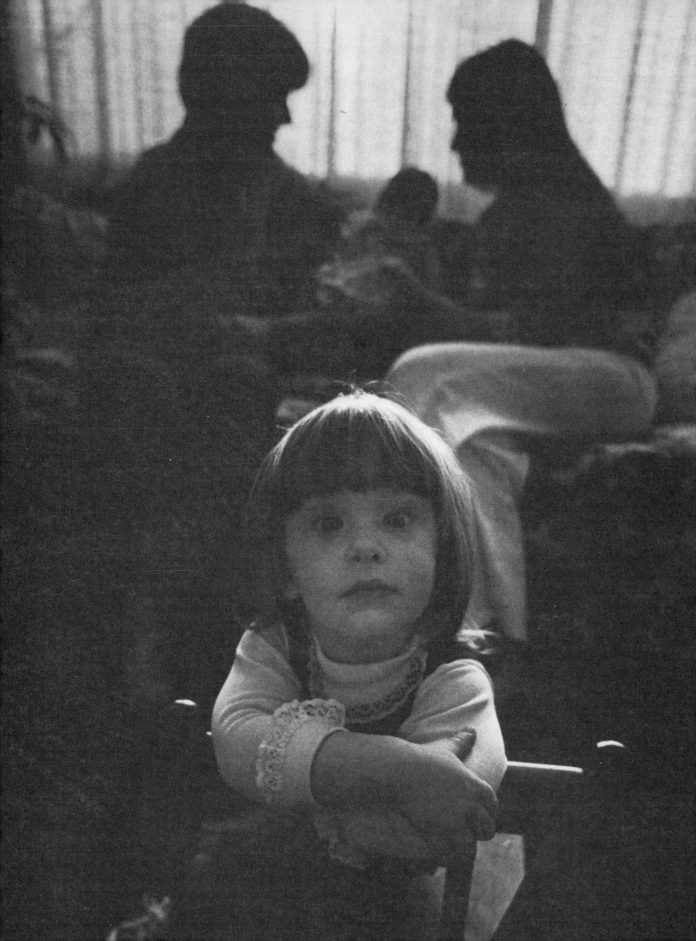

19

Options During and After Childbirth

This chapter discusses the possible options you can select from during and after your childbirth experience. As you read about these options, decide which are important to you, and ask your clinician which ones are permitted and encouraged in your birth setting. If there are procedures you wish to avoid—such as an IV (intravenous fluid) in early labor—you may need to sign a statement releasing the birthing facility from medical liability should complications arise. It is important that both you and whoever delivers your baby feel comfortable with the options you choose or eliminate.

After you have read this chapter, look over Table 31. If any of these questions concern you or you want to know more about these topics, be sure to discuss them with your clinician.

Optional Procedures During Early Labor

An enema, IV, and perineal shaving are not always performed automatically. Some of the pros and cons of these procedures are discussed below.

Enema

Routine enemas for women in labor began in an effort to decrease the chance of maternal and infant infection during delivery. If the rectum is not emptied prior to childbirth, feces may be uncontrollably expelled at delivery. Some women feel more comfortable pushing at delivery if they know their rectum is empty.

An enema consists of a warm sudsy solution that is inserted into the rectum through a tube. The presence of this fluid stimulates a bowel movement. As the enema is administered, you may notice some mild discomfort from rectal pressure. You will use either the bedpan or the bathroom for expelling the solution. If you want to avoid an enema, ask your clinician during a prenatal visit about omitting this procedure. For many if not most women, this procedure is unnecessary.

IV (intravenous fluid)

Most physicians advise women, once labor has begun, not to eat, in order to prevent nausea. An IV is inserted into a vein in your hand or arm to provide the fluid replacement you and your baby require during labor. A most important advantage of the IV is that it provides immediate access for drugs, fluid, or blood should an emergency occur.

The main disadvantage of an IV is that it limits your movement to some extent and may be uncomfortable during the insertion of the needle. If you are in early labor and want to write or walk around, you could ask the staff to delay IV insertion. Suggest placing the IV in the arm you are less likely to use, that is, your left arm if you are right-handed.

The prep (perineal shaving)

Shaving the perineal area theoretically lessens the chance of infection stemming from contamination of the birth canal during childbirth. Its main practical advantage, however, is in allowing better visualization of the area for the clinician during repair of the episiotomy. There are some disadvantages to perineal shaving—itching may occur as the hair begins to grow back and razor nicks or abrasions may themselves be a source of infection. In addition, some women find the shaving procedure embarrassing. In fact, many clinicians consider the procedure completely unnecessary.

As far back as the 1950s, studies showed that unshaved patients had no greater chance of episiotomy infection than those patients who had been shaved. Some physicians now suggest clipping the hair to improve the view of the perineal area. Partial shaving, which includes just the area around the vagina (so-called mini-prep) or no shaving at all is more widely practiced in many hospitals. Where routine perineal shaving continues, its use may be a result of convenience or even ignorance of research concerning this practice. The perineal shave is also something to discuss with your clinician during a prenatal visit.

Drugs for Pain Relief in Labor and Delivery

Pain relief through drugs during labor are generally of two types: direct administration of painkillers (narcotics) or sedatives, and regional anesthesia in which a local anesthetic blocks pain sensation in a particular area of the body. For the relief of pain during delivery, there are five types of anesthetic available. These methods are summarized in Table 30.

Drugs used during labor

There are two types of pain relief used during labor. Both are described here.

Narcotics and sedatives: Sedatives, such as Seconal, may be used in early labor to decrease anxiety. Narcotics, such as Demerol, relieve pain in more advanced labor; these drugs decrease the perception of pain by acting on the central nervous system. Other effects may include euphoria, sleepiness, or restlessness. Sedatives and narcotics readily cross the placenta and, while having no apparent ill effects in usual dosages, can delay the newborn's ability to breathe fully. This occurs most often if the baby is born prematurely or has experienced *fetal distress* (see Chapter 21) during labor. Other possible short-term effects on newborns include decreased interest in breast-feeding, decreased temperature or muscle tone after delivery, and decreased responsiveness to visual and auditory stimuli. Research continues to focus on possible long-term problems in infants exposed to these and other anesthetic drugs during labor and delivery. These drugs appear to be safe, however, when used in recommended dosages and when pregnancy is not complicated by premature labor or signs of fetal distress.

Regional anesthetics: The two types of regional anesthetics used in labor are known as the *paracervical block* and *epidural anesthesia*. Both allow you to remain awake and be aware of your labor while experiencing little or no pain. Only minimal amounts of the drug reach the baby.

Paracervical block involves injection of a local anesthetic into the vaginal tissue around the cervix to block the nerves to the uterus. The physician performs paracervical block during the pelvic exam usually when you are dilated four or more centimeters. This method provides good pain relief for an hour or two and may be repeated. A separate anesthetic is needed at delivery since the paracervical block does not anesthetize the vagina. Fetal monitoring is recommended when the paracervical block is used since heart rate abnormalities occasionally occur briefly following this procedure.

Epidural anesthesia, one of the safest and most effective methods of pain relief, is usually performed by an anesthesiologist and thus may be available only at medical centers and large hospitals. Epidural anesthesia requires placement of a small tube into the outer covering of the spinal cord through which travel nerves that sense pain from the uterus. Local anesthetic medication injected through the tube relieves pain during both labor and delivery. (A *caudal anesthetic* uses the same place but is approached from a slightly lower level.)

Like paracervical block, epidural anesthesia is considered good reason for electronic fetal monitoring since this procedure is occasionally associated with brief drops in the baby's heart rate during contractions. The epidural is usually administered when you reach four or more centimeters of cervical dilation. When properly performed, an epidural does not slow your contractions; but if administered too early, an epidural sometimes prolongs labor. Also, a high dose of an epidural in late labor may decrease the urge to push, increasing the need for a forceps delivery.

Drugs used during delivery

Anesthesia for delivery may be one of five different types, including the epidural already described. The other four are described below.

Spinal anesthesia, a form of regional anesthetic performed by the obstetrician or anesthesiologist, involves injection of a local anesthetic into the spinal canal that surrounds the spinal column. Anesthesia in the lower half of the body is thereby provided. With "saddle block" spinal anesthesia, the procedure produces anesthesia in that area of the body that would be in contact with a saddle during horseback riding. In other words with a saddle block, the anesthesia is restricted to the vulva and vagina and does not extend to the lower abdomen and legs. Compared to an epidural, spinal anesthesia is more likely to cause headaches and a drop in blood pressure. This problem is usually solved by simply increasing your IV fluids. Despite disadvantages when compared to the epidural, the spinal remains a popular, rapid,

Table 30   DRUG METHODS OF PAIN RELIEF IN LABOR AND DELIVERY

Method	When Given	Advantages	Disadvantages	Possible Effects on Baby
Sedative drugs (e.g., Seconal, Valium)	Early labor (1 to 3 cm. dilated)	Decreases anxiety	May cause drowsiness	Decreased initial responsiveness; respiratory problems (especially if premature)
Narcotic drugs (e.g., Demerol)	Active labor (after 3 cm. dilation usually)	Decreases pain at start of active labor without slowing contractions	Drowsiness during labor; may cause nausea and vomiting; pain relief using lower dosages may be minimal	Decreased initial responsiveness; respiratory problems (especially if premature)
Paracervical block	Active labor (after 3 cm. dilation usually)	Does not cause maternal or fetal sedation	Lasts only 1 to 2 hrs.; not always effective	Occasional severe drop in fetal heart rate follows procedure (fetal monitoring recommended)
Epidural	Active labor (after 5 cm. dilation usually) or for cesarean section	Effective, safe anesthesia during labor and delivery	Requires trained personnel (usually anesthesiologist) so more expensive and less available than other methods; increased chance of forceps delivery	Occasional dips in fetal heart rate (fetal monitoring recommended)
Spinal	After completely dilated or at delivery	Effective, safe anesthesia for delivery	Risk of headaches (5%); increased chance of forceps delivery; increased chance of temporary drop in blood pressure	Drop in fetal heart rate may occur (especially in high-risk pregnancies)
Pudendal or local anesthesia	At delivery	Safe; provides relief of pain for episiotomy and from vaginal stretching at time of delivery; may be used with nitrous oxide (inhalation anesthetic)	No relief of uterine pain (from contractions)	Rare
General anesthesia	Rarely, except for cesarean section	Complete pain relief; fast anesthetic for an emergency delivery	Possible aspiration (vomiting into the lungs); no participation in delivery	Decreased initial responsiveness; respiratory problems (especially if premature)

and effective method of childbirth anesthesia. Since minimal amounts of drug reach the baby, fetal well-being can be assured by close monitoring of fetal heart rate and the mother's blood pressure.

A *pudendal anesthetic block*, administered by the clinician just prior to delivery, involves injecting a local anesthetic around the pudendal nerve, which supplies sensation to the lower vagina. This procedure, performed much like a paracervical block, anesthetizes the lower birth canal but does not eliminate the pain of contractions. Some clinicians combine a pudendal block with inhalation of nitrous oxide (so-called laughing gas). Brief exposure to this inhalation anesthetic is considered safe since low concentrations are used. Along with pain relief, nitrous oxide may produce temporary euphoria or confusion. This is why some women prefer to use breathing techniques rather than nitrous oxide to supplement the pudendal block during delivery.

Local anesthesia involves injecting a small amount of local anesthetic directly into the vaginal opening. The anesthetic effect is only slightly less than a pudendal block. Except for rare instances of allergy to local anesthetics, local and pudendal techniques provide safe methods of delivery anesthesia for both mother and baby.

General anesthesia is rarely used for vaginal deliveries today because of the greater risk of breathing difficulties in the newborn and the high maternal risks associated with aspiration (vomiting into the lungs). In emergency situations, however, general anesthesia is often the method of choice especially when immediate delivery is needed. In this situation, the mother can be put to sleep in a matter of seconds, allowing prompt intervention which may be lifesaving to the baby.

Fetal Monitoring

Electronic fetal monitoring (EFM) continuously records the infant's heart activity as well as the

External fetal monitoring during labor.

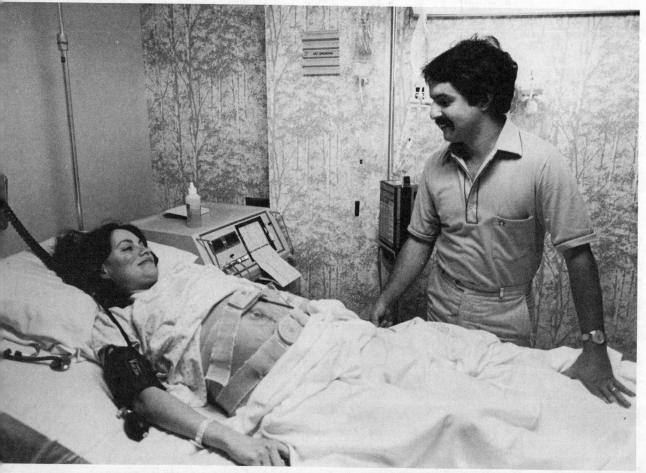

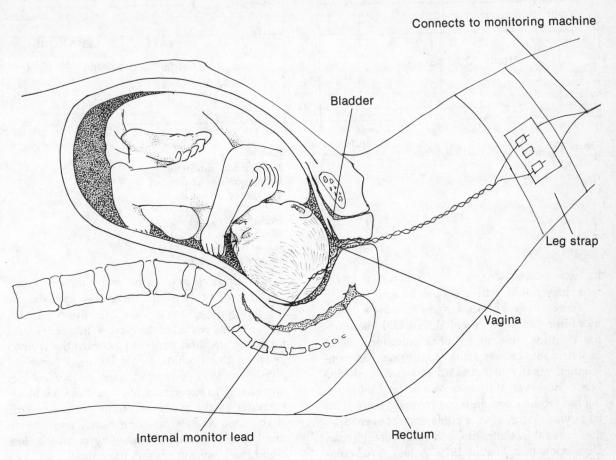

Connects to monitoring machine

Bladder

Leg strap

Vagina

Internal monitor lead

Rectum

Figure 18 *Fetal monitoring. The internal fetal monitor attaches to the fetal head. The other end of the lead attaches to the monitoring machine, which records the fetal heartbeat.*

frequency and duration of uterine contractions. There are two types of fetal monitoring: external and internal. One or the other may be used.

During internal fetal monitoring, a small wire electrode is attached to the fetal scalp to record fetal heart activity (see Figure 18). A second device, a thin, plastic tube, is passed into the uterine cavity to measure uterine contractions.

The external monitor consists of two straps placed around the woman's abdomen. The upper belt holds a device which measures the frequency and length of uterine contractions; the lower strap monitors the fetal heart rate. The two belts may have to be adjusted frequently during labor and may be slightly uncomfortable. External monitoring has the advantage of avoiding uterine or fetal scalp infections which occasionally occur with internal monitoring. The external monitor, however, may not record the fetal heart tracing clearly when mother or baby moves. For this reason, in-

ternal monitoring is preferred if there is any question of fetal heart abnormality.

Whether the internal or external monitor is used, it is attached to a machine next to your bed. This machine prints out a recording of fetal heart rate and uterine contractions. By looking at this paper, you can see when a contraction begins before you even feel it. The normal fetal heart rate ranges between 120 and 160 beats per minute. A heart rate slightly below or above these rates does not necessarily indicate fetal distress. The condition of the fetus is better judged by other aspects of the tracing, especially patterns in which the heart rate rises or falls during contractions. Both physicians and nurses recognize which patterns may indicate fetal distress. Figure 19 shows a typical normal fetal heart and uterine contraction pattern. Figure 20 depicts an abnormal tracing in which the fetal heart rate drops (*decelerates*) briefly during and after each contraction. This pattern,

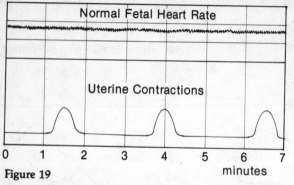

Figure 19

Contractions normally occur every two to three minutes.

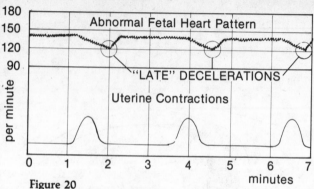

Figure 20

The fetal heart rate drops slightly with each contraction. This type of abnormal fetal heart pattern is called late decelerations *because the fetal heart rate does not return to normal until after each contraction (see circles).*

known as *late decelerations*, indicates that the fetus may not be getting enough oxygen.

There are no known dangers in using external monitoring and only minimal risks with the internal monitor (fetal and uterine infection). Most obstetricians believe fetal monitoring has contributed greatly to increased fetal safety during labor. However, the use of *routine* fetal monitoring has recently become a controversial issue. This issue was discussed at a conference convened by the National Institutes of Child Health and Human Development in March, 1979. A task force composed of health professionals, economists, lawyers, and consumers reviewed current findings on fetal monitoring. The panel concluded that present evidence does not show that routine EFM is beneficial in low-risk pregnancies, while its use in high-risk pregnancies should be strongly considered.

Some women feel that the monitor distracts their clinician or labor coach away from more direct participation in her care. Some see the monitor as highly restrictive (because of interference with movement) and an infringement on their control of the labor situation. Others view monitoring as beneficial in lessening anxiety about the baby's condition. Some couples participating in prepared childbirth use the monitor as a second "coach" which helps in timing breathing techniques.

Positions for Labor and Delivery

From the viewpoint of a woman's body structure, the squatting position offers the least resistance to the baby about to be born. Women delivering in many primitive cultures naturally assume a vertical squatting position. Hospitals approximate this position by having the woman lie on her back with her legs resting in stirrups. While convenient for physicians and nurses to examine the woman in labor, this position is not the most beneficial physiologically. A woman lying on her back is more likely to experience hypotension (low blood pressure) as the pregnant uterus compresses the large blood vessels near the heart, and even a small drop in blood pressure may mean that less blood (and oxygen) reaches the baby.

In many delivery rooms, the nurses encourage the mother to sit up and pull back on her knees while pushing. Some hospital labor beds can be cranked into the sitting position so you can assume a near squatting position during labor.

In other countries, such as England and New Zealand, a woman giving birth in a hospital traditionally delivers lying on her side. Some home-birth advocates encourage the side-lying position for delivery because it maximizes blood and oxygen flow to the baby. A study published in 1979 by Caldeyro-Barcia compared mothers using the traditional horizontal (lying flat on the back) position in labor to those using any position they chose, and it found the upright sitting position was preferred by 95% of women (see references at the end of this section). Labor in this vertical-preference group was 25% shorter than it was for the women in the traditional horizontal position because in normal, spontaneous labors, the vertical position increases the strength of contractions and the rate of cervical dilation.

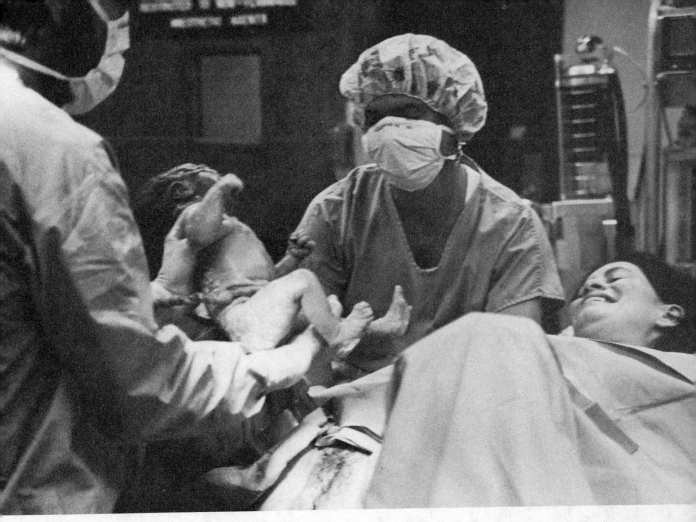

Father-attended birth.

Despite widespread discussion of different labor positions, the fact that there is not much data makes it difficult to conclude which position will be best for you and safest for your baby. You should find the position which is most comfortable whether it is sitting, squatting, or lying flat. Obviously certain limitations may be imposed by such factors as fetal monitoring, blood pressure cuffs, and so on. As a general rule, avoid lying on your back for long periods (although it can't be helped when pushing during delivery). If the baby has any difficulties such as fetal distress, many authorities recommend lying on your left side to maximize good circulation to the fetus.

Father-Attended Birth

Childbirth educators stress the importance of having the baby's father present during labor and immediately after birth when father-child attachment (see Bonding, discussed later in this chapter)

should begin. Hospitals that allow the father in the delivery room may require childbirth education classes as a prerequisite. The father can offer special support to the laboring mother; still, some women feel more comfortable not having their husband present. The hospital staff sometimes prefers that the husband not attend the birth because they worry that the father may faint, lose control of his behavior in the excitement of delivery, or interfere with the provision of care. In addition, should an emergency or complication arise, the father's presence may make the staff feel uncomfortable. However, these fears are rare exceptions, not the rule; and even in emergencies, the husband may provide valuable support for his wife.

In many hospitals, fathers now attend cesarean births. The mother usually has an epidural or spinal anesthetic so that she and her husband may share the first moments after delivery. Most hospitals don't allow fathers to be present if a general anesthetic is used. Support groups have become popular throughout the United States to

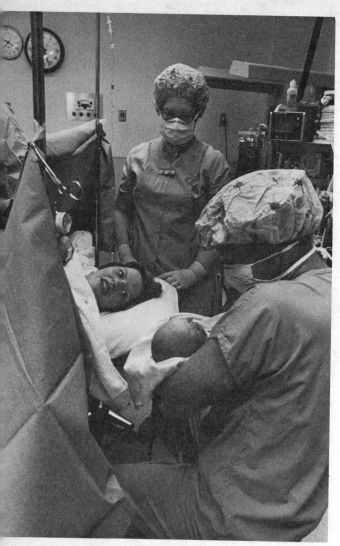

Father-attended cesarean birth.

children who attended childbirth reacted positively and with varying degrees of interest. Anderson (see reference list at the end of this section) feels that all children need to participate as much as possible in the birth of a sibling. Other researchers stress the importance of allowing children to see their mother promptly *after* delivery. If your child or children aren't allowed to visit you, be certain to talk with them on the phone and reassure them that you are all right.

Whether or not you choose to have siblings at the actual birth, their preparation for the arrival of a new baby is important. It's helpful to take your child to prenatal visits where he or she can hear the baby's heartbeat and see other pregnant women. If you know a family with a new baby, visit them so your child can realize how tiny the newborn baby will be. Show your child (or children) pictures of you when you were pregnant before and pictures of his or her birth, if available. Let the children help you fix the area for the new baby. Visit your local library for books about new babies and older brothers and sisters. This way you can help the child anticipate the feelings he or she will have after the newborn's arrival. Let the child select a present to give the new baby. Many parents buy a special toy for the older sibling and give it as a gift from the baby. Some parents also give the older child small items, such as coloring books, when the new baby receives gifts from visitors.

Even the most careful preparation can still not be enough for the young child to understand what

promote father attendance at cesareans. Special classes for preparation for cesarean childbirth are now available in most communities.

Inclusion of Siblings in the Birth Experience

With increasing emphasis on birth as a family event, more parents want their children to share in the labor and delivery experience. This may be an important reason for couples to choose a home or birth center setting over a hospital for childbirth. The response of children witnessing childbirth depends upon their age, family attitudes toward childbearing, and the manner of preparing the child for what will happen. Because only a few researchers have studied sibling-attended birth, the psychological effects of having children present at birth are not known. Several studies do indicate that most

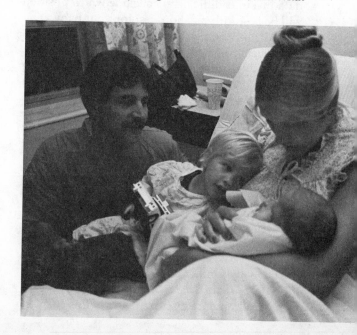

is about to happen. One three-year-old told us, "Yes, my mother's going to get a baby. They're on sale at the hospital. I saw them in the window there."

Episiotomy

An episiotomy is an incision that enlarges the vaginal outlet for the delivery of the baby. This incision is made when the baby's head is visible at the vaginal opening and the perineum is well distended or stretched. When it appears that the lower part of the vagina is not stretching adequately and a large perineal tear may result, an episiotomy is done. Normally some laceration (tearing) occurs during childbirth at the place where an episiotomy would be made, except in women with previous deliveries in which the vagina has been well stretched. Other indications for episiotomy are large babies, a premature baby (to prevent brain injury to the premature baby's extra-delicate nervous system), or abnormal position of the baby (for example, breech; see Chapter 21).

Some physicians routinely use an episiotomy in every woman having her first baby because of the greater chance of tearing. Whether or not this approach actually prevents problems later, such as a "dropped" uterus (uterine *prolapse*), is difficult to prove. Episiotomy stitches are uncomfortable and often itch. But a planned incision is sometimes easier to repair surgically than a ragged tear and heals with less scarring and discomfort. Another possible advantage of an episiotomy is that it avoids prolonged stretching of the vaginal muscles, thereby allowing better return of these muscles to their pre-delivery state. This may prevent vaginal muscle "looseness" during intercourse after childbirth.

There are two types of episiotomy: *midline* and *mediolateral* (see Figure 21). Ask your clinician to use the midline type because it heals more easily and causes *much* less discomfort.

Some childbirth educators and an increasing number of physicians question the practice of performing episiotomies routinely for childbirth. You may want to ask the clinician to perform an episiotomy only if he or she feels a tear is inevitable.

Leboyer Delivery (*Birth Without Violence*)

Dr. Frederick Leboyer, a French obstetrician, developed his techniques of "nonviolent birth"

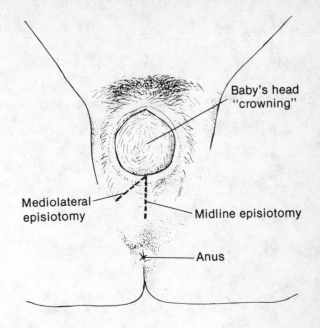

Figure 21
Types of episiotomy.

because he believed birthing is traumatic for the newborn. He saw birth from the newborn's viewpoint as a painful separation from a secure, comfortable environment where all the baby's needs were met. This shocking separation from the womb, Leboyer believed, is imprinted upon one's unconscious for life. His illustrated discussion of this method is presented in *Birth Without Violence* (see Appendix C).

Theoretically, the Leboyer technique, which has been modified in the U.S., reduces the contrast between the intrauterine environment and the outside world. The delivery room lights are dimmed and everyone present is encouraged to remain quiet or speak softly. The baby is placed on the mother's stomach immediately after birth. She strokes the baby and talks to the baby gently, providing the warmth of skin-to-skin contact. The umbilical cord is cut five to ten minutes after delivery. The baby is treated as a person from birth and is not slapped or held upside down by its feet to "encourage" crying. After observation of the newborn for possible problems, the baby is gently put into a warm tub of water, about body temperature, in an effort to mimic the baby's former, intrauterine world. In some hospitals, the father bathes the baby. In other settings, a portable tub is brought to the delivery table so both

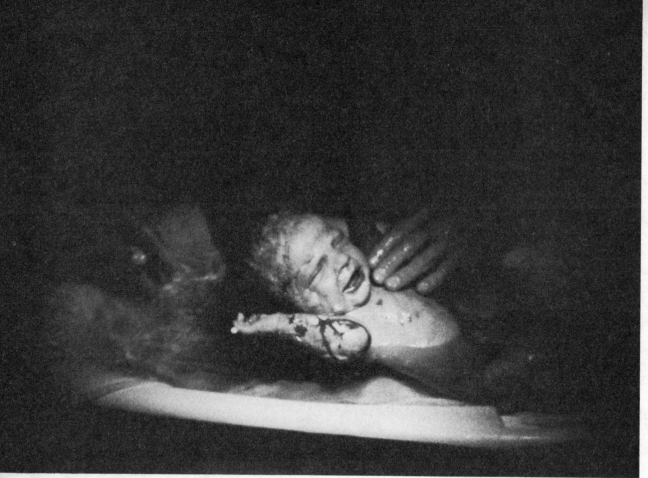

Newborn being bathed following Leboyer delivery.

parents can participate. After five to ten minutes in the bath, the baby is gently dried, wrapped, and returned to the mother.

One advantage of the Leboyer technique is that it increases immediate contact between the parents and child. The quiet delivery room provides a respectful atmosphere for welcoming a new human being into the world. Many babies delivered in this manner seem alert and calmer than usual. Claims that Leboyer delivery produces permanent behavioral or personality characteristics have not been substantiated, however. Some women believe that the Leboyer philosophy overstates the traumatic aspects of childbirth and that the initial separation of the baby from the mother's body is not nearly so painful as the hospital ritual of separation of mother and baby after birth.

Some physicians have raised questions about the safety of Leboyer delivery and expressed concern that infants bathed after delivery may be exposed to heat loss or inadequate monitoring. However, physicians in hospitals where Leboyer

delivery is often used have reported very favorably on the safety of the technique. One study by Kliot reviewed 1200 Leboyer childbirths, including some high-risk patients, and found no adverse effects from the use of the Leboyer techniques (see references at the end of this section). Advocates of Leboyer have pointed to such studies and suggested that if the child should appear in distress, lights can be turned on immediately and appropriate emergency techniques followed.

Bonding

Bonding refers to the internal process by which a mother or father forms a loving relationship with her or his offspring. It may begin when a mother first feels her baby move or the first time a father-to-be hears the fetal heartbeat. Or bonding may begin during or after childbirth. Although parents want to love their new baby right away, he or she is a little stranger to them, and it takes a while for each to get to know the other, to feel comfortable, and to develop love. "Mother's instinct" refers to a woman's natural desire to nurture and care for her baby. It is often through caring for the newborn that bonding, or feeling love toward the child, develops.

The first hour after birth is an especially critical time for bonding. Klaus and Kennell (see reference list at the end of this section) call this time the "early sensitive period" when mother and infant are mutually receptive to each other. At this time most babies are active and able to focus well on their surroundings. The mother is feeling happy with completion of childbirth and anxious to get to know her newborn. As the mother and father touch, kiss, hold, and care for their baby, they begin to become attached to the infant. Watching the child respond to caresses and having eye-to-eye contact with the baby evokes the stirrings of parental love. Though no one knows what a newborn feels, the baby seems to look closely at his or her parents and to enjoy close contact with them.

The idea of bonding is as old as childbirth itself. In years past, when home births were common, the bonding experience between parents and child

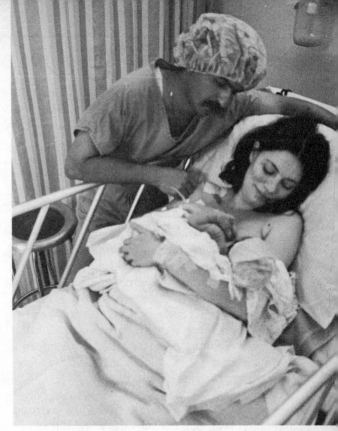

Parents and newborn share the first moments after childbirth as part of the bonding process.

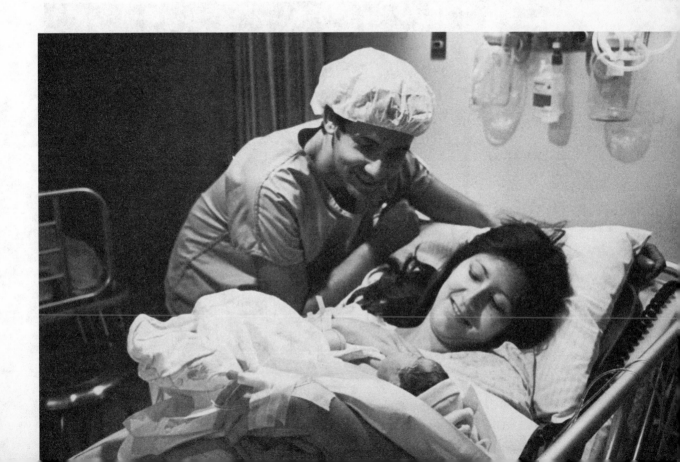

occurred naturally and often encompassed the entire family. Today many hospitals encourage parents to spend the first hour or two after delivery with their newborn. In fact, the American Medical Association endorses the concept of providing a bonding experience for the new mother and her newborn baby.

Awareness of the possible significance of bonding began in the intensive care nursery. Through various follow-up studies researchers discovered that a higher rate of child abuse existed among parents of prematurely born infants with prolonged hospitalization (and decreased maternal contact) than among parents of healthy newborns. Whether or not a postpartum bonding experience has permanent beneficial effects on the newborn or on the parents is unclear. Nevertheless, an early bonding experience between parents and child is becoming more and more popular and is an important element in a more humanistic, family-centered approach to childbirth.

Bonding, as the term which refers to an early experience of close contact between the parents and child, is an option to discuss with your clinician prior to labor. For the maximum effect of bonding, the child should receive silver nitrate eye

drops *after* the bonding experience, because these drops cloud the baby's vision and his or her ability to see the parents. When there is no evidence of maternal venereal disease, this delay will not harm the infant. For more information about bonding read *Maternal-Infant Bonding* by M. H. Klaus and J. H. Kennell.

Breast-Feeding

The American Academy of Pediatrics strongly recommends breast-feeding for all infants during the first four to six months of life. More and more women have been breast-feeding in the last decade probably because numerous studies indicate that breast milk is nutritionally superior to manufactured formulas or cow's milk. Breast-feeding is especially important for the premature or low birth weight infant who has special nutritional needs. In addition, breast milk has antibodies that help protect your infant against infection until he or she can produce his or her own antibodies (at about six months of age).

If you decide to breast-feed your baby, there are several things you can do in preparation.

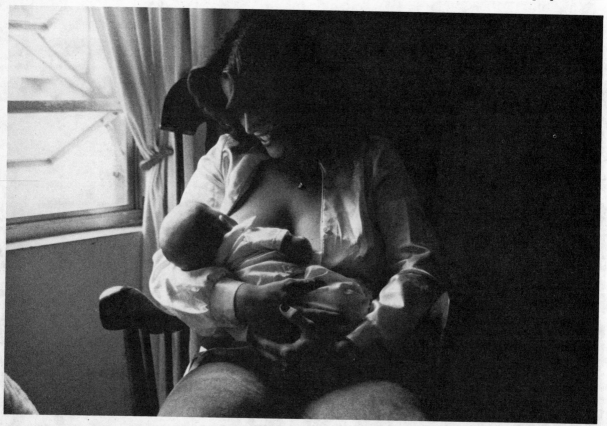

You'll need several supportive nursing bras to wear during the latter part of pregnancy and for nursing, because your breasts will be increased in size as long as you nurse. Once you stop nursing, your breasts will return to normal size or only slightly larger than before pregnancy. During the last two months of pregnancy, rub your nipples with a rough towel after bathing, and periodically massage your nipples between your thumb and forefinger to help toughen them for breast-feeding. Breast cream or A and D Ointment applied daily will help to prevent dryness around the nipple. Even before childbirth, your breasts may leak enough fluid to require the use of breast pads.

When you begin nursing, you can continue eating the same well-balanced diet as you did throughout pregnancy, although you need to increase your total fluid intake to a total of two to three quarts per day. At least one quart (four 8-oz. glasses) of these fluids should consist of whole or low-fat milk or skim milk for extra protein and calcium (see Chapter 46, Nutrition). If you don't like milk, substitute another dairy product, such as cheese or ice cream. Producing milk takes extra energy, so make an effort to get enough rest. Emotional tension may temporarily decrease your milk flow but will not affect its quality. See Chapter 31 for discussion of drugs and breast-feeding.

Begin nursing gradually to prevent sore nipples. Feed your baby on demand, but no more often than every two hours. Don't be surprised if it takes a few days to establish a regular breast-feeding schedule. Relax. It *will* happen. A newborn takes three or four hours to empty his or her stomach and will naturally regulate himself or herself to a schedule. Fortunately, infants eat more frequently during the day and less often at night. Alternate breasts and gradually build up to nursing no longer than ten minutes on the first breast and twenty minutes on the other. If your baby does not want to nurse twenty minutes on the second side, don't worry, because the baby sucks harder on the first side, getting about ninety percent of the milk in that breast in five to ten minutes. A pacifier may be helpful for babies who want to suck longer than twenty minutes. Release the baby from your breast by inserting your forefinger between the baby's mouth and your breast. Remember that your baby will get enough milk because whenever your infant sucks more, your breasts produce more milk.

Some working mothers breast-feed by using a breast pump or hand-expressing their milk during lunch hour to provide milk for the child's feedings when they are away from home. Breast milk can be safely stored in a refrigerator for forty-eight hours. Other mothers use formula milk when they are not at home to breast-feed their babies themselves. The working mother and other mothers often find total breast-feeding very demanding, and it is important to work out an arrangement that is comfortable for you. Some mothers have their babies fed jello-water (ungelled gelatin and water mixture), sugar water, or Gatorade rather than formula for the feeding when they are not with the babies. Some mothers use these liquids when they feel their baby is thirsty as opposed to hungry. Discuss this situation with your pediatrician and decide what best meets your family's needs. There are many resources, such as the La Leche League, that help breast-feeding mothers. For information about the La Leche League consult your telephone directory or write to:

La Leche League International
9616 Minneapolis Avenue
Franklin Park, Illinois 60134

Nursing Your Baby, by Karen Pryor, is only one of the good books currently available on this subject.

Bottle Feeding

Despite the current popularity and benefits of breast-feeding, bottle feeding is preferred by many mothers. The advent of disposable bottles, bottle liners, and nipples have made bottle feeding easier now than ever before. Today's manufactured formulas are safe and, if used properly, will keep your baby strong and healthy. A particular advantage of bottle feeding is that anyone can feed the baby, thereby freeing the mother for other activities. The mother who bottle feeds often feels satisfied that her child is getting adequate nutrition because she knows exactly how much formula the baby takes.

Pediatricians differ in their approach toward bottle sterilization, tending more toward "clean" as opposed to "sterile." Cleaning and rinsing the bottles thoroughly and washing or perhaps boiling the nipples is adequate for formula preparation. Some pediatricians still insist that bottles be sterilized for the first three months of the baby's life. You can buy formula as powdered milk formula (the cheapest), concentrated formula, or

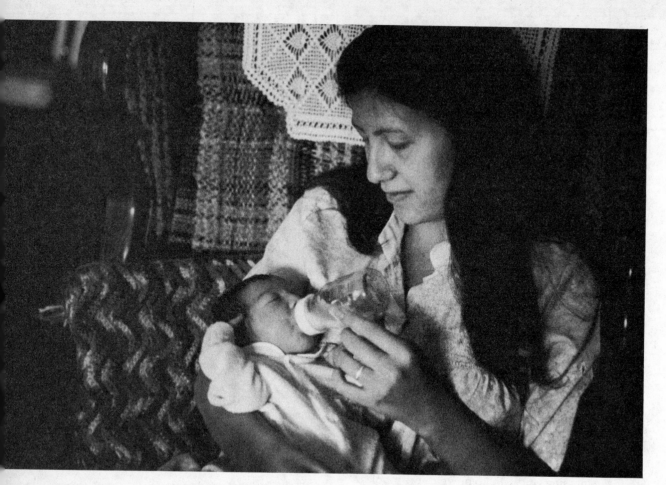

ready-to-use formula. All of these are easy to prepare for individual bottles.

It is better to avoid propping up a bottle because the infant may choke on the formula while lying on his or her back. Besides, the comfort the baby feels from being held close to you while you feed him or her is also very important.

It is a demanding experience for a mother to feed her new baby often during the day. As in breast-feeding, try to keep the baby awake long enough to complete the feeding. Newborns fall asleep easily after feeding. Make sure the nipple is not clogged. Feed your baby no more often than every two hours and preferably every three or four hours since it takes that long for the baby's stomach to empty. The baby will let you know when he or she is hungry and will naturally establish his or her own schedule. Newborns should be fed formula for the first four to six months of age, as this is the nutrient best absorbed in the intestinal tract. After six months, you can start your baby on solids, but be sure to keep the baby on formula (rather than whole cow's milk) throughout the first year.

Rooming-In

Rooming-in, now available in most hospitals, means that the baby stays in the mother's room where she can provide care and feeding on demand. The baby's crib may be at the mother's bedside or in a nursery nearby. With rooming-in, the father usually has unrestricted visiting privileges, and some institutions allow grandparents and siblings to hold and feed the baby as well. Ideally, rooming-in is available twenty-four hours a day though the mother may return the baby to the nursery whenever she needs to rest or wants to see visitors (called partial rooming-in).

Rooming-in programs stress parent education. A nurse usually works closely with the family, offering advice and support in newborn care. The mother practices bathing her baby and other skills, such as taking the baby's temperature in this reassuring environment. Rooming-in promotes bonding and prepares the mother for what to expect at home. The experience is often more popular with first-time mothers who are anxious to learn all they can, although some second-time mothers eagerly approach rooming-in as the only time they will have alone with their new child unhampered by older children at home.

Opponents of rooming-in say it is hard on mothers who are already exhausted after labor and delivery. They feel the mother needs the time now to rest and will have plenty of time to learn to care for the baby at home. New parents sometimes resent paying the high cost of hospitalization and then doing all of the baby care themselves. Mothers who already have one child may welcome their hospital stay as a chance to rest and take a break from child care.

Circumcision

Circumcision (a "cutting around") is the surgical removal of the *prepuce* (also called *foreskin*), which is the loose skin around the head of the male newborn's penis. Many parents don't realize that circumcision, the most common surgical procedure performed on American newborns, is no longer a routine procedure. Traditionally, the circumcision is done by the obstetrician, though this practice varies, especially when done for religious reasons. According to the American Academy of Pediatrics, there is no valid medical reason for newborn circumcision. Parental consent is needed prior to the operation, and often the parent has little chance to consider the advantages and disadvantages of the surgery.

At the end of the penis, the skin folds over and covers part of the glans, which is the name for the smooth head of the penis. This loose skin, called the prepuce, protects the meatus, which is the opening into the urethra, the tube through which urine passes from the bladder. When the prepuce is removed through circumcision, the glans is exposed and is therefore easier to clean. As the uncircumcised male grows and the penis develops, the foreskin eventually separates naturally from the glans. At this time the skin can be gently pulled back and effective hygiene accomplished.

Aside from hygienic considerations, there are also social and religious reasons that some parents choose infant circumcision. Sometimes a father feels that since he was circumcised, his son should be, too. Parents may feel that it is the "proper" thing to do, or simply that it "looks" better. In the past, a major reason for circumcision was to reduce the incidence of cervical cancer in women. A study, found since then to be faulty, showed a direct relationship between cervical cancer in women and husbands who were uncircumcised. Now, it is generally accepted that there is no increased risk of cervical cancer in women who have intercourse with uncircumcised males.

Hospitals or staff personnel may encourage circumcision promptly after delivery for reasons of efficiency. However, immediate circumcision may interfere with other birthing options, such as a Leboyer birth. An important reason to delay circumcision is to permit nurses and others to observe the newborn during the first critical hours.

When circumcision is performed by a skilled practitioner several hours or more after birth, the risks of complications are minimal although hemorrhage or infection can occur. Removal of too much tissue may be uncomfortable during later life; and narrowing of the end of the urethra may occur, requiring surgery to widen the urethral opening.

The long-term psychological effects of circumcision on the newborn, if any, are unknown. Delaying circumcision until later preschool years or adolescence, when a child is more acutely aware of his penis, could be seen by him as threatening. If circumcision is to be done, any psychological effects of this procedure would probably be less during the first few months of life.

If you have your baby circumcised, be certain to request that it be done at least a day after birth to make certain the baby is healthy. After circumcision the penis may be cleansed with mild soap and water. In the first few days after circumcision diapers should be changed often to avoid irritation to the glans. If your baby is not circumcised, gently retract the foreskin and clean the glans when you give him his bath.

Table 31   QUESTIONS TO CONSIDER WHEN YOU BECOME PREGNANT*

As your pregnancy progresses, you will probably have many questions about what to expect during childbirth. This may be particularly true if you're having your first baby. Listed below are questions about some aspects of labor and delivery which women are often curious about. Some of these questions may have been answered by the information in this chapter, and others you may want to ask your clinician.

1. Do I want to attend childbirth education classes for a so-called prepared childbirth?

2. If I've prepared for natural childbirth, can I change my mind during labor and receive anesthetics and/or other drugs?

3. What types of anesthetic does my doctor usually use during delivery, and what effect might they have on me or the baby?

4. How much does my husband or partner want to participate during labor and childbirth? Is he willing to be my "coach" if I decide on a prepared labor and delivery?

5. What kinds of alternative birth setting are available to me? What are the risks and benefits of each?

6. How do I know if I'm having a normal, low-risk pregnancy? What are the chances that I'll have a cesarean birth?

7. Are enemas and prepping—or shaving of the pubic area—always necessary?

8. Will I automatically be given an IV during labor?

9. When is it necessary for labor to be induced artificially?

10. What is a fetal monitoring machine? Is fetal monitoring necessary?

11. Are forceps likely to be used during delivery?

12. Is an episiotomy performed routinely? How will my doctor decide on whether to give me one?

13. Do I want to know more about so-called gentle birth, with dim lights, music, a quiet delivery room, and a warm bath for the baby?

14. Is a parent–infant bonding experience available? Do I have to prepare for this?

15. Will I get to see my baby as often as I like, for as long as I like, while I'm still in the hospital?

16. How long will I have to stay in the hospital?

---

* Modified with permission of Syntex Laboratories, Inc. (Effective Communication Series #8, 1978).

20

Complicated Pregnancies

Sometimes doctors talk about *high-risk pregnancies* when factors related to such things as age, smoking, or chronic illness are present. This labeling only serves as a warning to be especially careful about your pregnancy because you have a higher chance of developing complications. A high-risk pregnancy does *not* mean you won't have a normal pregnancy, labor, and delivery.

This chapter discusses some of the common medical conditions that may cause problems during pregnancy. We also include a discussion of tests that the high-risk mother may undergo to evaluate the fetus. Most conditions, if recognized quickly, can be managed safely.

Toxemia of Pregnancy

High blood pressure in pregnancy, sometimes known as *toxemia*, occurs in 6% to 7% of all pregnancies. This condition, while more common during a first pregnancy, can also affect a woman who has previously given birth, especially if she has a prior history of high blood pressure.

The first sign of toxemia may be a weight gain of five to ten pounds within a week, as a result of fluid retention. Although leg swelling in pregnancy is normal, prominent swelling of the hands, face, and fingers is not. Report these or other possible symptoms of excessive water retention, such as severe headaches or blurred vision, to your doctor.

Fetal complications of high blood pressure include inadequate fetal growth (see Chapter 16) and premature labor as well as possible fetal distress during labor (see Chapter 21 for both). Because of these complications, the physician often starts fetal testing (see High-Risk Pregnancy

Testing below), including estriols and fetal monitoring, as early as 32 to 34 weeks when toxemia is present. Abnormal tests sometimes indicate the need for early delivery. In most pregnancies associated with high blood pressure, however, the fetus is not in serious danger and can be delivered at about 37 weeks of pregnancy, or as soon as fetal maturity is confirmed.

A woman with severe toxemia may be hospitalized to control high blood pressure or for fetal testing. More often, these tests are done on an outpatient basis. Extra rest, especially done lying on your left side, improves circulation and is one of the most beneficial measures for a woman with high blood pressure. The use of a salt-free diet and so-called water pills have possible fetal hazards and are infrequently used today.

Rh Disease

The Rh factor is a substance in the blood of approximately 85% of white people and 95% of blacks. These individuals are known as *Rh positive*. The people who have no Rh factor in their blood are called *Rh negative*. Having Rh negative blood in no way affects your general health. However, a condition called Rh disease (hemolytic disease of the newborn) can occur in babies born to Rh negative women when the father and the baby are both Rh positive. A few cells of the fetus's Rh positive blood (inherited from the father) may "leak" into the mother's circulation during pregnancy, usually at delivery. The mother's system, because it is Rh negative, acts on the Rh positive cells as a foreign substance and produces antibodies (see glossary). These antibodies can cross the placenta and destroy some of the fetal red blood cells, producing anemia, which can lead to serious or even fatal brain damage. This condition rarely occurs in a first pregnancy.

Rh disease is uncommon today even in subsequent pregnancies because a drug called RhoGAM, developed in 1968, prevents the formation of antibodies when given to Rh negative women within seventy-two hours after delivering an Rh positive baby. Rh negative women should also receive a "mini-dose" RhoGAM injection after a miscarriage, therapeutic abortion or ectopic pregnancy. In November 1983, the American College of Obstetricians and Gynecologists began recommending RhoGAM for all susceptible Rh negative women *during* pregnancy as well as postpartum. New evidence suggests that administering the drug near the twenty-eighth week of pregnancy will benefit a few women who will otherwise develop Rh antibodies in late pregnancy. Despite the availability of RhoGAM, nearly one out of ten women for whom the drug is indicated do not receive it for one reason or another. Once developed, Rh antibodies are permanent and RhoGAM is of no benefit. Such antibodies represent a continuing risk of Rh disease in subsequent pregnancies if the fetus is Rh positive.

Rh blood typing and antibody testing are routinely done at the initial office visit. If you are Rh positive, you need not worry about Rh disease even if the father is Rh negative. If you are Rh negative, however, the father's blood type should be checked. If both you and he are Rh negative, your baby will also be negative and, therefore, unaffected by Rh disease. If the father, however, is Rh positive and you are Rh negative, then you are susceptible to Rh disease. In such susceptible Rh negative women, the clinician repeats the blood test, to check for antibodies, in the sixth and eighth months of pregnancy as well as at delivery.

If antibodies are detected in your blood during pregnancy, the physician may perform an amniocentesis (see later in this chapter and also Chapter 11) to assess the condition of the fetus by analyzing the amniotic fluid. When fetal blood cells are broken down by maternal Rh antibodies, the cells release bilirubin, a substance which shows up in the amniotic fluid. High bilirubin levels may indicate the need for early delivery to protect the fetus from further antibody damage. This approach is usually lifesaving to the fetus.

Viral Infection in Pregnancy

Two viral illnesses—German measles and herpes—can cause serious fetal damage. Vaccination against German measles (rubella) *prior to* pregnancy completely protects you from this disease. At present, there is no such vaccine against herpes.

Rubella (German measles)

Birth defects, including mental retardation, heart disease, hearing loss, and blindness, occur up to

50% of the time when rubella is contracted by the mother in the first eight to twelve weeks of pregnancy. Symptoms of rubella may mimic the common cold and include skin rash, swollen neck glands, and a slight fever. Blood tests can detect if you have had recent or past rubella infection, based on the presence in the blood of antibodies. Typically a high level of antibodies (or a rising level based on successive blood tests two weeks apart) indicates recent infection. A low antibody level indicates past infection and thus present immunity to (protection against) rubella. Absence of antibodies means you have not had rubella. Fortunately, a vaccine can be given *prior to* pregnancy to prevent the disease in such women. Nearly 20% of women entering childbearing age have not acquired immunity either from having had the disease or from the vaccination and are therefore susceptible to rubella. It's best to have your blood tested for rubella antibodies three months before you plan to get pregnant. This way, if your antibody level is too low (less than 1 to 20), you can get the rubella vaccine for complete protection. Although physicians routinely screen pregnant women for rubella, you cannot be vaccinated once you are pregnant or within three months before you become pregnant, because the vaccine itself could be harmful to the fetus. This is why you should avoid pregnancy for three months following vaccination. Vaccination is recommended *following* pregnancy in women found not to have immunity.

Herpes infections (herpes genitalis, genital herpes)

Herpes genitalis, a sexually transmitted disease (see Chapter 24), causes painful sores around the vaginal opening. The newborn may acquire this virus by direct contact with the sores at the time of vaginal delivery. (The virus almost never infects the fetus by crossing the placenta prior to delivery.) Fortunately, fewer than one out of every 2,000 newborns is affected by herpes. But since this disease in the newborn may be life-threatening, obstetricians take aggressive measures to prevent the baby from acquiring herpes at delivery.

If you have an active genital herpes infection within two to four weeks of delivery, you will probably be delivered by cesarean birth to reduce the risk of transmitting the infection to your baby. Since it isn't always possible to diagnose genital herpes by examination alone, laboratory tests help confirm the diagnosis. Fortunately the newborn's risk of acquiring a herpes infection that is present in the mother may be less than previously expected. In a study published in July, 1981, J. H. Grossman and coworkers reported on fifty-eight pregnancies complicated by known herpes infections. Mothers were examined and tested frequently in the final weeks of pregnancy; and if infection was present, cesarean delivery was performed when labor began. None of the infants had signs of herpes infections in this series of cases.

If you think you have herpes, see your doctor while the lesions (sores) are present so appropriate testing can be done. A woman with a history of herpes should have frequent examinations from the end of the seventh month on. This requires a speculum exam to look for symptomless lesions that may be on the cervix.

Premature Rupture of Membranes

Spontaneous leakage of amniotic fluid, usually in a gush, before the onset of labor occurs in 10% of pregnancies. Such leakage, called *ruptured membranes*, is usually not a problem unless it occurs several weeks before your due date when premature labor and early delivery could occur. When membranes rupture, delivery should normally occur within twenty-four hours to decrease the risk of infection to you and your baby. For this reason, you should go to the hospital when your membranes rupture.

If labor does not begin shortly after your membranes have ruptured, the physician will induce labor unless you are several weeks early. When ruptured membranes occur before about thirty-four weeks, the risks of prematurity from early delivery may outweigh the risk of infection. In such instances, the obstetrician often elects not to induce labor unless you show signs of infection.

Post Maturity—When Your Baby Is Overdue

The newborn is considered overdue, or *post mature*, when delivery occurs two weeks or more after your due date. No one knows why this occurs in 10% of all pregnancies. In late pregnancy, as the placenta ages, transfer of oxygen and other nutrients to the baby normally diminishes. Postmature babies, especially those three or more weeks overdue, have an increased risk of fetal distress (see Chapter 21) in labor. This risk is further compounded when the woman is over the age of thirty-four or is having her first baby. Post maturity also imposes greater likelihood of a difficult delivery as a result of large fetal size since over 70% of overdue newborns weigh more than 8½ pounds. In the nursery, post-mature infants have a slightly higher rate of low blood sugar, jaundice (see glossary), and respiratory problems.

Today obstetricians usually induce labor in women who are more than two weeks overdue. A so-called unfavorable cervix—when your cervix is hard, thick, and completely closed—may make induction of labor difficult or impossible. In this case, your doctor may perform an amniocentesis (see below) or other tests to assure fetal well-being. Abnormal fetal tests are indications for prompt delivery. If the tests are normal, you will be seen in the office frequently to determine when your cervix is favorable to inducing labor.

High-Risk Pregnancy Testing

Several tests evaluate the fetus during the last few weeks of a complicated or high-risk pregnancy.

Figure 22 *Amniocentesis. Amniotic fluid is withdrawn from the "bag of waters" surrounding the fetus and sent to a laboratory for various tests.*
Modified with permission of G. D. Searle and Co. (The Female Reproductive System. San Juan, Puerto Rico, 1976).

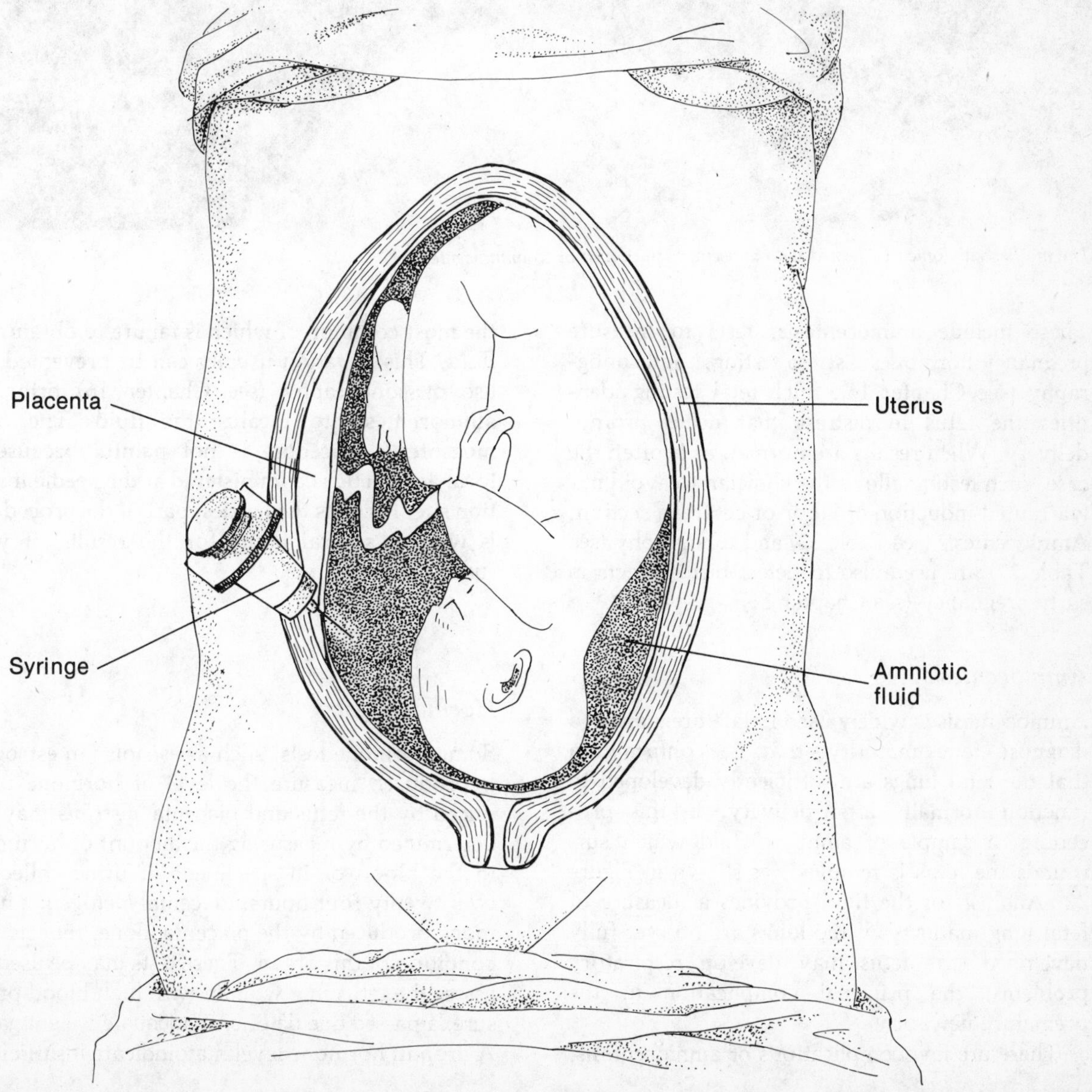

Placenta

Syringe

Uterus

Amniotic fluid

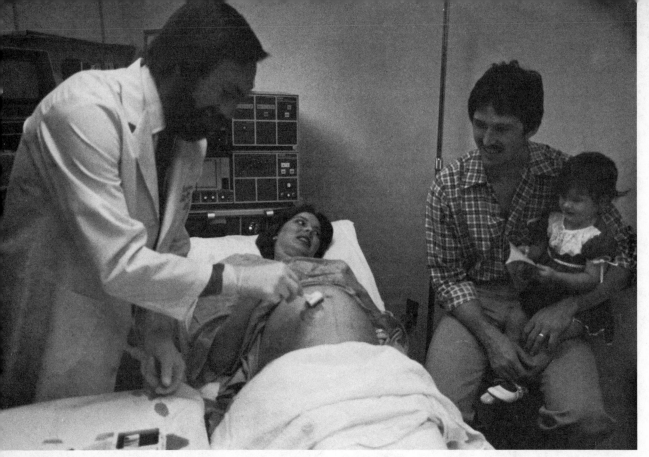

The mother's abdomen is cleaned with antiseptic solution prior to amniocentesis.

These include amniocentesis, tests to measure pregnancy hormones, "stress testing," and sonography (see Chapter 16). Such fetal testing identifies the fetus in distress that needs prompt delivery. When results are normal, as is often the case, such testing allows the clinician to avoid unwarranted induction of labor or cesarean section. Amniocentesis (see Table 32) and sonography (see Table 27) are used also to detect birth defects in early pregnancy (see Chapter 11).

Amniocentesis

Amniocentesis is widely used in late pregnancy to diagnose fetal maturity—that is, confirmation that the fetal lungs are sufficiently developed to function normally after delivery. In this procedure, a sample of amniotic fluid which surrounds the fetus is removed, as shown in Figure 22. Analysis of the fluid provides a measure of fetal lung maturity. If the lungs are not yet fully developed, the fetus may develop respiratory problems, the principal complication in the premature newborn.

There are few complications of amniocentesis,

the most common of which is failure to obtain the fluid. This situation usually can be prevented by use of sonography (see Chapter 16) prior to amniocentesis to localize the fluid. The amniocentesis procedure is not painful because a local anesthetic is administered at the needle insertion site. Perhaps the hardest part of the procedure is waiting several hours for the results, if you suspect a problem.

Hormone tests

Some hormone tests, such as estriols (an estrogen byproduct), measure the level of hormone produced by the fetus and placenta. *Estriols* may be determined by measuring the amount of hormone in the blood or in specimens of urine collected over twenty-four hours. Placental *lactogen*, a hormone produced by the placenta alone, reflects the condition of this organ. These tests may be used to assess the fetus in a woman with high blood pressure, a passed due date, or inadequate weight gain. A drop in hormone level may indicate insufficient

Table 32 **POSSIBLE REASONS FOR AMNIOCENTESIS**

Reason	When Usually Performed*
Evaluation for certain specific birth defects	16 to 18 weeks
Evaluation for fetal maturity when repeat cesarean section is planned	38 to 39 weeks
Evaluation for fetal maturity in high-risk pregnancies (e.g., high blood pressure, diabetes, Rh disease, overdue more than two weeks, inadequate fetal growth)	34 to 39 weeks

* Weeks of pregnancy counting from the first day of the last menstrual period (term pregnancy is 40 weeks).

transfer of oxygen to the fetus and require early delivery. Hormone tests are often used together with fetal monitoring in evaluating high-risk pregnancies, thereby increasing the accuracy of

fetal assessment and thus minimizing the need to prematurely deliver a fetus at high risk for fetal distress (see Chapter 21).

"Stress testing"

This test is a new means of assessing the high-risk fetus, utilizing *electronic fetal monitoring* (EFM), described in Chapter 19. EFM works because an oxygen-deprived fetus shows abnormal heart rate patterns. Unlike the hormone tests, EFM gives immediate results that are not subject to laboratory or patient error. The major drawback of EFM is the high number of false positive tests; that is, tests which appear to show a fetal problem when in fact the fetus is healthy. However, there are very few false negatives (negative means normal); so when monitoring is normal, fetal well-being for the next week is almost always assured.

There are two types of EFM: the *non-stress test* (NST) and the *contraction stress test* (CST). In general, the NST is used as a screening test; and, if there are abnormalities, then the CST is performed.

Non-stress testing (NST), which is completely safe, evaluates the fetal heart rate during fetal movement or spontaneous (Braxton-Hicks) uterine

Performing an amniocentesis.

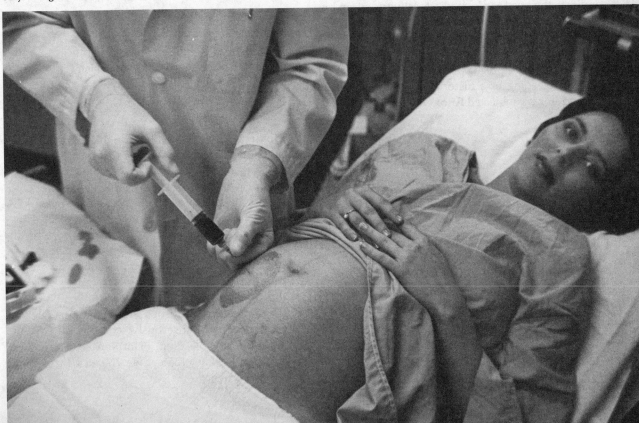

contractions. The heart rate normally increases slightly (accelerates) during either a contraction or fetal movement. During this test, you are connected to the fetal monitor, and you push a button to indicate when you feel the fetus move so the nurse or physician can evaluate the monitor's printout. A normal, or *reactive*, test almost always means the fetus is in a healthy condition. An abnormal, or *nonreactive*, test indicates the need for a contraction stress test. There are many falsely abnormal tests in NST testing, so an abnormal test does not necessarily mean the fetus is in danger.

The *contraction stress test* (CST) evaluates the fetal heart rate during contractions that occur spontaneously but usually require stimulation using a drug called oxytocin. In a normal, or negative, test, the fetal heart rate will remain unchanged or may increase slightly during contractions (as in the normal NST). In definitely abnormal, or positive, tests, the fetal heart rate drops slightly (decelerates) during and after each contraction (see Figure 20). Most CSTs are negative. In that case, it is safe to wait one week at which time the NST or CST is usually repeated. The suspicious test (neither positive nor negative) is usually repeated in twenty-four hours. The positive test, found in 5% to 10% of high-risk pregnancies, may indicate the need for immediate delivery, often by cesarean section. Compared to the NST, the CST is costlier, requires the use of hospital facilities, and often requires the use of intravenous oxytocin. Women who are pregnant with twins or who have vaginal bleeding or a history of premature labor should not be subjected to oxytocin.

Sonography

This procedure is widely utilized and not restricted to high-risk pregnancies (see Chapter 16).

Risk Factors in Pregnancy

A minority of women are subject to risk factors and are more likely to have complications during pregnancy, labor, or delivery. Risk factors related to maternal age, nutrition, smoking, and alcohol and other drugs are discussed elsewhere in this book (see index). In order to help predict whether problems may develop during labor, a scoring system has been developed to identify high-risk

Table 33	IDENTIFYING HIGH-RISK PREGNANCIES ACCORDING TO RISK FACTORS *

Risk Factor	Point Score **
High blood pressure (moderate or severe, often requiring hospitalization in pregnancy)	10
Severe kidney or heart disease	10
Diabetes (requiring insulin)	10
Previous stillbirth, premature or low birth weight infant, or newborn death that occurred within one month of birth	10
Overdue three or more weeks	10
Twins	10
Baby in breech position (in the last six weeks of pregnancy)	10
Previous multiple miscarriages (three or more)	10
Age older than 35 or younger than 15	10
Excessive drug use, including alcohol	10
Moderate alcohol intake	10
Previous kidney (not bladder) infection	5
High blood pressure (mild, not requiring hospitalization in pregnancy)	5
Pregnancy diabetes (diabetes developing in pregnancy, not requiring insulin)	5

table continues

mothers. Table 33 identifies high-risk pregnancies according to risk factors, with a point score assigned to each risk factor according to its potential for causing problems. Women with ten points or more total score can be considered high risk. A score of less than ten points total indicates low risk. Unfortunately, high-risk scoring systems do not identify all women who will develop complications during labor. Some women who are low risk during pregnancy may develop risk factors during labor, such as a prolapsed cord (in which the umbilical cord "drops" into the vagina where it may become dangerously compressed by the baby's head), bleeding, or prolonged labor. Your clinician will evaluate these factors throughout your pregnancy.

Table 33 Continued

Risk Factor	Point Score **
Previous cesarean section	5
Previous delivery of baby weighing more than 10 pounds	5
Have been pregnant five times or more	5
Severe flu, bronchitis, or viral illness	5
Severe anemia (hemoglobin less than 9 grams)	5
Weight less than 100 or more than 200 pounds	5
Height less than five feet	5
Previous child with a birth defect	5
Vaginal spotting	5
Smoking more than one pack of cigarettes a day	5
Emotional problems	5
Bladder infection	1
Previous high blood pressure in an earlier pregnancy	1
Family history of diabetes	1

 * Adapted from Hobel, C. J., Prenatal and Intrapartum High-Risk Screening, *American Journal of Obstetrics and Gynecology,* 117(1):1-9, 1973.
** Score of 10 points or more = high risk
  Score of less than 10 points = low risk

21

Complications of Labor and Delivery

At any time during labor, complications may arise and lead to inadequate oxygen supply to the fetus. This problem is particularly prevalent in women whose pregnancies have been complicated by such factors as high blood pressure, diabetes, or poor nutrition. Unexpected events, such as a prolapsed cord or severe bleeding in a previously normal pregnancy, may also complicate labor and delivery. For these reasons, close observation of your condition and that of your baby is very important throughout labor and delivery.

The fetus normally experiences mild oxygen deprivation during birth due to the stress of labor. When oxygen deprivation is moderate to severe in labor—a condition called *fetal distress*—the newborn is likely to be less responsive at birth as measured by what is called Apgar scores. These scores measure the general condition of the fetus at one minute and five minutes after birth by evaluating muscle tone, color, cry, respiration, and heart rate. Most healthy newborns score seven to ten. Although low Apgar scores are not necessarily cause for alarm—most of these babies grow up to be perfectly healthy, too—early detection of fetal distress may increase the newborn's chances for a healthy outcome.

Determining Fetal Distress

Except for a crisis such as a prolapsed umbilical cord (in which the cord "drops" into the vagina where it may become dangerously compressed by the baby's head), fetal distress in labor usually develops gradually and can be evaluated in three ways:

1. *Amniotic fluid*, normally clear, may become brown or green-colored from fetal stool, which is called *meconium*. This condition is a sign of fetal distress, except when the fetus is in breech position, and is an early warning that demands careful observation of the condition of the fetus.
2. *Fetal heart rate* is evaluated intermittently with a stethoscope or continually with electronic fetal monitoring (EFM) (see Chapter 19). With a stethoscope, the clinician can recognize a sustained drop in heart rate. But with the electronic fetal monitor the clinician is aware of brief, less severe drops in heart rate as well as more subtle patterns of fetal heart irregularity related to decreased oxygen flow to the baby. Thus, EFM may lead to earlier detection of fetal distress.
3. *Fetal blood oxygen levels* are obtained through fetal scalp sampling, which means the doctor obtains a tiny drop of blood from the fetal scalp during labor and analyzes the oxygen content. Fetal scalp sampling can

either confirm or prove false the apparent fetal distress indicated by fetal monitoring. The most accurate method of assessing fetal distress in labor combines fetal monitoring and fetal scalp sampling. When physicians base their decisions to do a cesarean section on an abnormality that shows up in both these assessment methods and not fetal monitoring alone, the cesarean birth rate is lower.

Premature Labor

Premature labor, one of the most common serious complications of pregnancy, occurs in approximately 8% of all pregnancies. Nearly half of all newborn deaths are associated with prematurity. Although prematurity is often associated with vaginal bleeding in late pregnancy, high blood pressure, and other medical complications, the cause is unknown over half the time. An increase in prematurity has been associated with a previous history of premature labors, with twins, and in pregnancies occurring before age seventeen or after age thirty-five. There is a slightly increased chance of prematurity in individuals who smoke,

A mother visiting her premature baby at the newborn intensive care unit.

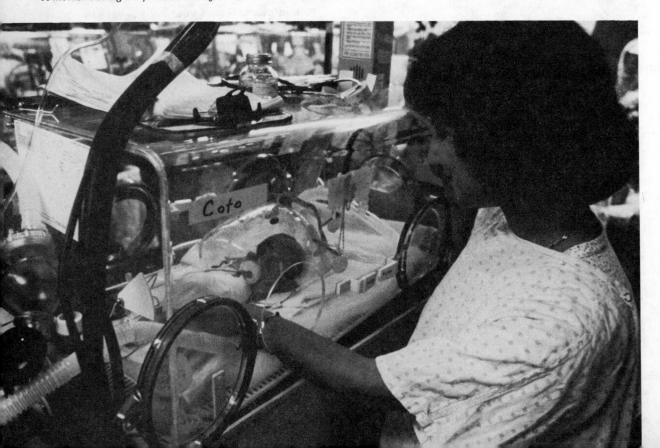

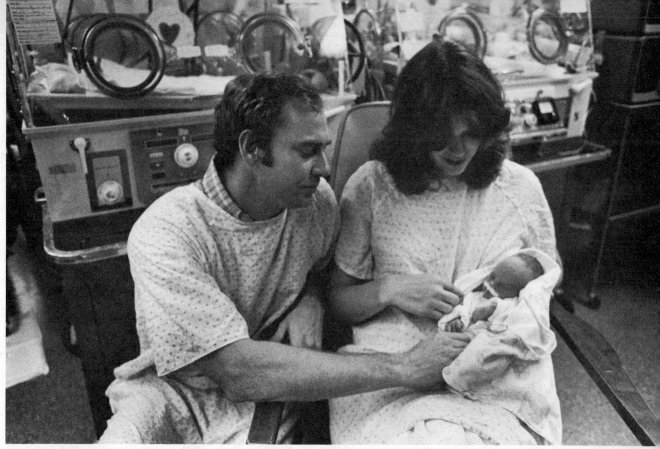

Parents holding their premature baby in the newborn intensive care unit.

abuse drugs, are poorly nourished, or have a previous history of two or more therapeutic abortions.

A strenuous job and long working hours are other factors which may contribute to premature birth, according to reports from the 1983 Anglo-American Conference on Pregnant Women at Work. One of the studies at this conference reported on the experience of 1,900 pregnant women employed in a wide variety of occupational categories. Working itself was not found to be a risk factor for premature birth, since housewives and pregnant workers showed similar rates of premature labor. But the study noted that as the number of working hours per week increased, prematurity rose from 3.6% for women with a part-time job to 10% or more for those who worked over forty hours a week.

Premature labor used to be defined as labor resulting in either the delivery of an infant weighing less than 5½ pounds at birth or an infant being delivered before 37 weeks of pregnancy. This definition failed to differentiate between babies born before 40 weeks (*premature*) and those born at 40 weeks but with low birth weight (*growth retarded*). Low birth weight babies born

Feeding a premature infant may require the help of both parents. In this photo, mother feeds while father holds the oxygen supply close by.

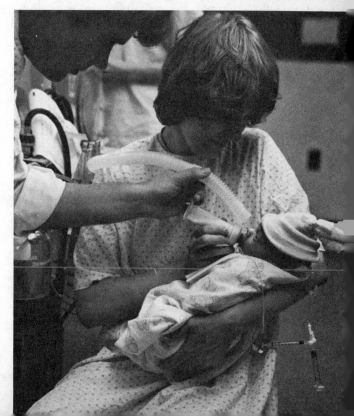

on schedule have fewer newborn complications than premature infants. When growth retardation coexists with prematurity, the risk to the newborn is greater than that for premature babies.

Treatment of premature labor

Premature labor is usually treated with strict bed rest. The success of this treatment alone has been less then 50% without drugs such as intravenous alcohol, the most widely used drug for this purpose until recently. Alcohol relaxes the uterus and blocks the body's release of oxytocin, a hormone that plays a role in the continuation of labor. Although alcohol therapy is often effective, upsetting side effects may occur including nausea, vomiting, and headache.

The newest drug to stop labor, ritodrine (Yutopar), was approved for this purpose by the FDA in late 1980. Ritodrine has been extensively tested and appears to be the most promising drug available to stop premature labor. Drug therapy may be used when labor starts between 24 and 36 weeks of pregnancy. Once your cervix dilates more than four centimeters or membranes rupture, drug therapy will probably be unsuccessful.

Drug therapy to stop labor, while promising in selected individual circumstances, is not likely to change the overall picture of prematurity. Recognition of early signs of premature labor is equally important. When in doubt, see your clinician promptly. A pelvic exam can tell whether you have started labor, and external monitoring can help in the evaluation of persistent contractions even before your cervix has begun to dilate.

Induction of Labor

There are several medical reasons (listed in Table 34) for inducing labor. Your physician can induce labor by rupturing the fluid-filled sac which surrounds the fetus (this procedure is called an *amniotomy*) or by giving synthetic *oxytocin*, a hormonal drug which stimulates contractions. Rupturing these membranes initiates labor within twenty-four hours in over 75% of women. When both methods of inducing labor are combined, 98% of women deliver within twenty-four hours. Some clinicians start oxytocin at the same time as amniotomy, while others wait for contractions to start on their own after the membranes have been ruptured. At other times, oxytocin may be started without breaking your waters when your cervix is

so-called unfavorable—that is, when your cervix is hard, thick, and completely closed—and delivery is unexpected for at least twelve hours.

Amniotomy, the safer and simpler of the two techniques, also allows assessment of the baby's amniotic fluid as noted earlier in this chapter. Once performed, amniotomy commits the clinician to delivery within twenty-four hours because of the increasing chance of infection after this time.

Oxytocin is a powerful drug, a synthesized form of the same hormone found in the brain, which works by stimulating the uterus to contract. It is usually given intravenously. The flow of oxytocin is increased very slowly to prevent overstimulation of the uterus since too frequent contractions may reduce the baby's oxygen supply. The major maternal risk of oxytocin, uterine rupture, is a rare occurrence. Although uterine contractions induced by oxytocin are identical to the contractions of normal labor, it is theoretically possible that improper use of the drug could cause fetal distress or uterine rupture. Some mothers who have experienced both types of contraction have felt that the induced labor is more painful.

Induction of labor may be either elective or medically indicated. Elective induction of labor, for the convenience of choosing your labor day, may subject the fetus as well as the mother to unnecessary risks during labor and delivery. Some studies associate elective induction of labor with a slightly increased incidence of prematurity (due to miscalculation of the baby's gestational age) and of cesarean births.

Medical reasons for inducing labor, which occur in fewer than 8% of all pregnancies, are listed in Table 34. In high-risk pregnancies, medically indicated inductions improve the chances of a healthy outcome for both mother and baby. The success of an induction, whether medical or elective, depends upon the readiness of the cervix. A cervix that is soft, thin, and already dilated two to three centimeters responds more readily to oxytocin than an unfavorable cervix, which is undilated, thick, and firm.

Augmentation of Labor

Stimulation, or augmentation, of labor means that the doctor attempts to enhance uterine contractions that have already begun, either by amniotomy or by administering oxytocin, or by a

Table 34   POSSIBLE MEDICAL REASONS FOR INDUCING LABOR

Reason	Comment
High blood pressure (toxemia)	Timing of induction depends on severity of toxemia. Labor is induced near term (40 weeks) if toxemia is mild but earlier if severe or if fetal tests are abnormal.
Diabetes (requiring insulin)	If you take insulin, labor may be induced three or more weeks early.
Rh disease (you are Rh negative and have had a blood test showing the presence of Rh antibodies—see Chapter 20)	Rare today; timing of induction depends on amniocentesis, which tells how severely fetus is affected.
Overdue (more than two weeks past your due date if this date is definitely established)	Amniocentesis may be done first to confirm fetal maturity if there is uncertainty about your due date.
Inadequate fetal growth	Depends on severity of growth problem as determined by successive sonograms and fetal tests.
Ruptured bag of waters (amniotic fluid leaking)	Labor is usually induced within 12 hours of rupture if 34 to 36 weeks or more, or if signs of infection are present (see Chapter 20) regardless of gestational age.

combination of both methods. The oxytocin method is used only if labor is not progressing properly. Amniotomy, however, is often performed routinely whether contractions are normal or not. This is because, in addition to facilitating regular contractions, the procedure enables the clinician to evaluate the condition of the fetus by noting whether the amniotic fluid is clear or stained with meconium (see glossary). Amniotomy is usually performed after you reach about four centimeters of cervical dilation.

Oxytocin is generally indicated when labor contractions are weak or irregular. When contractions are strong and regular, yet labor does not progress, oxytocin is of no benefit and cesarean section may be a more appropriate intervention.

Once the active phase of labor begins (usually after four centimeters dilation), prolonged labor may be of three types:

1. stoppage of labor (there is no change in cervical dilation for two hours or more);
2. slow labor (cervical dilation occurs at a rate slower than one centimeter an hour); and
3. failure of descent (the baby's head does not drop progressively deeper into the birth canal).

All types of prolonged labor are abnormal and may indicate a small pelvis, a large or abnormally positioned baby, or inadequate uterine contractions. When oxytocin is used to stimulate labor which is not progressing normally, delivery usually occurs within two to six hours. If labor does not progress normally with oxytocin, then cesarean birth may be unavoidable.

Breech Birth

In approximately 3% of all deliveries, the baby is in the *breech* position, with the baby's bottom or feet entering the birth canal first rather than the head. Breech presentation is a high-risk condition because of the greater likelihood of prematurity, a prolapsed cord, or fetal injury at the time of delivery.

Because of the high risk associated with breech delivery, many physicians automatically perform a cesarean section when it is the woman's first baby or the baby's feet are entering the birth canal (*footling breech*), as opposed to the baby's buttocks alone (*frank breech*). In a breech, particularly a premature breech, the head is relatively large compared to the buttocks and may become dangerously trapped within the cervix during vaginal delivery. If delivery is thereby delayed for several minutes, the supply of oxygen to the baby can be threatened. Efforts to release the head when it becomes entrapped during delivery may result in damage to the baby's brain, spinal column, or soft internal organs.

Many physicians believe that if vaginal breech delivery is to occur successfully, it is most likely

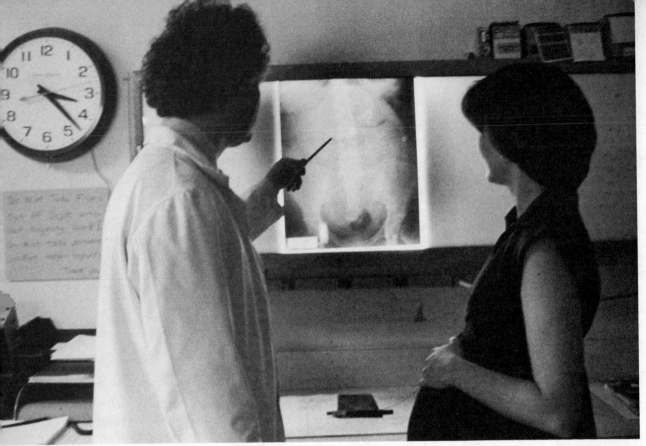

One of the few times that an X-ray may be helpful during labor is when the baby's position is breech (head up). The radiologist is pointing to the baby's head, seen in the upper part of the X-ray.

Opposite page—cesarean birth.

to be accomplished safely in a woman who has previously given birth and who has an average-size baby positioned as a frank breech where the buttocks alone enter the birth canal. The current approach toward delivering more breech babies by cesarean birth seems justified. One long-term study (reported by W. E. Brenner) of breech-delivered infants revealed that by nine years of age, 24.5% had repeated one or more grades in school, possibly indicating a high percentage of subtle, possibly unrecognized injuries at birth (see the references for Chapter 21 at the end of this section).

To prevent breech births, some obstetricians are returning to external version, a once-popular procedure in which the baby is manually "turned" from the breech to the normal head-first position. To aid in performing this maneuver, the doctor first gives an intravenous medication to the mother which temporarily relaxes the uterus. The procedure usually is done before labor begins, around the thirty-seventh week, and most often in a hospital where fetal monitoring is available.

Cesarean Section

A cesarean section, performed if the health of the mother or baby is threatened by vaginal delivery, is an operation to deliver a baby through an incision in the abdomen. Two types of abdominal incision can be used. The horizontal Pfannenstiel incision, which may be preferred for cosmetic reasons, is made at or just above the pubic hairline. This incision may require several additional minutes to make and thus is not used in an emergency. The other type of incision, called *midline* or *vertical*, starts just below the bellybutton and extends downward. (These two types of incision are shown in Figure 38, in Chapter 42.) The usual time from initial skin incision to delivery ordinarily takes only a few minutes. After the baby is removed from the uterus, the baby breathes normally and cries just like babies born vaginally.

The incision in the *uterus*, unlike the abdominal incision, is almost always one that runs horizontally across the lower part of the uterus, the so-

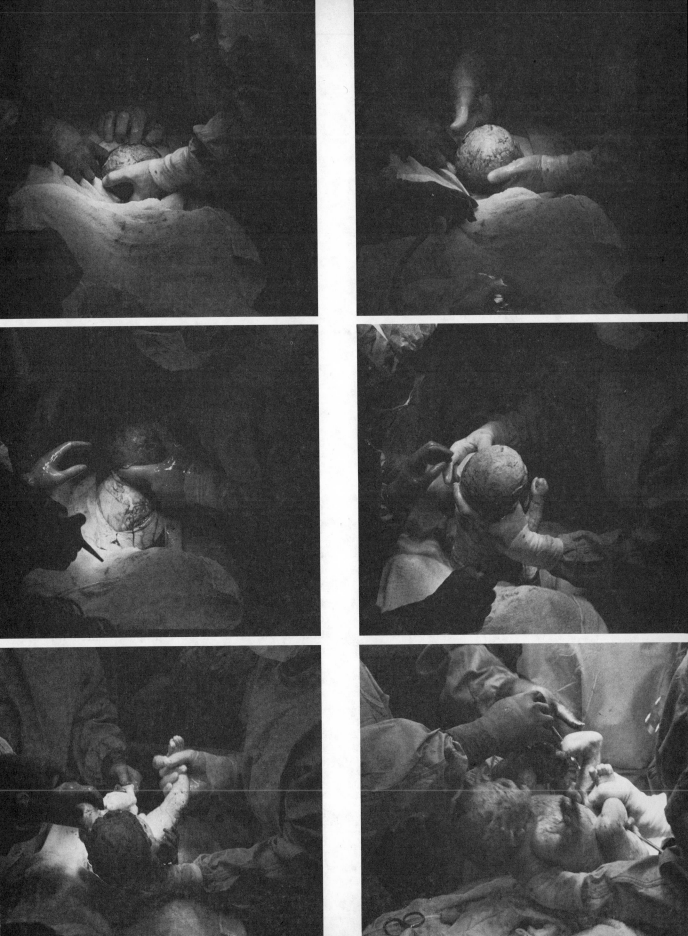

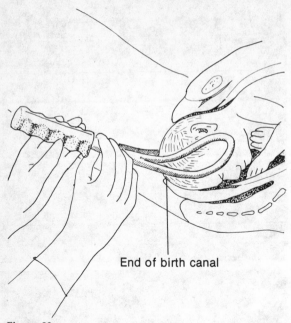

End of birth canal

Figure 23

Low-forceps delivery. The baby's head has reached the lower end of the birth canal before the forceps are applied.

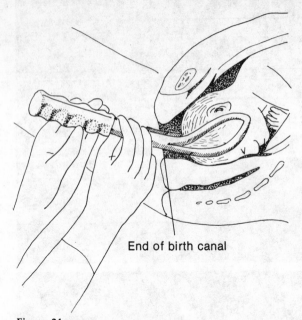

End of birth canal

Figure 24

Mid-forceps delivery. The baby's head still has not reached the lower end of the birth canal when the forceps are applied. In this situation considerably more traction may be required to deliver the baby vaginally compared to a low-forceps procedure.

called *low-transverse* incision. Although there are exceptions, this incision is almost always used because of its minimal association with infection, bleeding, and subsequent uterine rupture.

Cesarean births are more painful, more disabling, and more expensive than vaginal deliveries. Hospital stays for cesareans average five days as opposed to three days or less for normal deliveries. The most common complication of cesarean births, uterine infection, occurs 15% to 20% of the time, ten times the rate for vaginal deliveries. Although mortality associated with cesarean delivery is extremely low, approximately four to eight per ten thousand, this risk is several times that of normal deliveries. Cesareans have also been linked to prematurity and an increased risk of breathing problems in the newborn, especially when the operation is carried out without a medical reason.

Why the increase in cesarean births?

It is difficult to identify a single reason for the rising cesarean section rate in the United States, from an overall rate of 5% in 1970 to 10% in 1975, and more than 15% in 1981. Opponents of the rising cesarean birth rate cite fear of lawsuits as a cause and argue that the cesarean is easier for the doctor than performing a complicated delivery involving the use of forceps. Nevertheless, many obstetricians have abandoned the *mid-forceps* delivery that is usually more dangerous to the baby than delivery by cesarean section. A mid-forceps delivery is very different from the more common *low-forceps* procedure. With the low-forceps delivery, the baby's head is already visible and the instruments gently guide the head out of the lower vagina with little or no traction (see Figure 23). A mid-forceps delivery, on the other hand, may require significant traction (pulling) as well as rotation of the head into the proper position for delivery (see Figure 24).

The question of rising cesarean births was the subject of a recent National Institutes of Health (NIH) task force, which basically concluded that the number of cesarean deliveries could be safely decreased. The NIH panel met after months of intensive research and data collection dealing with medical, economic, and ethical considerations surrounding cesarean childbirth. One of the most significant recommendations of the panel of experts was to challenge the general rule, not applied outside the U.S., that once a woman has a cesarean delivery, all subsequent childbirths must be by cesarean. The NIH task force suggested that obstetricians should not automatically reject vaginal delivery in women who have had a previous cesarean section so long as the physician is prepared to perform immediate surgery in an emergency.

The "once-a-cesarean-always-a-cesarean" dictum originated in 1914 when most obstetricians performed a cesarean delivery by making a vertical incision in the upper part of the uterus, the so-called classical cesarean section. Labor in a subsequent pregnancy *is* a significant hazard after this technique has been used since the uterine scar is more likely to rupture. The risk of this complication is much less today since the classical operation is rarely performed. Instead, a low horizontal uterine incision (called *low-transverse* or *low-segment* cesarean section) is used, which minimizes the risk of the uterus rupturing during labor in a subsequent pregnancy. In light of data from national and international sources, the NIH panel suggested "labor and vaginal delivery after a previous cesarean birth [of the low-transverse type] are of low risk to mother and fetus in properly selected cases." Several studies indicate that about 50% of women who have previously delivered by cesarean birth may safely deliver vaginally.

The NIH task force also suggested that obstetricians use less liberal reasons for performing first-time cesarean births. Seventy-five percent of these primary cesarean deliveries are now done for one of three reasons: abnormal labor progress (*dystocia*), breech presentation, and fetal distress. On the controversial issue of *breech presentation*, the panel cautiously asserted that some of these babies may be delivered vaginally if the mother's pelvis is normal (that is, not too small) and the baby is of average size. The task force reviewed studies evaluating the relationship between electronic fetal monitoring (used to diagnose *fetal distress*) and cesarean deliveries and did not find a general cause and effect relationship. Most cesareans among women having monitoring appear to result from risk factors that required monitoring in the first place, and not to the procedure itself.

The panel expressed some doubt about the need for performing as many cesareans for the reason of abnormal labor progress, or dystocia, especially since it found no evidence that normal weight babies were healthier if delivered by cesarean. Dystocia, the number one reason given for first-time cesarean births, may be due to any combination of weak contractions, a small pelvis, or a large baby. Dystocia may be associated with long

A father holds his new baby moments after cesarean birth.

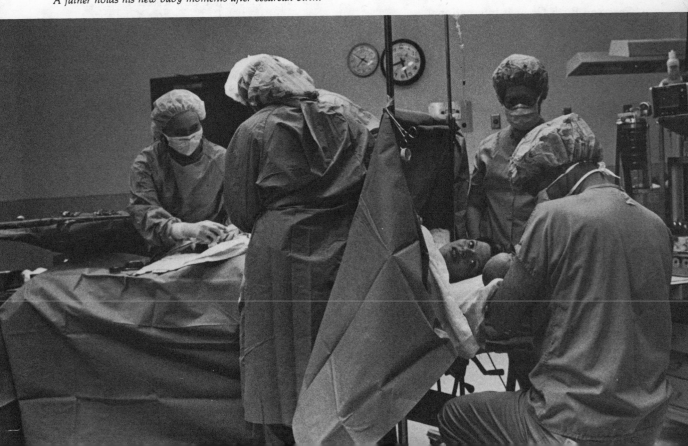

labor, especially in women who are overdue or who are less than five feet tall (and usually have smaller pelvic bones).

Options with cesarean birth

Even if you have your baby by cesarean birth, you can still experience a number of birth options in many hospitals. Fathers are more frequently being allowed in the operating room, and, in a few institutions, if you don't have general anesthesia, you can observe the birth procedure by means of a mirror so you can see the moment of your baby's birth. Even though you cannot immediately hold your baby, you should be able to hold and breast-feed your baby in the recovery room if you and the baby are progressing normally.

Resources

Some communities have cesarean support groups or special classes for repeat cesarean mothers. Find out what is available in your area from the local childbirth education association. Resources providing information on cesarean birth include:

C/SEC, Inc.*
66 Christopher Road
Waltham, Massachusetts 02154

Cesarean Birth Council International
P.O. Box 6081
San Jose, California 95150

Two well-written books about having a cesarean birth are:

Donovan, Bonnie. *The Cesarean Birth Experience.* Boston: Beacon Press, 1978 (paperback).

Hausknecht, Richard, and Heilman, Joan. *Having a Cesarean Baby*, New York: E. P. Dutton, 1982 (paperback).

Write to C/SEC, Inc. for this pamphlet (address above): *Frankly Speaking: A Pamphlet for Cesarean Couples.* (Cost: $4.00.)

---

* Cesareans/Support, Education, and Concern

References for Section Four

Chapter 14—Childbirth Education

Baldwin, R. *Special Delivery - The Complete Guide to Informed Birth.* Millbrae, Calif.: Les Femmes Publishing, 1979.

Brazelton, C. Effect of maternal expectations on early infant behavior. *Early Child Development and Care* 2:259-273, 1973.

McQuarrie, H. G. Commercial diagnostic tests for office use. *Contemporary OB/GYN* (special issue) 14:39, 1979.

Rao, C. V. Pregnancy tests for office and home. *Contemporary OB/GYN* (special issue) 16:107-112, 1980.

Jimenez, S. Education for the childbearing year – comprehensive application of psychoprophylaxis. *Journal of Obstetric, Gynecologic and Neonatal Nursing* 9:97-99, Mar/April 1980.

Post, C., et al. A "good beginning" for families . . . patient group education – what? why? *Pediatric Nursing* 6:32-36, Jul/Aug 1980.

Mason, D. Parent support groups: a place to turn for help. *American Baby* 42:49+, Sept 1980.

Chapter 15—Hospital Birth and Its Alternatives

Faison, J. B., Pisani, B. J., et al. The childbearing center: an alternative birth setting. *Obstetrics and Gynecology* 54(4):527-532, 1979.

Chard, T., and Richards, M. *Benefits and Hazards of the New Obstetrics.* Philadelphia: Lippincott, 1977.

Anderson, J. Alternative birth center gives parents a new option. *Hospital Forum* 19:4-5, Jul 1976.

Gerris, C. The alternative birth center at Mt. Zion Hospital. *Birth and the Family Journal* 3:127-128, fall 1976.

Wertz, R. W., and Wertz, D. C. *Lying-in: A History of Childbirth in America.* New York: Free Press, 1977.

Lubic, R., et al. The childbearing center – an alternative to conventional care. *Nursing Outlook* 26:754-760, Dec 1978.

Jones, D. Home early after delivery. *American Journal of Nursing* 78:1378-80, Aug 1978.

Devitt, N. The transition from home to hospital birth in the U.S. 1930–1960. *Birth and the Family Journal* 4:47-58, summer 1977.

Freeman, M. H. Giving family life a good start in the hospital. *American Journal of Maternal Child Nursing* 4:51-54, Jan/Feb 1979.

Hardy, C., et al. Hospital meets patients' demand for "home-style" childbirth. *Hospitals* 52:73-74, Mar 1978.

Mehl, L., et al. Outcome of elective home births – a series of 1146 cases in northern California. *Journal of Reproductive Medicine* 19(5):281-290, 1977.

Editorial: Home birth. *Journal of the American Medical Association* 241(10):1039, 1979.

Freeman, R. K., et al. Where will your patient deliver – at home? in the hospital? in an alternate birth center? *Contemporary OB/GYN* 12:104-130, Dec 1978.

Countryman, B. A. Alternative styles for childbirth – why parents aren't satisfied with the status quo, part I. *Journal of Nursing Care* 11:16-17, Aug 1978.

American College of Obstetricians and Gynecologists: Alternative birthing centers – a survey and bibliography. Nov 1980.

Sumner, P. E., and Phillips, C. R. *Birthing Rooms – Concept and Reality*. St. Louis: C. V. Mosby Co., 1981.

Dobbs, K. B., et al. Alternative birth rooms and birth options. *Obstetrics and Gynecology* 58(5):626-630, 1981.

Chapter 16—Pregnancy

Speroff, L. Exercise during pregnancy. *Contemporary OB/GYN* 23(6):25-29, June 1984.

Queenan, J. T. Advising pregnant and postop working patients. *Contemporary OB/GYN* 23(4):82-94, Apr 1984.

Charles, D., and Larsen, B. How colostrum and milk protect the newborn. *Contemporary OB/GYN* 24(1):143-166, July 1984.

Buytaert, G., et al. Iron supplementation during pregnancy. *European Journal of Obstetrics, Gynecology and Reproductive Biology* 15:11-16, 1983.

Jarrett, J. C., II, and Spellacy, W. N. Jogging during pregnancy: an improved outcome? *Obstetrics and Gynecology* 61(6):705-709, 1983.

Winick, M. Nutrition and pregnancy. *The Female Patient* 9(2):21-27, Feb 1984.

Friederich, M. A. Psychological changes during pregnancy. *Contemporary OB/GYN* 9:27-34, Jun 1977.

Brenner, P., and Greenberg, M. The impact of pregnancy on marriage. *Medical Aspects of Human Sexuality* 15-21, Jul 1977.

Notham, M., and Nadelson, C. (eds.) *The Woman Patient: Medical and Psychological Interfaces,* Vol. 1. Plenum Press: New York, 1978.

Pritchard, J. A., and MacDonald, P. C. *Williams Obstetrics,* ed. 16. New York: Appleton-Century-Crofts, 1980.

Martin, L. L. *Health Care of Women.* Philadelphia: Lippincott, 1978.

Benson, R. C. *Handbook of Obstetrics and Gynecology,* ed. 8. Los Altos, Calif.: Lange, 1983.

Manning, F. A., et al. Ultrasound in pregnancy. *The Female Patient* 72-79, Mar 1981.

Chapter 17—Labor and Delivery

Flowers, C. E. Psychological preparation for childbirth. *The Female Patient* 49-55, Feb 1978.

Benson, R. C., et al. *Current Obstetrics and Gynecologic Diagnosis and Treatment,* ed. 4. Los Altos, Calif.: Lange, 1982.

Pritchard, J. A., and MacDonald, P. C. *Williams Obstetrics,* ed. 16. New York: Appleton-Century-Crofts, 1980.

Chapter 18—Your First Weeks as a Mother

Gruis, M. Beyond maternity: post-partum concerns of mothers. *The American Journal of Maternal Child Nursing* 2:182-188, May/Jun 1977.

Braverman, J. Postpartum depression. *The Female Patient* 88-91, Feb 1978.

Peterson, G. H., and Mehl, L. E. Some determinants of maternal attachment. *American Journal of Psychiatry* 135:1168-1173, 1978.

L'Esperance, C. M. Pain or pleasure – the dilemma of early breastfeeding. *Birth and the Family Journal* 7(1):21-26, 1980.

Affonso, D. D. Missing pieces – a study of postpartum feelings. *Birth and the Family Journal* 4:159-64, winter 1977.

Sweeny, S., and Davis, F. Transition to parenthood – a group experience. *Maternal Child Nursing Journal* 8:59-64, spring 1979.

Jones, F., et al. Maternal responsiveness of primiparous mothers during the postpartum period – age differences. *Pediatrics* 65:579-84, Mar 1980.

Frate, D., et al. Behavioral reactions during the postpartum period: experiences of 108 women. *Women & Health* 4(4):355-377, winter 1979.

Neifert, M. R. Returning to breast-feeding. *Clinical Obstetrics and Gynecology* 23(4):1061-1072, Dec 1980.

Chapter 19—Options During and After Childbirth

Joint position statement on *The Development of Family Centered Maternity/Newborn Care in Hospitals,* Interprofessional Task Force on Health Care of Women and Children, Jun 1978, American College of Obstetricians and Gynecologists.

Mahan, C. S., and McKay, S. Preps and enemas—keep or discard? *Contemporary OB/GYN* 22(5):241-248, Nov 1983.

McKay, S., and Mahan, C. S. Laboring patients need more freedom to move. *Contemporary OB/GYN* 24(1):90-119, July 1984.

Pelosi, M. A., and Apuzzio, J. Making circumcision safe and painless. *Contemporary OB/GYN* 24(1):42-56, July 1984.

Goodlin, R. C. On protection of the maternal perineum during birth. *Obstetrics and Gynecology* 62(3):393-396, Sept 1983.

Grad, R. K. Breaking ground for a birthing room. *Maternal Child Nursing* 4:245-249, Jul/Aug 1979.

Klaus, M., and Kennell, J. *Maternal-Infant Bonding.* St. Louis: C. V. Mosby Co., 1976.

Hughey, M. J., McElin, T. W., et al. Maternal and fetal outcome of Lamaze-prepared patients. *Obstetrics and Gynecology* 51(6):643-647, 1978.

McClellan, M. S., and Cabianca, W. A. Effects of early mother-infant contact following cesarean birth. *Obstetrics and Gynecology* 56(1):52-55, 1980.

Klass, K., and Capps, K. Nine years' experience with family-centered maternity care in a community hospital. *Birth and the Family Journal* 7(3):175-180, 1980.

National Institute of Child Health and Human Development: National Institutes of Health Consensus Development Conference on *Antenatal Diagnosis,* March 1979, Dept of HEW, Bethesda, Maryland.

Berger, G. S., and Maynard, L. How routine should fetal heart rate monitoring be? *Contemporary OB/GYN* 12:35-41, Sep 1978.

Krebs, H. B., et al. Intrapartum fetal heart rate monitoring. *American Journal of Obstetrics and Gynecology* 133:762-772, Apr 1, 1979.

Pritchard, J. A., and MacDonald, P. C. *Williams Obstetrics,* ed. 16. New York: Appleton-Century-Crofts, 1980.

Mateo, C., et al. Anesthesiologists meet the demands of modern obstetrics. *Contemporary OB/GYN* 12:117-160, Nov 1978.

Committee on Technical Bulletins of the American College of Obstetricians and Gynecologists: Obstetric Anesthesia and Analgesia, Technical Bulletin #57, 1980, American College of Obstetricians and Gynecologists.

Puma, S. A family-centered event? – Preparing a child for sharing in the experience of childbirth. *Journal of Nurse-Midwifery* 24:5-10, May/Jun 1979.

Anderson, S. Siblings at birth: a survey and study. *Birth and the Family Journal* 6:80-7, summer 1979.

Caldeyro-Barcia, R. Influence of maternal position on time of spontaneous rupture of the membranes, progress of labor, and fetal head compression. *Birth and the Family Journal* 6(1), spring 1979.

Kliot, D. A., and Lilling, M. I. Parent-newborn bonding resulting from modifications of traditional birth techniques using the Leboyer approach. *Emotion and Reproduction* 20(B), Academic Press, 1979.

Leonard, C., et al. Preliminary observations in the behavior of children present at the birth of a sibling. *Pediatrics* 64(6):949-951, 1979.

deChateau, P. The importance of the neonatal period for the development of synchrony in the maternal-infant dyad – a review. *Birth and the Family Journal* 4:10-22, spring 1977.

Landry, K., and Kilpatrick, D. Why shave a mother before she gives birth? *The American Journal of Maternal Child Nursing* 189-190, May/Jun 1977.

Anderson, S. Childbirth as a pathological process: an American perspective. *The American Journal of Maternal Child Nursing* 240-244, 1977.

Cupit, L. Helping expectant parents understand the fetal monitor. *Pediatric Nursing* 6:21-23, May/Jun 1980.

American Academy of Pediatrics, Committee on Nutrition: Commentary on breast feeding and infant formulas, including proposed standards for formulas. *Pediatrics* 57:278-285, Feb 1976.

Woodruff, C. The science of infant nutrition and the art of infant feeding. *Journal of the American Medical Association* 240(7):657-661, 1978.

Gibbons, M. B. Why circumcise? *Pediatric Nursing* 5:9-12, Jul/Aug 1979.

Reeder, S., et al. *Maternity Nursing,* ed. 14. Philadelphia: Lippincott, 1980.

Novak, J., et al. Sibling preparation and participation in childbirth: implications for family development. *The Cybele Report* 2(3), spring 1981.

Chapter 20—Complicated Pregnancies
Chapter 21—Complications of Labor and Delivery

Sabbagha, R. E. Ultrasound in obstetrics and gynecology. *The Female Patient* 9:129-135, Jan 1984.

Quetel, T. A., and Bezjian, A. A. Obstetrical ultrasound: an overview and update. *Journal of the Florida Medical Association* 70(9):732-738, Sept 1983.

Patel, Y. A., et al. Changing trends in the incidence of caesarean section. *Journal of Obstetrics and Gynecology* 3:253-257, 1983.

Berkowitz, G. S., et al. Early gestational bleeding and pregnancy outcome: a multivariable analysis.

International Journal of Epidemiology 12:165-173, 1983.

Amirikia, H., et al. Cesarean section: a 15-year review of changing incidence, indications, and risks. *American Journal of Obstetrics and Gynecology* 140(1):81-86, May 1981.

Benson, R. C., et al. *Current Obstetrics and Gynecologic Diagnosis and Treatment*, ed. 4. Los Altos, Calif.: Lange, 1982.

National Institute of Child Health and Human Development: National Institutes of Health Consensus Development Conferences on *Antenatal Diagnosis*, March 1979, and on Cesarean Childbirth, Sep 1980; Dept of HEW, Bethesda, Maryland.

Hughey, M. J., LaPata, R. E., et al. Effect of fetal monitoring on the incidence of cesarean section. *Obstetrics and Gynecology* 49(5):513-517, 1977.

Minkoff, H. L., et al. The rising cesarean section rate – Can it safely be reversed? *Obstetrics and Gynecology* 56(2):135-143, 1980.

Merrill, B. S., and Gibbs, C. E. Planned vaginal delivery following cesarean section. *Obstetrics and Gynecology* 52(1):50-52, 1978.

Druzin, M. L., Paul, R. H., et al. Current status of the contraction stress test. *The Journal of Reproductive Medicine* 23(5):222-226, 1979.

Freeman, R. K. Defining the role of antepartum monitoring. *Contemporary OB/GYN* 13:65-71, Mar 1979.

Garite, T. J., Freeman, R. K., et al. Oxytocin challenge test. *Obstetrics and Gynecology* 51(5):614-618, 1978.

Queenan, J. T. Ultrasound in obstetrics and gynecology. *Current Problems in Obstetrics and Gynecology* 1(8):3-33, 1978.

Anderson, S. G. Real-time sonography in obstetrics. *Obstetrics and Gynecology* 51(3):284-287, 1978.

Queenan, J. T. Ultrasound in obstetrics and gynecology. *Current Problems in Obstetrics and Gynecology* 1(8):3-33, 1978.

Committee on Perinatal Health: Toward improving the outcome of pregnancy – recommendations for the regional development of maternal and perinatal health services, 1976, published by The National Foundation – March of Dimes: White Plains, N.Y.

Clewell, W. H. Prematurity. *The Journal of Reproductive Medicine* 23(5):237-244, 1979.

Brenner, W. E. Improving the prognosis of the breech infant. *The Female Patient* 40-47, Nov 1978.

Centers for Disease Control: Current status of rubella in the United States, 1969-1979. *The Journal of Infectious Diseases* 142(5):776-9, 1980.

Hobel, C. J. Prenatal and intrapartum high-risk screening. *American Journal of Obstetrics and Gynecology* 117(1):1-9, 1973.

Grossman, J. H., III, et al. Management of genital herpes simplex virus infection during pregnancy. *Obstetrics and Gynecology* 58(1):1-4, 1981.

Whitley, R. J., Nahmias, A. J., et al. The natural history of herpes simplex virus infection of mother and newborn. *Pediatrics* 66:489-494, 1980.

five

Sexual Issues for Today's Woman

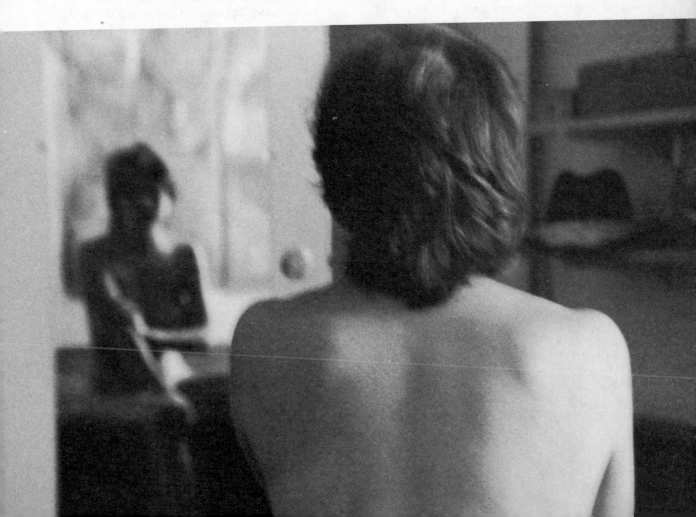

Female Sexuality

A woman's attitude toward her own sexuality is greatly influenced by the information and "messages" she received about sex while she was growing up. In spite of today's greater sexual freedom, sex still remains a hidden, secret, or even taboo subject much of the time.

Formal sex education in school, for example, fails to offer enough information to answer the questions young people may be too embarrassed to ask. In addition, parents often do not provide adequate sex information, either because they do not have enough information themselves or because they, perhaps like their own parents, feel uncomfortable discussing sex with their children. The message we may receive from all this is that sex is not a proper topic for open or easy conversation, and, hence, sex itself is to be suppressed.

The words people use to talk about sex and sexual parts of the body also give us clues about sexual attitudes. Terms that mean sexual intercourse are often vague ("doing it") or technical ("coitus") or evasive ("sleeping together"). Our sexual vocabulary seldom includes words that are plain and simple and human. No wonder people often feel embarrassed or nervous talking about sex!

So-called double messages are also abundant in our everyday lives, and it is easy to understand why many women (and men) feel confused about their sexuality. Your family or your religion may tell you to "be a virgin until you are married," while the media, through sexually explicit movies, for example, encourages sexual casualness. We may be torn between peer pressure for sexual freedom and our own determination of what is "right" and "wrong," "healthy" and "unhealthy," or "moral" and "immoral." Such conflicts may interfere with a person's ability to clarify his or her *own* values and needs.

If you feel uncertain about your own sexual

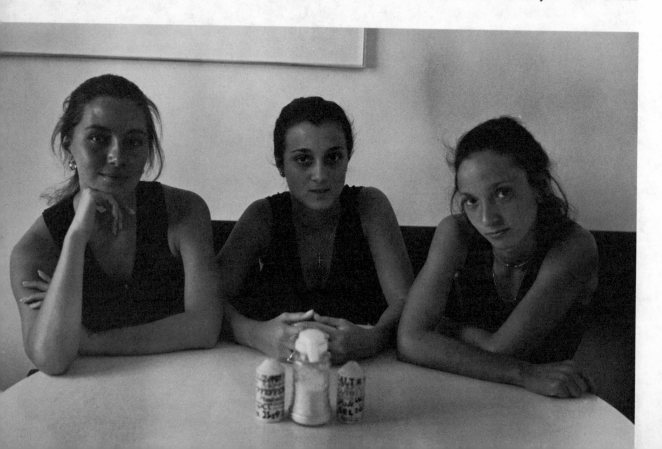

beliefs, you might try to review what you learned about sex from family, school, religion, peers, and society in general. Are there many conflicting messages? Try to decide which values are meaningful for you right now. You might find you have grown up with some sexual attitudes or beliefs you don't care to live with. Changing longstanding attitudes is not easy, but just being aware of them may help you substitute more desirable ones. Some people find that talking with partners, friends, or even a therapist may help them clarify or redefine their sexual goals.

Sexual Response Cycle

Our society often equates sex with intercourse. Though it is helpful to know about the sexual response cycle, there is nothing mandatory about having to go through the whole cycle each time. Kissing, hugging, and other acts of physical affection can be just as sexually satisfying as intercourse at times.

A woman responds to sexual excitement emotionally and physically. While the emotional response varies widely depending on several factors (your sexual attitudes, your relationship with your partner, the physical setting, and so on), the physical changes that the body goes through are similar in all situations. The *sexual response cycle* is the name given to these natural physical changes that a person experiences from initial sexual stimulation through orgasm and back to the original state. Although this cycle is divided into four basic stages—*excitement, plateau, orgasm,* and *resolution*—there isn't always a sharp line between the end of one stage and the beginning of the next. These changes result from two physiologic processes: engorgement (increased circulation of blood to certain parts of the body) and increased muscle tension.

When a woman becomes sexually aroused, whether from sexual fantasy, masturbation, or a sexual partner, the *excitement* state begins. The first response is vaginal lubrication; that is, the woman's vagina gets wet because vaginal blood vessels become engorged during excitement and force a mucuslike fluid into the vaginal canal. The amount of lubricant in the vagina can be affected by a number of different factors, including a woman's past sexual experience. When anxiety or pain is associated with previous intercourse, vagi-

nal lubrication may decrease. The older woman, too, usually finds that vaginal fluid naturally decreases. If you need additional lubrication, simply use a water-soluble lubricant, such as K-Y or Transi-Lube, which you can find in most drugstores. Contraceptive creams, jellies, and foams also provide extra lubrication. Avoid using a petroleum jelly (such as Vaseline) as a vaginal lubricant, however; a greasy jelly (that is, one that is not water soluble) does not wash out of the vagina by itself and can thus become a breeding place for bacteria.

During the excitement stage, increased blood circulation to the genital area deepens the color of the vulva to deep pink or reddish and makes the labia puffy and thicker. (You may want to refer at this point to Chapter 3, on female anatomy.) The clitoris also swells. Meanwhile, muscles in the woman's uterus begin to tense.

As sexual stimulation continues, the woman moves into the *plateau* stage of the sexual response cycle when the vaginal lips become even more engorged and puffy. The clitoris moves closer to the body and tucks itself up under its hood. Directly stimulating the sensitive clitoris at this time might be painful, but touching the hood with the clitoris underneath it only heightens the pleasurable sensations. During plateau, muscles all over your body tense up. Your heartbeat, blood pressure, and breathing rate increase with continued stimulation. The breast nipples become erect, and the breasts themselves become somewhat larger.

Women need continued sexual stimulation to reach the *orgasm* phase, the third stage in the response cycle. Orgasm, physiologically a reflex, occurs when the engorgement and muscle tension reach a peak and then release. Fewer than half of American women have orgasm during intercourse. Different women need different kinds of stimulation to produce an orgasm. Some women prefer breast stimulation or whole-body contact, while others like frequent touching of the clitoral area, and still others enjoy some other form of stimulation. Most women require at least some clitoral stimulation to achieve orgasm.

How women react to orgasm depends on the specific situation: whether or not you are alone or with a partner, the physical setting, the intensity of the orgasm, and so on. Some women tremble, some thrash a bit, others remain still. Some people are quiet, others may moan or weep or cry out. The important thing is to recognize that there is no "right" pattern to follow, and the amount of noise or movement a person makes does not necessarily show how much pleasure she is experiencing.

During the *resolution* stage of the sexual response cycle, engorgement subsides, the muscles relax, and you may perspire as your body returns to its pre-excitement state. The swollen clitoris and other parts of the body return to their normal state, as does your heart rate and blood pressure. A woman's body goes through the resolution stage whether or not she reaches orgasm. If she did not have an orgasm, the resolution stage lasts a bit longer.

Sexual Responsiveness

You probably find that you enjoy various approaches to sexual experiences. Sometimes, while becoming very excited, you may want to alter the pace of activity, slowing down and then building up to intense excitement once or several times to prolong the warm, tingly sensations. Or you might enjoy moving rapidly and directly into a state of higher excitement and orgasm. At other times, you may prefer the warmth of hugging without the goal of intercourse in mind.

Cultural beliefs about female sexual responsiveness have changed over the years. During the early part of this century many people did not believe that women had sexual urges and satisfactions comparable to a man's, so no one expected women to have orgasms. When researchers found that women did indeed experience orgasms, they believed orgasms were possible only during intercourse. Later, it was believed that women had two distinct kinds of orgasm: the "clitoral" type from clitoral stimulation and the "vaginal" type, which was believed to occur in the vagina during sexual intercourse. It is now known, however, that there is only one kind of orgasm, in which the clitoris and vagina each play a part: the clitoris *receives* the stimulation, and the vagina *reacts* to this stimulation with muscular contractions during orgasm. Although this physical reflex always happens in the same way, women may experience the feelings of orgasm in different places. Sometimes a woman may be more aware of the orgasmic feelings in her vagina, sometimes around the clitoris, sometimes in the entire genital area, with these feelings sometimes "spreading" to other parts of the body. Some women experience several orgasms at a time; others have one orgasm. Having multiple orgasms, however, does not neces-

sarily make the experience any more enjoyable. Only you can measure your own sexual satisfaction and thereby determine what is personally satisfying.

Sexual Expression

The variety of activities we take part in as we respond to our sexual needs is limited only by the imagination. This part of the chapter discusses common forms of sexual expression.

Although it is one of the most common and frequent sexual practices, masturbation, or self-stimulation, is a subject surrounded by ignorance and shame. Masturbation is in no way harmful, and some sex therapists even suggest masturbating techniques to increase body awareness, which often helps overcome certain sexual problems. Many individuals continue to masturbate even when involved in long-term sexual relationships.

When women masturbate, they generally stimulate the area of the clitoris, moving their fingers in small circles or using a pressing motion. These strokes gradually become more intense as a woman reaches orgasm, and most women continue to stimulate themselves through the orgasm. Some women find that tensing the muscles in their thighs or in their genitals increases sexual stimulation. Others use electric or battery-operated vibrators for stimulation. Many people have sexual fantasies while they are masturbating. The content of these fantasies, which may include, say, having sex with someone not available as a partner in reality, is limited only by the imagination.

When women are involved in sexual relationships with men, there are any number of sexual activities in which the two partners may engage, depending upon their shared interests, desires, and values. For a helpful book about female sexuality refer to: *For Yourself: The Fulfillment of Female Sexuality*, by L. Barbach, published in 1976 by Doubleday, Garden City, New York.

Some women prefer to have sexual relationships with other women. Although our society has a history of prejudice against relationships between two people of the same sex, such relationships are becoming more commonly accepted as valid expressions of the individual's sexual and emotional needs. *Our Right To Love* (edited by Ginny Vida, Englewood Cliffs, N.J., Prentice-Hall, 1978) is an informative resource book about female homosexuality.

Some people in our society are bisexual; that is, they have relationships with partners of both sexes. Many bisexuals choose a partner on the basis of personality rather than on gender. That is, the woman is attracted to others on the basis of their personal qualities, and, for her, such relationships with either a man or a woman might become sexual. Other women feel they can have different kinds of experiences with a woman from what they can have with a man, and they like to experience both of these relationships.

Another sexual option is celibacy: the voluntary decision not to have sexual partners for a given period of time. A person might choose to be celibate for many different reasons—to take time to heal after a relationship has ended, or to concentrate one's time and energy on other things.

Sexual Problems

The natural bodily responses to sexual stimulation do not always occur exactly as you might think they should or just in the way that you want. This brings up a sensitive question: when, if ever, does failure to achieve a desired response mean you have a sexual problem? There are times in everyone's life when they just are not feeling sensual or sexual. Illness, financial worry, and stressful work demands are only a few of life's crises that naturally decrease sexual interest and responsiveness.

There may also be times when you feel ready for a sexual experience but your body does not respond as expected—you just don't feel aroused. Such events happen to everyone from time to time and are not problems unless they begin to interfere with your relationship or occur with increasing frequency. In this sense, you are the one to decide whether or not there is a problem. This part of the chapter discusses the causes of some sexual difficulties.

Anxiety causes many sexual problems. The kind of anxiety that interferes with a person's ability to function sexually is very common and has many sources. Conflicting or inadequate information about sex is an important factor. Women are often brought up to repress or ignore their sexuality. They may, for example, be discouraged from the natural childhood activity of exploring their genitals, and they may not even be taught about their anatomy. If a woman does not understand how her body functions sexually, she

may experience difficulty or simply may not know what to do in a sexual situation. Sometimes uncertainties about sexual values underlie nervousness about sex if your partner wants to engage in a certain sexual activity but you do not. Other things that may make us anxious include unrealistic expectations about ourselves or our partners or too much emphasis on technique. Guilt feelings about sexuality, possibly because of what we have been taught about sex as children, can easily cause anxiety. Or a woman may be afraid that she is not a "good lover," or that her partner will reject her. If you have a sexual problem related to anxiety, it's important to explore the roots of your sexual attitudes and values on your own or with your partner or a therapist, so you will be able to clarify your own sexual needs, values, and goals. This self-exploration alone may relieve the anxiety and therefore the problem.

Anxiety about a sexual situation can make you do "sex-watching." That is, you begin watching yourself as if you were watching an actress in a movie. You may look at yourself and say, "I look too fat," or "What am I doing here?"and so on. Watching the "movie" as it plays in your head reduces your anxiety, because you are so preoccupied with the "movie" that you do not experience your feelings of anxiety. However, this means that you do not allow yourself the full benefits of your pleasurable feelings either. A person cannot completely enjoy the sexual experience while sex-watching; your energy cannot go both ways. It is fairly common to engage in sex-watching; and, if you find yourself doing it, try to refocus your attention and get into the experience, or maybe take time out to talk with your partner about how you are feeling.

Sex-watching is not the same as having a sexual fantasy. In a fantasy, you think sexual thoughts and imagine sexual activities. Sex-watching takes you and your feelings out of the sexual situation, while fantasy can be a way to get even more deeply involved.

Another major source of sexual difficulties is poor communication between sexual partners. Some people will not talk to their partners about sexuality, fearing, for example, that talking during sex will "spoil the mood." Or sometimes sexual preferences go unexpressed because one partner assumes that the other already knows which manner of touching, for example, gives the greatest pleasure. At other times you may feel shy or nervous about telling your partner what you like because you are afraid that he may think you are criticizing him. In all of these situations, the partners need to talk with each other. It may help to begin by acknowledging feelings such as fear, shyness, or embarrassment. Such open communication may make it less threatening to discuss sexual problems.

Sexual problem areas

There are three basic areas in which a person might experience sexual problems: sexual desire, sexual arousal (excitement), and orgasm.

Lack of desire is a very common sexual problem. While everyone experiences variation in sexual interest from time to time, a problem may arise when lack of desire persists. People who experience a lack of desire do not initiate sexual activities and may have few sexual fantasies. Such individuals may participate in sex but do not find the experience very satisfying.

Occasionally, lack of sexual desire has a physical cause, such as chronic illness or drugs, like sedatives or alcohol. More often this problem results from psychological factors. Anxiety, depression, and guilt, and any of the situations which produce these symptoms, may contribute to a lack of sexual desire. The problem may be a relationship conflict, especially where differences in attitudes or values exist or where an underlying power struggle between partners leads to resentment or hostility. Other relationship problems such as unresolved anger or fear of intimacy can lower an individual's sexual desire.

Some therapists use what might be called relearning methods to treat lack of sexual desire. The therapist may, for example, help the client learn positive attitudes about sexuality. However, the underlying causes of this problem are usually more complicated than other sexual problems. Thus, treatment for lack of sexual desire often requires the use of more traditional counseling methods to explore relevant individual and/or relationship conflicts.

In the second problem area—sexual arousal—a woman has sexual desires and wants to be sexual, but her vagina will not lubricate. The woman and her partner may not know how to trigger stimuli for lubrication, or the woman may have that information but not know how to share it with her partner. Sometimes even when a woman wants to be sexual, her anxiety about sex prevents her body from functioning normally. This situation might

occur in a woman who was told as a child that sex is "bad" and has not unlearned this message as an adult.

Related to lack of sexual arousal is the problem of painful intercourse, called *dyspareunia*. Sometimes a woman has intercourse when she has not had enough time to become aroused or when she is not getting aroused because of psychological reasons. In such cases, her vagina may not lubricate, and intercourse will be painful or uncomfortable. But most of the time, dyspareunia is due to a physical problem. A vaginal irritation or infection is a very common cause. Quite simply, if there is an infection in the vagina, movement of the penis inside will hurt. An allergic reaction to a douche or a contraceptive product may also cause painful intercourse. There is a difference between vaginal discomfort during intercourse caused by vaginal infections or allergic symptoms, and deep

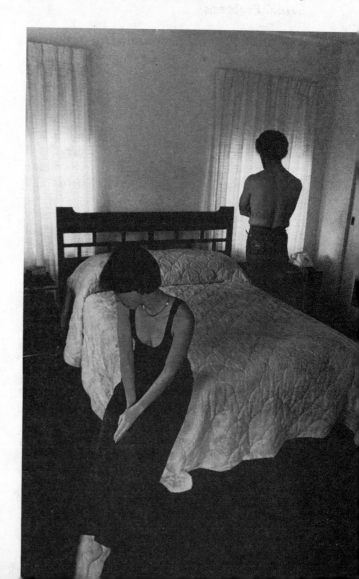

dyspareunia which is felt as pain or discomfort in the lower abdomen during intercourse. Deep dyspareunia is sometimes caused by a pelvic infection, endometriosis, or scarring after previous surgery (see Chapter 81 on pelvic pain). Once the symptoms of the physical problem are treated, dyspareunia typically disappears. As long as painful intercourse continues, however, anticipation of discomfort may lead to decreased vaginal lubrication and further contribute to the pain.

One of the most common sexual complaints of American women is the third sexual problem area—difficulty in reaching orgasm. As discussed earlier, a majority of women do not reach orgasm during intercourse. Sometimes a woman may have orgasms through masturbation but never with her partner. Or she may be able to experience orgasm with one partner but not with another. If a woman can have orgasms by, for example, self-stimulation or when a partner touches her, lack of orgasm during intercourse need not be defined as a sexual problem. If, however, a woman does not reach orgasm by means of any type of sexual stimulation, and if failure to have an orgasm disturbs her or her relationship, then she and her partner may want to consider sex therapy (see below).

In general, the causes of difficulties with orgasm are similar to the reasons for other sexual problems. Frequently, a woman simply does not receive either enough stimulation or the kind of stimulation she needs. Sometimes a woman is so eager to have an orgasm that she tries too hard, and she is so busy being anxious about this orgasm that her body cannot respond.

Treatment for failure to experience orgasm involves dealing with any anxiety that may be present and having the couple learn the appropriate and adequate stimulation needed. This often involves exercises to learn how the female body responds, along with an understanding that this process takes some time to unlearn old responses and learn new ones.

Sex Therapy

What are your options if you decide you have a sexual problem? You might begin by getting more information. There are a number of useful books available that focus on specific topics, for example, offering women information with which they can teach themselves how to have orgasms.

Sometimes, especially if self-help does not work, you might want to seek professional help from a person who has been specially trained in the field of sex therapy.

Barring physical causes most sexual problems are not "individual" problems but are problems of the couple. Most sex therapists approach sexual problems with this view and work only with the couple. In other words, contrary to what may be expressed by a woman's partner (implicitly or explicitly), he is part of the problem.

Sex therapy today approaches sexual problems as learned behavior patterns. We are born with the ability to be sexual, but such factors as ignorance, guilt, cultural attitudes, and other contributing factors may place roadblocks in the way of normal sexual responsiveness. In this approach, the therapist helps the couple identify and remove these roadblocks by a process of relearning while also helping them to explore any problem areas in their relationship that might have a bearing on the sexual difficulty.

Sex therapists often give couples exercises in what is called *sensate focus* to practice at home between sessions. Sensate focus refers to a massage technique that teaches you to focus on the pleasurable sensations you feel when your body is being touched. The first set of exercises involves your partner massaging your body but without touching your breasts or genitals. Only later is direct genital stimulation permitted. In this way, you can experience pleasurable feelings without worrying about either sexual performance or having an orgasm.

What constitutes a qualified sex therapist? Unfortunately, many people call themselves sex therapists but are not qualified as such. Moreover, authorities within the profession do not agree on the qualifications for a competent sex therapist. There is some consensus, however, as to certain base lines that should be used to evaluate a sex therapist. These base lines include the following:

1. The therapist should have a terminal (or advanced) degree in his or her profession: for example, M.D. (psychiatrist), Ph.D. (psychologist), MSW (social worker), M.A. or M.S. (Marital and Family therapist), M.S. (nurse).
2. He or she should be competent in doing marital therapy or marital counseling—that is, working with couples who have marriage problems.

3. The therapist should be trained both in human sexuality (including the physiology of the sexual organs) and in the treatment of sexual dysfunctions. This training should include supervised experience in sex therapy.

State licensure is not always a good measure of competence; not all States have licensing programs for certain professions, like social workers. Affiliation with a professional association may or may not be a good indicator of competence in this area. There are, throughout the country, organizations that certify sex therapists according to certain standards. One such group is the American Association of Sex Educators, Counselors, and Therapists (AASECT). AASECT demands, for certification, 100 hours of individual supervised experience or 150 hours of group supervision. Such certification alone may not ensure competence, but that in combination with the base lines described above may be a good indicator of qualification.

How do you find a qualified sex therapist?

1. Look for a clinic that is sponsored by a university, medical school, or social agency. Such clinics are geared to education and training and often charge lower fees.
2. Call the nearest university department of psychology or social work or medical school department of psychiatry for a referral.
3. Check the list of sex therapists certified by AASECT (see Resources below).
4. Do not simply accept a referral from a doctor, clergyman, friend, etc. Check out the person's qualifications as suggested above.

Before you make an appointment with a prospective therapist, don't be afraid to ask questions about his or her qualifications as a sex therapist. The following questions are appropriate to ask: Do you have special training in sex therapy techniques? Where did you receive your training? How long was the training? Did you have supervised experience? If the person is qualified, he or she will not mind answering your questions.

Resources

This organization will provide information about qualified sex therapists in your area:

American Association of Sex Educators, Counselors, and Therapists
600 Maryland Avenue, S.W.
Washington, D.C. 20024

Write for a list of publications available from this organization:

Sex Information and Education Council of the U.S.
80 Fifth Avenue, Suite 801
New York, New York 10011

23

Sexuality and Pregnancy

A woman's sexual feelings during pregnancy can be affected by previous sexual attitudes, her relationship with her partner, and how she feels about the pregnancy itself. Some women feel markedly more sensual and free, and they even experience more intense orgasms than when they are not pregnant. It is natural for a pregnant woman to have more vaginal secretions, and the added lubrication may enhance the sexual pleasure of both partners. Other women feel more inhibited by feelings of unattractiveness or out of a sense of protectiveness toward their unborn. Changes in hormones, too, may increase or decrease sexual drive as can your partner's response to your new appearance.

It is helpful to realize that some fluctuation in sexual appetite normally accompanies pregnancy. Fatigue and nausea may dampen one's ardor during early pregnancy. From most accounts, sex appears most satisfactory during the second trimester when a woman is generally feeling very well. Many couples find that pregnancy encourages sexual experimentation at this time. Positions with the woman on top or entry from the side or rear are often more comfortable. During the last few months of pregnancy, sexual activity often declines as a result of increasing physical discomfort.

Many pregnant women experience a greater need for affectionate body touching as opposed to sexual intercourse. During pregnancy, as at any other time of lovemaking, it is important to communicate your concerns and needs to your partner. Otherwise, expression of a need to be touched, for example, may confuse your partner, who may infer that your behavior indicates a desire for intercourse. Satisfying sexual activity can be an experience of mutual pleasuring through a variety of means, not just genital stimulation.

Despite misconceptions that the penis can rupture the membranes or hurt the fetus, sexual activity may continue up to the time of labor in a normal pregnancy. In a woman with a history of premature labor, however, many physicians recommend abstinence during the last few months of pregnancy. Conditions causing bleeding (see Chapters 52 and 53) may also require sexual abstinence. If you have questions pertaining to sexual activity, discuss them with your clinician. If your clinician recommends abstinence, find out exactly what that means—in most situations, sexual activity outside of intercourse can continue. Mutual fondling or masturbation may relieve tension in the event that sexual intercourse is limited.

Following childbirth, it is wise to abstain for two to three weeks since the cervix remains partially open during this time, thus increasing susceptibility to infection. Episiotomy stitches vary in degree of discomfort they produce. Many women are understandably apprehensive about experiencing painful intercourse after childbirth, and this fear alone creates tension that may cause some discomfort. Exercising extra gentleness, sometimes with the aid of lubricants such as K-Y or Transi-Lube, makes intercourse more comfortable. Sometimes pain persists even though nothing is wrong. That is a signal to relax, slow down, and concentrate on enjoying pleasurable sensations that accompany each step along the way to intercourse. The postpartum period is a time of stress in general, and it is often hard for a new parent to find time to relax and enjoy sex.

If you are breast-feeding, you may find that you are more sexually stimulated. Your breasts and genitalia are apt to be more sensitive, requiring more gentleness in sexual play. Nursing also tends to decrease vaginal secretions so you may need added lubrication. Some women find the fullness of their breasts increases their sexual self-image, making them feel more erotic and sensual. A husband's sexual response to his wife's breast-feeding varies, and it is important to share these feelings with each other.

Some couples find that childbirth changes the vaginal size, resulting in decreased sexual feeling. This may result from stretching or tearing of vaginal muscles during childbirth. Special exercises can help (see Chapter 28).

For more information, read *Making Love During Pregnancy*, by Elisabeth Bing and Libby Colman (see Appendix C). This candid book covers many of the sexual feelings and fears that women commonly experience during pregnancy.

24

Sexually Transmitted Diseases

Venereal disease—infections transmitted from one person to another during intercourse or other intimate contact—is the second most common type of infection in the U.S. today, surpassed only by the common cold. In 1984, more than ten million Americans visited doctors and clinics because of venereal disease (VD). The VD epidemic is often attributed to more liberal attitudes and changing patterns of sexual behavior. Other factors include our increasing population and the development of modern contraceptive methods, which decrease the use of traditional methods (the condom and diaphragm) that offer some protection against VD. Finally, some types of VD recur despite treatment and require multiple office visits, while other forms of sexually transmitted disease cause little or no symptoms, allowing the infected person to remain unaware that he or she is passing the disease. A woman's symptoms may seem minor and not irritating enough to warrant medical attention. For this reason and because their symptoms are less noticeable than symptoms in the male, women are especially susceptible to complications of venereal infections.

In addition to the classic sexually transmitted diseases—gonorrhea and syphilis—newer forms of venereal infections have emerged. Two prominent examples, genital herpes and nongonococcal urethritis, now rival gonorrhea and syphilis as major health problems in women. Any of these four diseases, if acquired during pregnancy, may harm the fetus.

Another new disease which has received widespread public attention is AIDS, which stands for Acquired Immune Deficiency Syndrome. Although the exact cause and mode of spread is uncertain, AIDS is suspected of being a viral infection which can be sexually transmitted. Out of a total of 4,861 cases of AIDS reported to the Centers for Disease Control by June 1984, the groups at highest AIDS risk continue to be homosexual or bisexual men and intravenous drug users. Only 7% of all cases reported have involved women.

The shame, fear, or embarrassment which has surrounded VD for centuries is still present today. You may feel that only "dirty" or "immoral" people get these diseases. But an individual's social or economic status, race, religion, or creed confer no immunity against venereal disease. Even when one is "selective" about a partner, the risk of exposure to symptomless infection may be present.

In any event, there are ways to minimize the risk of getting a sexually transmitted infection. These ways include the following:

1. Avoid sexual activity if you or your partner has possible symptoms of VD (a genital rash, sore(s), or discharge) or if you or your partner is symptomless but one of you thinks you may have been exposed to a sexually transmitted infection.
2. Urinate immediately after intercourse.
3. Be choosy about your partner; your chances of acquiring VD increase if your partner has had other partners recently.
4. Use a barrier method of contraception. The condom offers the most, the diaphragm intermediate, and spermicides the least protection against VD, but all offer more than either the pill or the IUD.

In this chapter we discuss the symptoms, diagnosis, and treatment of sexually transmitted infections. Vaginal infections and skin infestations (lice and scabies), which may be transmitted sexually, are included in separate chapters (see Chapters 85 and 70).

Table 36, which appears at the end of this chapter, lists some things you should do and should not do if you think you have been exposed to a sexually transmitted disease.

For information on all aspects of VD, write for a list of current pamphlets to:

Technical Information Services
Center for Prevention Services
Centers for Disease Control
Atlanta, Georgia 30333

Table 35   EARLY SYMPTOMS OF SEXUALLY TRANSMITTED DISEASES

Disease	Symptoms in Men	Symptoms in Women
Gonorrhea	None in 10% to 15%; usually thick discharge from penis or painful urination	Often none; slight vaginal irritation, itching, or discharge; burning with urination
Nongonococcal urethritis (NGU)	May be none; slight discharge from penis or mildly painful urination; eyes, when involved, become red and irritated	Usually none; may be slight vaginal irritation, itching, or discharge; burning with urination; eyes, when involved, become red and irritated
Trichomonas vaginitis	Usually none; sometimes burning with urination	May be none; usually foul-smelling vaginal discharge with itching; burning or painful urination
Condylomata acuminata (venereal warts)	Small wartlike growths around genital area	Small wartlike growths around genital area
Genital herpes	May be none; usually painful ulcers in and around genital area	May be none; usually painful ulcers in and around genital area; painful urination
Syphilis	Painless ulcer around genital area or mouth; may be unnoticed	Painless ulcer around genital area or mouth; may be unnoticed
Parasitic skin infections: lice ("crabs"), scabies	Intense itching and sometimes rash around the pubic area	Intense itching and sometimes rash around the pubic area

or write to American Social Health Association:

VD
P.O. Box 100
Palo Alto, California 94306

Gonorrhea

Gonorrhea, the best known and most widely reported venereal infection, affects three million people annually. Gonorrhea is caused by a bacterial organism, called *Neisseria gonorrhoeae*, which thrives in a warm, moist environment, such as the mucous membranes. In women, this organism is usually found in the cervix or urethra. Rectal infections can also occur (without rectal intercourse), and gonorrhea can infect the throat of men or women after oral sexual activity with an infected person.

Symptoms

Twenty percent of women with gonorrhea have nonspecific symptoms of vaginal discharge or irritation or slight discomfort urinating. These symptoms usually occur within two to seven days after exposure. Eighty percent of women with gonorrhea, however, have no symptoms at all. In contrast, the majority of men with gonorrhea will have painful urination or a discharge from the penis. Women exposed to gonorrhea often become aware of their infection only when notified by their respective partners. Symptomless infections in both men and women (known as the *carrier* state) make this disease difficult to control. In less than three percent of individuals, gonorrhea may spread to the blood, causing fever, rash, and arthritis. The most serious complication of gonorrhea, pelvic inflammatory disease (see later in this chapter), occurs in approximately seventeen percent of women with this infection and is a major cause of sterility in women.

Diagnosis

The clinician cannot tell by examination whether or not you have gonorrhea, and there is no blood test for this infection. Sometimes a gram stain, a special slide test of cervical secretions, may suggest this diagnosis. A firm diagnosis, however, requires a laboratory technique known as a culture, in which a cotton-tipped swab is dipped into the cervix and then sent for evaluation to the pathology lab. The diagnosis is confirmed if, in twenty-four to seventy-two hours, bacterial growth of the specific gonorrhea organism is identified.

Effect in pregnancy

Gonorrhea acquired early in pregnancy slightly increases the risk of premature labor, stillbirth, and postpartum uterine infection. Also, the newborn may acquire serious eye infection if gonorrhea is present during delivery. To prevent this infection, newborns routinely receive silver nitrate eye drops after delivery. In pregnancy, most gonorrhea infections remain in the cervix and rarely spread to the uterus or tubes. This is probably due to the cervical mucus plug which acts as a barrier to infection.

Treatment

The physician treats gonorrhea by prescribing penicillin in a single injection or a one-time oral dose. If you are allergic to penicillin, the doctor will prescribe a five-day course of tetracycline. Tetracycline may have the additional advantage of curing other sexually transmitted infections such as nongonococcal urethritis (see below). Treatment is the safest approach if you suspect exposure to gonorrhea regardless of whether a positive culture is confirmed, because in a small percentage of cases the gonorrhea culture is a "false negative"—that is, for some reason the organism cannot be grown and cultured.

A gonorrhea attack confers no immunity to subsequent infection. "Ping-pong" gonorrhea—successful treatment, reinfection, and repetition of the cycle—is common. If you suspect your sexual partner may be a carrier (if symptoms or a positive culture persists after you have had treatment), encourage him to use a condom and to seek medical attention. Condoms, while not one hundred percent effective, do decrease the probability of infection. Whether or not your symptoms persist, you should obtain a repeat gonorrhea culture after treatment to make sure the infection is gone.

Syphilis ("bad blood," lues)

Syphilis occurs far less often than most other sexually transmitted diseases but is potentially the most dangerous. Left untreated, syphilis can lead to blindness, mental deficiency, or some other serious problem. Approximately 20,000 cases of syphilis are reported annually in women.

Symptoms

Symptoms of syphilis are classified into three stages. In the *primary* stage, the microorganism (*Treponema pallidum*) causing this disease causes formation of a hard, oval-shaped, painless sore known as a *chancre* (pronounced "shanker") from two to twelve weeks after exposure. If the chancre occurs in the vagina, a woman may not even notice this painless ulcer, which disappears on its own two to four weeks later. Although the majority of chancres affect the genital area, five percent occur on the lips, breasts, or mouth. If primary syphilis is untreated, *secondary* syphilis (the second stage) develops one to two months later, when the organism spreads into the bloodstream. At this time, a painless rash (often involving palms of the hands and soles of the feet), swollen lymph glands, and fever may occur. These symptoms, too, may go unnoticed and subside by themselves. During *latent* syphilis, the secondary symptoms have subsided and the only evidence of infection is a positive blood test. After one year of latent syphilis, the person is not likely to be infectious, an exception being the pregnant woman, who may infect her unborn child. The most serious stage, *tertiary* syphilis (the third stage), develops from one to twenty-five years after the secondary stage. In tertiary syphilis, serious, irreversible damage to the liver, bones, brain, heart, and other organs may occur.

Diagnosis

Syphilis, like gonorrhea, cannot be diagnosed by examination alone. The diagnosis requires laboratory tests involving either the use of a special microscopic technique (*dark-field examination*) or, more commonly, a blood test. Blood tests for syphilis include one called the VDRL (which stands for Venereal Disease Research Labs) and another called the RPR (rapid plasma reagin). These so-called *screening* tests may not become positive for up to six weeks after exposure to syphilis or for three weeks after the chancre appears; therefore, a blood test immediately after exposure to this disease may not be positive for syphilis and should be repeated several weeks later if the initial test comes back negative. The clinician orders a *specific* blood test for syphilis if you have a positive *screening* test to make sure the original test is not a "false positive"—that is, the test is positive as a result of conditions (viral infections, for example) not caused by syphilis. A scraping of the lesion (performed like a Pap smear) can immediately diagnose syphilis. However, this test requires a special dark-field microscope, which is not available in most doctors' offices.

Effect in pregnancy

Untreated syphilis in the pregnant woman may result in miscarriage, stillbirth, birth defects, or severe infection of the newborn. For this reason, clinicians routinely check the mother for syphilis at the beginning of pregnancy and sometimes in the last three months of pregnancy as well. Unlike gonorrhea and herpes, which rarely affect the newborn prior to delivery, syphilis may directly infect and damage the fetus during pregnancy, especially in the second half.

Treatment

Penicillin, the standard treatment for syphilis, is very effective in the primary and secondary stages of this disease. Penicillin treatment for syphilis requires an injection containing a special, long-acting form of this drug. It is important to realize this fact since oral forms of penicillin prescribed to treat gonorrhea may not be effective against syphilis, if you happen to have syphilis as well. For this reason, a woman treated with oral penicillin for gonorrhea should be tested six weeks later for syphilis. Anyone with primary or secondary syphilis should not have sexual intercourse for one month after receiving treatment. Condoms, while usually protective against gonorrhea, do not offer adequate protection against syphilis.

Genital Herpes

Genital herpes, now the third most common sexually transitted disease, afflicts at least 500,000 new individuals each year.

Herpes often causes severe physical problems. In addition, depressed feelings related to a sense of loss of control and anxiety from fear of transmitting herpes to a partner may lead to prominent and sometimes persistent psychological symptoms.

Herpes infections are due to viruses that may be of two types. The herpes simplex virus type I (HSV-I) generally causes cold sores or fever blisters on the lips and mouth. HSV-I is rarely acquired by sexual contact. Herpes simplex virus type II (HSV-II) generally occurs in the genital area. Although either virus strain can spread to other parts of the body, nearly ninety percent of genital herpes is due to HSV-II, which is usually acquired by sexual contact.

Genital herpes is highly contagious whenever the blisters (see below) are present, both at the time of an initial attack and at the time of a recurrence. In addition to infection by sexual transmission, the virus can spread from one area to another on the same person (autoinoculation). Fingers and eyes are especially vulnerable.

Symptoms

Genital herpes appears three to twenty days following sexual contact with an infected person. At first, one or more fluid-filled blisters form in or around the genital area and burst in two or three days, becoming extremely painful ulcers (sores). In a woman painful urination is characteristic at this time. The sores heal by themselves in two to three weeks. If herpes involves only the cervix or upper vagina, symptoms may be minimal or nonexistent. However, during the first infection, generalized symptoms usually occur, including fever and swollen lymph glands in the groin. In the absence of symptoms, the herpes virus is believed to lie dormant along the course of the affected nerve.

Some people never have recurrences, some have a few, and others have recurrences on a regular basis. A recurrence of herpes is characteristically shorter and less severe than the first attack. Some women experience burning, itching, or tingling at the place of previous infection just before the herpes sores reappear. In rare instances recurrences may involve the cervix alone and may not be apparent to a woman or her partner, but she may nevertheless be infectious. Men, too, have been noted in a few case reports to be infectious in the absence of external sores, for a day or two just prior to or following a recurrence. A variety of factors may trigger genital herpes recurrences: colds, fever, menstrual periods, emotional stress, tightfitting clothing, and vaginal infections. Sexual contact is not necessary for a recurrence.

Diagnosis

The physician usually diagnoses genital herpes during a pelvic examination by the appearance of sores. This diagnosis is not always clear-cut, however, especially after the sores begin to heal. Three tests can confirm your clinician's diagnosis: 1) a Pap smear of open sores detects cell changes characteristic of herpes 60% of the time; 2) special herpes cultures—the most accurate means of diagnosis—also require material from early, non-healed sores; and 3) blood tests can measure herpes antibodies (see glossary) and confirm previous or present HSV-II infections. Once antibodies form—about two weeks after a first-time herpes infection—they remain permanently in the blood. However, blood testing may not be particularly helpful (*unless the result is negative*), since current methods frequently don't distinguish between HSV-I and HSV-II antibodies.

Effect in pregnancy

Serious newborn infection may occur if vaginal delivery is performed during or shortly after the active stage of the disease when blisters are present (see Chapter 20).

Treatment

Unlike other sexually transmitted diseases, there is no cure for genital herpes. Present treatment of herpes aims to provide symptomatic relief and to prevent a bacterial infection from developing alongside the one caused by the herpes virus. Warm tub baths to which are added Betadine douche or solution (three tablespoonfuls) or Domeboro powder or tablets may provide relief. And you can sprinkle your underwear with cornstarch or talcum powder to keep the area dry. Your physician may prescribe a topical (applied locally) anesthetic or pain medication as well as antibiotics to prevent infection. It is important to avoid sexual activity for as long as sores persist and until they completely heal.

A new drug (acyclovir), brand-named Zovirax, has become available. This drug may lessen the intensity and duration of symptoms of herpes, but it will not prevent recurrent attacks or cure the disease.

Long-term effects of herpes

A definite increased risk of cervical cancer (see Chapter 36) exists in women who have had herpes infections. Therefore, women with a history of genital herpes should have a Pap smear every six to twelve months. Through such screening, any atypical cells (cells that do not look normal) may be detected early and easily treated.

Resources

A nonprofit service of the American Social Health Association publishes a newsletter with the latest research and other information about genital herpes. For more information, write:
Herpes Resource Center
P.O. Box 100
Palo Alto, California 94302

Nongonococcal Urethritis (Nonspecific Urethritis)

Nongonococcal urethritis (NGU) refers to several newly discovered types of sexually transmitted infections which are largely symptomless in the female and may cause mild burning on urination or a urethral discharge in the male, resembling gonorrhea—hence the term *nongonococcal urethritis*, which means inflammation of the urethra not due to gonorrhea. (In women, since the cervix rather than the urethra is the principal place affected, the term *urethritis* is somewhat misleading.) Several types of bacteria are suspected of causing NGU although only one, *Chlamydia trachomatis*, has been positively identified.

NGU is now becoming one of the most common sexually transmitted diseases. The Center for Disease Control estimates that NGU now occurs twice as often as gonorrhea. Chlamydia infection often coexists with other sexually transmitted disease and is present in the cervix in approximately forty percent of women with gonorrhea. When it spreads beyond the cervix, chlamydia infection can affect the Fallopian tubes and lead to pelvic inflammatory disease (see below).

Symptoms

NGU symptoms develop up to three or four weeks after exposure but are usually mild or nonexistent in women. Men often have mild burning with urination or a thin urethral discharge similar to a mild case of gonorrhea. Women may have mild vaginal irritation, burning, or discharge but more often a woman does not realize she is infected unless her partner mentions symptoms. NGU may affect the eyes by direct contact with an infected area and produce redness, mild itching, or irritation (conjunctivitis). Eye infection does not require sexual contact.

Diagnosis

This sexually transmitted disease is one of the most difficult to diagnose. NGU cannot be detected by pelvic exam and may be confused with other infections which produce vaginal discharge. A specific diagnosis for chlamydia requires a culture (obtained as for a gonorrhea culture); unlike other bacteria, however, the chlamydia organism is not easy to grow and takes special cell-culture techniques which are not widely available. However a simpler, quicker test ("enzyme immunoassay") is now available. The test requires a pelvic exam to obtain cells from the cervix using a cotton swab. In women with persistent vaginal discharge, NGU is considered likely whenever a slide test is negative for vaginitis (see Chapter 85) and the gonorrhea culture proves negative.

Effect in pregnancy

The fetus is not likely to be affected before delivery. During childbirth, however, direct contact of the newborn with chlamydia bacteria causes a minor eye infection nearly fifty percent of the time or pneumonia in a much smaller percentage of cases.

Treatment

The doctor treats NGU with tetracycline for one to three weeks. During pregnancy, since tetracycline is contraindicated, erythromycin is used. In women, early treatment is important to prevent spread of the disease to the ovaries and tubes. Treatment of chlamydia infection is often complicated by the fact that this infection may be misdiagnosed as or coexist with gonorrhea. In either case, penicillin, if prescribed, will not kill chlamydia organisms. For this reason, if your partner has a persistent discharge diagnosed as NGU, both of you need a course of treatment with tetracycline. You should be treated even if you have no symptoms, since over fifty percent of women exposed to men with NGU become infected. Even following appropriate tetracycline

therapy, NGU may become a recurrent problem requiring further therapy.

Pelvic Inflammatory Disease

Inflammation or infection within the tubes (salpingitis) or ovaries (oophoritis) is known as *pelvic inflammatory disease* (PID). Such an infection occurs in at least 850,000 women annually and partially explains the increasing rates of infertility and tubal pregnancy which have more than doubled in the last two decades. PID leads to sterility in approximately 60,000 young women every year. It is estimated that seventy-five percent of all pelvic inflammatory disease is initially sexually transmitted, involving a gonorrhea or chlamydia infection in most cases. At other times, PID follows infection associated with childbirth, abortion, or surgery involving the pelvic organs. More recently, intrauterine contraceptive devices (IUDs) have been associated with an increased chance of PID, especially in a woman with a prior history of tubal infection.

PID usually starts with a cervical gonorrhea infection which then spreads into the uterine cavity and extends into the tubes (see Figure 25). Pus formation may remain in the tubes or extend to the ovaries. The result is adhesions and scar tissue within and around the tubes (see Figure 26). When infection is severe or inadequately treated, the chances for permanent tubal damage and sterility increase.

Not all infections respond to the initial antibiotic treatment; sometimes stronger drugs requiring hospitalization are needed. If the initial attack of PID is not controlled, chronic infection may develop with recurrent episodes of pain and infection not necessarily brought on by sexual activity. The development of chronic PID seriously threatens a woman's childbearing potential as the chance of infertility doubles with each new attack.

Symptoms

Pelvic inflammatory disease, even in its early stages, can make a woman acutely ill with symptoms of low abdominal (pelvic) pain, vaginal discharge, and fever. Pelvic pain is moderate to severe and frequently occurs within one week of a menstrual period. Infection often follows the menstrual period, a time when the cervix dilates and facilitates passage of gonorrhea and other bacteria from the cervix into the uterine cavity.

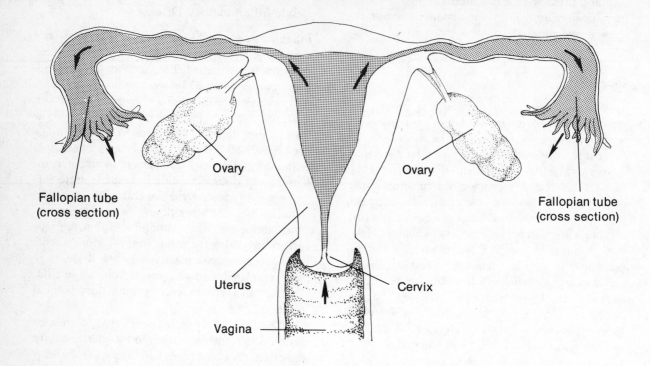

Figure 25   *Pathways of pelvic infection. Gonorrhea and other types of VD can cause tubal infections (pelvic inflammatory disease).*

Diagnosis

The clinician usually diagnoses PID by pelvic exam. Few specific diagnostic tests are available, aside from a culture of the cervix, which reveals gonorrhea up to fifty percent of the time. The physician can, however, confirm or rule out a diagnosis of PID by laparoscopy (see glossary).

Treatment

In its earlier stages, physicians successfully treat PID with oral antibiotics. In more advanced cases, the doctor may hospitalize you in order to give the antibiotics by IV (that is, intravenously), which allows higher blood levels of these drugs. Only if you have recurrent bouts of PID that are unresponsive to medical treatment, or a pelvic mass indicating abscess formation, will you require surgery. If the infection is localized, the surgeon may need to remove only the affected tube and ovary. Frequently, especially if both tubes are affected, removal of tubes, ovaries, and uterus is the only means of definitive treatment.

Effect in pregnancy

PID is a major cause of ectopic (tubal) pregnancies (see Chapter 81). Tubal scarring from previous infection makes a woman more susceptible to this complication of early pregnancy. Thus, ectopic pregnancy is at least twenty times more common in women with a history of tubal infections. However, during a normally progressing pregnancy, acute attacks of pelvic infection rarely occur, partly because of the mucus plug which acts as a barrier to infection.

Venereal Warts (Condylomata Acuminata)

Venereal warts, small growths caused by the papilloma virus, commonly accompany other sexually transmitted infections, such as gonorrhea. The incubation period for condylomata is much longer than for most other sexually acquired infections, averaging one to three months or more. Two-thirds of the women who come into direct contact with venereal warts contract this disease.

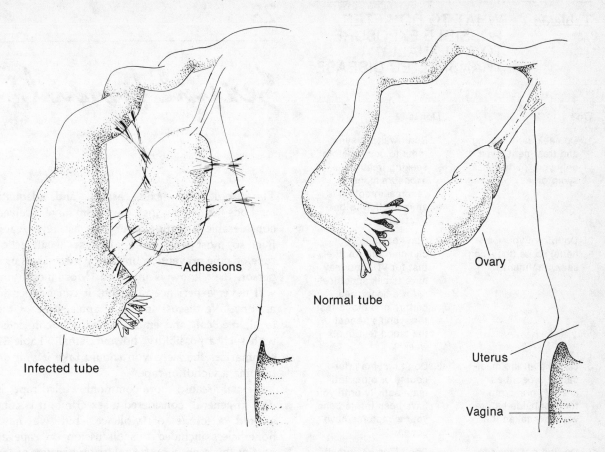

Figure 26 *The left tube shows signs of infection, swelling, and adhesions to the ovary. The right tube and ovary are normal.*

Symptoms

Venereal warts are painless, fleshy growths, often no larger than the tip of a pencil. When in clusters, these warts give a cauliflower appearance. They are symptomless aside from occasional mild irritation or itching.

Diagnosis

Diagnosis is based on the appearance of these growths. Because of the possibility of confusing them with syphilitic lesions, your clinician may order a blood test for syphilis. Biopsy to confirm the diagnosis of condylomata is rarely necessary. You should, however, have a vaginal slide and culture tests for trichomonas and gonorrhea since these infections often occur simultaneously with condylomata.

Effect in pregnancy

In pregnancy, venereal warts tend to grow in size, bleed, or become infected. In rare cases, they may block the birth canal, making a cesarean section inevitable. There have been case reports of condylomata growths on the newborn's larynx, but otherwise no adverse effect on the infant has been noted.

Don't take podophyllin treatments (described below) during pregnancy because they may harm the newborn.

Treatment

The clinician treats these growths in the office by applying a chemical called podophyllin around the affected area. Occasionally several treatments may be necessary. You should apply petroleum jelly to the skin around the edge of the area to be treated because podophyllin is caustic to normal skin. To prevent burns wash off the podophyllin in a warm bath four to six hours after application by the clinician. The warts usually go away within two weeks. After treatment, warm tub baths followed by dusting with cornstarch may help get rid of the warts faster by keeping the area dry. Until the warts

Table 36

WHAT TO DO AFTER POSSIBLE EXPOSURE TO A SEXUALLY TRANSMITTED DISEASE

Do's	Don'ts
1. Do seek early testing and treatment (even if only your partner has symptoms).	1. Don't wait for symptoms to occur before seeking treatment—*exposure* alone to venereal infection is an indication to be treated.
2. Do inform your partner(s) so he (they) can seek treatment.	2. Don't assume your clinician will routinely test for VD. You may have to ask specifically for a gonorrhea culture or a blood test for syphilis (repeat the blood test in six weeks).
3. Do take all the medication prescribed even if your symptoms subside before you have taken it all.	3. Don't resume intercourse or other intimate activity until you have been treated and your symptoms have gone.
4. Do find out when to return for a follow-up visit to be sure you have been cured.	4. Don't blame yourself; sexually transmitted infection may produce little or no warning symptoms in either partner.

disappear you are better off not wearing girdles, pantyhose, or nylon-crotch underpants and not swimming or having sexual intercourse. When venereal warts persist or recur despite podophyllin treatment, the doctor may excise them surgically or use cryosurgery (see glossary).

Recently laser surgery (see Chapter 36) has been used successfully to remove venereal warts from the vulva in patients who don't respond to other methods of treatment. The laser may be especially useful when large amounts of condylomata are present or in pregnancy when podophyllin is contraindicated.

Sexual Assault

The problem of sexual assault and adequate methods for helping the rape victim have received considerable attention over the last few years. Even so, most people do not discuss the subject of rape or rape prevention until they themselves or a person they know is involved. Most likely you will never experience rape, but it can happen to anyone. We discuss in this chapter some of the legal, medical, and emotional aspects connected with such a possibility, however small. Table 37 summarizes the steps you should take if you do become a victim of rape.

Sexual assault, more commonly called rape, is not, in general, considered a sex crime; it is considered a crime of violence. But we have nonetheless included this discussion on rape as part of this section on sexual issues because of the related problems—the possibility of venereal disease and pregnancy—and because for many women there exists a real concern that needs to be dealt with.

Most communities have a twenty-four-hour crisis hot line, with people available who can advise you about obtaining medical care and about the police procedures involved in reporting rape. Write down, in a place where you can quickly find it, the telephone number of the nearest rape or other crisis center in case you ever need it.

Legal Aspects

If you are raped and you decide to press charges, you will need medical evidence to show that you were raped. You do not have to make the decision to press charges immediately, however. Have an examination by a physician trained to treat rape victims. This procedure is an involved one, not so much medically as legally, in order to adequately prepare medical findings for evidence at a later date. Legally, all evidence can be obtained only by a physician, as opposed to a nurse practitioner or another care provider.

Whether or not to bring charges against the attacker is your decision. The attack may be reported anonymously through your rape crisis center. Pressing charges in person is a lengthy process, and some women feel it is too traumatic emotionally. Women who do press charges against their attacker frequently do so on the basis that charging him with assault may prevent him from attacking again.

Unfortunately, rape is the only crime in our society in which the victim may be dealt with as if she were an accessory. Police officers or examining personnel may act as if you somehow "provoked" the rape. In general, people react uncomfortably toward rape victims, and this uneasiness may make your immediate medical examination more difficult. It is helpful to have a supportive person with you during this time.

Medical Care

If you have physical injuries, the physician will care for these injuries first. All injuries, no matter how slight, will be recorded. A pelvic examination is performed to search for evidence of recent trauma or intercourse and to test for gonorrhea, which may be detected in semen. Since evidence of sperm disappears from your cervix in approximately eight to ten hours, have your pelvic exam done as soon as possible. The vaginal secretions are tested for sperm cells as well as acid phosphatase, a substance produced by the male prostate gland.

The physician also checks for possible physical evidence, including hairs, bits of skin, dirt, blood, or grass stains on your clothing, under your fingernails, or on any other part of your body. (Because you may be feeling very vulnerable after a rape, this meticulous physical exam can be upsetting.) Your pelvic hair may be combed to further search for evidence of your attacker. Each piece of evidence will be labeled and sealed, in case you decide to press charges.

The risk of sexually transmitted disease (VD) is relatively high after rape, and you will be tested and possibly treated for gonorrhea and syphilis. Because these diseases cannot be completely ruled out immediately, you should return for repeat tests—in two weeks for a gonorrhea test and in six to eight weeks for a syphilis test. A follow-up exam at the time of the syphilis test is also advisable to check for the presence of the other venereal diseases that may not show up until then.

The chance of pregnancy occurring as a result of rape is small. You will be given a pregnancy test to determine if you are already pregnant. If not, you may want to consider using the "morning-after" pill, which prevents conception when taken within seventy-two hours after intercourse (see Chapter 9). You should have a repeat pregnancy test at six to eight weeks, perhaps at the time of the follow-up exam mentioned above. Also, if you do not take the "morning-after" pill, you should avoid intercourse (or use some form of birth control) until you know this repeat pregnancy test is negative.

Emotional Reactions

Most attackers use a weapon to force their victims to submit to rape. When faced with the threat of possible death, most women feel they have no

---

Table 37   WHAT TO DO IF YOU ARE A RAPE VICTIM

1. Call someone close to you. This isn't a time to be alone.

2. Don't take a shower or bath, don't douche, and don't change clothes until after you have been examined by a physician, even though you may want to.

3. Call the nearest rape crisis center. They can help you through the next few hours *in a way no one else can.*

4. Go with your friend and perhaps someone from the rape crisis center to the nearest medical facility that handles rape victims. Bring extra clothing in case your clothing may be needed as evidence.

5. Don't feel you must decide now whether you will press charges. Take every legal precaution so that you can take legal action later if you decide to do so. You can report the rape immediately to the police and decide later if you want to press charges. Or you can have the rape crisis center report the rape, with or without using your name.

6. Return to a physician or medical facility for follow-up VD and pregnancy tests.

---

choice but to submit in order to stay alive. After it is over, you may feel both shock and relief for having survived this act of violence.

Later you may find yourself feeling depressed, angry, and helpless. Some women, for weeks or months, deny it ever happened, but eventually the anger surfaces. You may feel ashamed, used, and bitter that this attack happened to you. Most women have the inner strength to work through the crisis of rape. It will help if you can acknowledge these feelings gradually and talk with a few close friends about what happened. Use a rape crisis center if available. Seek competent professional counseling if possible. The long-term psychological impact of rape should not be underestimated, especially when it involves a child or it is an initial sexual experience. A rape experience can be an underlying cause of sexual problems in later life.

Rape Prevention

Many communities have rape prevention classes or lectures sponsored by the community, a women's center, or a local service organization. If you do not have access to such a service or you do not wish to attend, here are some things you can do to minimize the risk of rape.

1. *In your car:* Keep your doors locked at all times, even if you are leaving your car for only a short time. If you have car trouble and must stay with your car (as on a limited access highway), raise your hood, get into your car, lock your doors, and wait for the police; it's usually safer not to accept help from a stranger. At night park in well-lighted areas. When you approach your parked car, have the key in your hand and look around and inside the car before you get in. Don't pick up hitchhikers.

2. *At home:* Keep your doors locked (and, when possible, use a deadbolt) at all times even if you leave for just a moment. If possible, use a 180-degree peephole on your entry door; and avoid letting in anyone you don't know or aren't expecting (for example, service repairmen). Use initials rather than your first name on your mailbox and in the telephone directory.

3. *On the telephone:* Avoid giving out personal information or confirming your telephone number to someone you don't know. Report any obscene telephone calls you receive to the telephone company and any personal threats you receive to the police.

4. *Out-of-doors:* Avoid walking or jogging alone at night; if you do, follow well-lighted, well-traveled routes. Carry protective items such as mace, where State laws permit, and a whistle. Avoid conversation with strangers even to give directions, especially if you are in a position where you could be cornered. Don't hitchhike. Don't accept rides from strangers. If you frequent recreational places alone or with other women, especially at night, be careful who you leave the place with.

How to Help a Friend Who Has Been Raped

When you know someone close to you has been raped, you will undoubtedly want to help her. The best kind of support you can give is the same as if she were the victim of any other kind of crisis. You can play an important role by providing the reassurance and support she needs. You can help by encouraging her to seek medical care and remaining with her, if she prefers, throughout the entire examination procedure. If you can, encourage her to talk about her feelings, but only after she is ready to do so. Sometimes a rape victim is afraid to talk about the attack for fear her family or friends will change their attitudes toward her. She may blame herself and think of what she could have done to prevent it. But this is not the time to reproach or reprimand her, which may reinforce her own self doubts. Perhaps the best help you can give her is to see that she gets competent medical care and to reassure her that it *is* possible to survive such a traumatic event.

Resources

For further information about rape, write to:

National Center for the Prevention and Control of Rape
5600 Fishers Lane, Room 15-99
Rockville, Maryland 20857

References for Section Five

Chapter 22—Female Sexuality

Osofsky, H. J., et al. Gynecologic aspects of sexual

dysfunction. *The Female Patient* 9(2):100-109, Feb 1984.

Sandler, J., Myerson, M., and Kinder, B. *Human Sexuality: Current Perspectives.* Tampa, Florida: Mariner Publishing Co., Inc., 1980.

Kaplan, H. S. *The New Sex Therapy.* New York: Brunner/Mazel, 1974.

Kaplan, H. S. *Disorders of Sexual Desire and Other New Concepts and Techniques of Sex Therapy.* New York: Brunner/Mazel, 1979.

Teeters, C. *Women's Sexuality - Myth and Reality.* San Jose, Calif.: Women, Inc., 1977.

LoPiccolo, J., and LoPiccolo, L. (eds.). *Handbook of Sex Therapy.* New York: Plenum, 1978.

Masters, W. H., and Johnson, V. E. *Human Sexual Response.* Boston: Little, Brown, 1966.

Chapter 23—Sexuality and Pregnancy

Sandler, J., Myerson, M., and Kinder, B. *Human Sexuality: Current Perspectives,* Ch. 7, 90–92. Tampa, Florida: Mariner Publishing Co., Inc., 1980.

Naeye, R. L. Coitus and associated amniotic fluid infections. *New England Journal of Medicine* 301(22):1198–1200, 1979.

Kyndely, K. The sexuality of women in pregnancy and postpartum: a review. *Journal of Obstetrics and Gynecological Nursing* 7:28–32, Jan/Feb 1978.

Wales, E: The impact of childbirth on sexual functioning. *The Female Patient* 44–51, Sep 1979.

Chapter 24—Sexually Transmitted Diseases

Jacob, A. J., et al. Genital herpes infection in pregnant women near term. *Obstetrics and Gynecology* 64(4):480-484, 1984.

Reichman, R. C., et al. Treatment of recurrent genital herpes simplex infections with oral acyclovir. *Journal of the American Medical Association* 251(16):2103-2107, Apr 1984.

Harger, J. H., et al. Characteristics and management of pregnancy in women with genital herpes simplex virus infection. *American Journal of Obstetrics and Gynecology* 145:784-791, 1983.

Straus, S. E., et al. Suppression of frequently recurring genital herpes: a placebo-controlled double-blind trial of oral acyclovir. *The New England Journal of Medicine* 310:1545-1550, 1984.

Washington, A. E., et al. Hospitalizations for pelvic inflammatory disease: epidemiology and trends in the United States, 1975-1981. *The Journal of the American Medical Association* 251:2529-2533, 1984.

Noble, R. C. *Sexually Transmitted Diseases - Guide to Diagnosis and Therapy.* New York: Medical Examination Publishing Co., 1979.

Luger, N. M. Spotting and treating "the other" sexually transmitted diseases. *Modern Medicine* 47–52, Jan 30, 1978.

Blough, H. A., and Guintoli, R. L. Successful treatment of human genital herpes infections with 2-deoxy-d-glucose, *Journal of the American Medical Association* 241:2798–2801, 1979.

Adam, E., Kaufman, R., et al. Persistence of virus shedding in asymptomatic women after recovery from herpes genitalis. *Obstetrics and Gynecology* 54(2):171–173, 1979.

Wilbanks, G. D. How to diagnose and treat genital herpes. *Contemporary OB/GYN* 16:81–85, Aug 1980.

Committee on Technical Bulletins of the American College of Obstetricians and Gynecologists: Sexually Transmitted Diseases Other Than Gonorrhea and Syphilis, Technical Bulletin #51, 1978, American College of Obstetricians and Gynecologists, Washington, D.C.

Washington, A. E., and Morton, R. S. Nongonococcal urethritis. *Current Prescribing* 35–41, Oct 1979.

Rakel, R., Candib, L., et al. Forum highlights: vaginal infections. *The Female Patient* 21-29, Apr 1981.

Sexually transmitted diseases. *The Harvard Medical School Health Letter* 6(6):1–2, 1981.

McCormack, W. M., et al. Sexually transmitted conditions among women college students. *American Journal of Obstetrics and Gynecology* 139(2):130–133, Jan 1981.

Chapter 25—Sexual Assault

Sandler, J., Myerson, M., and Kinder, B. *Human Sexuality: Current Perspectives,* Ch. 13, 167–169. Tampa, Florida: Mariner Publishing Co., Inc., 1980.

Brownmiller, S. *Against Our Will—Men, Women, and Rape.* New York: Simon and Schuster, 1975.

Boston Women's Health Book Collective: *Our Bodies, Ourselves,* Ch. 8. New York: Simon and Schuster, 1976.

Bode, J. *Fighting Back - How to Cope With the Medical, Emotional and Legal Consequences of Rape.* New York: Macmillan, 1978.

Ipema, D. K. Rape - the process of recovery. *Nursing Research* 28(5):272–275, 1979.

Sexual Assault. Office of the Attorney General, Tallahassee, Florida: Jun 1977.

168

six

Health Concerns During and After Menopause

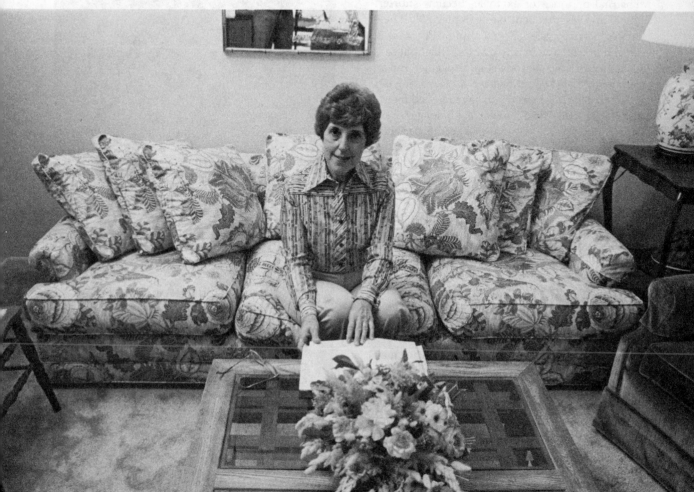

Menopause

Menopause marks the time in a woman's life when menstrual periods cease. The hormone changes that occur at this time and the symptoms that may be produced as a result are discussed in this chapter. Elsewhere in this book we have touched upon other medical concerns of the middle-aged and older woman that are not related to the menopause.

Although the average age for menopause is fifty-one, menopause may occur anywhere between ages forty-one and fifty-five. For several years before menopause, hormone levels gradually decline, causing changes throughout your body. Menstrual periods, for example, become shorter, lighter, and less frequent (see Chapter 76). These changes in your cycle reflect a gradual decrease in estrogen production by the ovaries. Menopause is reached once your periods stop altogether for an entire year. It is helpful to keep a record of your periods to determine when you have reached menopause. After this time, you can no longer have children but you can continue to lead a perfectly normal life sexually and in every other way.

Menopause and Midlife Crisis

The end of the reproductive period constitutes a crucial developmental step in the life cycle of many women. During this period of time a woman may experience a so-called midlife crisis and become preoccupied with aging or serious illness despite the fact that at this time she has about thirty percent of her life span ahead of her. During this time, too, women may feel "caught between generations"—between their children who may still need their help and their own parents who may increasingly depend upon them.

Social and cultural factors may also contribute to problems experienced during menopause. Our society's preoccupation with youth and childbear-

ing helps condition women to expect menopause to be a time of crisis or depression. The woman who has dedicated her life to bearing and caring for children may feel hardest hit by the menopause and be the most vulnerable to depression when her children grow up and leave home. The woman who has enjoyed her children but now is glad to have time for her own interests may not be as concerned with the onset of menopause. Actually, some women feel relieved when they are sure of avoiding pregnancy and the nuisance of a monthly period.

Symptoms of Menopause

The range and intensity of emotional responses and physical signs associated with the climacteric (the several years before menopause) vary tremendously. Although many women experience depression, others are hardly affected. It is worth noting

Photograph by Joanne Swanson.

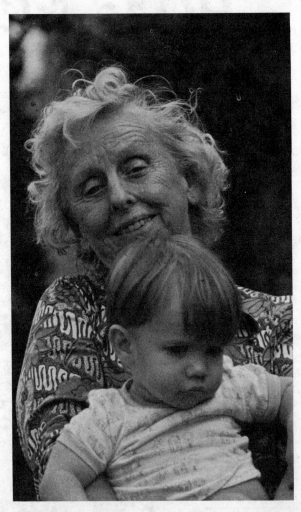

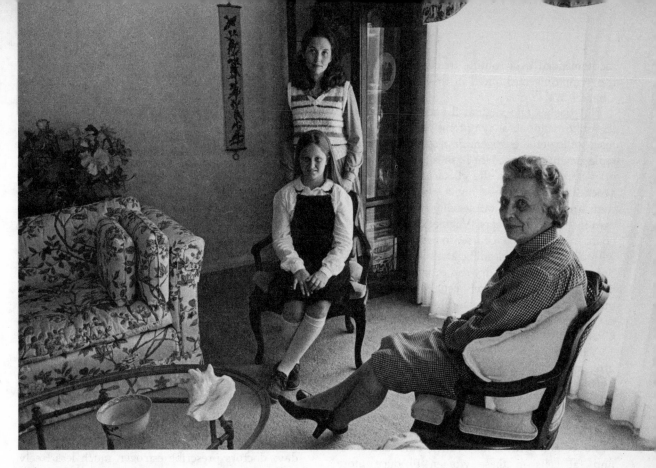

that the frequency of severe depression requiring psychiatric treatment is not higher for menopausal women than for other age groups. Loss of sleep and the fatigue associated with menopausal symptoms such as hot flashes is sufficient reason for a mild case of the blues in many people. How you react depends somewhat upon the way you have coped with change in the past and perhaps upon your mother's menopausal experience. If you do have bouts of depression, it is reassuring to note that most women experience an increased sense of emotional well-being as the physical symptoms of menopause diminish. Sharing your feelings with friends can often greatly reduce your concerns about the normal symptoms accompanying menopause and aging.

Most women have very little difficulty with hot flashes and other menopausal symptoms. In fact, 50% of all women undergoing menopause have little in the way of symptoms aside from cessation of menses. Symptoms are more pronounced if menopause occurs abruptly (for example, as a result of surgery) as opposed to gradually over a period of one to two years. If hot flashes or other symptoms are present, they often last only a few months while the body adjusts to lower estrogen levels. Declining estrogen levels cause physical changes—muscles lose some strength and tone, the bones become more brittle, and there is a loss of elasticity of tissue, including the tissue of the genitalia. Vaginal lubrication may decrease noticeably, and the vaginal tissue becomes thinner and more susceptible to irritation or infection. These gradual changes vary in severity, depending on the individual woman. Painful intercourse may be lessened by the use of water-soluble vaginal lubricants (such as K-Y lubricating jelly) and regular sexual activity. Painful and/or frequent urination is also a common experience in postmenopausal women. This condition is not caused by an infection but by changes in the urinary system as part of the aging process.

Only about 15% of menopausal women have symptoms severe enough to require treatment. The many nonspecific symptoms accompanying or preceding menopause include headaches, skin changes, insomnia, irritability, depression, palpitations, and fatigue. None of these symptoms is due strictly to hormone changes (low estrogen). The cause is probably a combination of psychological stress, poorly understood hormonal changes, and the aging process itself. Estrogens are *not* recommended as a routine treatment for any of the symptoms mentioned in this paragraph (see Chapter 27).

Hot flashes and vaginal dryness or irritation, the only menopausal symptoms that are a direct result of lowered estrogen, *do* respond to estrogen replacement therapy. Hot flashes (see Chapter 68) may appear early in the climacteric along with generalized sweating at night; these two symptoms are self-limited and usually subside on their own in one to two years. Vaginal dryness can account for painful intercourse, sometimes associated with discharge or bleeding after sexual activity. Symptoms of vaginal dryness or irritation related to lowered estrogen levels usually do not occur until after the menopause and, unlike hot flashes, may persist and require periodic treatment (see Chapter 27).

Various hormone tests obtained during and after menopause show that not all women have a decline in estrogen below normal levels. Even after the age of sixty, up to 10% of women maintain normal or near-normal levels of estrogens. This maintenance of a normal estrogen level occurs in some women because the ovaries, adrenal glands, and fat cells in these women produce more estrogen than usual for reasons not understood. This individuality in body chemistry explains some of the variation in menopausal symptoms among different women.

Tests for the Menopause

Sometimes a woman experiencing hot flashes or lighter, less frequent periods wants to know whether or not she is approaching menopause. The most accurate way to answer this question is by a blood test to measure the brain hormones FSH and LH (see glossary). These hormones indirectly reflect the amount of estrogen produced by the ovaries. This test confirms if you have reached menopause and no longer need to use contraception. Other blood tests to measure estrogen levels directly are less reliable since estrogen blood levels can vary widely each day. The *maturation index* is the simplest and least costly way to evaluate estrogen levels. The maturation index evaluates vaginal cells to determine your estrogen level. The cells are obtained like a Pap smear at the time of a pelvic exam. This test, too, is much less accurate than FSH in determining whether you have reached menopause.

27

Estrogen Replacement Therapy

The practice of prescribing estrogen-containing drugs to replace the amount of estrogen no longer being supplied by the ovaries at and after menopause is known as *estrogen replacement therapy* (ERT). In the past, physicians frequently prescribed estrogen to relieve any menopausal symptom. Today, doctors prescribe estrogen much less freely than they did just a few years ago. Long-term estrogen therapy, once heralded as the answer to the so-called empty nest syndrome and the midlife crisis, has been almost completely abandoned. Reports of serious adverse effects, including uterine cancer, associated with years of ERT have produced widespread concern among women. Women now know better than to take estrogen without solid medical indications.

This chapter provides a summary on the controversial question of estrogen replacement therapy. In order to present the information as objectively as possible, we have tried to avoid taking sides on the subject of ERT since generalizations may oversimplify issues or may not apply to the needs of individual women. After reading this chapter, you will be able to weigh the pros and cons and can then decide for yourself.

When to Use Estrogen

Recent evidence linking prolonged use of estrogens* to uterine cancer (see Chapter 39) has led,

---

Not the combination of estrogen and progesterone as found in most birth control pills. Birth control pills have not been associated with uterine cancer.

more than any other factor, to increasingly restricted use of estrogen replacement therapy. In light of this concern, many women want to know when the benefits of ERT may outweigh the risks. It is worth remembering that most recent studies confirm a definite increased risk of uterine cancer only when estrogen is used *for two years or more*.

There are three FDA-accepted indications for ERT in menopausal women: treatment of hot flashes, treatment for symptoms of vaginal atrophy, and prevention of osteoporosis.

Hot flashes

Although hot flashes are not life threatening, they may be weakening to some women, producing secondary symptoms such as insomnia. Treatment of moderate to severe hot flashes and/or night sweats should include periodic attempts to decrease and gradually discontinue ERT within one to two years. Although estrogens do relieve these symptoms, hot flashes subside on their own in most women in a matter of months.

Vaginal atrophy

Vaginal atrophy refers to thinning of the vulvar and vaginal tissue which may become easily irritated and susceptible to vaginal infection (see Chapter 85, on atrophic vaginitis). As a result of these changes, painful intercourse or bleeding after intercourse may occur. When symptoms of vaginal atrophy occur in the absence of hot flashes, use estrogen creams rather than pills so that a smaller amount of the drug will be absorbed. Estrogen treatment can reverse the symptoms of vaginal atrophy.

Osteoporosis

Osteoporosis, which results in progressive degeneration of the spine, occurs in approximately 50% of postmenopausal women, many of whom may then develop fractures of the backbone or hip with increasing age. Osteoporosis eventually produces nonradiating low back pain (see Chapters 46 and 49), curvature of the spine, and diminished height. The FDA classifies estrogens as "probably effective" in the prevention of osteoporosis. Several recent studies have concluded that estrogen therapy, when given at the beginning of menopause, can slow osteoporosis. A

1984 NIH panel agreed that cyclic estrogen therapy, preferably in combination with progesterone, currently represents the most effective single modality for preventing osteoporosis in women. Once this disease has begun, however, ERT will not reverse the condition.

In addition to estrogen, regular weight-bearing exercise and a well-balanced diet containing sufficient calcium and vitamin D are also considered important measures for controlling osteoporosis. Two to three glasses of vitamin D–enriched milk per day are recommended for women over forty. Women at greater risk for developing osteoporosis—thin, white women as well as those with a family history of this disease, a sedentary life style, or a diet low in calcium—should also take a calcium supplement to maintain positive calcium balance and develop as much bone density as possible before menopause. Most women need some calcium supplementation, since dietary needs for calcium—about 1,000 milligrams for women before menopause and 1,200–1,500 milligrams daily after menopause—are unmet by the average American dietary intake of about 500 milligrams per day. Many bone specialists recommend a form of calcium carbonate (for example, OsCal or its generic equivalent).

Present studies suggest but do not prove that estrogen therapy prevents osteoporosis-related fractures. Nevertheless, many authorities now consider prevention of osteoporosis the primary reason for the menopausal woman to use estrogen. Those who favor ERT note that mortality from hip fractures (which are often osteoporosis-related) greatly exceeds mortality due to uterine cancer. Several tests which measure bone density are being investigated to identify women at risk for developing osteoporosis. Although no single screening test has reached widespread acceptance, a technique called photon absorptiometry (see glossary) appears promising and can be performed in an office setting.

Premature or surgical menopause

In addition to the three conditions above, a woman who has experienced premature menopause (before age forty) or surgical menopause (removal of the ovaries) also may need estrogen therapy. Following removal of the ovaries in women under the age of forty, estrogen replacement therapy is particularly recommended because estrogen delays or minimizes the increased risk of heart disease in the young woman whose ovaries have been surgically removed. This protective effect does not work for postmenopausal women. Controversy exists as to the appropriate length of time for which estrogen should be prescribed following premature menopause or surgical menopause before age forty. In order to obtain the beneficial effects unique to these circumstances, most clinicians prescribe ERT at least until a woman reaches her forties, and some physicians recommend estrogen therapy to age fifty, especially in a woman who has had a hysterectomy.

Contraindications to ERT—
When to Avoid Taking Estrogen

Avoid estrogen use for treatment of menopausal symptoms if any of the following conditions apply to you:

1. You have a previous history of blood clots associated with estrogen use (including estrogen in birth control pills). Blood clots that you previously had include any that occurred in the leg (thrombophlebitis), in the lung (pulmonary embolus), in the brain (stroke or cerebrovascular accident—called a CVA), or in the heart (heart attack or coronary thrombosis). A history of blood clots *unrelated* to taking estrogens is not an absolute contraindication to ERT (that is, such a history does not mean you absolutely cannot have ERT) but rather an indication to use caution and to discuss your previous condition fully with your doctor before starting to take estrogen. Confusion exists here because birth control pills—a more potent form of estrogen—have been linked to an increased risk of blood clots, a history of which *is* an absolute contraindication to taking birth control pills. But estrogen use to treat menopause symptoms is not known at this time to cause blood clots, heart attacks, or strokes, perhaps because the dosage of estrogen in ERT is less than that in birth control pills. Some doctors believe, however, that future studies will show that ERT does cause blood clotting disorders in a tiny percentage of cases.

2. You *presently* have a condition involving a blood clot in the leg (thrombophlebitis) or elsewhere in the body.

3. You are pregnant or you may be pregnant. Estrogen may cause birth defects especially when taken in early pregnancy.

4. You have a history of breast or uterine cancer. There have been reports that in special circumstances the growth of *already-established* cancers of this type may be stimulated by estrogen. There is presently no clear evidence showing that estrogen *causes* breast cancer. However, estrogen's role in causing uterine cancer in some women is clear. The relationship between long-term estrogen therapy and a possible increased risk of *developing* uterine cancer is discussed in Chapter 39.

5. You have unexplained or abnormal vaginal bleeding.

Precautions About the Use of ERT—
Possible Reasons to Avoid Taking Estrogen

Some conditions, while not absolute reasons to avoid estrogens, are likely to be made worse by taking this drug. Estrogen may stimulate the growth of *uterine fibroids* and produce symptoms of heavy menstrual bleeding or cramping. When these things happen and then ERT is stopped, symptoms, including fibroid growth, usually subside without the need for surgery. *Jaundice* is also more likely to develop especially when estrogen is taken by a woman with a history of liver disease. *Gallbladder problems*, too, are more frequent. One study indicates a twofold to threefold increased risk of surgically confirmed gallbladder disease in women on ERT. Estrogens, by increasing fluid retention, may worsen or increase recurrences of certain conditions, such as *migraine headaches*, *epilepsy*, or *heart disease*, the control of which is dependent upon preventing excessive fluid accumulation in certain parts of the body.

Estrogen is suspected, but not proven, to have a worsening effect on certain conditions, such as *high blood pressure* and *diabetes*. You may have to increase the dose of medication you take for these conditions if you also take estrogen. In addition, if you have risk factors for breast or uterine cancer (see Chapters 33 and 39), use particular caution about taking estrogen; discuss the situation with your doctor before deciding on ERT.

Side Effects of ERT

The most common side effects of ERT are nausea, breast tenderness, and fluid retention. Infrequent effects which you should report to your doctor include vomiting, headaches, depression, pigmentation of facial skin, loss of hair, hair growth, skin rash, breast secretions, and intolerance to contact lenses. Also, be sure to notify your clinician of any abnormal or unscheduled vaginal spotting or bleeding.

Some women normally experience a period each month two to three days following the last estrogen pill (or the last progesterone pill in the case of combined estrogen and progesterone treatment). It is abnormal, however, to have spotting or bleeding during the days when the pills are taken; this condition is sometimes called breakthrough bleeding (see glossary) and may require a change in estrogen dosage. Any such abnormal bleeding should be evaluated by your physician. Abnormal bleeding in a woman over forty is best investigated either by endometrial biopsy (an office procedure; see glossary) or by dilatation and curettage (D & C; see glossary).

Different Types of Estrogen

The particular estrogen drug prescribed matters little since all estrogens act in the same way. But the dosage and duration of estrogen use can be very important both in reducing side effects and in practically eliminating the risk of developing uterine cancer. The smallest dose, used for the shortest period of time necessary to relieve symptoms, is recommended. In the case of Premarin, for example, the low dosage forms—0.3 or 0.625 mg as opposed to 1.25 or 2.5 mg—might be used just for six to twelve months and then stopped to see if the symptoms no longer persist.

Many authorities now recommend the use of estrogens in combination with a progesterone drug such as Provera, Amen, Norlutin, or Norlutate. Recent research shows that taking progesterone during the second half of each month may decrease the risk of uterine cancer from ERT. It is believed this protective effect is due to progesterone's ability to counteract estrogen and prevent estrogen "overstimulation" of the uterine lining. Such overstimulation, when prolonged over a period of years, may be an important factor in the subsequent development of uterine cancer.

The same precautions that apply to oral estrogen (pills taken by mouth) apply to injectable hormone shots which contain estrogen and to estrogen creams. Injectable estrogen offers no advantages over oral forms, is more likely to produce irregular bleeding, and may be more costly. Estrogen creams (see Table 102) may be used instead of pill forms in some women with symptoms of vaginal itching or irritation (atrophic vaginitis) associated with estrogen deficiency (see Chapter 85). Some forms of estrogen contain tranquilizers and should be used with caution and awareness of potential sedative side effects. Other estrogen preparations contain small amounts of the male sex hormone testosterone, which may cause hair growth or hoarseness in some women. Among unproven theories for taking testosterone-containing drugs is that they provide "get up and go" and increased sexual drive.

Table 38 summarizes the common estrogen preparations used in ERT.

While estrogen use has been more restricted in the past five years, certain women will need and benefit from estrogen (and possibly progesterone) therapy. Certainly women who have had hysterectomies and women for whom low-dose, short-term estrogen therapy is prescribed have the least risk. The risks must be compared to the expected benefits if you have severe symptoms which affect the quality of your life. You should avoid the use of estrogen for nonspecific menopausal symptoms such as depression, fatigue, headaches, or age-related changes in the skin, hair, and breasts. Estrogen is of no benefit for these particular symptoms. Remember there is no medical evidence that estrogen slows the aging process. Although certain menopausal symptoms may be relieved by ERT, thus helping you adjust more easily to what may be a difficult time in life, menopause itself is no longer an indication for estrogen. Consult your physician about the risks and benefits, but remember: the decision is ultimately yours to make, after you carefully consider both sides.

Table 39 gives the answers to some common questions about estrogens.

Table 38   COMMON BRANDS OF ORAL ESTROGEN-CONTAINING DRUGS

Plain Estrogen	Estrogen Products Containing Testosterone	Estrogen Products Containing a Tranquilizer
Estinyl	Estratest	Menrium
Estrace	Mediatric	Milprem
Estratab	Premarin with Methyltestosterone	PMB
Estrocon		
Evex		
Menest		
Ogen		
Premarin		

Table 39   QUESTIONS COMMONLY ASKED ABOUT ESTROGENS

Question	Yes	No	Comment
Are the estrogens commonly prescribed for hot flashes as strong as estrogens in birth control pills?		X	They are much less potent.
Are estrogens used in treating the menopause associated, like birth control pills, with blood clots, heart attacks, or stroke?		X	Estrogens used in treating menopausal symptoms are not known to cause blood clots. However, until this area is fully studied, the possibility of a very small risk of blood clots cannot be ruled out even in women without known risk factors.
Are heart attacks prevented by taking estrogen after the menopause?		X	But estrogen may protect against heart disease in women who have had their ovaries surgically removed, especially under age 40.
If hormones (ERT) are stopped in a woman who has gone through menopause, will hot flashes subside eventually?	X		Usually in less than six months.
Are thyroid tests affected by estrogens?	X		Some thyroid tests are affected, but the amount of thyroid in the bloodstream is unchanged.
Are blood fatty substances (triglycerides) elevated in women taking estrogens?	X		This fact is important especially in women with risk factors for heart disease.
Should estrogen be stopped one month prior to elective surgery such as hysterectomy?	X		Stopping estrogen may decrease risk of blood clots associated with surgery.
Is estrogen helpful for the treatment of depression?		X	Only if depression is directly associated with hot flashes or other symptoms of estrogen deficiency.
Is the most common side effect of estrogen weight gain?		X	Nausea is more common.

Gynecologic Problems Related To Menopause

In preparing this section, we were surprised to find in the popular literature very little emphasis on health problems of the middle-aged and older woman. Most women's health books focus on health issues of the childbearing years and contain a short chapter on menopause with barely a mention of related problems like osteoporosis (see Chapter 27), prolapse of the uterus, and urinary stress incontinence. These last two gynecologic conditions and others that sometimes follow menopause as a result of decreasing estrogen levels are discussed in this chapter.

Around the time of menopause many women first notice certain symptoms that are associated with hormone changes that may affect the pelvic organs. These symptoms, known collectively as *pelvic relaxation*, may include frequent urination, vaginal or lower abdominal pressure, low back pain, or a feeling that "something is falling out." Pelvic relaxation refers to a gradual weakening of the vaginal muscles that support the uterus, bladder, and rectum. Weakening of these muscles may give rise to vaginal protrusions or hernias (see below), a "dropped" uterus (prolapsed uterus), or difficulty with bladder control (urinary stress incontinence; see glossary). Sometimes these problems begin before menopause, especially in women who have had difficult childbirth. Repeated childbirth, genetic factors, obesity, and conditions such as a chronic cough that continually strain pelvic muscles also cause a susceptibility to pelvic relaxation

problems. Unless symptoms are severe, most women do not need surgical treatment. Surgery for any of the conditions is an elective procedure, the timing of which depends on the severity of the symptoms.

Vaginal Hernias (Cystoceles and Rectoceles)

Vaginal hernias (see also Chapter 86) appear as a bulge in the vaginal wall; your physician can diagnose them on pelvic examination. These painless protrusions represent a weakness in the muscles separating the vagina from the bladder (this one is called a *cystocele*) or the rectum (a *rectocele*). When these organs push against and bulge into the vaginal wall, completely emptying your bladder (in the case of a cystocele) or having a bowel movement (with a rectocele) sometimes becomes difficult. Symptoms of vaginal pressure and frequent urination (see Chapter 83) are common with cystoceles. Rectoceles cause symptoms less often but account for chronic constipation when a bowel movement becomes trapped in the rectocele and hardens.

About half of all postmenopausal women have at least mild degrees of these vaginal hernias, but fewer than 10% require surgery. You may need surgery for a cystocele if it causes chronic discomfort, frequent urination which interferes with daily activities, or incontinence (a condition where you are unable to hold in your urine). A rectocele may require surgical repair if you have frequent difficulty having a bowel movement. Rectoceles, even small ones, are sometimes associated with vaginal muscle damage, which gives rise to a sensation of vaginal looseness during intercourse, a problem that may also be surgically repaired.

Uterine Prolapse ("Dropped" Uterus)

Most women who have given birth have some degree of uterine prolapse, which is most often symptomless. Your partner may be the first to notice a more advanced prolapse if he feels "blockage" during penetration in intercourse. Moderate or severe prolapse may cause pressure or heaviness in the lower back or lower abdomen. Complete prolapse in which the uterus extends outside the vagina when the woman bears down is rare.

The clinician diagnoses uterine prolapse if the cervix visibly moves downward in the vaginal

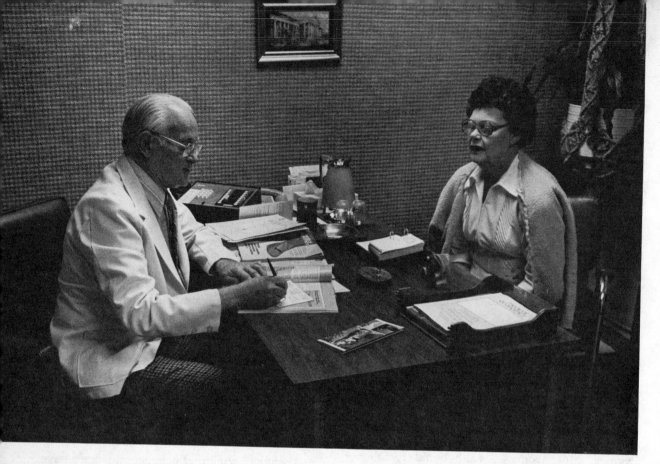

canal when he or she asks you to strain down during the speculum part of the pelvic examination. A dropped uterus in itself is not an indication for surgery especially if you have few or no symptoms and no related condition such as a vaginal hernia. However, this condition is one of the most common reasons given for hysterectomy. Vaginal hysterectomy (see Chapter 44) may be indicated, however, when prolapse causes severe backache or pelvic discomfort. To confirm this diagnosis, the clinician may attempt to reproduce your symptoms during the pelvic examination by pulling down on the uterus with a special clamp which attaches to the cervix. Another way to help establish that backache or other symptoms are due to prolapse and not to some other cause is to use a *pessary* (see below). If symptoms are then reduced, surgery is likely to relieve the discomfort.

A hysterectomy for mild prolapse is performed when other related surgery (such as for a vaginal hernia) is needed. In this case, hysterectomy improves the results of the associated surgery and prevents the need for a second operation in case prolapse symptoms become worse later. Hysterectomy also may be done if a woman desiring sterilization has symptoms of prolapse.

An alternative to surgery as a treatment for

uterine prolapse is the use of a pessary, a rubber device which the clinician places into the vagina to support the uterus. Though not a permanent cure for the problem, a pessary prevents prolapse symptoms in women who do not want definitive surgery. The clinician removes and cleans the pessary every month or every two months to prevent vaginal infections, one of the complications of this device.

Urinary Stress Incontinence

Urinary stress incontinence is the involuntary loss of urine during sudden activity that increases pressure inside the abdomen, like coughing, laughing, or sneezing. From time to time, every woman normally experiences this problem and it may occur more frequently during pregnancy. Severe or frequent urinary stress incontinence results from muscle weakness around the urethra and bladder. The term *urethrocele* refers to a displaced urethra, which often accompanies urinary stress incontinence. This condition may be associated with urethrocele, cystocele, or uterine prolapse.

The physician diagnoses urinary stress incontinence on the basis of a history of the sudden loss of urine upon coughing, sneezing, laughing, or some other sudden strain. It is important for the clinician to differentiate this problem from other conditions affecting the urinary tract, such as infections, which are detectable by urinalysis or urine culture (see Chapters 83 and 84). If there is any doubt about the diagnosis, a urologist is usually consulted. This specialist may perform a cystoscopy, an office or outpatient procedure to examine the inside of the bladder to look for signs of inflammation or infection.

You may prevent the progression of this condition by doing an exercise (called Kegel's exercise) that will eventually strengthen your vaginal muscles. To do this exercise: Slowly contract (pull in) the muscle you use to control urination (as though you were going to stop the urine flow); hold it for three seconds and then gradually relax the muscle. Do this tightening-relaxing sequence as often as possible. The more often you do it, the better will be the result. Over a period of several months, you can build up your vaginal muscle tone and strength. Like any exercise, this program requires persistence and patience to get results. In the long run, this exercise will control mild degrees of urinary stress incontinence. (A possible added benefit is greater sexual satisfaction brought about by increased vaginal sensation and snugness during intercourse.)

When urinary stress incontinence becomes so severe that you need to wear a pad, or the problem becomes socially inconvenient or embarrassing, surgical treatment usually becomes necessary. This treatment involves a special operation performed through either the abdomen or the vagina to reposition the bladder and urethra. If the vaginal approach is used and the woman has completed her family, vaginal hysterectomy is often performed as well as the bladder surgery to improve the surgical results. Both the abdominal and the vaginal operations have the same goal: to reposition the displaced urethra so that it functions normally. With either operation, there is a recurrence of symptoms within five years at least 30% to 40% of the time. If there is a recurrence of symptoms, the need for additional surgery may then be evaluated.

References for Section Six

Chapter 26—Menopause

Chapter 27—Estrogen Replacement Therapy

Committee on Technical Bulletins of the American College of Obstetricians and Gynecologists: *Estrogen Replacement Therapy.* Technical Bulletin #70, 1983, American College of Obstetricians and Gynecologists, Washington, D.C.

Committee on Technical Bulletins of the American College of Obstetricians and Gynecologists: *Osteoporosis.* Technical Bulletin #72, 1983, American College of Obstetricians and Gynecologists, Washington, D.C.

Gambrell, R. D., Jr., et al. Decreased incidence of breast cancer in postmenopausal estrogen-progesterone users. *Obstetrics and Gynecology* 62(4):435-443, 1983.

Hammond, C. B., et al. Effects of long-term estrogen replacement therapy. *American Journal of Obstetrics and Gynecology* 133:525-36, Mar 1, 1979.

National Institute on Aging: National Institutes of Health Consensus Development Conference on *Estrogen Use and Postmenopausal Women.* Sept 1979. Bethesda, Maryland: Dept. of HEW.

Quigley, M. M., and Hammond, C. B. Estrogen replacement therapy - help or hazard? *New England Journal of Medicine* 301: 646-648, Sept 1979.

Kistner, R. W. The menopause. *The Female Patient* 31-37, Sept 1979.

Notelovitz, M. Estrogen, lipids and heart disease. *The Female Patient* 18-24, Aug 1980.

Tataryn, I. V., et al. Objective techniques for the assessment of postmenopausal hot flashes. *Obstetrics and Gynecology* 57(3):340-344, 1981.

Lender, M., and Spencer, H. Postmenopausal osteoporosis. *The Female Patient* 5(9):15-19, 1980.

Erlik, Y., Tataryn, I. V., et al. Association of waking episodes with menopausal hot flushes. *Journal of the American Medical Association* 245(17):1741-1744, 1981.

Albanese, A. A., et al. A new screen for asymptomatic bone loss. *Diagnosis* 71-75, Nov 1980.

Mosher, B. A., and Whelan, E. M. Postmenopausal estrogen therapy: a review. *Obstetrical and Gynecological Survey* 36:467-475, 1981.

Chapter 28—Gynecologic Problems Related to Menopause

Mattingly, R. F. (ed.) *TeLinde's Operative Gynecology,* ed. 5. Philadelphia: Lippincott, 1977.

Kistner, R. W. *Gynecology - Principles and Practice,* ed. 3. Chicago: Year Book Medical Publishers, 1979.

seven

The Woman Consumer and Drugs

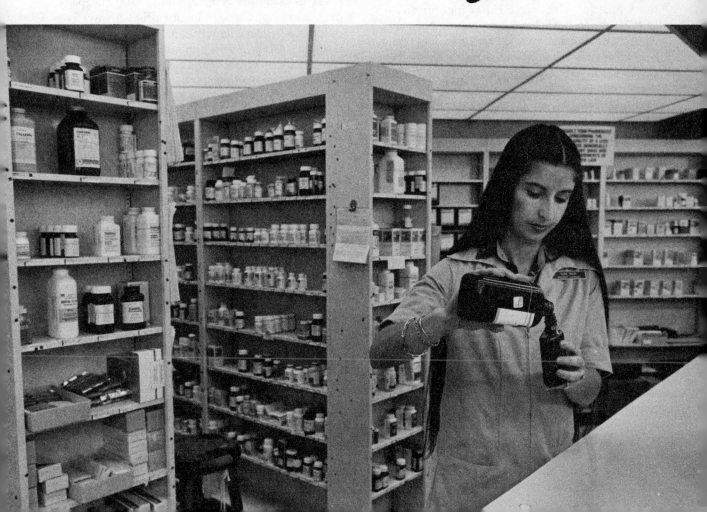

29

Understanding the Drugs You Take

In 1978, U.S. doctors wrote a total of 1.4 billion prescriptions; the majority were for women. Historically, women have been the major users of both prescription and nonprescription (also called over-the-counter) drugs. It follows from this fact that women are also at greater risk for drug abuse. In 1978, the House Select Committee on Narcotics Abuse and Control revealed that twice as many women as men are using minor tranquilizers such as Valium or Librium; fifty percent more women than men are using barbiturates (sleeping pills) and three times as many women as men are using amphetamines (in some diet pills) for medical purposes. As the principal consumers of both prescription and nonprescription drugs, women have a personal responsibility to know the effects of the drugs they take and a financial stake in knowing some rules about medicine shopping. This section of the book will help you understand both of these areas.

Generic Versus Brand Name Drugs

Every drug has a *generic*, or chemical, name. A *brand* or *trade* name is a name given to a drug product by the manufacturer who first developed the drug. The brand name is designed to be short and easy to remember. For example, the brand name of a common tranquilizer, Librium, is far easier to spell and to recall than its generic name, chlordiazepoxide. These brand name drugs are allowed to be manufactured and sold only by the manufacturer that developed the drug, since that company usually acquires patent rights for seventeen years. During this period of time, the company that introduced the product has exclusive manufacturing rights and other manufacturers are prevented from marketing a drug with the same chemical structure. After the patent period has ended, the product can be manufactured by other drug companies and sold under its generic name or under the new manufacturer's own trade name.

Generic drugs cost you less than brand name drugs because they can be manufactured by competing drug companies and this competition lowers prices. At the present time, ninety percent of all prescriptions are written by brand name. Although more generic name prescriptions could be written, not all brand name drugs are available by generic name, because the patent rights have not yet expired. The same Food and Drug Administration (FDA) standards apply to the manufacture of both generic and brand name drugs.

One of the most significant trends nowadays in prescribing practices is the substitution of generic drugs for brand name drugs. Generic substitution refers to using the generic, and usually cheaper, drug instead of the brand name drug. Always request the generic equivalent drug if one is available. This substitution can be done by the physician who writes the prescription or, in some States, by the pharmacist. If your State does not allow the pharmacist to substitute the generic drug when your physician has prescribed a brand name drug, ask your pharmacist to call the physician to authorize the substitution.

Nonprescription Versus Prescription Drugs

Over-the-counter (OTC) drugs differ from prescription drugs because they require no prescription for you to obtain them and they are generally cheaper and less powerful. No doubt, you take nonprescription drugs for relief of minor problems such as headache, diarrhea, and indigestion. Studies have shown that most consumers get their information on over-the-counter drugs from advertising rather than from labels on the drug itself. Currently drug advertisements are not regulated by the FDA; however, drug labels must provide all the directions needed by the average person. It is important that you carefully read the label as well as any accompanying information in the package.

Chronic use of OTC drugs for long periods, especially when they do not relieve your symptoms, can mask underlying illness, possibly delaying diagnosis and treatment. For this reason, you should avoid chronic self-medication. Use the two-week rule-of-thumb: If you have been taking, say, aspirin every day for two weeks for headaches and you still have headaches, make an appointment with your doctor. If you have questions about side effects or adverse (unfavorable) reactions of any OTC drugs you are taking, ask your pharmacist these questions.

Before You Take Prescription Drugs

1. If you regularly use antacids, laxatives, pain relievers, or diet aids, mention this use to your physician before he or she prescribes a drug for you. Many OTC drugs don't "mix" with prescription medicines.
2. Tell the clinician about any allergic reactions (such as itching, rash, vomiting, or difficult breathing) you have had to drugs in the past. Allergic reactions to certain drugs like penicillin tend to get worse each time you take the drug. You may want to take a special skin test to safely determine if you are allergic to penicillin (or any of its forms, such as Ampicillin).
3. Inform your clinician of any past health problems as this may influence his or her choice of drugs for you. For example, certain drugs are dangerous for a person with chronic liver or kidney disease, since these organs are involved in eliminating the drug from your body. Some drugs affect chronic conditions in a harmful way. Birth control pills, for instance, may make migraine headaches, epilepsy, or heart disease worse because of increased fluid retention.
4. If there is any possibility of pregnancy, avoid drugs altogether unless specified by your doctor. (See Chapter 31, *Drugs and the Pregnant Woman.*) Seemingly harmless drugs, even aspirin, may be harmful to the fetus.
5. If you are breast-feeding, avoid using drugs if possible because almost all drugs can pass into the breast milk. Subtle drug effects on the newborn's growth, development, or behavior are difficult to measure and in most cases are unknown.

When You Are Given a Prescription Drug

Here are some questions you should ask your clinician when he or she has prescribed a drug for you.

1. What is the purpose of the drug? Has a diagnosis been made? If not, find out if drug treatment is really necessary or if the symptoms are likely to subside on their own. For example, birth control pills are often prescribed for adolescents to "regulate" their cycle although some menstrual irregularity is perfectly normal among teen-age women.
2. Are less costly OTC drugs available? For instance, for nonpregnant women, prescriptions for multiple vitamins and iron are practically never necessary and almost always more costly than OTC equivalents.
3. What are possible side effects to watch for? What should be done if they occur?
4. How often should the drug be taken? When a prescription reads "four times a day," does that mean this amount is the necessary dosage to get a curative effect, as with antibiotics, or does that indicate the maximum dosage per day for a drug to be taken only "when needed" as with pain medication?
5. For how many days should the drug be taken? Until this entire prescription is used up or less? Should I have the prescription refilled?
6. Could this drug interact harmfully with other prescription or OTC drugs I am taking? What are the symptoms to watch for? Find out if food or alcoholic beverages will affect the way the drug should be taken. For example, is it better to take this drug on an empty stomach, before meals, after meals? How many hours before or after I take the medication can I drink alcohol?
7. Can the generic equivalent be prescribed if one is available?

When Taking a Prescription Drug

1. Keep a record of the drug, dosage, and the time of day you take each dose. This record will accomplish at least two things: 1) it will remind you of when you took your last dose; and 2) if you are taking more than one drug and they shouldn't be taken at the same

time, you can remember to separate the times you take them. Put the record where it will remind you to take the drug.

2. Ask your pharmacist for a copy of the manufacturer's package insert that accompanies prescription drugs. These inserts provide detailed information about the drug although not in layman language since they are intended primarily for the pharmacist or physicians. Other pamphlets written for patients may be available with certain prescription drugs.

3. Know how to store the drug. Some drugs have to be refrigerated and others have to be kept in a tight, dry container. Keep them safely out of the reach of small children—perhaps in a locked medicine cabinet or, when necessary to be refrigerated, in a part of the refrigerator that a child cannot reach.

4. Take the full course of the drug prescription if that is what your doctor's instructions are. Sometimes symptoms improve before the drug therapy has been completed and it is tempting to stop taking the drug. A relapse of symptoms can occur, as with certain vaginal infections.

5. Be familiar with harmful side effects. If they occur, stop the drug and inform your doctor.

6. If you are taking a drug chronically, get periodic checkups. Women taking prescription medication chronically for high blood pressure, thyroid conditions, contraception, or any chronic health problem should have a checkup at least annually.

7. If surgery is scheduled, review your prescription drugs with your physician. Oral contraceptives, for example, should be stopped one or two months prior to elective surgery, since blood clots after an operation are more common in users of birth control pills.

8. Discard drugs that you have not used. It can be dangerous to take old, outdated drugs.

30

Avoiding Drug Abuse

Currently one of the most urgent health problems facing women is the overuse of psychoactive prescription drugs and some nonprescription drugs. Psychoactive drugs are drugs which affect the mind, such as tranquilizers, sedatives, and antidepressants. These drugs are often referred to as mood-altering drugs. Although alcohol is not a prescription drug, it is considered a mood-altering drug. In fact, alcohol is the most commonly abused drug in the U.S.

You don't have to be on heroin to be an addict. Drug abuse covers a spectrum from addiction, in which stopping the drug leads to physical withdrawal symptoms, to psychological dependency alone. According to the National Institute on Drug Abuse (NIDA), nearly 1% of U.S. women may have a dependency problem or an outright addiction to legally available medicines. Data collected in 1977 from twenty-four metropolitan areas by the Drug Abuse Warning Network show that women comprise 59% of all drug-related emergency room visits and account for 43% of all drug-related deaths.

Why are women more prone than men to abuse psychoactive drugs? This situation may be related to the fact that women are more likely than men to acknowledge psychological distress and to seek medical aid for it. Physicians' prescribing practices may also contribute to legal abuse depending on how the problems of male and female patients are perceived. Physicians who accept the sexual stereotype of women as "weak and helpless" may be more likely to prescribe tranquilizers for female symptoms of anxiety and depression.

Some drug companies may indirectly encourage drug abuse through advertisements that depict drugs as a solution to normal life stresses. Stereotyped

Table 40   SYMPTOMS OF DRUG ABUSE

	Symptoms of Excessive Use or Overdose	Symptoms of Withdrawal
Narcotics	extreme drowsiness or confusion	nausea, vomiting, stomach cramps
	loss of appetite	excessive nervousness
	slow, shallow breathing	sweating
	cold, clammy skin	hand tremor
	seizures	watery nose and eyes
	coma	yawning
Barbiturates, Sleeping Pills, Tranquilizers, and Alcohol	slurred speech, staggering gait	excessive nervousness
	disorientation	insomnia
	extreme drowsiness, falling asleep at work	hand tremor
	slow, shallow breathing	confusion
	cold, clammy skin	seizures
	coma	
Stimulants (Diet Pills)	agitation or extreme nervousness	depression, apathy
	excitation or irritability	confusion
	hallucinations, dilated pupils	irritability
	seizures	

sex roles often appear in these advertisements: the women suffer from anxiety, nervousness, and depression, while the men are more often troubled with physical symptoms.

Whatever the cause, the problem of misuse of mood-altering drugs is real.

What Is Drug Abuse?

Drug problems are so complex that even experts sometimes have difficulty making accurate diagnoses. Drug abuse occurs when a drug is taken routinely by an individual to "get through the day." When the individual depends upon taking the drug in order to function, this situation constitutes drug abuse. Stopping chronic use of many psychoactive drugs, even tranquilizers like Valium, can result in withdrawal symptoms, such as delirium, trembling, psychotic behavior, and exaggeration of reflexes. The effects of overdose and withdrawal of the various kinds of mood-altering drugs are listed in Table 40. Early signs of drug abuse—warning signals—are listed in Table 41.

The use of multiple drugs (*polypharmacy*) is common in individuals who have drug abuse problems and may cause a variety of unexpected serious side effects from drug interactions. Alcohol, as mentioned earlier, is the most commonly abused drug in the U.S. If you take any type of medication, check with your doctor to see if it's safe to drink alcoholic beverages during the time you are taking the medication. There may be additive effects that can impair heart and respiratory functions when alcohol is taken.

Although limited research has been done in the area of women and drugs, the available literature indicates significant differences between the male and female drug abuser. Characteristics of the female drug abuser that are frequently mentioned

Table 41   WARNING SIGNALS OF DRUG ABUSE

If you answer yes to any of the questions below, you may have a problem with drugs, alcohol, or both.

1. Are you defensive if a friend or relative mentions your drug or alcohol use?

2. Are you sometimes embarrassed or frightened by your behavior under the influence of drugs or alcohol?

3. Have you ever gone to see a new doctor because your regular physician would not prescribe the drug you wanted?

4. When you are under pressure or feel anxious, do you automatically take a tranquilizer or a drink or both?

5. Do you take drugs more often than recommended by your doctor or for purposes other than those recommended by your doctor?

6. Do you mix drugs and alcohol?

7. Do you regularly drink or take drugs to help you sleep?

8. Do you have to take a pill to get going in the morning?

include: problems with sexual identity; difficulty handling anger directly, resulting in passive, indirect, and acting-out behavior; intense feelings of personal inadequacy; fear of close relationships. There are certain critical times in a woman's life when drug abuse is more likely to occur: early in a marriage, the birth of the first child, an unwanted pregnancy, divorce, widowhood, menopause, or major surgery. Just being aware that you might be more susceptible to drug abuse during these times of crisis will, it is hoped, help you avoid letting drugs become a crutch. In such highly stressful times, you may want to consider seeking out extra support from family or friends; or you might want to consult a competent therapist.

The Controlled Substances Act

Legal drugs subject to abuse are regulated by the Controlled Substances Act. This Federal law specifies several different categories of prescription and nonprescription drugs according to how likely the drugs are to cause addiction and harmful effects as a result of excessive use. We have arranged these so-called controlled drugs by highest, intermediate, and lowest drug abuse potential in Tables 42, 43, and 44, respectively.

Table 42   DRUGS WITH HIGHEST POTENTIAL FOR ABUSE*

Drug Family	Generic Name	Common Brand Names Containing This Drug	Medical Use
amphetamine (stimulant)	amphetamine	Dexedrine, Biphetamine, Desoxyn	lose weight**
amphetamine (stimulant)	phenmetrazine	Preludin	lose weight**
analgesic (narcotic)	codeine	codeine tablets (15, 30, 60 mg) (various brands)	pain relief cough suppression
analgesic (narcotic)	oxycodone	Percodan, Percocet, Tylox	pain relief
analgesic (narcotic)	meperidine	Demerol	pain relief
barbiturate (sedative)	amobarbital	Amytal	promote sleep
barbiturate (sedative)	secobarbital	Seconal	promote sleep
barbiturate (sedative)	pentobarbital	Nembutal	promote sleep
sleeping pill	methaqualone	Quaalude	promote sleep

* Controlled Substances Act
** Not approved for this use in some States.

Table 42 includes the strongest of all prescription pain killers (analgesics), cough suppressants, sleeping pills, and diet pills. Table 43 encompasses less potent and lower dose pain pills and cough suppressants. Also, milder barbiturates and sleeping pills, tranquilizers like Valium, and the least toxic diet pills are included in this group. Table 44 includes mainly drugs for cough and a few drugs for diarrhea. Many of the products in Table 44 may be purchased over-the-counter in most States

Table 43 DRUGS WITH INTERMEDIATE POTENTIAL FOR ABUSE*

Drug Family	Generic Name	Common Brand Names Containing This Drug	Medical Use
amphetamine-like (stimulant)	phentermine	Fastin, Ionamin	lose weight
amphetamine-like (stimulant)	diethylpropion	Tenuate, Tepanil	lose weight
amphetamine (stimulant)	phendimetrazine	Prelu-2	lose weight
analgesic (narcotic)	codeine	Empirin with Codeine (#1, #2, #3, & #4) Empracet #3, #4 Fiorinal with Codeine (#2 & #3) Phenaphen with Codeine (#2, #3, & #4) Tylenol with Codeine (#1, #2, #3, & #4) Synalgos-DC	pain relief cough suppression
analgesic (narcotic)	hydrocodone	Tussend Liquid Tussionex	cough suppression
analgesic (narcotic)	opium	Paregoric	pain relief relief of intestinal spasm and diarrhea
analgesic (narcotic)	propoxyphene	Darvon Darvon Compound Darvocet-N Wygesic	pain relief
analgesic (nonnarcotic)	pentazocine	Talwin	pain relief
barbiturate (sedative)	butabarbital	Butisol	relief of anxiety promote sleep
barbiturate (sedative)	phenobarbital	Luminal	relief of anxiety
sleeping pill	chloral hydrate	Noctec	promote sleep
sleeping pill	ethchlorvynol	Placidyl	promote sleep
sleeping pill	flurazepam	Dalmane	promote sleep
tranquilizer	meprobamate	Equagesic	pain relief
tranquilizer	meprobamate	Equanil, Miltown	relief of anxiety
tranquilizer	chlordiazepoxide	Librium, Limbitrol	relief of anxiety
tranquilizer	lorazepam	Ativan	relief of anxiety
tranquilizer	oxazepam	Serax	relief of anxiety
tranquilizer	chlorazepate	Tranxene	relief of anxiety
tranquilizer	diazepam	Valium	relief of anxiety
tranquilizer	prazepam	Centrax	relief of anxiety

* Controlled Substances Act

Table 44 DRUGS WITH LOWEST POTENTIAL FOR ABUSE*

For Diarrhea *Contain small amounts of paregoric:*

Parepectolin, Donnagel PG

For Cough *Contain small amounts of codeine:*

Actifed C Expectorant

Ambenyl Expectorant

Capital with Codeine Suspension

Dimetane Expectorant DC

Novahistine DH and Expectorant

Phenergan VC Expectorant with Codeine

Robitussin AC and DAC

Triaminic Expectorant with Codeine

Tylenol with Codeine Elixir

* Controlled Substances Act

simply by signing the pharmacist's register, specifying the type and amount of medication purchased. The ready availability of drugs in this group may make them subject to more frequent abuse compared to some of the more potent drugs in the other tables.

In the past decade, the problem of women and substance abuse has received increasing attention by government agencies, such as HEW (the former Department of Health, Education, and Welfare). The Program for Women's Concerns (PWC) was established in 1974 within the office of the National Institute on Drug Abuse (NIDA) as a special advocate for women's interests. The Program for Women's Concerns, in addition to its advocacy role within NIDA, provides educational pamphlets and nationwide resource information concerning drug abuse treatment services available to women.

Resources

Local drug abuse or women's health centers: see your telephone directory.

For information about drug abuse prevention, write:

National Institute on Drug Abuse
Prevention Branch
5600 Fishers Lane, Room 10A-30
Rockville, Maryland 20857

For information about drugs, write:

National Clearinghouse on Drug Abuse
P.O. Box 416
Kensington, MD 20795

The Clearinghouse also maintains an updated directory of women's drug abuse treatment programs throughout the United States.

For information about alcohol, write:

National Clearinghouse for Alcohol
Information
P.O. Box 2345
Rockville, Maryland 20852

Resource groups for alcohol abuse:

If you are having a problem with alcohol abuse, no matter what your age is, you can contact:

Alcoholics Anonymous
P.O. Box 459
Grand Central Station
New York, N.Y. 10163

For local meetings see your local telephone directory under Alcoholics Anonymous.

If a member of your family (any age) or a friend is having a problem with alcohol abuse, write:

Al-Anon Family Group Headquarters, Inc.
P.O. Box 182
Madison Square Station
New York, N.Y. 10159

For local Al-Anon meetings see your local telephone directory under Al-Anon Family Group. If you are a teen-ager (or younger) and a family member or friend is having a problem with alcohol abuse, *you* can get help with how to deal with the problem. Look under Alateen, or Al-Anon-Alateen, in your telephone directory.

For all of these alcohol programs (Alcoholics Anonymous, Al-Anon, and Alateen) you do not have to give your last name; you can attend meetings and can remain, as the name implies, anonymous.

31

Drugs and The Pregnant Woman

The subject of drug use during pregnancy is beset with conflicting reports and controversy. The shocking realization of the effect of drugs on the fetus occurred in the 1960s following the thalidomide tragedy. Thalidomide was prescribed widely in Europe as a sedative for four years before it was found to cause profound limb deformities in the fetus when the drug was taken in early pregnancy. Although the drug had not been approved by the FDA for use in the U.S., the thalidomide story led to stricter drug regulation within the U.S. by the FDA. Today there is increasing concern about possible biochemical and long-term behavioral effects on the fetus of drugs taken during pregnancy as well as for physical malformations of the fetus.

Women are presented with new press reports every day about drugs potentially harmful to the unborn. At the same time a constant barrage of advertisements in the media encourage women to consume drugs for a variety of symptoms, many of which are common to pregnancy. The ready availability and lack of labels warning against use in pregnancy on most over-the-counter drugs may help account for the widespread use of these remedies by pregnant women. Recent studies show that American women consume an average of four to nine drugs, mostly nonprescription, during a typical pregnancy.

You should ask your physician about *any* drug you are routinely taking when you become pregnant. The use of most drugs during pregnancy is associated with some risk to the fetus; this risk must be weighed against the expected benefits of the drug. There are several points to be considered when you make this choice:

1. Approximately 2% to 5% of all pregnancies result in birth defects. It is believed that most of these defects are due to a variety of interacting causes of which drugs are only one factor. In fact, it is estimated that drugs cause only 1% to 3% of these birth defects.

2. Extremely few drugs are known to cause malformations. These include thalidomide (no longer marketed), sex hormones, and certain drugs used to treat cancer.

3. Some drugs are considered safe in pregnancy either because they are not absorbed or because long-term use has not been associated with harmful effects on the newborn (see Table 45).

4. The placenta is not a barrier. Most drugs travel across the placenta and reach the fetus. For this reason, it is difficult to completely exclude the possibility of harmful fetal effects for most drugs. Some effects may take years to show up, as in the case of DES (see Chapter 37), a drug now believed to cause vaginal cancer in young women who were exposed before birth, when their mothers were pregnant with them and were given this drug to prevent miscarriage.

5. The effect of a drug on the fetus depends partly on the stage of pregnancy. In early pregnancy, especially during the first two

---

Table 45   DRUGS PRESENTLY CONSIDERED SAFE TO USE DURING PREGNANCY

Symptom	Drug
Pain (e.g., headache)	Acetaminophen (e.g., Tylenol, Datril)—after second month
Diarrhea	Kaopectate
Constipation	Certain laxatives (see Chapter 58 on constipation)
Heartburn	Antacids (but avoid antacids containing aspirin)
Itching; insomnia	Diphenhydramine (Benadryl*)
Hay fever; sinus congestion	Chlorpheniramine (Chlor-Trimeton)

* Requires prescription.

months after conception, the fetal organs are forming, and unnecessary drugs should be avoided. This is the stage when drug-induced malformations usually occur (see Table 46). In middle and late pregnancy, drugs may be harmful to the fetus's chemical functioning, which could result in adverse effects such as internal bleeding or growth retardation (see Table 47). Just prior to labor, drugs may affect the baby's capacity to adjust to life outside the uterus. Breathing difficulty may be encountered at birth in newborns exposed in late pregnancy to tranquilizers, sedatives, or excessive alcohol.

6. Certain medical conditions may necessitate the taking of drugs in pregnancy. Often the

---

Table 46   DRUGS WHICH MAY CAUSE FETAL ABNORMALITIES IN EARLY PREGNANCY

Not all drugs listed here are definitely known to cause birth defects in humans. However, the available evidence, including animal research, indicates the advisability of avoiding these drugs in pregnancy particularly in the first three months.

Drug	Comment
Alcohol	see text and Table 51
Aspirin	
Barbiturates	
Caffeine (?)	known to cause birth defects in animals but not in humans; FDA recommends avoiding caffeine-containing products or using them sparingly in pregnancy
Some diet pills	amphetamines
Vitamin A or D	excessive use (megavitamin dosage; see Chapter 46)
Some hormones	includes birth control pills and progesterone pills for pregnancy testing
Librax	contains Librium (see below)
Sleeping pills	for example, Dalmane
Tetracycline	for example, Achromycin, Sumycin, Vibramycin, Minocin
Tranquilizers	for example, Valium, Librium, Tranxene

Table 47   DRUGS WHICH MAY CAUSE ADVERSE FETAL EFFECTS IN LATE PREGNANCY

Drug	Comment
Alcohol	see text and Table 51
Antibiotics (some)	chloramphenicol, nitrofurantoin (for example, Macrodantin), sulfa (for example, Azogantrisin, Azogantanol, Bactrim, Septra), streptomycin, tetracycline (for example, Achromycin, Sumycin, Vibramycin, Minocin)
Aspirin	
Barbiturates	
Caffeine (?)	see Table 46
Thiazides (water pills)	
Tranquilizers	

advantages of taking these medicines outweigh the fetal risks involved (see Table 48).

7. Drug use during breast-feeding may be associated with certain risks to the newborn although the quantity of most drugs in breast milk is very low (see Tables 49 and 50).

Remember, it is important to consider carefully before you take any drug while you are pregnant. Because new research studies are constantly uncovering new information, it is a good idea to consult with your clinician on any new findings that would make advisable or inadvisable the use of any drug you plan to take while you are pregnant. This responsibility is yours; you owe it to yourself and your unborn.

Drinking Alcohol During Pregnancy

Infants born to women who drink heavily during pregnancy are likely to have a definite pattern of physical and mental abnormalities recently described by researchers as the *fetal alcohol syndrome*. Some or all of the conditions listed in Table 51 may be present with variable severity. The complete syndrome probably occurs with a frequency of one to two out of one thousand live births.

Table 48 DRUG USE DURING PREGNANCY FOR CERTAIN MEDICAL CONDITIONS

Condition	Comment
Asthma	Continue most medications; avoid drugs containing iodides as iodides may be harmful to the fetus; avoid steroids such as Prednisone and Aristocort unless advised by physician; safety of Cromolyn (new drug) not established.
High blood pressure	Continue medications under physician supervision.
Diabetes	Avoid all oral medication—possibly harmful to fetus; use insulin only—dosage of insulin will increase during pregnancy.
Seizures	Dilantin and other drugs used in treating seizures have been associated with an increased risk of fetal malformations. However, the benefits of these drugs in women taking them to prevent seizures outweigh the risks. A neurologist's consultation may be advisable.
Hypothyroidism (low thyroid)	Frequent thyroid blood tests are necessary to determine correct dosage.

Both animal and human research studies have singled out alcohol apart from smoking, poor nutrition, or other risk factors as the major influence in the development of the fetal alcohol syndrome. Alcohol readily crosses the placenta. The fetus receives as much alcohol as the mother; but since the fetus burns up alcohol half as fast as the mother does, the alcohol remains in the fetal system longer. Although we don't know how much alcohol is required to endanger the developing fetus, it is now believed that a woman who drinks more than six hard drinks per day, particularly in early pregnancy, clearly risks harm to the fetus. At this level of alcohol consumption, the risk of a serious problem in the fetus has been reported at between 30% and 50%. The effect on a fetus of consuming two to six drinks per day is associated with a *lesser* risk (about 20%), and the level below which *no* risk is present is unknown.

In 1977, the National Institute on Alcohol Abuse and Alcoholism issued a warning concerning the potential adverse effects of alcohol on the developing fetus. The Institute recommended an absolute maximum of two one-ounce mixed drinks or two five-ounce glasses of wine or two twelve-ounce cans of beer during any one day during pregnancy or when pregnancy is planned. Since the effects of episodic or binge drinking are unknown, you should not "save up" drinks for several days. The safest advice would be to avoid alcohol completely in pregnancy.

For more information on alcohol and pregnancy, write to:

National Clearinghouse for Alcohol
  Information
P.O. Box 2345
Rockville, Maryland 20852

Table 49 DRUGS TO AVOID IF YOU BREAST-FEED

If you are breast-feeding and you take—	your baby may develop—
aspirin (high doses)	bleeding problems
atropine (antispasmodic drug)	constipation or more serious reactions
barbiturates (high doses)	drowsiness (baby will nurse less easily)
birth control pills	(long-term effects unknown)
ergotamine (antimigraine drug)	nausea, vomiting, or diarrhea
Flagyl (for vaginitis)	low blood count
laxatives (stimulant type except milk of magnesia and Dulcolax)	diarrhea
sleeping pills	drowsiness (baby will nurse less easily)
sulfa (antibiotic)	jaundice
tetracycline (antibiotic)	tooth discoloration (rare)
thiazides (water pills)	jaundice or bleeding (rare)
tranquilizers (for example, Valium, Tranxene, Miltown, Equanil)	drowsiness (baby will nurse less easily)

Smoking During Pregnancy

While pregnancy is one of the most important times to stop smoking, it is also one of the most difficult times to quit. It is estimated that nearly one-third of women of childbearing age smoke and that many of these women continue to do so during pregnancy. In 1979, the Surgeon General's update on smoking came down hard on pregnant women who smoke, warning that cigarettes may slow fetal growth, double the chance of a low birth weight baby, and increase the risk of having a stillborn child. These findings confirm data collected from the U.S. Collaborative Perinatal Project, which examined more than 50,000 pregnancies at twelve hospitals. Some of the most valuable information came from 227 women who were studied during two pregnancies but who smoked during only one of them. These women had smaller babies in the smoking pregnancy, a finding which tends to prove wrong the claims that constitutional differences between women who smoke and those who don't smoke affect the baby rather than the smoking itself.

Table 50   DRUGS PRESENTLY CONSIDERED SAFE TO TAKE IF YOU BREAST-FEED*

Drug	Comment
Alcohol	
Antacids	
Antiarthritics	
Antibiotics (some)	ampicillin (for example, Principen, Omnipen, Polycillin), cephalosporins (for example, Keflex, Kafocin), erythromycin
Iron	
Laxatives (mild)	Dulcolax, milk of magnesia, Metamucil
Pain relievers	both nonnarcotic and narcotic in recommended doses
Stool softeners	
Vitamins	

* Newborn allergic reactions may occur but are uncommon. Newborns with problems such as prematurity may accumulate drugs and more readily develop side effects.

Table 51   POSSIBLE EFFECTS ON THE NEWBORN FROM ALCOHOL ABUSE* DURING PREGNANCY

1. Low birth weight.
2. Abnormally small head.
3. Facial or joint deformity.
4. Heart defect.
5. Poor coordination.
6. Hyperactivity.
7. Learning disability.
8. Poor growth before and after birth.
9. Mental retardation.

* See text under Drinking Alcohol During Pregnancy.

One of the reasons assumed for the slower growth of the fetus in smoking mothers is the effect of carbon monoxide, one of the substances in cigarette smoke. This gas inhaled by the mother forces oxygen out of her blood and, after crossing the placenta, does the same thing to the fetus's blood. In a heavy smoker, the fetal oxygen supply may be reduced by as much as fifty percent. Another ingredient in cigarette smoke, nicotine, has been shown to pass freely across the placenta where it constricts blood vessels and thereby diminishes the supply of nourishment to the fetus.

Although smoking is associated with the many adverse conditions listed in Table 52, these conditions affect nonsmokers as well. For this reason, the magnitude of the smoking risk in a given woman is difficult to judge. Conditions such as miscarriage and premature labor are known to be associated with a variety of factors of which smoking is only one. Since the number of cigarettes smoked directly affects the degree of impairment of the fetus, cutting back would be beneficial to the woman who feels she cannot quit completely.

Resources

For further reading:
DATA: Drug, Alcohol, Tobacco Abuse During Pregnancy. Write to:

March of Dimes Birth Defects Foundation
Box 2000
White Plains, N.Y. 10602

Table 52 POSSIBLE EFFECTS ON THE NEWBORN FROM SMOKING DURING PREGNANCY

1. Low birth weight of newborn.
2. Premature labor.
3. Miscarriage.
4. Stillbirth.
5. Birth defects.
6. Premature rupture of membranes.
7. Bleeding in late pregnancy.
8. Sudden infant death syndrome.
9. Infant respiratory illness, including pneumonia.

"Drugs and Pregnancy," by Pauline Postotnik. In *FDA Consumer*, October 1978. Write:

HFI 20
Food and Drug Administration
5600 Fishers Lane, Room 15B-32
Rockville, Maryland 20857

References for Section Seven

Chapter 29—Understanding the Drugs You Take

Baum, C., et al. Drug use in the United States in 1981. *Journal of the American Medical Association* 251(10):1293-1297, Mar 1984.

Hecht, A. Generic drugs: how good are they? *FDA Consumer* 17-20, Feb 1978.

Lehmann, P. Food and drug interactions. *FDA Consumer* 20-23, Mar 1978.

Griffenhagen, G. B. (ed.) *Handbook of Nonprescription Drugs*, ed. 5. Washington, D.C.: American Pharmaceutical Association, 1977.

Physicians' Desk Reference, ed. 38. Rutherford, N.J.: Medical Economics, 1984.

Physicians' Desk Reference for Nonprescription Drugs, ed. 5. Rutherford, N.J.: Medical Economics, 1984.

James, J. D., et al. *A Guide to Drug Interactions*. New York: McGraw-Hill, 1978.

Chapter 30—Avoiding Drug Abuse

Wolcott, I. Women and psychoactive drug use. *Women and Health* 4(2):199-202, 1979.

Nellis, M., et al. *Drugs, Alcohol and Women's Health: An Alliance of Regional Coalitions*. Report prepared for National Institute on Drug Abuse, Dept. of HEW, 1978.

Mellinger, G. D., Balter, M. B., et al. Psychic distress, life crisis, use of psychotherapeutic medications: national household survey data. *Archives of General Psychiatry* 35:1045-1050, 1977.

Davidson, V., and Bemko, J. International review of women and drug abuse (1966-1975). *Journal of the American Medical Women's Association* 33:507-512, 1978.

Drug Enforcement Administration, Office of Compliance and Regulatory Affairs: *Physician's Manual - An Informational Outline of the Controlled Substances Act of 1970*, April 1978, U.S. Dept. of Justice, Washington, D.C.

Drug Enforcement Administration, Office of Compliance and Regulatory Affairs: *Controlled Substances Inventory List*, Jan 1979. U.S. Dept. of Justice, Washington, D.C.

Hollister, L. E., et al. Benzodiazepines 1980: current update. Supplement to *The Journal of the Academy of Psychosomatic Medicine* 21(10), Oct 1980.

Chapter 31—Drugs and the Pregnant Woman

Bergman, H. D. Drugs during pregnancy. *Southern Pharmacy Journal* 11-15, Mar 1979.

Yaffe, S. J. Drug use during pregnancy. *Drug Therapy* 137-146, Jun 1978.

Shaywitz, B. A. Fetal alcohol syndrome: an ancient problem rediscovered. *Drug Therapy* 95-108, Jan 1978.

Scialli, A. R., and Fabro, S. What drugs are safe during nursing? *Contemporary OB/GYN* 23(6):211-222, June 1984.

Hanson, J. W. Preventing the fetal alcohol syndrome. *The Female Patient* 38-44, Oct 1979.

Meyer, M. B. How does maternal smoking affect birth weight and maternal weight gain? *American Journal of Obstetrics and Gynecology* 131:888-893, 1978.

Kretzschmar, R. M. Smoking and health: the role of the obstetrician and gynecologist. *Obstetrics and Gynecology* 55(4):403-406, 1980.

Rudolph, A. M. Effects of aspirin and acetaminophen in pregnancy and in the newborn. *Archives of Internal Medicine* 141(3):358-363, 1981.

eight

Diseases of the Female Reproductive System

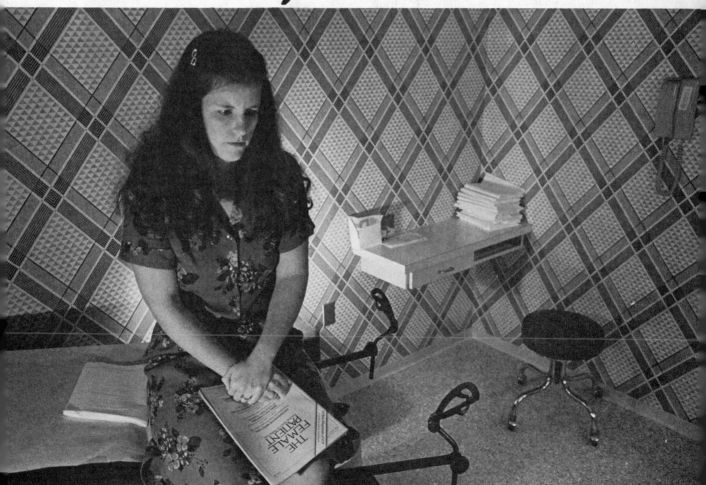

32

Toxic Shock Syndrome

The use of tampons has recently been associated with a rare and sometimes fatal disease called *toxic shock syndrome* (TSS). This mysterious illness first received wide public attention in early 1980 when the Centers for Disease Control reported several studies linking the use of Rely brand tampons with an increased risk of developing TSS. Despite the absence of proof that Rely actually causes TSS, enough evidence accumulated to prompt the manufacturer to withdraw Rely from the market. Cases of TSS have also occurred with tampons produced by all the other major manufacturers, although the risk appears to be lower than with Rely. The convenience and comfort of tampons are a high priority to many women, and the current concern regarding the safety of tampons now on the market has led the FDA to propose that all tampon manufacturers place warning labels on their packages.

Toxic shock syndrome is a name given to a disease characterized by a collection of symptoms experienced most often by women during their menstrual period. Although the exact cause of TSS is unknown, a bacterium called *Staphylococcus aureus* has been identified in many women experiencing this disease. It has been theorized that tampon use may favor the growth of this bacterium in the vagina because the natural flow of blood is blocked by the tampon. Once absorbed into the bloodstream from the vagina, the staph bacteria or their toxins (poisonous substances) may then cause the symptoms of toxic shock: rash, high fever, vomiting, and diarrhea followed by a sudden drop in blood pressure. Penicillin drugs are usually effective in treating TSS, but in some cases the bacteria are resistant to the antibiotic.

Knowledge of TSS is still very limited. Although initial reports emphasized the link between TSS and tampon use, other cases of confirmed TSS have been found in nonmenstruating women, in children, and in males. The proportion of nonmenstrual TSS cases reported to the Centers for Disease Control increased from 7% of all cases in 1980 to 22% in 1982. Sixteen cases of TSS have been reported in diaphragm users and four cases in users of the vaginal contraceptive sponge (Today) as of early 1984. Users of the vaginal sponge who have difficulty removing it should consult a physician, while postpartum women, who may be at increased risk for TSS, should seek medical advice before using the sponge.

Additional research is needed to determine the extent to which TSS is associated with tampon use. Although at least 70% of menstruating women in the U.S. use tampons, only 2,401 cases of TSS have been reported to the Centers for Disease Control as of January 1984. The frequency of TSS in actuality may be somewhat higher because of incomplete reporting of cases.

The American College of Obstetricians and Gynecologists has offered these guidelines for women using tampons:

1. Change tampons often—at least as frequently as every six to eight hours.
2. Use medium or regular tampons instead of super-absorbent ones (often designated as "Super" or "Super Plus").
3. Alternate tampon use with sanitary napkins (or mini- or maxi-pads) during a given menstrual period.
4. If symptoms of high fever, vomiting, diarrhea, or sunburnlike rash occur, discontinue tampon use and immediately consult your physician.

Based on the theory that certain tampons may scratch the mucosal lining (surface) of the vagina and thus lead to the staphylococcal infection, Dr. S. A. Kaufman from Lenox Hill Hospital, New York City, has added the following guidelines:

1. On days when secretions in the vagina are scanty, use a water-soluble lubricating jelly on the tampon applicator to avoid nicking the vaginal mucosa.
2. Use tampons with no applicators or with cardboard applicators, because plastic applicators may be more likely to cause mucosal scratches.

33

Breast Diseases

Benign Breast Conditions

Fibrocystic disease, sometimes called cystic mastitis (see also Chapters 56 and 57), is the most common breast disorder and the most frequent cause of a breast lump in a woman under the age of twenty-five. Characteristic symptoms include lumpy, tender breasts, particularly during the week before menses. Occurring predominantly in women between thirty and fifty, fibrocystic disease usually involves both breasts. When the woman or her doctor feels a distinct lump, the doctor usually tries to withdraw fluid from the involved area or performs a breast biopsy (see Chapter 56).

Most authorities now consider fibrocystic disease a slight risk factor for breast cancer and a possible indication to have periodic mammograms after the age of thirty-five, particularly if you have a family history of breast cancer. The use of birth control pills in women with fibrocystic disease is controversial (see Chapter 9). Recent studies now indicate that a diet low in foods containing caffeine may relieve the symptoms of this condition (see Chapter 57).

A relatively new hormonal drug, danazol, has been approved by the FDA for treating severe fibrocystic breast disease. Symptoms improve in nearly 80% of women after two to eight months of treatment. Although danazol appears to be one of the most promising treatments for this condition, disadvantages are its cost (presently about $25 to $80 a month, depending upon dosage) and possible unwanted side effects including absent menstrual periods, acne, and slight weight gain. Symptoms return in approximately 50% of women within one year of stopping the drug. Some form of birth control (other than the pill) should be used during danazol therapy since the drug is contraindicated in pregnancy.

The most common breast tumor in women younger than twenty-five is the benign (non-cancerous) fibroadenoma. Most predominant in women fifteen to thirty, this tumor produces a firm, movable, nontender lump. Fibroadenomas are removed both to confirm the diagnosis and to prevent damge to breast tissue from localized tumor growth.

Breast Cancer

In the last decade, the frequency of breast cancer, the most common cancer in women, has increased by about one percent each year. In 1984, this tumor was the most common cause of death in women forty to forty-four years old. (See Table 63 for information on frequency statistics and other factors associated with breast cancer.

Approximately one woman in eleven will develop breast cancer. The disease, however, is rare before the age of thirty-five; 85% of the tumors occur in women over forty.

The five-year survival rate for this disease (68%) has changed little in the past thirty years because of the tumor's tendency to spread rapidly before it is large enough to be felt. Early detection of cancer when it is still confined to the breast results in up to a 90% cure rate. When the tumor spreads to nearby lymph nodes under the arm, the proportion of women still alive after five years decreases to approximately 45%. Most clinicians believe that the best hope for attacking this disease is through early diagnosis, which can be achieved through more aggressive efforts to screen and identify women at risk for breast cancer (see Table 53).

Screening for breast cancer

Since early breast cancers rarely cause pain or other symptoms, the importance of screening techniques cannot be overemphasized. A monthly breast self-examination, periodic examination by your clinician, and selective use of mammography (X-ray) are your best preventive health measures.

The American Cancer Society recommends that women over twenty-five examine their breasts monthly after menses. For women past menopause the examination should be done on a regularly scheduled monthly basis. In fact, over 90% of breast cancers are detected by women themselves. Table 54 indicates abnormal breast changes you should report to your doctor. Symptoms of breast

Table 53   RISK FACTORS ASSOCIATED WITH BREAST CANCER

Highest Risk Factors:

1. Personal history of breast cancer.
2. Family history of breast cancer in a close relative (mother or sister).
3. History of breast biopsy showing "proliferative" or "atypical" cell changes.
4. History of mammogram suspicious for breast cancer.

Other Risk Factors:

1. First pregnancy after age thirty (or never had children).
2. Family history of breast cancer in a distant relative (maternal aunt or grandmother).
3. History of menstrual periods before age twelve.
4. History of fibrocystic breast disease.
5. Obesity or a high-fat diet.
6. History of an abnormal thermogram.
7. Previous endometrial cancer.
8. Menopause after age fifty.

Possible Risk Factors—Not Proven:

1. Estrogen hormones, including the pill.
2. Being a DES mother (see Chapter 37).
3. Plastic surgery to enlarge breasts using implants*.

---

* Risk not associated with implants but with possible decreased ability to detect breast lumps through physical examination after such surgery.

---

disease include breast discharge and breast lumps (see Chapters 55 and 56).

Breast X-rays (mammography)

It is now believed that most breast cancers are present for six to eight years before they become larger than a pea and can be felt. Mammography, an X-ray technique that provides a picture of the breasts, is the best screening method currently available for detecting nonpalpable tumors (ones that can't be felt). *Xeroradiography*, a relatively new technique developed by Xerox Corporation, records the X-ray images from your mammogram on paper, rather than on X-ray film. Some radiol-

ogists believe that this process provides a clearer picture of the breasts than the X-ray itself.

Currently, the National Cancer Institute and the American Cancer Society Breast Cancer Demonstration Projects have detected increasing numbers of nonpalpable small breast cancers, using mammography. Mammograms accurately identify breast cancer 85% of the time. Compared to tumors found by physical examination alone, those detected through mammography are more likely to be in an earlier stage and not yet spread beyond the breast.

There is general agreement that women over fifty and certain high-risk women under fifty should receive periodic mammograms to screen for breast cancer. The benefits of mammography are less clearly established for women under fifty without symptoms. The American Cancer Society, as of July 1983, recommends periodic mammograms for all women beginning at age *forty*, while the American College of Obstetricians and Gynecologists recommends this routine screening beginning at age *fifty* (see Table 55). Women between thirty-five and forty should have at least an initial mammogram and more frequent mammographic screening if they are at high risk for breast cancer. Large-scale studies have clearly shown about a 30% decrease in breast cancer mortality among women over fifty who receive annual mammograms.

Table 54   BREAST CHANGES TO REPORT TO YOUR DOCTOR

The following are possible signs of breast cancer:

Change	Comment
Breast lump or lumps	especially if painless and involving only one breast and if lumps do not become smaller following menses
Breast discharge	especially if bloody or involving only one breast
Skin changes	flaking, crusting, or "weeping" eruptions around the nipple; dimpling or retraction of skin over a portion of one breast

---

The furor in recent years over breast X-rays stems from the possibility that, theoretically, *radiation exposure* during the mammography could itself cause breast cancer. When mammography is performed repeatedly in women under fifty over a prolonged period (such as twenty years), concern is warranted—at least until the benefits of routine breast X-rays in young, *symptomless, low-risk* women are proved or disproved. This issue, however, should not obscure the value mammograms have in other situations where the risk/benefit ratio is clearly in the woman's favor. In diagnosing a breast mass or nipple discharge or in evaluating women with risk factors for breast cancer, mammograms are clearly beneficial.

In the past few years, two significant developments in mammography—lowered radiation dosage and improved X-ray imaging (which provides a clearer picture)—have shifted the risk/benefit ratio in the direction of greater safety. In 1963, when mammograms first came into widespread use, the radiation dosage ranged from 6 to 8 rads. Today, the dosage for a breast X-ray may range from 0.5 to 1 rad, or about ten times less than what was used in most of the earlier studies to calculate radiation risk. With modern equipment delivering lower dosages of radiation to the breast, risks from breast X-rays are far outweighed by their value in early detection of breast cancer. In fact, breast cancer screening projects in the 1970s have shown that for every breast cancer detected solely by physical examination in women under fifty, another six such cancers were detected solely by mammograms.

Thermography

Some breast cancers (as well as a number of other, benign conditions) cause an increase in the breast's skin temperature. Thermography, a relatively new technique, provides a photographic image of heat patterns on the breast surface. A heat-detecting device maps and records hot spots or areas of increased blood distribution. While it avoids X-rays, thermography has somewhat limited usefulness since it does not easily distinguish between cancer and other breast diseases. The result is a high percentage of false-positive thermograms. The majority of women with abnormal thermograms do not have or develop breast cancer. Nevertheless, a woman with an abnormal thermogram has several times the risk of developing breast cancer. Despite its technical limitations,

Table 55 PERIODIC MAMMOGRAMS

When are periodic* mammograms (breast X-rays) recommended for women without symptoms of breast disease?

Under 35 years	Not generally recommended unless highest risk factors are present (see Table 53).
35 to 50 years	May be recommended if one or more risk factors are present.
	If no risk factors are present, initial mammogram recommended between ages 35 and 40.
	Not recommended for women who received DES in pregnancy (see Chapter 37) unless a personal or strong (mother or sister) family history of breast cancer is present.
Over age 50	Generally recommended for all women.

* Annually or less often as determined by your physician. *Note:* These recommendations are consistent with the September, 1979, guidelines of the American College of Obstetricians and Gynecologists.

thermography is a safe screening technique, which may be used in combination with mammography to detect early breast disease more accurately than either method alone.

Treatment of breast cancer

Mastectomy (breast removal) is usually the primary treatment for breast cancer. In the past ten years, there has been considerable debate as to the best method. Most surgeons now agree, however, that there are relatively few indications for the classical procedure known as *radical mastectomy*, in which the entire affected breast, the chest muscles underneath, and the lymph nodes under the arm are removed. A less extensive procedure, the *modified radical mastectomy* (also called *total mastectomy*), without removal of the chest wall muscles, is now the standard operation for most breast cancers. With cure rates comparable to more radical operations, the total mastectomy allows for better cosmetic results and less immobility and swelling of the arm because the chest wall muscles are preserved.

Other types of mastectomy include *simple mastectomy* (complete removal of the breast but not the lymph nodes under the arm *or* the chest wall muscles), and *segmental mastectomy* (or *lumpectomy*) in which only a portion of the breast is removed, including the cancer and a surrounding margin of breast tissue. Lumpectomy, with or without radiation therapy, is a controversial approach now under study in a number of cancer centers to determine whether this less radical surgery can achieve results comparable to total mastectomy. Preliminary results in women with early tumors have been quite favorable; but before definite conclusions can be reached, there must be long-term follow-up for ten to twenty-five years.

Other treatment, used singly or in combination, includes anticancer drugs (chemotherapy), hormone therapy, and radiation. Radiation therapy is used before surgery to shrink the tumor or after to eliminate any remaining cancer cells. Hormones and anticancer drugs are usually used to stop more advanced breast cancer from spreading. Hormone manipulation may include removal of the ovaries to eliminate the natural source of estrogens that could stimulate tumor growth in women with this cancer.

Because technical knowledge affecting treatment of breast cancer changes so rapidly, any woman with this disease should consider referral to a major cancer center, which will have the latest, specialized methods to diagnose and treat the disease.

Rehabilitation after breast surgery

During rehabilitation, physical therapy may be necessary. Some women may want to select a prosthesis (artificial replacement) at this time. Sometimes plastic surgery can be performed to reconstruct the breast. Following less radical forms of surgery, breast reconstructive surgery may be relatively easy. At other times, the plastic surgery may involve taking skin and other tissue from another part of the body, such as the thigh, and grafting it onto the breast.

After the initial crisis of a mastectomy has passed, there is a continuing need for emotional support. Support groups, such as the American Cancer Society's Reach to Recovery Program, composed of women who have experienced mastectomy, help women cope with the emotional problems associated both with the loss of a breast

and with being afflicted with a serious disease. It is encouraging to note that a recent study assessing psychological and social adjustment to mastectomy found that 70% of the women studied felt they had made a satisfactory emotional adjustment one year after their surgery.

For information about the Reach to Recovery Program, write to:

Reach to Recovery
19 W. 56th Street
New York, New York 10019

or telephone: (212) 586-8700.

Resources

For more information about all forms of cancer, including breast cancer, contact the following groups:

1. Cancer Information Service, telephone 800-638-6694. This is a national, toll-free telephone network which provides information about cancer and cancer-related resources to the general public.
2. Office of Cancer Communications. This organization provides information on all aspects of cancer research, operates the Cancer Information Service, and distributes free publications on cancer to the general public. Write to:
    Office of Cancer Communications
    National Cancer Institute
    Building 31, Room 10A-18
    9000 Rockville Pike
    Bethesda, Maryland 20205
3. Your local chapter of the American Cancer Society. The A.C.S. can provide helpful educational material as well as information on local and regional resources. Or write to:
    American Cancer Society, Inc.
    777 Third Avenue
    New York, New York 10017
    or telephone (212) 371-2900.

Uterine Fibroids

Uterine fibroids are the number one cause of an abnormally enlarged uterus and one of the most common reasons for hysterectomy. Fibroid tumors, composed of muscular and fibrous tissue, originate in the wall of the uterus (see Figure 27). The size, shape, location, and symptoms of uterine fibroids are tremendously variable, sometimes making it difficult or impossible to differentiate them from an enlarged ovary. Fibroids, single or multiple, usually grow slowly, if at all. They may increase in size under the influence of estrogen produced during pregnancy or from birth control pills or estrogen taken to treat menopausal symptoms. When estrogen production stops following menopause, fibroids tend to decrease in size.

Less than one out of two hundred uterine fibroids becomes cancerous. An enlarged uterus where the enlargement is due to a fibroid is unlikely to be cancerous in the absence of abnormal bleeding or rapid growth. Although usually symptomless, large fibroids may contribute to chronic backache, pelvic pain, and heavy or prolonged periods. When uterine fibroids are located within the uterine cavity, they may also contribute to impaired fertility, repeated miscarriage, or premature labor.

Diagnosis

Uterine fibroids are usually detected during a routine pelvic exam because they result in an enlarged, irregular uterus. Once an irregularity has been found, the clinician often employs several techniques to localize and identify fibroids: sonography (to differentiate between ovarian and uterine masses), hysterosalpingography (to identify fibroids located within the uterine cavity), and regular abdominal X-rays (refer to the index for more information about these procedures). Fibroids are sometimes detected inadvertently at the time of a D & C (see glossary). The fibroids produce an irregular surface along the uterine cavity that the doctor can feel during this procedure. These tumors cannot be removed, however, during the D & C since they are embedded in the uterine wall.

Treatment

At present, there is no medical treatment to shrink fibroids. Fortunately, surgery is not necessary for the woman who has small fibroids (smaller than four inches in diameter) that cause few or no symptoms. However, she should have checkups at least every six months to check for rapid fibroid growth, which may indicate malignancy.

Surgery is indicated (see Table 56) if the fibroids cause chronic or severe pain or bleeding. Surgery is also usually performed for symptomless fibroids that are four to five inches or more in diameter or for those that are growing rapidly. Surgery involves removing either the fibroid alone (myomectomy) or the entire uterus (hysterectomy).

When it is impossible to determine from tests whether a pelvic mass is an enlarged ovary or an enlarged uterus, surgery may also be needed to

Figure 27
Different types of fibroid tumor.

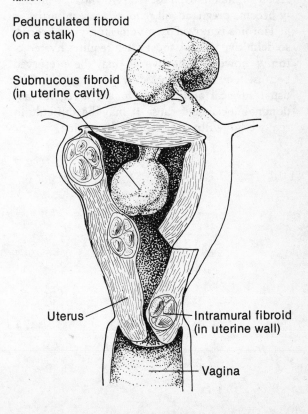

Pedunculated fibroid (on a stalk)

Submucous fibroid (in uterine cavity)

Uterus

Intramural fibroid (in uterine wall)

Vagina

Table 56　POSSIBLE REASONS FOR FIBROID SURGERY

1. Persistently heavy periods, often with anemia, despite a D & C.

2. Persistent pain, backache, or severe menstrual cramps.

3. Increase in fibroid growth especially in a woman not taking the pill or other estrogen-containing drug.

4. Large fibroids (four to five inches or more in diameter; that is, uterine enlargement to about 12-weeks size or more).

5. When the diagnosis is in doubt making it impossible to distinguish between a uterine and an ovarian tumor.

---

clarify the diagnosis. The more conservative surgical procedure, myomectomy, is usually performed only on women who want to retain their childbearing potential. Myomectomy is most likely to be successful when there is a single, isolated fibroid which does not involve a large amount of the uterine wall. Following myomectomy and repair of the uterus, most women who subsequently become pregnant will require cesarean births.

Fibroids removed by myomectomy may recur, so definitive therapy most often requires hysterectomy; however, the ovaries may be preserved because they are unaffected by this condition. The usual surgical approach is to use a regular abdominal incision because it may be difficult to remove large fibroids through the vagina.

35

Endometriosis

Sometimes the tissue that lines the uterine cavity (this lining is called the *endometrium*) implants at other places, such as the ovaries, the tubes, or outside the uterus. When this condition occurs, the disorder is called *endometriosis*. A chronic, characteristically progressive condition, endometriosis occurs only during the premenopausal years and is most prevalent among women in their thirties and forties.

Exactly how endometrial tissue gets to these places is unknown, but it is believed that during menstruation, portions of the endometrium are displaced from the uterine cavity into the Fallopian tubes and from there into the abdominal cavity. These endometrial deposits adhere to the surfaces of other organs, such as the ovaries and intestines, and sometimes form large cysts.

Because endometrial tissue responds to hormonal influences during the menstrual cycle, women who have this disorder often feel pain just prior to or during menstruation. The character and severity of endometriosis pain, however, varies considerably, depending on where the endometrial tissue is deposited. Although some women have no pain at all, others chronically experience pelvic pain or painful intercourse. Aside from pain, the other important health problem associated with endometriosis is infertility, which is found in about 10% of women with this condition. Endometriosis may contribute to infertility by interfering with ovulation or by causing tubal blockage.

Pregnancy tends to prevent or lessen the symptoms of endometriosis, while delayed childbearing may predispose to this disease. With more and more working women postponing pregnancy until their thirties or even later, the incidence of endometriosis—often called the "working women's disease"—is expected to rise during the 1980s.

Diagnosis

A doctor often presumes a woman has endometriosis if, during a pelvic examination, he or she feels nodular, tender areas behind or beneath the cervix. No laboratory tests are available to confirm the diagnosis, however. Only by seeing the pelvic organs during surgery can a doctor be certain that endometrial deposits exist. (Even when a woman with endometriosis experiences severe chronic pelvic pain, there may be no abnormal physical findings.)

The first step in the surgical diagnosis of endometriosis is often laparoscopy. In this procedure, the doctor views the pelvic organs with a small, telescopelike instrument. Laparoscopy eliminates the need at this point for the traditional abdominal incision. When significant disease is not found, often the doctor can remove small endometrial implants by cauterizing (see glossary) them through the laparoscope.

Treatment

In the early stages of endometriosis, pregnancy, which interrupts menstruation, is a form of preventive therapy. Most authorities agree that pregnancy tends to lessen the symptoms of this disease. Breast-feeding may also benefit women with endometriosis since it can extend the menses-free interval.

Standard initial treatment for endometriosis consists of hormone drugs, usually containing either progesterone or a combination of estrogen and progesterone (as found in most oral contraceptives). The woman who has not started or completed her family should not delay treatment for endometriosis since the disease is often progressive with symptoms of pain increasing and greater likelihood of impaired fertility. Hormone drugs dissolve endometrial deposits in many women; however, symptoms may recur when therapy stops.

A new hormonal drug, danazol, is increasingly used and is rapidly becoming the standard nonsurgical treatment for moderate to severe forms of endometriosis. Although danazol is costly (presently about $160 a month), the drug appears to offer the most effective hormonal treatment for women with severe pain or infertility due to endometriosis. Danazol's side effects may include weight gain, acne, and, on rare occasions, increased hair growth. Danazol must be taken for three to six months to be effective, and pregnancy is contraindicated during this time. Approximately 70 to 90% of the women taking danazol obtain relief from pain symptoms and nearly 70% of the women taking it to overcome infertility may become pregnant following danazol therapy, if no other infertility factors are present.

When hormonal drugs fail to relieve symptoms or if an undiagnosed pelvic mass is suspected of being an endometriosis cyst, a woman may require surgical evaluation. There are at least three different ways to approach this surgery. Your gynecologist should discuss the alternatives with you so you can select the option that best suits your needs.

The most conservative approach is laparoscopy to confirm the diagnosis, establish the extent of the disease, and remove small endometrial deposits. Further surgery is put off until you have the opportunity to discuss the surgical findings and possible alternatives with your doctor.

The second approach involves limited surgery. Through a regular abdominal incision, the surgeon removes endometrial cysts, adhesions, or other evidence of endometriosis which cannot be removed during laparoscopy. In addition, certain pelvic nerves may be cut by means of a rather extensive but beneficial pain-relieving operation known as a *presacral neurectomy*. With this approach, potential fertility may be preserved and enhanced. It is unclear how fertility is restored by these procedures because it is unknown how endometriosis causes sterility.

The most definitive as well as radical surgery for endometriosis involves a complete hysterectomy, that is, one involving removal of both tubes and ovaries. Although this surgery eliminates childbearing potential, this alternative may be the best one for the woman who has already completed her family since, after limited surgery, endometriosis can recur.

Recently a new technique, the carbon dioxide laser (see Chapter 36), has been introduced for the surgical treatment of endometriosis. The laser uses a high-intensity light beam for precise destruction of abnormal tissue—in this case, small areas of endometriosis. The laser technique can be combined with either laparoscopy or limited surgery through a regular abdominal incision. The latter approach may be used with microsurgery (see Chapter 13). Only time will tell whether laser surgery will prove to be an effective alternative to more traditional surgical methods of treating endometriosis.

36

Cervical Abnormalities and the Pap Smear

What You Should Know About Your Pap Smear

Cervical abnormalities can be detected early, thanks to Pap smear screening. The Pap smear is a painless procedure for obtaining cells from the cervix which are then sent to a laboratory for microscopic analysis. The technique, however, is just a screening device, and only a cervical biopsy can establish a firm diagnosis if the Pap smear is abnormal. The Pap smear is an effective screening tool because precancerous changes usually occur over a number of years before cervical cancer develops. Pap smears also can detect about 50% of endometrial (uterine) cancers and a much lesser percentage of other tumors in the female reproductive tract. Approximately 45 out of every 1,000 women screened have abnormal Pap smears, but many of these are due to infections, not to cancer or precancerous changes. Such precancerous changes are called *dysplasia.*

Dysplasia is classified as *mild, moderate,* or *severe.* Severe dysplasia is the most likely of the three to become cancerous, while milder forms sometimes go away on their own. Over a period of many years, about one-third of the women with moderate or severe dysplasia will develop cervical cancer if the condition is not treated. Severe dysplasia characteristically progresses first to surface cancer, or *carcinoma-in-situ*, involving only the outer layer of the cervix. Both dysplasia and carcinoma-in-situ, readily diagnosed by Pap smears, can be cured nearly 100% of the time with appropriate therapy.

According to more recent terminology, dysplasia and carcinoma-in-situ are sometimes referred to collectively as cervical intraepithelial neoplasia (CIN). In the "CIN" classification the different grades of dysplasia are given a number based on severity—for example, mild dysplasia would be equivalent to "CIN_1" and carcinoma-in-situ would be equivalent to "CIN_3."

Table 57   PAP SMEAR CLASSIFICATIONS

Number	Name	Descriptive Term*	Is Cervical Biopsy and/or Colposcopy Indicated?
I	normal	"negative," sometimes "mild inflammation"	no
II	atypical	usually "inflammation," occasionally "dysplasia"	yes, if repeat Pap smear is still abnormal after treatment of infection
III	suspicious	usually "dysplasia," sometimes "carcinoma-in-situ" (surface cancer), rarely "invasive carcinoma" (cancer)	yes
IV	positive	usually "carcinoma-in-situ" (surface cancer), sometimes "invasive carcinoma" (cancer)	yes
V	positive	usually "invasive carcinoma" (cancer)	yes

* New terminology may refer to dysplasia or carcinoma-in-situ as *cervical intraepithelial neoplasia* (CIN).

Pap smears are classified by number, name, and descriptive term indicating the most likely cause for an abnormality when there is one (see Table 57). Most people have a *normal*, or Class I, so-called negative, smear. All other classes denote an abnormal condition, which is not necessarily a cancerous or precancerous one. The second most common Pap smear result is a Class II smear, often called *atypical* and described in the report as "inflammation" to reflect underlying cervical or vaginal infection. Class III smears are usually labeled *suspicious*, since up to 50% of the women in this category may have cervical cancer (usually the early surface type). Most of the other 50% have varying degrees of dysplasia. Class IV and V smears are usually called *positive*. "Carcinoma-in-situ," or early surface cancer, usually describes Class IV smears. And "invasive carcinoma" is the descriptive term for those in Class V, denoting that the tumor extends into deeper layers of tissue.

The American Cancer Society (A.C.S.) now recommends that all women over the age of twenty who are sexually active have a Pap smear at least once every *three* years (see Table 3, in Chapter 4). This guideline applies only after you have had two negative (normal) Pap smears one year apart. If risk factors for cervical cancer (see Table 58) apply to you, you will need to have this test performed more frequently. The A.C.S. still recommends annual breast and pelvic examinations for women over forty but has relaxed this recommendation to every three years for those under forty.

The American Cancer Society's change to the three-year frequency represents a major shift from the previous recommendation that a woman should have a Pap smear every year. The change is based partly upon the rationale that cancer of the cervix usually passes through detectable precancerous stages over a period of years. But cost effectiveness is also a major concern. According to the A.C.S., the new recommendation represents a compromise between risk and cost benefits which will provide a twofold cost savings while delivering about 97% of the increase in life expectancy achieved by an annual Pap smear.

The American College of Obstetricians and Gynecologists (ACOG) has expressed strong opposition to the cancer society's new policy. In a policy statement dated June, 1980, ACOG noted that approximately 5% of cancers of the cervix progress from a symptomless stage detectable by Pap smear to an advanced invasive cancer in three years or *less*. Many obstetricians have concerns

---

Table 58 **RISK FACTORS ASSOCIATED WITH CANCER OF THE CERVIX**

1. First intercourse, marriage, or pregnancy at an early age.
2. Multiple sex partners.
3. Herpes vaginal infection.
4. Large family size (many pregnancies).

---

about the new guidelines since most of the background work on which the guidelines are based was done in Scandinavian countries and Iceland, which have smaller, more homogeneous populations with fewer high-risk women. It is estimated that 50% to 80% of American women are in the high-risk category for cancer of the cervix. Because of such facts and concern that lengthening the screening interval may result in an increase in untreated cancers, ACOG has recommended that most women continue to have Pap smears on an annual basis.

Evaluation of Abnormal Pap Smears

When a minor vaginal or cervical infection is responsible for a Class II classification, the smear frequently reverts to Class I two or three months after treatment of the infection. In cases like these, no other immediate tests are necessary. If a *repeat* Class II Pap smear occurs, however, or a Class III, IV, or V smear is obtained initially, the doctor will perform a cervical biopsy to evaluate the abnormal Pap smear (see Figure 28). He or she may first do a *colposcopy*, a relatively new and painless office procedure using a colposcope. The colposcope is a special type of microscope which allows the doctor to examine the cervix and vagina more closely by magnification. This instrument also permits the doctor to take a more accurate cervical biopsy. When combined with cervical biopsy, colposcopy may eliminate the need for the more extensive and costly surgical procedure, the cone biopsy (see below). A cone biopsy, however, may still be necessary if the findings up to this point cannot explain the abnormal Pap smear.

Evaluation of the Cervical Biopsy

Ultimate treatment of an abnormal Pap smear depends upon what the cervical biopsy reveals—

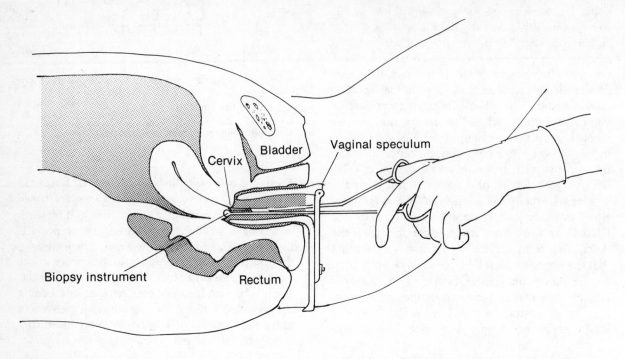

Figure 28 *Biopsy of the cervix. The doctor uses an instrument to biopsy, or remove a small piece of tissue from, the cervix.*

inflammation, precancerous changes (dysplasia), or, rarely, cancer. Inflammation of the cervix (cervicitis) may be associated with a vaginal infection or discharge that requires only local treatment with vaginal creams or suppositories. Therapy for dysplasia depends upon its severity and usually consists of either cryosurgery or cone biopsy. A new procedure, laser therapy, is also available for the treatment of dysplasia at some university centers; however, the technique is costly and still somewhat experimental.

Cryosurgery

Cryosurgery, or so-called cold cautery, destroys tissue by freezing rather than by burning with an electric current (electrocoagulation or so-called hot cautery). In recent years, cryosurgery has become more popular than electrocoagulation to treat cervical infections, benign cervical growths, such as polyps, and some forms of dysplasia. Cryosurgery is most often used to treat mild or moderate dysplasia. A few clinicians, who rely heavily on their expertise as colposcopists, also treat severe dysplasia or even surface cervical

cancers with cryosurgery. This latter approach is controversial because its long-term effectiveness has not been studied. Many gynecologists believe severe dysplasia and surface cervical cancer call for a cone biopsy.

As compared to electrocoagulation, cryosurgery has the advantage of producing little or no discomfort. It also poses the least risk of complications, such as bleeding, further infection, or (rarely) infertility from scarring. Cryosurgery also avoids the hazards of cone biopsy, when this more extensive procedure is not necessary.

Following either hot or cold cautery, a watery vaginal discharge may occur for about two weeks. Most clinicians recommend avoiding intercourse, douching, and the use of tampons during this time.

Cone biopsy (conization)

A cone biopsy is an extended form of cervical biopsy, which derives its name from the cone-shaped wedge of tissue that is removed from the lower cervix (see Figure 39, in Chapter 44). Although a cone biopsy removes the same tissue as would be destroyed by cryosurgery, the biopsy usually removes a *deeper* section of tissue. The procedure is performed under general anesthesia in a hospital or an outpatient care facility.

The most common complication of cone biopsy is postoperative bleeding; it occurs about 10% of the time and it may develop as late as two weeks after surgery. Much less often the procedure leads to narrowing or blockage of the cervical canal, thereby resulting in impaired fertility. An extensive or deep cone may weaken the cervix's ability to remain closed during pregnancy and, on rare occasions, may cause a woman to be more susceptible to miscarriage or premature labor.

Unlike cryosurgery, a cone biopsy provides additional tissue for evaluation. Thus, the pathologist can confirm the original biopsy diagnosis and be more certain that an additional or more serious abnormality has not been overlooked.

Most gynecologists perform cone biopsies as initial therapy when the cervical biopsy shows severe dysplasia or carcinoma-in-situ. The procedure may also be necessary for mild or moderate dysplasia when colposcopy is unavailable or does not give full results. If the cone biopsy reveals nothing more than mild or moderate dysplasia, then no further treatment is indicated. If severe dysplasia or carcinoma-in-situ is found from the cone biopsy, however, hysterectomy is the definitive treatment. This surgery is often put off temporarily, however, in a woman who desires future childbearing until after she completes her family. Finally, if invasive cancer of the cervix is found, prompt treatment, either surgery or radiation therapy, is the recommended approach (see below).

A woman with a history of dysplasia or carcinoma-in-situ should have regular Pap smears at least every six months or more frequently, as individual circumstances dictate. Following a cone biopsy or cryosurgery, a woman should not have her next Pap smear until three to four months later since the surgical procedures may cause temporary cell changes that could produce falsely abnormal Pap smears.

Laser Surgery

A new technique called laser surgery has received widespread publicity and increased use in the treatment of dysplasia and carcinoma-in-situ. The laser uses a high-intensity light beam for precise destruction of abnormal tissue. The procedure is usually performed on an outpatient basis. Although most gynecologists have not been trained in laser surgery, residency programs in obstetrics and gynecology now usually include such training. Special courses involving hands-on experience in the use of the laser have recently become popular among practicing gynecologists anxious to become skilled in the latest surgical technology. While no generally accepted standard exists for giving physicians hospital privileges to perform laser surgery, in many hospitals credentials committees are now establishing guidelines for competency in the use of lasers.

In experienced hands the laser appears to be as effective in treating dysplasia and carcinoma-in-situ as the other methods—cryosurgery and cone biopsy. The laser may not offer a significant advantage over cryosurgery, since laser surgery is more costly without offering greater effectiveness. Compared to traditional cone biopsy, the laser reportedly has fewer complications such as infection and bleeding, but again may be more costly.

Cancer of the Cervix

Cervical cancer is one of the most common pelvic cancers in women. The incidence of invasive cervical cancer, where the tumor extends into deeper tissue layers or spreads to other organs, has decreased about one half in the past twenty years. However, the incidence of carcinoma-in-situ, which involves only the outer portion (surface layer) of the cervix, has risen steadily. Overall survival from cervical cancer has steadily improved over the past ten years, more so than for any other malignancy in women. The statistics have been attributed in part to early detection of precancerous changes through Pap smear screening. (See Table 63 for information on frequency statistics and other factors associated with cervical cancer.)

Invasive cancer rarely occurs in women who have regular checkups. But when it does, it may cause a blood discharge between periods or spotting after intercourse. By the time carcinoma-in-situ has become invasive, there is likely to be an abnormal growth on the cervix. Cervical biopsy is then performed to establish the diagnosis. Carcinoma-in-situ alone usually does not produce symptoms or abnormal physical findings.

Cervical cancer is sometimes referred to as a venereal disease because risk factors consistently relate to sexual intercourse and the cancer rarely occurs in the absence of regular intercourse. The disease hardly ever occurs, for example, in nuns, other celibate women, or lesbians. Risk factors for cervical cancer include multiple sex partners, first intercourse at an early age, early marriage, large family size, and possibly long-term use of birth control pills (more than five years). Although the sexually transmitted agent in cervical cancer has yet to be identified, the herpes virus has been suspected of playing a role since women with herpes vaginal infections have an increased risk of developing this malignancy. The rising rate of vaginal herpes infections in recent years is becoming a major concern to thousands of young women who have a history of this viral disease. Women with one or more risk factors (see Table 58) should have Pap smears at least annually. With regular checkups, invasive cancer—even in high-risk women—should be completely preventable.

Treatment

Treatment of cervical cancer depends on the tumor's stage when diagnosed. Carcinoma-in-situ may be treated with cone biopsy in a woman who has not completed her family. However, definitive treatment of carcinoma-in-situ requires hysterectomy because surface cancer can recur in approximately 10% of the women treated with cone biopsy alone.

Invasive cancer may be treated by a more extended hysterectomy, called *radical hysterectomy*, in which the upper portion of the vagina and the pelvic lymph nodes are also removed, or by radiation therapy. Most women with cervical cancer can be cured, including up to 95% of those with early invasive cancers and nearly 100% of those with carcinoma-in-situ.

The DES Story

During the 1940s and 1950s, in an attempt to prevent miscarriages, thousands of expectant mothers took synthetic estrogen drugs called DES, which stands for diethylstilbestrol. (DES and DES-related drugs are listed in Table 59.) Twenty years later, seven young women developed vaginal cancer called *clear cell carcinoma*, a malignancy hardly ever reported before. An investigation of the women and their families showed a definite relationship between treatment of pregnant women with DES-type drugs and the development in their daughters of a variety of uterine and vaginal abnormalities, including vaginal cancer. Fortunately, the incidence of this cancer has turned out to be much lower than originally feared, the estimated frequency being between 1.4 per 1,000 and 1.4 per 10,000 of exposed daughters.

Benign Changes in DES Daughters

Up to 80% of DES daughters have benign changes involving the cervix or vagina as a result of exposure to this drug. These abnormalities include slight, symptomless anatomical changes involving the upper vagina and cervix. These would go unnoticed if pelvic examinations were not done. An examination may reveal that the cervix is surrounded by a fold of vaginal tissue, sometimes known as a *vaginal collar*. In addition, the glands normally found only in the cervix appear in small numbers in the vagina as well. This condition, called *adenosis*, occasionally leads to a slight increase in vaginal discharge.

It has been theorized that vaginal cancer may develop in areas of adenosis since 90% of the women who have vaginal cancer have adenosis as well. At present, however, there is not a single documented case of vaginal cancer developing in a previously identified area of adenosis.

Several investigators report a possible link

Table 59   DES-TYPE DRUGS*

Amperone	Diethylstilbestrol Dipropionate	Menocrin	Oestromon	Stilpalmitate
Benzestrol		Meprane	Orestol	Stilphostrol
Chlorotrianisene	Diethylstilbenediol	Mestilbol	Pabestrol D	Stilronate
Comestrol	Digestil	Methallenestril	Palestrol	Stilrone
Cyren A	Domestrol	Metystil	Restrol	Stils
Cyren B	Estan	Microest	Stil-Rol	Synestrin
Delvinal	Estilben	Mikarol	Stilbal	Synestrol
DES	Estrobene	Mikarol forti	Stilbestrol	Synthoestrin
DesPlex	Estrobene DP	Milestrol	Stilbestronate	Tace
Di-Erone	Estrosyn	Monomestrol	Stilbetin	Teserene
Diestryl	Fonatol	Neo-Oestranol I	Stilbinol	Tylandril
Dibestil	Gynben	Neo-Oestranol II	Stilboestroform	Tylosterone
Dienoestrol	Gyneben	Nulabort	Stilboestrol	Vallestril
Diethylstilbestrol Dipalmitate	Hexestrol	Oestrogenine	Stilboestrol DP	Willestrol
	Hexoestrol	Oestromenin	Stilestrate	
Diethylstilbestrol Diphosphate	Hi-Bestrol			

* From *DES Exposure in Utero*, (former) Department of Health, Education, and Welfare, Publication No. (NIH) 76-1119.

between DES exposure in utero (that is, a woman's exposure to the drug when she was a fetus in her mother's uterus) and certain malformations of the daughter's uterus that may make the daughter susceptible to complications during pregnancy, especially premature labor. To date, however, there is no conclusive evidence that exposure to DES makes women more susceptible to having problems conceiving or delivering their babies normally.

DES Daughters and Cancer

In October, 1978, a task force on DES (formed by the former Department of Health, Education, and Welfare (HEW)) verified the link between DES exposure in utero and increased risk of vaginal cancer. In fact, approximately 360 DES daughters have been found to have cancer of the vagina. The disease may be symptomless in its early stages, or a woman, as young as a teen-ager, may experience abnormal bleeding.

Considerable controversy surrounds the question of whether cancer of the *cervix* or precancer-ous cervical changes (dysplasia) are related to DES exposure. A definite relationship is yet to be established, and the increased risk of *cervical* cancer, if present, is believed to be extremely small.

Overall, the chances of a DES daughter developing vaginal or cervical cancer are slight. But, because the long-term effects of DES exposure are unknown, the DES task force currently recommends that DES daughters minimize their exposure to estrogen, whether in the form of birth control pills, postmenopausal estrogens, or postcoital (after intercourse) contraceptives. Estrogens are not absolutely forbidden, but they should be taken only after careful discussion of alternatives with your clinician.

Evaluation of DES Daughters

If a woman was possibly exposed to DES-type drugs before birth, an attempt should be made to verify the information from medical records. The physician who cared for the mother during her pregnancy should have them. A DES daughter should, starting at the age of fourteen (or earlier if there is abnormal vaginal bleeding or discharge), have a pelvic exam at least once a year (see Table 60). Her checkup should include a regular Pap smear, as well as a Pap smear of the upper vagina since this is where vaginal cancer would arise. She should also have an iodine staining of her vagina and cervix to identify abnormal areas and possible adenosis. If adenosis is suspected, a biopsy (removal and examination of tissue) is necessary to confirm this diagnosis. Such biopsies cause very little discomfort. To help identify suspicious cervical or vaginal areas, many gynecologists will also perform colposcopy (see Chapter 36, under Evaluation of Abnormal Pap Smears). This procedure is not essential, however, because most, if not all, DES-related abnormalities are easily seen or felt on pelvic exam or by iodine staining. If the clinician does find benign cervical or vaginal abnormalities, including adenosis, no specific therapy is indicated. The woman should, however, have frequent checkups, usually about every six months, depending on the severity of the findings. These checkups should include both the Pap smear and iodine staining. Abnormal Pap smears should, of course, be evaluated and treated as discussed in Chapter 36.

DES Mothers

There is controversy about the relationship between DES exposure during pregnancy and the development of breast cancer in mothers who were treated with this drug. The DES task force reported two studies on this issue: one found no association whatsoever while the other suggested a possible, but statistically insignificant, association. Still, DES mothers should have regular annual breast and pelvic examinations and perform self-examinations of their breasts every month. In addition, the DES task force suggests that until the issue of DES and gynecologic cancer is clarified further, DES mothers should avoid *routine* mammograms before age fifty, unless they have significant risk factors, such as a strong family history of breast cancer.

DES Sons

Recent studies have shown an increase in genital and possibly urinary tract abnormalities in males

Table 60   RECOMMENDATIONS FOR DES DAUGHTERS

1. Have an annual pelvic examination, including Pap smear and iodine staining of the vagina, starting at age 14.

2. If your Pap smear is abnormal, make sure that a colposcopic examination is performed. You'll also need more frequent examinations—every six months.

3. Report abnormal or irregular vaginal bleeding to your clinician.

4. Avoid or restrict use of estrogen for birth control (the pill), menopause symptoms, and after-intercourse contraception.

5. If you become pregnant, be especially alert for signs of premature labor. Ask your clinician to perform frequent pelvic examinations during your pregnancy to check for early dilation of the cervix.

exposed to DES. The abnormalities include lowered sperm counts, undersized penises, small or undescended testes, and testicular cysts. Young men and boys who were exposed to DES in utero should have their primary care physician or a urologist examine them to determine if they have any of the problems associated with DES exposure.

Resource

Further information about DES is available from the National Cancer Institute. Request the booklet entitled *Questions and Answers about DES Exposure before Birth* (80-1118). Write to:

Office of Cancer Communications
National Cancer Institute
Building 31, Room 10A-18
9000 Rockville Pike
Bethesda, Maryland 20205

38

Ovarian Cysts and Tumors

An enlarged ovary may result from a variety of different kinds of tumors. A tumor is a swelling or an abnormal tissue growth, and the great majority are benign. Some tumors are solid, while others, known as *cysts*, consist of a thin-walled sac filled with fluid (see Figure 29). In children or in women over forty, *neoplasms* (new growths) usually cause the tumors. In women of childbearing age, however, an enlarged ovary usually results from ovarian cysts which are nonneoplastic—not representative of new growth. Rather, these ovarian cysts are the byproducts of hormone changes that occur during the normal functioning of the ovaries.

Each time the ovary produces an egg, a small cystlike structure (the *follicle*) forms. Typically, the follicle ruptures at ovulation when the ovary releases the egg. Occasionally, the follicle fails to rupture and instead continues to grow, forming a *follicle cyst*. Follicle cysts rarely require treatment. Most regress (return to normal) or occasionally may rupture later on. Sometimes multiple tiny follicle cysts are found in both ovaries. This fairly common condition, known as *polycystic ovary syndrome* (see Chapter 76), occurs because of a hormone imbalance associated with infrequent or absent menstruation. After ovulation, the follicle normally becomes a small hormone-producing structure, known as the *corpus luteum*. Occasionally, the corpus luteum continues to grow, forming a *corpus luteum cyst*.

Ovarian cysts and neoplasms may produce pelvic pain if they rupture, twist, bleed, or become infected. Most of these tumors, however, are symptomless and are first detected during a pelvic examination.

Evaluation of an Enlarged Ovary

Evaluation of an enlarged ovary depends on a woman's symptoms, age, and the characteristics of the tumor at the time of examination. Most ovarian cysts found in women of childbearing age tend to be small (usually less than two inches in diameter) and, in the absence of pelvic pain, can be reevaluated after the next menstrual period. Some clinicians recommend hormones (often birth control pills) to suppress cyst growth for one or two months. If the cyst does not regress during this time, surgery is indicated.

Women with tumors that are larger than three inches in diameter are usually operated on without delay. In a woman past menopause, any ovarian enlargement is abnormal and considered an indication for surgical diagnosis. Only by means of biopsy (tissue removal) can a clinician determine the exact cause of an enlarged ovary. Sometimes a doctor cannot clearly differentiate an ovarian enlargement from a uterine enlargement during the pelvic examination. This distinction is important because uterine growths are less likely to be malignant. Sonography (see glossary) has now replaced the abdominal X-ray as the best means to distinguish the two. If an ovarian tumor can be ruled out, surgery may be unnecessary.

Many ovarian tumors require exploratory surgery (laparotomy) performed through an abdominal incision. The physician may also attempt to establish a diagnosis through laparoscopy, a much less involved procedure, which may be performed on an outpatient basis (see glossary). Laparoscopy is commonly done to assess cystic growths in women under forty or in situations where the clinician cannot determine from the pelvic examination or sonography whether the enlargement originates from the ovary or from the uterus. Sometimes the laparoscopy procedure uncovers unsuspected disease, such as pelvic infection or endometriosis. These conditions may account for symptoms of pelvic pain previously attributed to an ovarian cyst.

An ovarian tumor which appears suspicious at the time of surgery is biopsied to find out if the tissue is cancerous. The surgeon may remove a small area of tumor at the time of laparoscopy. If a regular incision has been made, the biopsy usually consists of removal of the entire tumor. Either way, the tissue is sent to the hospital pathologist for an immediate preliminary evaluation, known as *frozen section*. If the tissue is cancerous, further surgery can be done without delay.

Nonmalignant tumors may require no further treatment, depending somewhat on the woman's

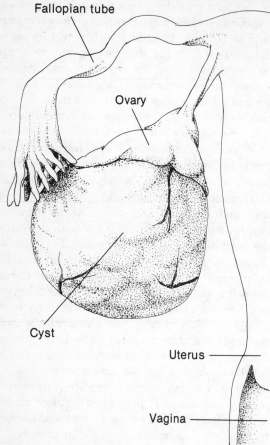

Figure 29
*Noncancerous cyst involving
the left ovary.*

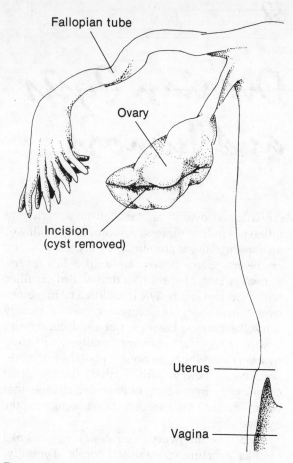

Figure 30
*Many benign ovarian cysts
can be surgically removed
without removing the entire
ovary. Normal hormone
production continues in the
remaining part of the ovary.*

age and childbearing plans. During the childbearing years, most benign ovarian cysts can be removed without damaging the affected ovary (see Figure 30), and no further surgery need be done. However, if you are over forty or if you have completed your family, your doctor may recommend more aggressive treatment, depending upon the tumor's microscopic appearance. The problem is that certain types of ovarian growths cannot be classified as strictly benign or malignant. These types are sometimes described as having "intermediate," or borderline, potential for becoming cancerous later and are sometimes managed by removal of one or both ovaries (oophorectomy; see glossary) as well as the tumor itself. For this reason desire for future childbearing is a particularly important issue that a woman should

discuss thoroughly with her surgeon *before* the operation. In a young woman, removal of just the affected ovary is often done for treatment of these borderline tumors if future childbearing is desired.

Ovarian Cancer

Although less common than cancers of the uterus or cervix, ovarian cancer has become the leading killer among gynecologic malignancies in the last five years, accounting for an estimated 11,000 deaths in 1983. Approximately one woman in seventy may develop ovarian cancer, although rarely before the age of thirty. The overall five-year survival rate of about 35% has improved only slightly in the past thirty-five years. (See Table 63) for information on frequency statistics and other factors associated with ovarian cancer.)

Although at present specific screening tests are unavailable for early detection, periodic pelvic examinations provide some assurance that ovarian cancer will not go undetected. Ovarian cancer characteristically spreads silently and rapidly to other organs within the abdominal cavity and is discovered in a late stage approximately two-thirds of the time. Unlike breast and uterine cancer, ovarian malignancy is associated with a very few known risk factors. Women who have never given birth or have a family history of gynecologic cancer or a personal history of chronically irregular periods may be at slightly increased risk.

Early symptoms of ovarian cancer may include pelvic pressure, abdominal swelling, gas pains, indigestion, and vague abdominal discomfort. Rarely are any of these symptoms, however, attributed to an ovarian tumor since they are usually due to other, benign causes.

The treatment for ovarian cancer is surgery. Occasionally young women who have early tumors involving just one ovary and who have not completed their families may be treated by removal of just the tube and ovary on the affected side. Definitive treatment, however, requires removal of the uterus as well as both tubes and ovaries. (Most clinicians recommend removing the ovaries during elective pelvic surgery being done for some other reason in women over the age of forty-five (some recommend forty) since the 1% risk of ovarian cancer in this age group outweighs the hormonal benefits of preserving the ovaries.)

Few ovarian cancers, even the most advanced, are inoperable. Even if the tumor spreads beyond the abdominal cavity, survival is related directly to the amount of cancerous tissue removed, even if all of it cannot be reached. Following surgery, chemotherapy has been increasingly used to lessen the symptoms and improve the prognosis for women with this disease.

Uterine Cancer

Because uterine cancer begins inside the womb in the tissue lining the uterine cavity (endometrium), the tumor initially cannot be seen or felt during a pelvic examination. While the Pap smear can detect cervical cancer at least 90% of the time, it is unlikely to uncover uterine cancer in more than 50% of the women tested.

Characteristically, uterine (endometrial) cancer afflicts a woman at or past menopause. It is rare before age forty, but about 25% of these cancers do occur in premenopausal women, causing abnormal bleeding between periods or heavy, prolonged menses.

The incidence of endometrial cancer rose sharply in the 1970s, with 37,000 reported cases in 1979, more than double the incidence ten years before. It is not clear to what extent rising uterine cancer rates reflect an aging population, nutritional factors, or the enthusiasm for long-term estrogen administration prior to the 1970s. However, death from this disease has remained constant at about 3,000 cases annually for the past five years, perhaps because an increasing proportion of these tumors are being detected at an early, curable stage. (See Table 63 for information on frequency statistics and other factors associated with uterine cancer.)

There are various factors that increase a woman's chances of developing uterine cancer (see Table 61). But while one or more of these conditions apply for many women, only a very few women are likely to develop this malignancy. Still, some authorities now recommend that women of menopausal age who have one or more risk factors should be screened annually by means of one of the procedures for sampling endometrial tissue (see Diagnosis, below).

Estrogen and Uterine Cancer

The association between long-term estrogen use and the development of uterine cancer is now

Table 61   RISK FACTORS ASSOCIATED WITH UTERINE (ENDOMETRIAL) CANCER

1. Family history of uterine cancer.

2. Obesity.

3. High blood pressure.

4. Diabetes.

5. Polycystic ovaries.

6. Infrequent periods (less than four per year) or infertility due to lack of ovulation.

7. Menstrual periods continuing after age fifty.

8. Infertility or never pregnant.

9. Prolonged treatment with estrogen.*

---

* Not including oral contraceptives.

essentially proven. The effect of short-term estrogen therapy, however, is less clear. Since 1975, at least nine studies have revealed a strong association between estrogen treatment for menopausal symptoms and uterine cancer. Some of these studies seemed to suffer from design flaws, making it difficult to compare estrogen users and nonusers. Another source of possible bias includes the fact that women who have taken estrogen and then develop abnormal bleeding may receive more thorough diagnostic attention in the form of tests such as endometrial biopsies, whereas nonusers of estrogen might not be as likely to have these diagnostic tests done.

In an attempt to clarify the link between estrogen and uterine cancer, the National Institutes of Health (NIH) convened a task force in September, 1979. Comprising research scientists, practicing physicians, and consumers, the task force found that women who took estrogens in the usual daily dose increased their risk for uterine cancer severalfold after using the estrogen for two or more years. The NIH task force also noted that uterine cancer rates paralleled the number of prescriptions filled for estrogen compounds, which peaked in 1976 and then declined. While it's unclear what the risk is if a woman takes lower dosages for shorter periods, the risk is likely to be much less since the risk of developing endometrial

cancer decreases with shorter duration of hormone use and lower dosage. In any case, the task force concurred with recent reports that estrogen use is most likely to be associated with slower-growing uterine cancers, which are the easiest to detect early and to cure.

The NIH panel also noted that many studies suggest that the use of progesterone during several days of each estrogen treatment cycle might reduce the risk of endometrial cancer. Many clinicians now use this cyclic approach to estrogen treatment (see Chapter 27).

The NIH task force, in stating its final conclusions about the use of estrogen in menopausal women, did not say flatly that the drug should not be used. Rather, the task force noted that risks and benefits (from possible prevention of hip fractures, for example) may counterbalance each other and must be weighed for each woman individually. On this basis, an improvement in the quality of life through relief of severe menopausal symptoms or a desire to prevent osteoporosis might be important factors in deciding whether or not to take this drug. (See Chapter 27 for current indications for menopausal estrogen therapy.) Table 62 gives a number of recommendations that may help to minimize the risk of uterine cancer in postmenopausal women who use estrogen hormones. These recommendations are consistent with the final NIH report.

Table 62   RECOMMENDATIONS TO MINIMIZE UTERINE CANCER RISK IN WOMEN WHO TAKE ESTROGEN

If you take estrogen:

1. Ask your clinician to perform a periodic (for example, annual) endometrial biopsy or aspiration (see glossary) to evaluate the uterine lining.

2. Use the lowest possible dose which relieves symptoms (for example, 0.3- or 0.625-mg pills instead of 1.25 or 2.5 mg).

3. Ask your clinician about prescribing progesterone (for example, Provera) for several days each month.

4. Consult your clinician if abnormal vaginal bleeding occurs (any vaginal bleeding after the menopause is abnormal).

Diagnosis

Uterine cancer may be diagnosed by endometrial biopsy or endometrial aspiration (see glossary), two office procedures which evaluate the tissues and cells lining the uterine cavity. It may also be detected by dilatation and curettage (D & C), a surgical procedure performed in a hospital or an ambulatory care facility.

With an endometrial biopsy, the clinician removes samples of endometrial tissue with a curette. Endometrial aspiration is usually a less painful procedure during which the physician washes out the uterine cavity with a syringe that is connected to a small tube that contains a sterile solution. The fluid is then drawn back into the syringe for later laboratory evaluation of uterine cells.

In a woman over forty who is bleeding abnormally but exhibits no other physical symptoms, such as uterine enlargement, an endometrial biopsy or aspiration is usually performed first. These procedures are 80% to 90% reliable in detecting endometrial cancer. Since office procedures may miss 10% of uterine cancers, a D & C is also indicated in the postmenopausal woman when the office biopsy does not produce a diagnosis or is negative.

Sometimes the pathology report from a uterine biopsy or D & C will reveal *endometrial hyperplasia*, an overgrowth of the uterine lining. This condition is believed to result from a hormone imbalance in which the quantity of estrogen is excessive in comparison to the quantity of progesterone. Endometrial hyperplasia may occur by itself, or it may result from prolonged use of estrogen hormones. Estrogen-progesterone imbalance is a normal occurrence in women approaching menopause and is even more likely in infertile or obese women and in women with polycystic ovaries. Such hormone imbalance may account for the increased risk of uterine cancer in women with these conditions. Women who take birth control pills—which all contain a balance of estrogen *and* progesterone—do *not* have a greater risk of developing endometrial hyperplasia.

Endometrial hyperplasia occasionally progresses to uterine cancer. When described in a pathology report as "adenomatous" or "atypical," it is definitely considered premalignant. The condition can often be reversed by administering progesterone hormones. The progesterone counteracts the effect of excessive estrogen stimulation on the uterus. In women who are being treated with estrogen to alleviate postmenopausal hot flashes, endometrial hyperplasia can be prevented by administering progesterone for several days each month. (If endometrial hyperplasia develops and subsequently persists, estrogen should be discontinued.) Most authorities believe recurrent or precancerous types of endometrial hyperplasia are indications for hysterectomy, especially in women near menopausal age. For the woman who has not completed her family, progesterone therapy may be tried; but such therapy remains controversial for the older woman with a recurrent or precancerous form of hyperplasia.

Treatment

Because uterine cancer may spread rapidly, treatment for early stages of this disease involves removal of the uterus as well as both tubes and ovaries. More advanced tumors may be treated with radiation or chemotherapy, in addition to surgery. A gynecology cancer specialist (gynecologic oncologist) is usually consulted if uterine cancer spreads beyond the cavity of the uterus. In this case, the surgeon may have to perform a more extensive hysterectomy, known as a *radical hysterectomy*.

References for Section Eight

Chapter 32—Toxic Shock Syndrome

Centers for Disease Control. Toxic-shock syndrome and the vaginal contraceptive sponge. *Morbidity and Mortality Weekly Report* 33(4):43, Feb 3, 1984.

Toxic shock syndrome update. FDA Drug Bulletin 10(3):17–19, 1980.

Emergency/acute care tips. *The Female Patient* 46, Dec 1980.

High-absorbency tampons linked to toxic shock syndrome. *Physicians' Washington Report* 3(8):1, Feb 1981.

Davis, J. P., et al. Toxic-shock syndrome: epidemiologic features, recurrence, risk factors and prevention. *New England Journal of Medicine* 303:1429–1435, 1980.

Tofte, R. W., and Williams, D. N. Toxic shock syndrome: clinical and laboratory features in 15 patients. *Annals of Internal Medicine* 94(2):149–155, 1981.

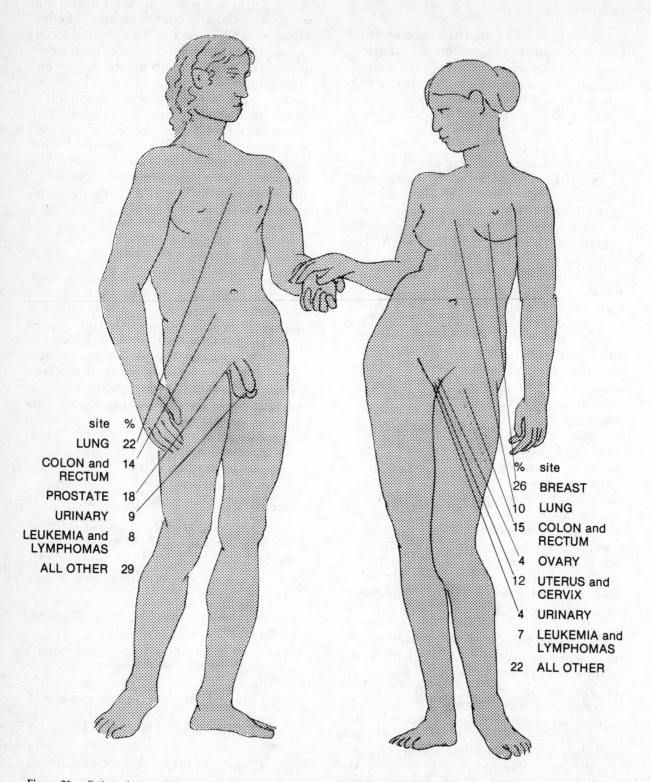

site	%
LUNG	22
COLON and RECTUM	14
PROSTATE	18
URINARY	9
LEUKEMIA and LYMPHOMAS	8
ALL OTHER	29

%	site
26	BREAST
10	LUNG
15	COLON and RECTUM
4	OVARY
12	UTERUS and CERVIX
4	URINARY
7	LEUKEMIA and LYMPHOMAS
22	ALL OTHER

Figure 31   *Estimated cancer incidence for 1984. The chart shows the distribution of the different types of cancer by sex. For example, breast cancer accounts for 26% of all cancers in women. Percentages are based on projections from the National Cancer Institute's Surveillance, Epidemiology, and End Results Program. Carcinoma-in-situ, or surface cancer, of the cervix is not included in the statistics.*

Table 63   FREQUENCY STATISTICS AND OTHER FACTORS ASSOCIATED WITH CANCER OF THE REPRODUCTIVE ORGANS*

	Location			
	Ovary	Uterus	Cervix	Breast
Estimated number of new cases in 1984 (U.S.)	18,300	39,000	16,000**	115,000
Estimated number of deaths in 1984 (U.S.)	11,500	2,900	6,800	37,300
Percent of all cancer deaths in women	6%	2%	4%	19%
Average age	62 (rare before age 40)	57 (rare before age 40)	46 (very uncommon before age 40)	54 (very uncommon before age 40)
Is tumor growth stimulated by estrogen drugs?	no	sometimes***	no	sometimes***
Do periodic examinations allow early detection?	sometimes	definitely	definitely	often
Frequently tumor is detected by:	routine pelvic examinations	endometrial biopsy for abnormal bleeding	Pap smear	self-examination

  * See also Figure 31.

  ** Not including surface cancer (carcinoma-in-situ).

*** However, no data has established that estrogen-containing drugs *cause* breast or uterine cancer.

Chapter 33—Breast Diseases

Leis, H. P., et al. Fibrocystic breast disease. *The Female Patient* 8:56-77, May 1983.

Office of Cancer Communications: *The Breast Cancer Digest – A guide to medical care, emotional support, educational programs and resources.* 1979, NIH Publication No. 80-1691, Dept. of HEW, Bethesda, Maryland.

National Institutes of Health: Consensus Development Conference on *The Treatment of Primary Breast Cancer: Management of Local Disease.* June 1979, Dept. of HEW, Bethesda, Maryland.

Strax, P. Mammography – a radiologist's view. *Ca–A Cancer Journal for Clinicians* 29(1):46–52, 1979.

Committee on Technical Bulletins of the American College of Obstetricians and Gynecologists: *Epidemiology and Diagnosis of Breast Disease.* Technical Bulletin, #71, 1983, American College of Obstetricians and Gynecologists, Washington, D.C.

Executive Board of American College of Obstetricians and Gynecologists: Statement of policy – Mammography. Sept 1979, American College of Obstetricians and Gynecologists, Washington, D.C.

Chapter 34—Uterine Fibroids

Mattingly, R. F. (ed.) *TeLinde's Operative Gynecology,* ed. 5. Philadelphia: Lippincott, 1977.

Novak, E. R., and Woodruff, J. D. *Novak's Gynecologic and Obstetrical Pathology,* ed. 8. Philadelphia: Saunders, 1979.

Chapter 35—Endometriosis

Fayez, J. A., and Taylor, R. B. Endometriosis: staging and management. *The Female Patient* 8:36/1-36/15, Nov 1983.

Kelly, R. W., and Roberts, D. K. CO_2 laser laparoscopy: a potential alternative to danazol in the treatment of stage I and II endometriosis. *The Journal of Reproductive Medicine* 28:638-640, 1983.

Buttram, V. C., Jr., and Betts, J. W. Endometriosis. *Current Problems in Obstetrics and Gynecology* 2(11): 3–58, 1979.

Speroff, L., et al. *Clinical Gynecologic Endocrinology and Infertility,* ed. 3. Baltimore: Williams and Wilkins, 1983.

Greenblatt, R. B., and Tzingounis, V. Danazol treatment of endometriosis: long-term follow-up. *Fertility and Sterility* 32(5):518–520, 1979.

Chapter 36—Cervical Abnormalities and the Pap Smear

Schumann, G. B. Female genital tract cytology. *The Female Patient* 9(5):111–129, May 1984.

American Cancer Society Report on the Cancer-Related Health Checkup. *Ca–A Cancer Journal for Clinicians* 30(4):194–232, 1980.

Clark, E. A., and Anderson, T. W. Does screening by "Pap" smears help prevent cervical cancer? *Lancet* 2:1–4, July 7, 1979.

Executive Board of the American College of Obstetricians and Gynecologists: Statement of policy – Periodic cancer screening for women. June 1980, American College of Obstetricians and Gynecologists, Washington, D.C.

Nelson, J. H., Averette, H. E., et al. Detection, diagnostic evaluation and treatment of dysplasia, carcinoma-in-situ and early invasive cervical cancer. *Ca–A Cancer Journal for Clinicians* 29(3):174–192, 1979.

Lucas, W. E. Cervical cancer: what's the latest in diagnosis and therapy? *Contemporary OB/GYN* 14:19–24, Dec 1979.

Novak, E. R., and Woodruff, J. D. *Novak's Gynecologic and Obstetric Pathology*, ed. 8. Philadelphia: Saunders, 1979.

Rich, W. M. The abnormal Pap – a rationale for management. *The Female Patient* 5:14–18, Nov 1980.

Chapter 37—The DES Story

Braly, P. S., and Berman, M. L. Managing problems of DES daughters. *Contemporary OB/GYN* 24(1):61–72, July 1984.

DES Task Force: *Summary Report*. NIH Publication No. 79-1688, Sept 1978, Dept. of HEW, Washington, D.C.

Herbst, A. L. (ed.) *Intrauterine Exposure to Diethylstilbestrol in the Human*. Proceedings of Symposium on DES, 1977. American College of Obstetricians and Gynecologists, 1978 (monograph).

Herbst, A. L. DES update. *Ca–A Cancer Journal for Clinicians* 30(6):326–332, 1980.

Cousins, L., Karp, W., et al. Reproductive outcome of women exposed to DES in utero. *Obstetrics and Gynecology* 56(1):70–76, 1980.

O'Brien, P. C., et al. Vaginal epithelial changes in young women enrolled in the national cooperative DES adenosis (DESAD) project. *Obstetrics and Gynecology* 53:300–308, Mar 1979.

Rotterdam, H., et al. Vaginal and cervical abnormalities in DES daughters. *The Female Patient* 22–29, Mar 1979.

Herbst, A. L., and Scully, R. E. Update on DES daughters. *Contemporary OB/GYN* 17(5):55–70, 1981.

Chapter 38—Ovarian Cysts and Tumors

Committee on Technical Bulletins of the American College of Obstetricians and Gynecologists: *Cancer of the Ovary*. Technical Bulletin #73, 1983, American College of Obstetricians and Gynecologists, Washington, D.C.

Barber, H. R. Ovarian cancer: part II. *Ca–A Cancer Journal for Clinicians* 30(1):2–15, 1980.

Kistner, R. W. *Gynecology - Principles and Practice*, ed. 3. Chicago: Yearbook Medical Publishers, 1979.

Barber, H. R. Management of borderline malignant ovarian tumors. *The Female Patient* 15–19, March 1981.

Chapter 39—Uterine Cancer (see also references for Section Six, Chapter 27)

Richart, R. M., et al. Screening for endometrial cancer. *Contemporary OB/GYN* 23(6):223–232, June 1984.

Gusberg, S. B. An approach to the control of carcinoma of the endometrium. *Ca–A Cancer Journal for Clinicians* 30(1):16–22, 1980.

Antunes, C. M., et al. Endometrial cancer and estrogen use: report of a large case-control study. *New England Journal of Medicine* 300:9–13, Jan 4, 1979.

Barron, B. A. Exogenous estrogen and endometrial cancer: a statistical problem. *Contemporary OB/GYN* 11:135–142, Feb 1978.

Kistner, R. W. *Gynecology - Principles and Practice*, ed. 3. Chicago: Year Book Medical Publishers, 1979.

Walker, A. M., and Jick, H. Declining rates of endometrial cancer. *Obstetrics and Gynecology* 56(6):733–736, 1980.

Jones, H., III, et al. Early diagnosis of gynecologic cancer. *The Female Patient* 6(5):14–22, 1981.

Davies, J. L., et al. A review of the risk factors for endometrial carcinoma. *Obstetrical and Gynecological Survey* 36(3):107–116, Mar 1981.

nine

Gynecologic Surgery

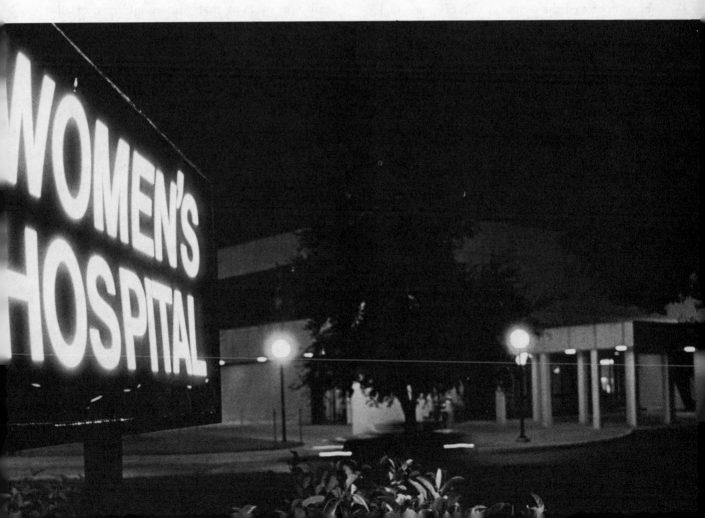

40

Deciding About Surgery

Between 1966 and 1976, the number of surgical operations per 1,000 persons increased from 78 to 95; and, in the fifteen to forty-four age group, women had more than twice as many surgical operations as men. Surgery involving the female pelvic organs is now safer than ever before. Better anesthesia, newer antibiotics, and increased numbers of board-certified obstetrician-gynecologists have improved the technical side of gynecologic surgery. And by obtaining second opinions and becoming better informed before surgery, women have learned to avoid unnecessary operations. This chapter will help you decide whether or not you need surgery and what to expect if you do.

Getting a Second Opinion

It is estimated that nearly ten percent of all surgeries performed in 1977 were unnecessary. Second surgical opinion programs have been established all over the country in an effort to curtail unnecessary surgery and thereby reduce health costs, surgical complications, and loss of life. The former Department of Health, Education, and Welfare, for example, set up a nationwide network of over 100 referral centers that provide names of physicians who participate in second surgical opinion programs. You can obtain information about the center nearest you by calling toll free 800-638-6833; in Maryland call 800-492-6603. You should also contact your insurance agent to see if your health insurance policy, like that of many insurance companies, includes the cost of second opinions in its coverage. Some insurance companies now *require* second opinions on the need for surgery before they will pay benefits.

Seeking a second opinion may be one way to make sure you get the best possible care. A second opinion is especially desirable if your diagnosis is uncertain, if the need for surgery is not clear to you, or if the problem is a chronic one for which surgery was not previously advised. If you want a second opinion, simply call the number listed above or ask your doctor or your local medical association to refer you to a board-certified obstetrician-gynecologist. You need not worry about offending your physician if you ask for a referral for a second opinion. Today physicians have come to expect such requests as a standard precaution against unnecessary surgery.

Informed Consent

Before you decide to have surgery and sign a legal-consent form, you need to know the answers to the five questions listed below. These make up the elements of what is called *informed consent*, a legal term meaning that you are informed of all the relevant facts surrounding your surgery and, on that basis, you consent to have the operation.

1. Why is surgery necessary?
2. What alternative treatment is available?
3. What exactly is to be done?
4. How can I expect to benefit from this surgery?
5. What complications may occur?

Even though you sign an operative consent, you can always change your mind, right up until the moment before surgery.

People differ as to how much they want to know about risks and complications, depending on how they cope with stress and whether they like to consider all aspects of a problem or put details out of their minds. However, it's a good idea to discuss specific worries about surgery with your doctor. You should have a clear understanding of the proposed operation and be able to summarize in your own words what exactly is to be done. Be sure you know the operation's likelihood of accomplishing what it is intended to do. For example, a hysterectomy may not always cure symptoms of pain, but the same operation relieves symptoms of abnormal uterine bleeding one hundred percent of the time. You may also want to ask your surgeon what kind of recovery period

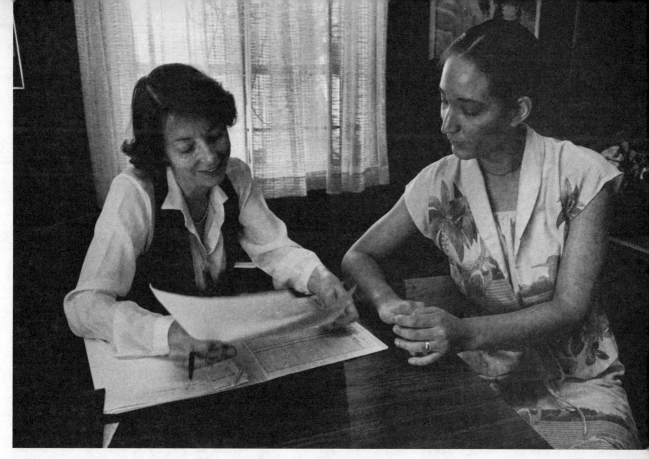

Obtaining a second opinion—an option to consider before you have surgery.

you can expect. And, finally, you should discuss with your surgeon what you would want if *unexpected findings* occurred. In deciding how to approach this issue, consider these questions:

1. Do you want to become pregnant in the future?
2. How important to you is maintaining childbearing potential relative to the discomfort caused by your symptoms?
3. If surgery to relieve these symptoms unexpectedly required, for example, a hysterectomy, would you still want the surgery?
4. If it also required removal of your ovaries, would you still want it?

Answering these questions will help you make a sound and rational decision about surgery.

When You Enter the Hospital

Bring only essentials with you to the hospital. If you will be staying overnight, these items include your toothbrush, slippers, robe, nightgown, less than five dollars including change for phone calls

and snacks, your medical insurance cards, and perhaps a book or magazine. Leave valuables, such as jewelry (including rings) and credit cards, at home.

After you arrive on the floor, a nurse (and perhaps a resident physician if your hospital is affiliated with a medical school) will visit you and take medical histories. The nursing history is taken and used by the nurses to develop a plan which aims at personalizing your hospital stay.

This is a good time for you to get to know the nursing staff, especially the head nurse on your floor, since they will take care of you after surgery. The licensed practical nurses (LPNs) and nurse's aides will provide most of the bedside nursing, including periodic checking of your blood pressure, pulse, temperature, and so on. Registered nurses (RNs) are responsible for the care given on their floor and are always available should a problem arise. RNs can answer many questions about your surgery and often teach preparatory classes beforehand. If you have a problem after surgery—anytime, day or night—it is the RN's job to contact your physician and explain the problem. If you have requests, such as a particular diet or room change, tell any of the nurses. If the problem persists or you have difficulty making your needs known, ask to speak with the head nurse on your floor. Keep in mind that many hospitals are somewhat understaffed because of nationwide nursing shortages—this factor might be responsible for a problem going unrecognized. Most nurses will help you once they know you have a problem.

You will spend most of the day before surgery having tests and other procedures necessary to get you ready for surgery. A complete blood count (see glossary), urinalysis (see glossary), and pregnancy test are routine. Other blood tests, a chest X-ray, and a cardiogram are often ordered for women over age thirty-five.

The evening before your surgery, the anesthesiologist stops by and usually asks the same questions you answered before. This repetition, though perhaps annoying, usually works to your advantage, especially if it uncovers previously overlooked details such as a drug allergy. Be sure to mention *medications* you are currently taking, *drug allergies*, *past serious illnesses*, and any *present* or *chronic conditions* you have, especially any involving your heart or lungs. These areas may influence the type of anesthetic drug used. You can usually choose the type of anesthesia you want unless you have a particular medical problem. Discuss with the anesthesiologist your feelings about being awake or asleep during the operation. Keep in mind that the anesthesiologist you see the night before surgery may not be the same one who gives you your anesthesia since, in most hospitals, they work rotating shifts. Your own doctor will probably come by sometime before surgery, but if you have any last-minute questions, mention to the nurses that you want to see your doctor to ensure that he or she does stop by.

The night before major surgery you will receive an enema to prevent difficulty having a bowel movement immediately after your operation. A douche, often ordered before major surgery, is intended to lessen the chance of postoperative infection within the abdominal cavity stemming from the bacteria normally inhabiting the vagina. If you are going to have general anesthesia, you won't be permitted to eat or drink anything after midnight the night before surgery because your stomach has to be empty.

The Morning of Surgery

The morning of surgery, someone will shave (prep) the skin surrounding the surgical area if you are to have abdominal surgery. Only the pubic hair is shaved for vaginal operations. Many physicians don't require a prep before minor procedures such as a D & C or laparoscopy; so discuss the prep beforehand with your surgeon.

You will be asked to remove all makeup and nail polish so that your skin color can be more closely observed in surgery. Remove contact lenses and any dentures as well. You will probably not be permitted to wear any rings during the surgery. A tube may be inserted into your bladder prior to surgery either in your hospital room or in the operating room after you are asleep. This tube, a catheter, prevents your bladder from filling up during surgery and thereby allows better visualization of your pelvic organs. About an hour before surgery the nurse gives you a sedative injection to make you drowsy and relaxed. Also you may notice your mouth becoming dry from the atropine which is usually given with the sedative. Atropine drugs dry up secretions in the lungs and keep the air passages free of mucus during administration of general anesthesia.

Just before surgery, you will be wheeled by stretcher to a holding area outside the operating room. At this time, a physician or nurse will start an intravenous infusion (IV). This involves inserting a small needle into a vein in your hand. The needle is connected by plastic tubing to a bottle containing the fluids you need during and after surgery. If blood is needed during the surgery, it is administered through the IV.

The Operating Room

Once in the operating room, which is significantly cooler than outside, you will notice that everybody wears surgical gowns, caps, masks, and gloves to prevent contamination of the sterile operating field. If you are having a general anesthetic, the anesthesiologist or nurse anesthetist usually administers sodium pentothal through your IV tubing to put you to sleep. After you fall asleep, an anesthetic gas which you breathe is administered either by mask or through a tube inserted into your windpipe. This so-called endotracheal tube, used for longer operations requiring deeper anesthesia or for surgical procedures like laparoscopy, prevents any stomach contents from reaching the lungs during surgery. If an endotracheal tube is used, don't be surprised if you have a sore throat for a day or two after surgery.

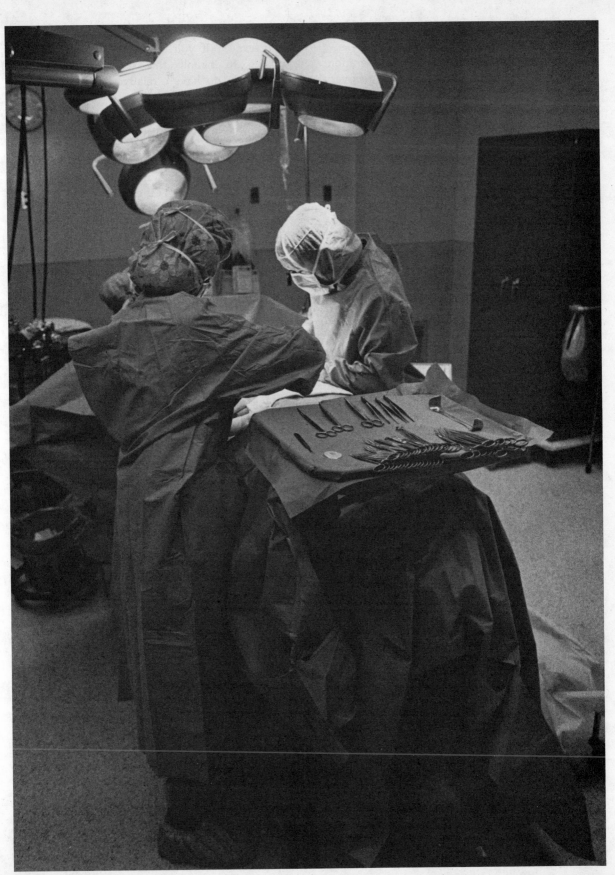

The Recovery Room

Depending on the length and type of operation, you spend about one or two hours in the recovery room, where visitors are not allowed. However, you can and should arrange for a close friend or relative to meet your surgeon after your surgery. Find out from your surgeon where this person should wait and when he or she can expect to hear from your doctor. After talking with your surgeon following the operation, this person can wait for you in your hospital room.

In the recovery room, specially trained nurses will monitor your physical condition closely and encourage you to "turn, cough, and deep breathe" frequently to expand your lungs, as well as to bend and move your legs to improve circulation. After major gynecologic surgery, you are likely to have two tubes attached: your IV and a urinary catheter tube. The catheter, which may produce a sensation that you have to urinate, continuously drains your urine into a portable bag that hangs on the side of your bed. After a general anesthetic, you are likely to be groggy and may not remember the recovery room at all. As anesthesia wears off, the nurse gives you pain medication to keep you comfortable. You may request this medication, ordered automatically by your surgeon, if you need it. After you are stable and you begin to awake from anesthesia, you will be transferred to your room, or sent home if you have had surgery as an outpatient.

Recovering in the Hospital

In the immediate postoperative period after major surgery (for example, vaginal hysterectomy or any operation requiring a regular abdominal incision), your surgeon will come around to check on your general condition and perhaps examine your lungs and abdomen. Your doctor will write orders in your chart concerning four areas: activity, diet, tubes, and medication.

It is a good idea for you to become familiar with what these orders are. Hospital nursing staffs are busy, and you should be aware of what's planned for you: what and when medication is to be given, what you are allowed and not allowed to eat and drink, what your activity limitations and your doctor's recommendations are. Don't be afraid or embarrassed to ask questions. You have a right to know, for example, what the medication is that you are taking, what it is for, and what side effects you may expect. If you think you will be physically unable to handle this responsibility, arrange beforehand to have a relative or close friend ask questions and monitor your recovery procedures.

Activity

If you have had a general anesthetic, you will be encouraged to cough and take deep breaths to help expand your lungs. You can expect to be out of bed and walking (with your IV and catheter if they are still in use) the day after surgery. Early walking and moving about helps your lungs expand after a general anesthetic and promotes good circulation. Walking also helps you pass intestinal gas, a discomfort accompanying most abdominal operations on the second or third postoperative day. The first time you walk, someone will assist you. As soon as you are walking comfortably and feeling stronger and your IV and catheter have been removed (about the third or fourth postoperative day), you can shower and wash your hair. If you have an abdominal dressing, it will need changing after your shower.

Diet

Your diet normally progresses from clear liquids for a day or two after surgery to a regular diet by the third or fourth postoperative day. Your diet can be progressed as fast as you are ready, but you should not force yourself if you are not hungry or if you feel nauseated. Gas pains often occur on about the second day, an expected sign that your intestines are starting to function normally. If gas pains are not relieved by walking, a mild laxative or enema may be ordered.

Tubes

The catheter (tube) draining the bladder, if a catheter is used, is usually removed the next morning. However, if bladder surgery was performed, the catheter remains for several days. Your IV is removed when you can tolerate a clear liquid diet and if you don't need the IV for drugs, such as antibiotics. When vaginal or abdominal drains are used, these soft rubber tubes designed to prevent infection are moved outward a little each day from their position just inside the incision and completely removed within a few days of your operation.

Medication

Pain shots are replaced by milder pain pills as soon as you are ready, usually on the second or third day after surgery. Pain medication is a common source of nausea; if nausea occurs, ask for a change of medication as well as something for the nausea. You may want to ask for a sleeping pill as well when you switch from pain shots to pain pills. If you experience something you think may be a side effect, tell one of the nurses. You might be having a bad reaction to some medication.

When You Go Home

We have outlined the basics of what to expect before and after surgery. Your situation may be different depending on your surgery and your doctor's routine. If you have questions about your diet, activity, or medications, don't hesitate to ask. Find out what limitations your doctor thinks you should have, as, for example, in the areas of climbing stairs, driving, and resuming your normal physical activities. If your physician is not immediately available, ask a nurse.

Recovery from major gynecologic surgery usually requires a hospital stay of four to six days after the operation. It takes most people this long to gain enough strength to begin to manage at home. Even then some help will probably be necessary for two to four weeks. Before you leave the hospital, certain medical requirements must usually be met: you must not have signs of infection, such as fever, within the twenty-four hours before you are discharged; you must have resumed normal bowel and bladder function and your normal diet; if you have an abdominal incision, it must appear clean and uninfected; and your blood count must be reasonably normal.

Upon discharge, you are normally given instructions as to what you can and cannot do; at this time you may get a prescription for pain or antibiotic drugs. If you have had an abdominal operation, you may have clips or stitches, which are usually removed from five to eight days after surgery. In vaginal operations, the stitches are absorbed and do not need removal. Before you go home, schedule your follow-up visit, ask about the purpose and side effects of any new medications, and ask if you should watch out for any particular symptoms that might necessitate a call to your physician.

Short-Stay Procedures

Outpatient surgery saves you time and money and minimizes the upset of your home life and employment. About one-third of all gynecologic operations that previously required overnight stays can now be performed safely and effectively in an outpatient surgical setting. Some insurance companies do not cover outpatient surgery; you may want to check your coverage before such surgery.

In short-stay surgery, you can still have general anesthesia and go home the same day, usually within six hours of your arrival at the hospital. You will need someone to take you home after outpatient surgery, and you should avoid driving for twenty-four hours from the time you leave the hospital if a general anesthetic is used. The same general procedures are followed before outpatient surgery as for major surgery; the difference is that the postoperative recovery is at home. Table 64 lists operations that can be performed on an outpatient basis.

Resources

For information about a second surgical opinion and for the referral center nearest you that can give you the names of physicians who participate in the second surgical opinion program, call toll free 800-638-6833; in Maryland call toll free 800-492-6603.

Table 64 OPERATIONS THAT CAN BE PERFORMED ON AN OUTPATIENT BASIS

1. Dilatation and curettage (D & C).
2. Therapeutic abortion.
3. Laparoscopy (for diagnosis).
4. Tubal sterilization by laparoscopy, mini-laparotomy, or vaginal tubal ligation.
5. Cone biopsy.
6. Breast biopsy.*
7. Breast plastic surgery.*

---

* Usually performed by general surgeons.

Dilatation and Curettage (D & C)

Gynecologists perform dilatation and curettage (D & C) more often than any other surgical procedure because it diagnoses and treats many pelvic problems. *Dilatation* is the gradual widening of the cervix, accomplished by placing progressively wider metal rods into the cervical opening (see Figure 32). *Curettage* refers to the insertion of a special, spoon-shaped instrument, called a *curette*, through the dilated cervix to curette, or scrape out, the tissue that lines the uterine cavity (see Figure 33). Another instrument shown in Figure 33, called a tenaculum, is used to grasp and steady the cervix during this procedure. Minimal anesthesia (usually a light general anesthetic, though a local or spinal may be used) is required for a D & C, which takes about fifteen minutes to perform and gives most women little or no postoperative discomfort. Shaving of pubic hair is no longer routinely done by many surgeons—check with your doctor.

When Is a D & C Indicated?

Dilatation & curettage provides the best method of diagnosing uterine causes of abnormal bleeding, including uterine cancer. Women over forty who have abnormally heavy or frequent periods often undergo a D & C to rule out the possibility of a malignant tumor. When vaginal bleeding occurs in the postmenopausal woman, a D & C is mandatory to diagnose the cause. In a woman of childbearing age, a D & C is often both diagnostic and therapeutic; the usual causes—benign growths (polyps) and hormone imbalance leading to an excess growth of uterine lining tissue—are often

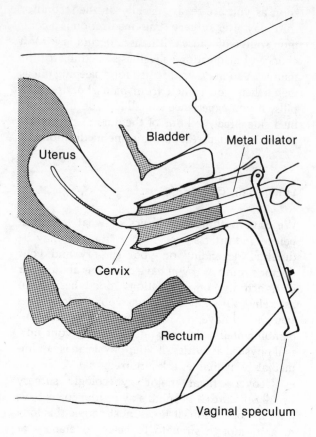

Figure 32
A metal dilator is used to widen, or dilate, the cervix during a D & C.

readily cured by this procedure. As a therapeutic measure, gynecologists perform a D & C most commonly after a miscarriage to prevent (or stop) hemorrhage or subsequent infection. Sometimes a D & C is needed after an abortion complicated by bleeding caused by retained tissue not removed during the abortion procedure.

Recovering from D & C

Recovery after a D & C is nearly immediate. You may experience slight vaginal bleeding and mild pelvic cramping for a few hours but rarely for more than a day. You can usually resume normal activity within a day or two. Most clinicians permit intercourse, douching, and the use of tampons within a week or two. Your first period after the operation may be earlier or later than expected. You should have a checkup a few days after the

Sterilization Options

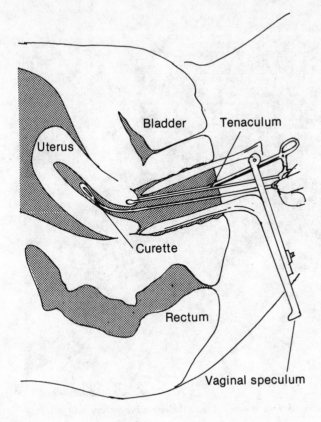

Figure 33

A curette is used to remove tissue from inside the uterine cavity during a D & C.

operation to discuss the surgical findings with your clinician.

Complications

D & C is associated with fewer complications than any other gynecologic surgical procedure. The main serious complication of a D & C is pelvic infection, which is more likely to occur if the procedure is performed while you *presently* have an infection of your reproductive system. (A sexually transmitted infection or any other infection of the uterus, tubes, or ovaries should be fully treated *before* you have a D & C.) After a D & C, immediately report to your clinician any symptoms of pelvic infection, such as pelvic pain, fever, or a bad-smelling vaginal discharge. Serious complications, such as bleeding from uterine injuries, are rare.

Currently in the United States, over twelve million men and women have opted for sterilization; that is, they have chosen by means of a surgical procedure to utilize a permanent method of birth control. And each year another million persons request it. In 1970, women accounted for only 20% of sterilizations. By 1978, this percentage had increased to 59%, making surgical sterilization the number one method of birth control for married women over the age of twenty-nine.

When your family size is complete or you have medical reasons to avoid pregnancy, voluntary sterilization appears to be the safest, least expensive, and most effective method of female contraception.

Deciding About Sterilization

The decision to become sterilized by means of a surgical procedure is a voluntary decision that you should be absolutely certain about making. Although you can change your mind at any time prior to surgery, it is the kind of choice that should leave no doubts in your mind as to whether to have it done. A decision about sterilization should be made only after careful consideration and only after you have had the opportunity to fully discuss your questions and concerns with your clinician, preferably more than once.

The reason you must be sure about your decision is because the operation is considered irreversible. Only a small percentage of women who ask to have the condition reversed (that is, to have their tubes "untied") can successfully become pregnant. If there is any possibility that you may want to become pregnant in the future, perhaps

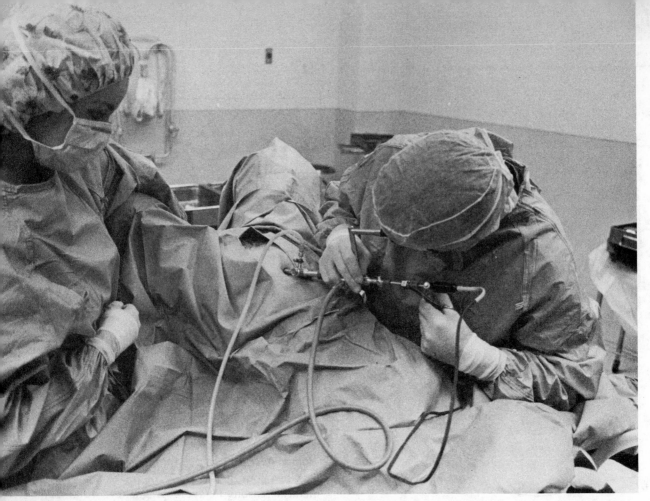

The surgeon looks through the eyepiece of the laparoscope. The Fallopian tube is grasped with the operating forceps held in the surgeon's left hand.

because of remarriage, then choose a reversible contraceptive method instead. If you are past childbearing age, say in your mid-forties, you, too, may want to use another method of birth control (excluding the pill; see Chapter 9), since fertility declines rapidly at this age, requiring contraception for only a few more years at most.

You and your partner or spouse may want to consider the option of male sterilization, called *vasectomy.* Keep in mind that vasectomy is slightly less risky, less costly, just as effective as female sterilization procedures, and just as irreversible. If, after considering all other forms of birth control, you decide on female sterilization, there are several operations from which to choose.

Operations for Female Sterilization

Female sterilization prevents pregnancy by blocking or dividing the Fallopian tubes and thereby preventing union of the sperm and the ovum, or

egg—that is, preventing the egg from being fertilized by the sperm. This blocking or dividing of the tubes is achieved surgically by what is known as *tubal ligation*—which means "tying" the tubes. There are various methods for accomplishing this "tying," which we will discuss below. Hysterectomy, a much riskier procedure than tubal operations, is not usually performed for purposes of sterilization unless other pelvic conditions also require this surgery.

Excluding hysterectomy, there are basically five different methods of female sterilization, discussed below.

1. *Laparoscopic tubal ligation* (so-called *Band-Aid* or *bellybutton surgery*), a relatively new outpatient procedure, is the most popular method of female sterilization in the United States because it has the shortest recovery period of any method and it leaves only a tiny scar just inside the navel (see Figure 34). (This procedure will be referred to as *laparoscopy* throughout this chapter.)

After giving the patient a general anesthetic, the surgeon makes a small (one-half inch) incision just inside the navel. Then the surgeon inserts a needle through the abdominal incision and slowly injects carbon dioxide gas, which repositions the intestines so that your uterus and tubes can be seen clearly. The surgeon then removes the needle and introduces the *laparoscope*, a telescopelike instrument with a light source, through the navel incision. Next, the surgeon inserts a second instrument through an opening within the laparoscope (see Figure 35). Or this second instrument may be inserted through another tiny incision just above the pubic hairline. This "sealer" instrument blocks the tubes by electrical or nonelectrical means. In the most common method, electrocoagulation, an electric current seals (burns) the tubes by "clumping" them together (see Figure 36). In nonelectric techniques, a metal clip or silicone rubber band constricts the tube by binding the tube around the outside of it. This method has the advantage of avoiding accidental burns to other internal organs and has greater potential for reversibility (that is, restoring fertility) than electrocoagulation. However, clips and bands seem to produce slightly more postoperative pain. After completing the procedure, the surgeon releases the carbon dioxide gas and places a band-aid over the tiny incision after closing it with a single suture.

Immediate postoperative side effects may include slight abdominal discomfort and distention (a bloated feeling) or shoulder pain, which usually subsides within forty-eight hours but may last for up to a week. The shoulder pain results from the pressure of any leftover gas. You may also experience slight vaginal bleeding for a few hours from the manipulation of the uterus necessary to visualize the tubes during laparoscopy. Occasionally redness and swelling occur around the incision several days later. You can clear up this condition rapidly by cleaning the area with peroxide and applying warm, moist gauze compresses four or so times a day. Most women who undergo laparoscopic sterilization resume their usual activities after a day or two.

In fewer than one percent of these operations, the surgeon finds unexpected pelvic

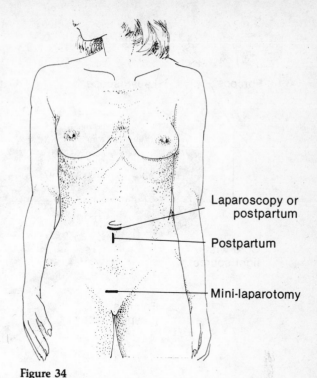

Laparoscopy or postpartum

Postpartum

Mini-laparotomy

Figure 34

Types of tubal sterilization incisions. The incision for the laparoscopic tubal ligation (laparoscopy) is made just inside the navel. Postpartum tubal ligations can be performed through a small incision just inside the navel or through a slightly longer vertical incision below the navel. The incision for the mini-laparotomy is made at or just above the pubic hairline. Not shown are incisions for abdominal tubal ligation (see Figure 38) and for vaginal tubal ligation.

adhesions during laparoscopy. If these adhesions dangerously obscure the surgeon's view of your tubes, he or she must make a regular abdominal incision to complete the operation safely.

Rare major complications of laparoscopy usually relate to anesthesia, internal bleeding, or damage to internal organs. Electrocoagulation, the most common laparoscopic method of tubal occlusion (blocking), has been associated with a very slight risk of accidental intestinal burns. If your surgeon does electrocoagulation, ask him or her to use *bipolar* coagulation forceps. The newer bipolar system uses less electric current than the unipolar type and decreases the

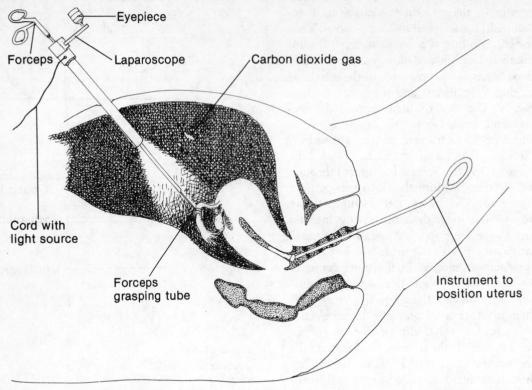

Figure 35   *Laparoscopy method of tubal sterilization. Laparoscopy alone, without use of the sealer instrument, is commonly used as a diagnostic procedure in the evaluation of pelvic pain, pelvic tumors, or infertility.*

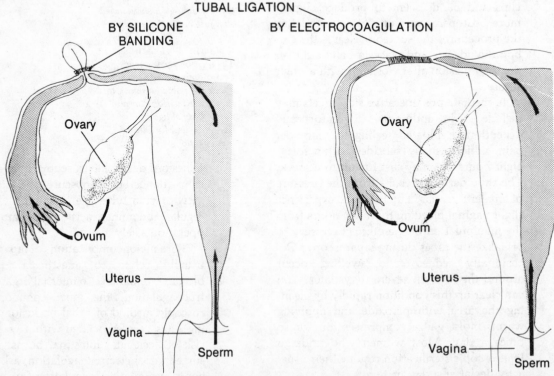

Figure 36   *Depending on the technique used, the tubes may be blocked in a number of ways. Shown above are the two commonest methods used during laparoscopy tubal ligation: banding and electrocoagulation.*

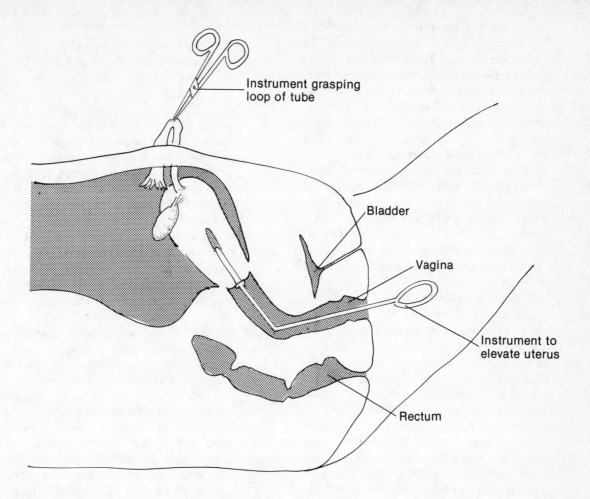

Labels on figure:
- Instrument grasping loop of tube
- Bladder
- Vagina
- Instrument to elevate uterus
- Rectum

Figure 37   *Mini-laparotomy method of tubal sterilization.*

risk of burns. Only one laparoscopy in three hundred requires major surgery to treat complications related to bleeding, burn injury, or damage to internal organs. If you have had previous abdominal surgery, especially with a vertical scar below the navel, you probably should not have this type of sterilization procedure performed because there is an increased risk of intestinal damage during laparoscopy. The possibility of intestinal damage results from the fact that after previous abdominal surgery the intestines are more likely to adhere to the abdominal wall and not fall back out of the way at the time of laparoscopy. Many laparoscopy complications can be prevented by avoiding the procedure when these relative contraindications exist: pronounced obesity (increases technical difficulty of laparoscopy), serious heart disease, or chronic respiratory illness (the carbon dioxide gas

may cause a tendency to irregular heartbeats or to breathing difficulties).

2. *Mini-laparotomy* differs from laparoscopy in that the surgeon uses no visualizing instrument. Although some women have local anesthesia for a mini-laparotomy, most surgeons recommend general anesthesia since many patients otherwise experience some discomfort. The physician begins the "mini-lap" with a small, one- to two-inch incision at or just above the pubic hairline (see Figure 34). With the help of an assistant who uses an instrument inserted through the vagina and positions the uterus and its tubes near this incision (see Figure 37), the surgeon simply lifts the tubes through this incision and blocks them by the desired method. Usually the tubes are tied (ligated) using a suture, although bands and clips sometimes are used.

Increasing in popularity in the United

States, the mini-laparotomy is considered by some authorities the safest procedure for female sterilization. This operation is ideally suited for women who cannot undergo laparoscopy because of previous abdominal surgery or serious heart or respiratory illness. The small incision utilized in mini-laparotomy allows rapid recovery within two to three days. Although the procedure may be performed on an outpatient basis, most patients stay overnight because of greater discomfort with this procedure compared to laparoscopy. The major drawback of mini-laparotomy is the technical difficulty of operating through a tiny incision. For this reason, if you weigh over 20% of ideal body weight (see Table 104) or have a history of tubal disease such as endometriosis or tubal infections, you should consider another method of sterilization.

3. *Vaginal tubal ligation (colpotomy)* may be best suited for women who have contraindications to laparoscopy, such as previous abdominal surgery, or who are not ideally suited for mini-laparotomy because they are overweight. However, many gynecologists have not been trained in this technique, which is technically more difficult than other sterilization procedures. For colpotomy, the surgeon makes a one- to two-inch incision in the vagina below the cervix. The surgeon then draws the tubes through this incision and ligates them with suture material. As with laparoscopy, the surgeon will resort to an abdominal incision if, as a result of scarring or adhesions, he or she cannot adequately visualize the tubes.

Compared to abdominal incision methods in which the skin is scrubbed with an antiseptic solution and made nearly sterile, the vagina's high bacterial count makes the patient more susceptible to infection. As a result of such infections about two to three percent of women experience painful intercourse up to several months following vaginal tubal ligation. Advantages of vaginal tubal ligation include the fact that the procedure can be performed under local or spinal anesthesia, instead of general anesthesia, and the absence of a visible scar. Recovery from vaginal tubal ligation, while less rapid than for laparoscopy, usually requires only one or two nights in the hospital,

and sometimes the procedure may be performed on an outpatient basis.

4. *Abdominal tubal ligation* (using *laparotomy*—an incision in the abdomen) usually requires an abdominal incision made either vertically below the navel or horizontally just at the pubic hairline (see Figure 38). The surgeon may recommend laparotomy if you require abdominal surgery for other reasons or have had recent or chronic tubal infections or endometriosis. These conditions often cause adhesions or scarring, making it technically difficult or impossible for you to undergo sterilization by one of the other methods. For most women, laparotomy represents the least desirable method of sterilization because of its greater risks, longer hospital stay (three to five days), and prolonged recovery period.

5. *Postpartum tubal ligation*, essentially a mini-laparotomy that follows childbirth, is the second most commonly requested sterilization procedure. In this method, the surgeon makes a one- to two-inch incision inside or just below the navel (see Figure 34), draws part of each tube through the incision, and ligates the tubes using suture. Laparoscopy is seldom used immediately following childbirth because of the increased risk of damage to the uterus, which lies directly underneath the bellybutton at this time.

Postpartum tubal ligation usually does not prolong your hospital stay. The operation may be performed any time during the first three days postpartum, but it is most often done immediately after you deliver—in which case the same anesthetic (for example, epidural) may be used. This operation is associated with the same general risks as mini-laparotomy.

Although postpartum tubal ligation is convenient and avoids an additional hospitalization later, many women prefer to wait six weeks or more before making their final decision. It is unwise to base a decision to be sterilized on assumptions about the newborn's condition at birth. Problems in an apparently healthy baby may not show up until a day or two later. If you and your husband are considering sterilization, it makes sense to consider your options during pregnancy rather than at the time of labor and

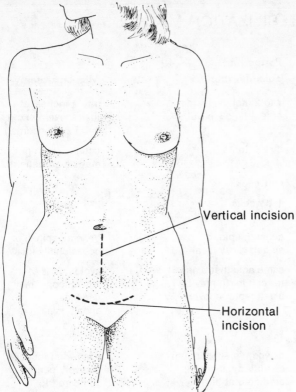

Vertical incision

Horizontal incision

Figure 38

Most gynecologic operations performed through the abdomen use either a vertical (midline) or a low horizontal (Pfannenstiel) incision.

delivery or during the stressful postpartum period. You don't want to have to make this choice just before an emergency cesarean section, in the middle of a stressful labor, or when you are adjusting to the demands of a tiny newborn. Such conditions may make sound, objective decision making difficult.

Safety of Female Sterilization

Although no surgical procedure is without risk, tubal sterilizations are among the safest operations performed. The risk of death from this one-time operation is extremely low and no more than the *yearly* risk involved from the use of the pill or an IUD. Major complications, such as infections, bleeding, and damage to the internal organs as well as complications from anesthesia, occur in fewer than one percent of all surgeries. Although the various sterilization operations have slightly different benefits and risks, the skill and experience of your surgeon has much more to do with a safe, successful result than the type of

operation you select. As with other surgeries, the safety of tubal sterilization depends somewhat upon your own health. If you tend to be overweight, smoke, or have serious medical problems such as heart disease, your chances of surgical complications increase. Also, if you have had previous tubal infections, any surgical procedure which manipulates the tubes can cause the infection to flare up.

Effectiveness of Female Sterilization

Because of inconclusive research, it is impossible to state precisely the exact effectiveness of each sterilization procedure. Although the chance of fertility is remote, pregnancy has occurred after tubal sterilization operations, at a rate of two to three per one thousand operations. Many of these pregnancies occur not as a result of surgical failure but because the woman was pregnant at the time of surgery. As a precaution, most hospitals perform pregnancy tests prior to any surgery. To be sure you are not pregnant—and to avoid the possibility of a "false negative" pregnancy test—it is advisable to have your sterilization operation within the first two weeks following a normal period.

After Female Sterilization

Since the ovaries are not involved in tubal sterilization, hormone production is not interrupted. You will therefore continue to menstruate and ovulate (the egg, after release, becomes absorbed inside the abdomen). Most authorities agree that abnormal bleeding following tubal ligation usually means that the woman had a prior tendency to have this problem and that it is thus not a direct effect of the operation itself. Sometimes, however, tubal surgery may lessen the blood supply to the nearby ovaries and may then account for subsequent hormone imbalance and the accompanying symptoms of irregular or heavy periods. Tubal ligation has no direct effect, bad or good, on aging or sexual functioning. The predominant psychological effect in a woman who comfortably made the decision is great relief from fear of unwanted pregnancy, a feeling which often facilitates sexual enjoyment and emotional well-being. However, a woman who rushed into the decision for sterilization may regret it and later experience some depression.

Table 65 COMPARISON OF TUBAL STERILIZATION METHODS

	Laparoscopic Tubal Ligation (Laparoscopy)	Postpartum Tubal Ligation	Mini-laparotomy
Incision	1/2 inch, inside the navel	1 to 2 inches; inside or just below navel	1 to 2 inches, at or just above pubic hairline (horizontal)
Hospital stay	outpatient	three nights	usually overnight; may be outpatient
Recovery period	24–48 hours	one week	one week
Intercourse may be resumed	24 hours	4–6 weeks	2–3 days
Anesthetic	general; rarely local	general, epidural, or spinal; rarely local	general, spinal, or occasionally local
Major advantages	rapid recovery	same anesthetic as for childbirth may be used; rapid recovery	avoids risks of laparoscopy; may use local anesthesia
Major disadvantages	rarely, serious complications may occur	newborn's subsequent condition cannot be predicted at birth, which may affect sterilization decision	somewhat longer recovery period compared to laparoscopy
Area shaved	around navel or not at all	around navel or below	only hair over pubic bone

Choosing the Right Operation

Which operation you choose depends upon individual circumstances—your physical condition, the type of anesthesia you want, and whether or not you plan to have the surgery immediately after childbirth. Among female sterilization procedures, the laparoscopy method and the mini-laparotomy method offer the greatest safety (assuming they are not inadvisable for you) and, when done on an outpatient basis, cost the least. If you are considering one of these newer methods, find a doctor who is experienced in one of these specialized techniques. If you plan to have your tubes tied after childbirth, you will avoid a second hospitalization later; but don't make this decision dependent on the baby's health at delivery.

Finally, if you have a history of pelvic disease, such as tubal infections or endometriosis, remember that you have a greater chance of medical complications with laparoscopy, mini-laparotomy, or vaginal tubal ligation. When you have planned to have any one of these three procedures performed, discuss in advance with your surgeon what you want done if unexpected findings occur. For example, if the surgeon finds adhesions, it may be necessary for the surgeon to terminate the procedure or to perform a regular incision in order to tie your tubes. In rare circumstances, the clinician may find a so-called frozen pelvis, where dense scarring or tubal damage makes tubal sterilization impossible, even through an abdominal incision. In the event that this occurs, you must make it clear in advance whether you want the original procedure stopped or you want to have more extensive surgery done, usually including a hysterectomy.

Table 65 summarizes the important factors concerning the various methods of tubal sterilization.

Resources

Resources for information on sterilization are the following:

Vaginal Tubal Ligation (Colpotomy)	Abdominal Tubal Ligation (Laparotomy)
1 to 2 inches, within the vagina	3 to 4 inches, horizontal or vertical abdominal incision
usually overnight; may be outpatient	three to five nights
1–3 weeks	2–6 weeks
4–6 weeks	2–6 weeks
general or spinal; rarely local	general or spinal
avoids any abdominal incision; alternative if laparoscopy or mini-lap is contraindicated	best visualization of pelvic organs
increased risk of infection	longest recovery period; highest number of complications
pubic hair around vagina	abdominal area of incision

1. Association for Voluntary Sterilization, Inc.
   122 E. 42nd Street, 18th Floor
   New York, New York 10168
   (212) 573-8350

The above association provides information on sterilization and referrals to qualified specialists.

2. Planned Parenthood Federation of America, Inc.
   810 Seventh Avenue
   New York, New York 10019
   (212) 541-7800

Write for literature on sterilization and the location of the office nearest you if it is not listed in your telephone directory.

43

Terminating Pregnancy

This chapter is for the pregnant woman who, after carefully examining her alternatives, chooses to have an abortion. Abortion, the voluntary termination of pregnancy, was legalized by the U.S. Supreme Court in 1973. Since that time, the number of women requesting this procedure has steadily increased while the mortality rate associated with abortion has decreased to less than one death per 30,000 abortions.

Emotional Effects of Abortion

When abortion is indicated for medical reasons or follows amniocentesis that diagnosed a birth defect, a woman's grief may be understandably profound. But regardless of the circumstances, most women feel varying degrees of ambivalence and emotional distress about the decision. Fortunately, severe depression happens to very few women after a pregnancy termination. Rather, after the initial conflicts, the majority soon return to their previous emotional balance. In fact, some women report a sense of great relief after abortion along with some of the same mixed feelings that went into making the decision.

It is normal after an abortion to experience feelings of depression and loss, and women vary in the intensity with which these emotions are felt, depending upon numerous complex factors. It is natural, perhaps even necessary, to feel sad at this time as you adjust to no longer being pregnant. However, it's usually better not to keep such emotions entirely to yourself as this may lead to a sense of isolation and further distress. It may help to share your feelings with a close friend, relative, or counselor who will help you acknowledge and accept these emotions, thereby starting the process of returning to "normal life."

In some circumstances, the emotional aftermath of abortion is more severe. Experience shows that later abortions, especially the saline type, tend to cause more prolonged grieving and other problems such as insomnia or intestinal upsets. Abortion may also be more stressful in the absence of a supportive family or partner, or when the woman feels she was forced because of external circumstances to make the decision to terminate pregnancy. If you feel you may need some help handling the conflicts associated with your abortion, you should seek abortion counseling *before* and *after* termination of pregnancy. Such counseling is usually provided by women's centers and Planned Parenthood centers as part of the overall cost of the procedure. Counseling or referral to a qualified counselor should be available through your clinician if he or she is performing the operation.

Methods of Terminating Pregnancy

Abortion becomes increasingly hazardous with each additional week of pregnancy after the first three months, so it's best to obtain early medical attention. Be sure that the clinical setting you choose (see Chapter 2) has adequate *follow-up care* in case you develop complications later. Women with serious health problems such as diabetes, heart disease, or bleeding disorders should seriously consider having the abortion in a hospital setting, where emergency equipment is immediately available.

When this operation is performed in the first three months of pregnancy, the doctor uses some type of suction (called *suction abortion*) to remove the embryo from the uterine cavity. If the woman is between 13 and 16 weeks pregnant, the operation performed is called *dilatation and evacuation* (D & E), a procedure to dilate the cervix and remove the fetus and placenta. After 16 weeks, most clinicians accomplish abortion by instilling a substance such as saline (a salt solution) into the amniotic sac around the fetus to stimulate labor and delivery (called *instillation abortion*).

Suction abortion, performed in women who are up to 12 weeks pregnant (first trimester), may be performed in a clinic, an office, an ambulatory care facility, or a hospital (usually on an outpatient basis). There are two types: *menstrual extraction* and *vacuum curettage*.

Menstrual extraction is an abortion procedure performed as early as one week after conception but no later than two weeks after a missed period. A woman considering this procedure must obtain a blood pregnancy test to verify pregnancy because a urine test is likely to be negative this early in pregnancy. (A negative blood test means that you are not pregnant and do not need the procedure.) Menstrual extraction, unlike other suction abortion methods, requires little or no dilation of the cervix. You may not need anesthesia if you have been pregnant before. In women with first-time pregnancies, however, injection of a local anesthetic around the cervix (paracervical block) prevents cramping. The physician performs menstrual extraction by placing a soft, flexible tube through the cervix and into the uterine cavity. The free end of the tube is connected to a hand-held syringe which provides suction as the doctor pulls back on it. Since this method has a failure rate of 2.5%, it is important to have a follow-up exam in one to two weeks so the clinician can confirm that you are no longer pregnant. Because of this failure rate, some doctors recommend waiting until seven or eight weeks of pregnancy when a standard suction abortion may be carried out with a failure rate of less than 1%.

Vacuum curettage, the usual method of first trimester abortion (also known as *suction curettage*, or *suction D & C*), is normally performed between 7 and 12 weeks of pregnancy, counting from the first day of your last menstrual period. Either local anesthesia (paracervical block) or general anesthesia is used. If the abortion is done under local anesthesia, the doctor may give you a sedative, such as Valium, a few minutes before the procedure to lessen your anxiety. Almost all women who are awake experience some degree of discomfort from the procedure, depending on how well the block "takes."

First the doctor will swab the vagina with an antiseptic. Shaving the pubic hair is unnecessary and you may specifically request that this be avoided. He or she then places a metal clamp on the cervix to steady the uterus and dilates the cervix using small, blunt, metal rods of progressively increasing diameter (see Figure 32). The cervix can also be dilated by means of laminaria (a kind of small, tubular marine plant); the clinician places a laminaria rod into the cervix the day before surgery and removes it at the time of the operation. The use of laminaria, which have been used widely in Japan and Europe, promotes slow, relatively painless, cervical dilation that results from the unique moisture-absorbing property of these rods that causes them to swell in diameter. After dilation, and removal of the laminaria, the doctor positions a plastic tube through the dilated cervix and attaches its free end to an electric suction pump. The suctioning empties the uterine cavity in three to five minutes. Most surgeons then examine the uterus with a metal instrument called a curette to ensure that no tissue remains. If you desire, the physician will insert an IUD following this abortion procedure. Recent reports indicate that immediate postoperative IUD insertion is safe and effective.

Dilatation and evacuation (D & E) is the procedure of choice between 13 and 16 weeks of pregnancy (second trimester). An abortion after 12 weeks usually involves significantly greater medical risk, emotional distress, and cost compared to procedures performed in the first three months of pregnancy. The physician often orders a sonogram (see Chapter 16) to determine the exact stage of gestation if you are more than 12 weeks by pelvic examination, because the bimanual examination cannot reliably evaluate uterine size after the first three months of pregnancy. D & E is usually performed in the hospital on an outpatient basis. General anesthesia is recommended although some clinics perform this procedure using local anesthesia. Many clinicians insert one or more laminaria rods the day before surgery. Since the cervix must be dilated more than with early abortions, the use of laminaria helps to prevent forceful cervical dilation using instruments that may damage the cervix. Such damage has been linked to subsequent pregnancy complications including an increased risk of premature labor and late miscarriage. The D & E is performed much like the D & C (see Chapter 41) but with special instruments to remove the larger volume of tissue encountered at more advanced stages of pregnancy.

Instillation abortion methods, performed between 16 and 24 weeks of pregnancy, initially involve injection of one of three substances: a salt solution (saline), a drug (prostaglandin), or a chemical compound (urea) into the amniotic fluid sac. To accomplish this, the clinician numbs the skin with a local anesthetic and then inserts a needle through the lower abdomen and *instills* (puts in drop by drop) the substance. Labor pains start within a few hours, and delivery of the fetus occurs from eight to seventy-two hours later (usually within twenty-four hours), so that a one- to two-day hospital stay is not unusual. The physician may shorten the time from instillation to delivery of the fetus by using laminaria to facilitate cervical dilation or by using an intravenous drug called oxytocin to stimulate uterine contractions. Delivery of the placenta is delayed in 30% to 40% of instillation abortions. If the afterbirth does not follow the delivery of the fetus within one to two hours, severe bleeding may occur. Therefore, if the doctor cannot manually remove a delayed placenta, he or she may perform a D & C to complete the abortion procedure.

Of the three substances used in instillation abortions, saline is used most widely. Because fluid retention often accompanies saline use, this type of instillation is potentially hazardous for women with serious heart or kidney disease. Compared to saline, prostaglandin instillation is associated with nearly twice as many major complications, including infections and bleeding, as well as with a high incidence of nausea, vomiting, and diarrhea. No woman with a lung disease, such as asthma, should undergo prostaglandin instillation, because this hormone may cause spasm of the breathing tubes (bronchi) in the lungs. A new chemical for use in instillation abortion is urea, which only recently was approved by the FDA, making comparisons to saline and prostaglandin difficult. Urea instillation is not contraindicated in women with heart or lung disease and may ultimately prove to be the safest method of the three.

Comparison of D & E with instillation abortion

Instillation abortion poses double the risk, greater costs, and more emotional trauma to the woman than does the D & E performed earlier in pregnancy. In the past, women beyond the 12-week cutoff date for standard suction abortions waited until 16 weeks or more when instillation methods became technically feasible to perform. Studies indicate that at 13 to 16 weeks an *immediate* D & E is safer than waiting until 16 weeks to have a saline abortion. D & E lasts only a few minutes and spares the woman several days of hospitalization and the emotional trauma of labor and delivery of the fetus. Also, fewer infections and bleeding complications are associated with D & E as compared to saline instillations. Despite the relative advantages of the D & E, not all physicians are trained to perform this procedure, an important consideration to keep in mind if you are more than 12 weeks along and require an abortion. Find a surgeon experienced in this procedure to lessen the risk of uterine damage, a possible hazard with D & E even in the most skilled hands. *After* 16 weeks of pregnancy, a D & E is no safer than other methods of abortion.

Other methods of second trimester abortion

Older methods of abortion after 12 weeks of pregnancy require major operations through an abdominal incision. These include hysterectomy (removal of the uterus) and hysterotomy, a surgical procedure in which the fetus is delivered through an incision in the uterus. Because of the greater frequency of medical complications, these operations are rarely used today for pregnancy termination.

A newer approach utilizes vaginal suppositories containing the hormone prostaglandin which stimulates uterine contractions and was approved for this use by the FDA in 1977. Prostaglandin suppositories cause a high rate of side effects, especially nausea, vomiting, and diarrhea, making them an unacceptable alternative for most second trimester abortions.

After Your Surgery

Following an abortion, you should expect the mild cramping and slight vaginal bleeding to subside almost completely within an hour. A nurse or another assistant will monitor your pulse, your blood pressure, and your general condition until you are ready to go home. If you are Rh negative, the physician or nurse will administer a small dose of RhoGAM at this time to prevent Rh complications in future pregnancies (see Chapter 20). The physician may prescribe pills to help your uterus contract, antibiotics to prevent infection, or analgesics to lessen pain. If you will be taking birth control pills, ask for the prescription at this time so that you can start taking them one week after your abortion.

Many clinics and physicians provide a checklist

Table 66   RECOMMENDATIONS AFTER A PREGNANCY TERMINATION

From the time of your abortion until your follow-up visit in one or two weeks:

1. Know the telephone number of the physician who will be available (or the clinic) if you have a problem.

2. Take your temperature four times a day for about the first three days. Report to your clinician a rise in your temperature to 100.4° or more that occurs at any time before your follow-up visit.

3. Report any of these warning signs to your clinician: heavy bleeding (more than three or four pads in twelve hours), prolonged bleeding (for three days or more), severe abdominal pain, chills, bad-smelling vaginal discharge.

4. Don't douche, use tampons, or have intercourse for two weeks.

5. Follow any specific instructions that may have been given you by your doctor or the clinic or hospital.

of *do's* and *don'ts* during the recovery period following abortion. Some information you will need to know until your follow-up visit in one or two weeks is provided in Table 66.

Your Follow-up Visit

At your follow-up visit, the clinician will examine your uterus, making sure there are no signs of infection or enlargement. At this time, in addition to any questions you may have concerning contraception or future pregnancy, be sure to ask about your pathology report, which is your assurance that pregnancy was successfully terminated. If the report fails to indicate *fetal tissue*, *products of conception*, or *chorionic villi* (the technical name for microscopic placental tissue), the likeliest explanation is that you still have a uterine pregnancy that was "missed" at the time of your procedure. In such instances, after conferring with the pathologist to make sure nothing was overlooked, the clinician would probably repeat the procedure or first obtain a sonogram to rule out tubal pregnancy (see Chapter 81).

Complications of Abortions

In general, an abortion is one of the safest procedures in medicine. Most complications are minor. *Major* complications, such as bleeding requiring a transfusion, occur least often for early suction abortion (0.6%), to a moderate degree for D & E (1%), and most often for instillation methods (2% to 3%).

Table 67 indicates mortality risks for various methods of abortion. The risk of death from early abortion is less than one-tenth the risk of childbirth, while the risk of instillation abortion methods is similar to that of having a baby.

Immediate complications

Early complications occurring within the first twenty-four hours of abortion include bleeding, uterine damage, and anesthesia-related problems. Incomplete emptying of the uterus causes bleeding and ultimately requires a D & C in less than 1% of all suction abortions and 10% of second-trimester procedures. Laceration (tearing) of the cervix from the clamp used to steady the uterus is easily treated by a single suture. Uterine perforation (passage of one of the instruments through the uterine wall), a potentially serious injury, occurs two to three times per one thousand abortions, with most patients requiring no more than careful overnight observation in the hospital. Anesthesia complications, though uncommon, can occur, and general anesthesia is just as safe as local anesthesia.

Table 67 — MORTALITY RISKS FOR VARIOUS METHODS OF PREGNANCY TERMINATION

Method	No. of Deaths Per 100,000 Cases, 1972–1980
Suction abortions up to 8 weeks	0.5
Dilatation and evacuation	6
Instillation methods (saline or prostaglandin)	7 to 13
Hysterotomies/hysterectomies	43

Delayed complications

The most frequent delayed complications are bleeding and uterine infections. Therefore, you should contact your doctor for these signs of uterine infection: pelvic pain, heavy bleeding, fever (100.4° or more), chills, or foul-smelling vaginal discharge. These symptoms, which may begin several days to two weeks after the abortion procedure, usually respond well to oral antibiotics. If you are not feeling better twenty-four to forty-eight hours after treatment or if bleeding is heavy for several days (strongly suggesting that some tissue still remains inside the uterus), the clinician will perform a D & C. In rare instances, infection following abortion may spread to your tubes and require hospitalization for intravenous antibiotic treatment to prevent serious tubal damage, which could lead to chronic pain or sterility.

Long-term Effects

Future fertility is rarely impaired after pregnancy termination. Most authorities presently agree that a single abortion performed in the first 12 weeks of pregnancy does not threaten future childbearing potential. There is some evidence, however, that *repeat* abortions pose some risk to future childbearing. A recent World Health Organization study reports that women who underwent two or more abortions had a two- to three-times-greater chance of miscarriage, premature delivery, or low birth weight infant. Considering its possible effects on reproductive potential, abortion as a means of contraception is very undesirable.

Resources

For information about abortion services in your area contact your physician or your local county health department, women's center, or Planned Parenthood office. For information about an abortion provider near you, write or call:

National Abortion Federation
110 E. 59th Street
New York, New York 10022
800-223-0618: toll free except in the State of New York; from New York State call collect (212) 688-8516.

44

Hysterectomy and Its Alternatives

In the past, fifty to sixty percent of all women in the United States have had a hysterectomy at some point in their lifetime. Hysterectomy is still the most frequently performed major operation in the U.S., although the frequency of this surgery has dropped since the late 1970s. According to the National Center for Health Statistics the nationwide rate of hysterectomies reached an all-decade high in 1977, but has steadily declined, with 702,000 of these surgeries performed in 1981. Today women are more aware of less drastic choices than hysterectomy for most gynecologic problems. This chapter tells you when hysterectomy is necessary and when you should avoid it, and it includes a discussion of the possible risks and a list of the medical alternatives to hysterectomy. Being better informed will help you ask crucial questions, evaluate alternatives, and feel more secure in whatever decision you make.

In our culture, the uterus has been seen as a symbol of reproductive ability or as an expression of femininity. The only physiologic function of the uterus, however, is to house the growing fetus during pregnancy. In fact, this operation has major *medical* impact only on the woman of child-bearing age because she will no longer menstruate or be able to conceive. Contrary to popular belief the uterus does not produce hormones, enhance sexual responsiveness, control weight, or prevent hair growth. Consequently, none of these factors

are affected by removal of the uterus. However, removing the ovaries (a separate procedure sometimes accompanying a hysterectomy) in premenopausal women may cause temporary hot flashes, which can be prevented by estrogen replacement therapy (see Chapter 27).

Depending on circumstances discussed later in this chapter, the surgeon removes the uterus either through the abdomen or through the vagina. Either method may involve additional surgery. Here are common terms that describe each type of hysterectomy and possible related surgery.

Total abdominal hysterectomy refers to removal of the uterus (and cervix) through an abdominal incision.

Vaginal hysterectomy refers to removal of the uterus (and cervix) through a small incision in the vagina.

Either total abdominal hysterectomy or vaginal hysterectomy is sometimes also referred to as *simple, incomplete,* or *partial hysterectomy.* Either operation is in reality a *total hysterectomy* since both the uterus and cervix are removed (see Figure 39) in both of these operations.

Bilateral salpingo-oophorectomy refers to removal of both tubes and ovaries and may accompany abdominal hysterectomy. Although the name is technically incorrect, the combination of these two procedures (removal of tubes and ovaries plus removal of the uterus and cervix) is often referred to as *total hysterectomy* (see Figure 39).

Unilateral salpingo-oophorectomy refers to removal of the tube and ovary on one side only.

Radical hysterectomy, an operation performed only for certain pelvic cancers, refers to extended hysterectomy, which includes removal of the uterus (along with the cervix) and upper vagina as well as the adjacent pelvic lymph nodes.

Regardless of the approach (abdominal or vaginal), the surgeon detaches the uterus from the Fallopian tubes and ovaries and from the upper vagina. The ovaries and Fallopian tubes remain basically in the same location as before hysterectomy since they retain their attachment to the pelvic side wall after this operation. The surgeon then closes the vaginal opening from which the uterus was detached, restoring the vagina to its original shape and position. The intestines then fill in the space where the uterus was.

Whether or not the surgeon removes your ovaries during hysterectomy depends largely on your age and the condition of your ovaries. Most gynecologists remove both ovaries if hysterectomy is

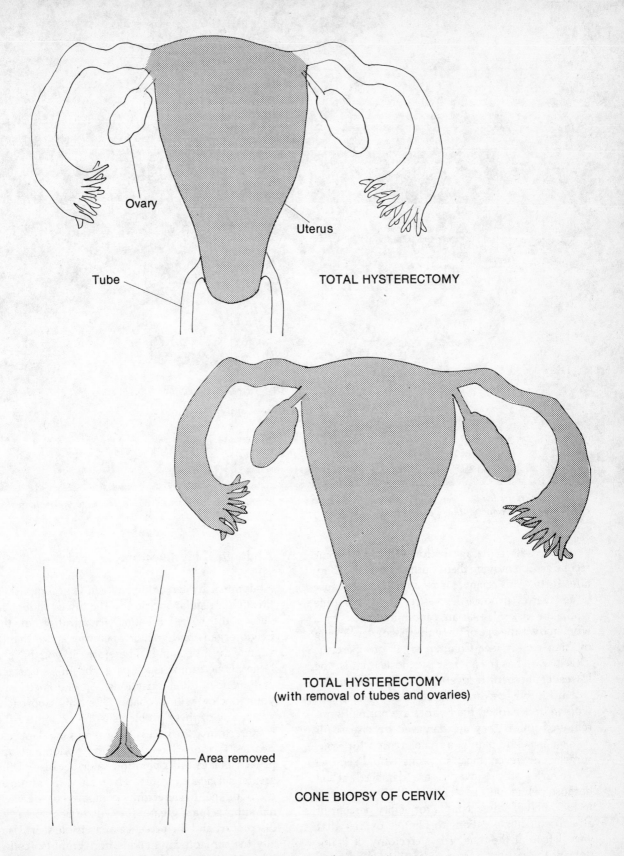

Ovary

Uterus

Tube

TOTAL HYSTERECTOMY

TOTAL HYSTERECTOMY
(with removal of tubes and ovaries)

Area removed

CONE BIOPSY OF CERVIX

Figure 39   *The shaded areas show what is removed in different gynecologic operations.*

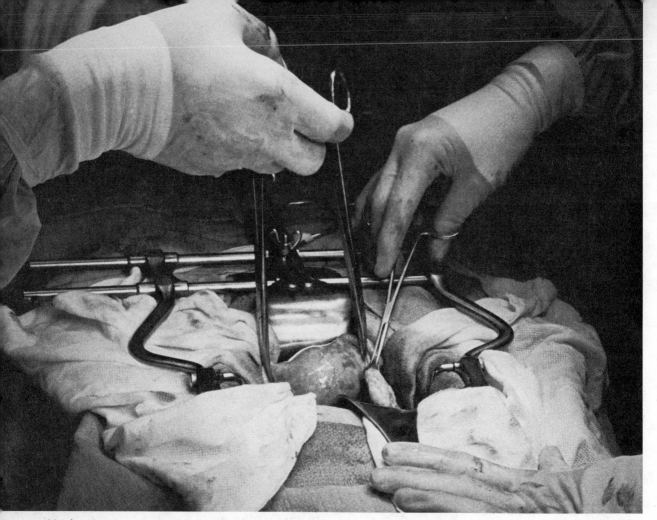

Metal retractors are used to keep an abdominal incision spread apart to provide the necessary exposure for surgery. The uterus can be seen in the center of the operating field.

performed after the age of forty-five, and some recommend removing them during a hysterectomy after forty. This removal is recommended because your ovaries produce less estrogen at this time while the risk of ovarian cancer increases. In a woman over the age of forty the risk of developing ovarian cancer (see Chapter 38) is one percent. This disease has the poorest prognosis (that is, the lowest chances for recovery) of any pelvic cancer, and no means of early detection is available. In women under forty, the ovaries are normally not removed unless they are damaged by disease. If persistent pelvic pain is a major reason for your surgery, however, most surgeons would remove the ovaries if the ovaries are damaged at all because pelvic pain is otherwise likely to persist. In fact, pelvic pain accounts for eighty percent of all subsequent operations to remove ovaries that were left in at the time of hysterectomy. It is important to discuss these considerations in advance with your surgeon.

Abdominal Hysterectomy

Abdominal hysterectomy, which is accomplished through a regular incision in the lower abdomen, allows the surgeon better visualization of the pelvic organs and greater operating space than a vaginal hysterectomy. Therefore, if you have a large pelvic tumor (such as a fibroid), suspected malignancy, tubal infections, or endometriosis, your doctor will probably use this approach. When any of these problems is the reason for the hysterectomy, the necessity of removing damaged ovaries is more likely; and the abdominal approach makes this operation safer because of the greater surgical exposure. The main disadvantages of abdominal hysterectomy compared to the vaginal approach are greater immediate postoperative discomfort and the presence of a visible scar. Usually the surgeon can make a horizontal (so-called bikini) incision which extends across the top of the pubic hairline. This incision is less noticeable than a vertical one which goes from below the navel to the top of the pubic bone.

Vaginal Hysterectomy

Compared to abdominal hysterectomy, vaginal hysterectomy is technically more difficult because of the limited space in which the surgeon has to operate. This approach is ideal when the uterus is not enlarged and ovarian disease is not expected. Your surgeon may recommend this approach especially when the uterus has "dropped" as a result of the weakening of surrounding muscles and ligaments (see Chapter 28). Often, vaginal surgery to repair a cystocele or rectocele (see glossary) can be done at the time of vaginal hysterectomy. If none of the reasons for an abdominal approach is present, most surgeons will choose vaginal hysterectomy because of the shorter operating time involved as well as the speedier, less painful recovery and cosmetic advantage since there will be no visible scar.

Indications for Hysterectomy

Urgent indications for hysterectomy may include pelvic cancers, severe pelvic infections, or uncontrollable bleeding. In these instances, a hysterectomy may be lifesaving. Most often, however, the timing of hysterectomy depends upon the severity of your symptoms. Table 68 indicates conditions which may require hysterectomy and possible alternative therapy. Remember that pelvic pain and vaginal bleeding—the most common symptoms leading to hysterectomy—do not necessarily mean that something is wrong with your uterus or

Table 68   CONDITIONS WHICH MAY REQUIRE HYSTERECTOMY

Condition	When to Consider Hysterectomy	Alternative Therapy
Fibroids	persistent, heavy menstrual bleeding, especially if severe anemia is present or if childbearing is not desired fibroid growth fibroids greater than 12-weeks size	myomectomy (surgical removal of fibroid tumor only) stopping all estrogen medication, including the pill iron for anemia due to blood loss
Bleeding problems	lack of response to alternative therapy, especially if severe anemia is present or if childbearing is not desired	hormones (e.g., progesterone, the pill) antibiotics for uterine infection IUD removal D & C or endometrial biopsy iron for anemia
Uterine prolapse ("dropped" uterus)	persistent or severe pelvic pain, pressure, or backache after other causes have been ruled out if surgery for urinary incontinence (e.g., bladder surgery) is planned and childbearing is not desired	pessary (see glossary)
Carcinoma-in-situ (CIS) or severe dysplasia	hysterectomy is *recommended* for CIS if childbearing is not desired	cone biopsy (see Figure 39) cryosurgery
Cancer of uterus, ovary, or cervix	hysterectomy is *recommended* unless radiation or chemotherapy is treatment of choice	often none (radiation or chemotherapy in select cases)
Pelvic inflammatory disease (tube or ovary infections)	if chronic pelvic pain or infection persists, especially if future childbearing is unwanted or is prevented by this disease	antibiotics
Endometriosis	if chronic pelvic pain persists, especially if future childbearing is unwanted or is prevented by this disease	hormones (e.g., progesterone, the pill)
Desire for sterilization	if any of the above conditions are present	tubal sterilization or vasectomy

Table 69   CONDITIONS WHICH DO NOT JUSTIFY HYSTERECTOMY

Avoid hysterectomy . . .	Because . . .	Unless . . .
to "prevent" cancer	the risks of surgery outweigh any so-called preventive benefits	you already have precancerous changes of the cervix (severe dysplasia) or uterus (atypical endometrial hyperplasia) (see Chapters 36 and 39)
for sterilization	the risks of hysterectomy surgery are much higher than for tubal sterilization or vasectomy	you also have one of the conditions named in Table 68 and hysterectomy is the treatment of choice
for bleeding problems if a D & C or endometrial biopsy is not done first	a uterine cancer requiring different treatment may be diagnosed	
for a "dropped" bladder or uterus if you have little or no discomfort or other symptoms	there is no indication for surgery	
for pelvic pain without a definite diagnosis	the pain may not be relieved by hysterectomy	diagnostic tests are first done, possibly including X-rays and laparoscopy (see Chapter 81)

that you need this surgery. For more information on the conditions and alternatives to hysterectomy listed in Table 68 refer to the index about the specific item in question.

When to Avoid Hysterectomy

Second opinion programs and greater consumer awareness about the risks of major surgery have reduced the number of unnecessary hysterectomies in recent years. One difficulty in deciding whether to have this operation is that the patient herself must supply some of the input as to the reasons for having it (for example, pain, bleeding) and must also consider the expected benefits to be derived. Truly informed consent (discussed in Chapter 40) is all-important: Will your pain be relieved? Will sexual enjoyment increase? Will you have more energy and more time free of disabling symptoms? The answers will most often be a qualified yes. In other words, there are a good many instances when the results of this surgery cannot be fully determined in advance.

There are, however, specific instances when you should avoid or delay having this operation. For example, to have a hysterectomy to prevent cancer of the cervix or uterus (in the absence of risk factors) makes no sense because the risks of

having this major surgery outweigh the so-called cancer-protection benefits. Similarly, hysterectomy is not considered the first choice for sterilization in most healthy women. One of the tubal ligation operations (or vasectomy) is cheaper, easier, and safer unless other gynecologic conditions are present. At other times, hysterectomy may be premature if your problem has not had adequate diagnostic evaluation. Pelvic pain, for example, may be due to conditions involving the urinary tract, skeletal system, or digestive system; but you won't know unless appropriate tests and X-rays have ruled out these possibilities (see Chapter 81). Even then, a diagnostic laparoscopy may identify a problem that can be solved with surgery short of hysterectomy. To name another example: hysterectomy should be avoided in a postmenopausal woman with bleeding until after a D & C (see Chapter 41) is first done. The D & C might indicate the need for therapy different from hysterectomy or might itself be sufficient therapy. Finally, medical conditions such as obesity, high blood pressure, and diabetes increase the risk of any major surgery, including hysterectomy. For this reason alone, some women should avoid exposure to such risks unless strong indications for hysterectomy warrant it (see Table 68). These and other examples of when to avoid hysterectomy are summarized in Table 69.

Deciding About Hysterectomy

Your decision regarding hysterectomy must take into account both the severity of the problem and your desire for future children. Although hysterectomy may improve your quality of life by relieving chronic symptoms such as pain or bleeding, where there is a choice some women are willing to tolerate these symptoms instead of having surgery. When deciding whether or not to have a hysterectomy, here are essential questions to ask your doctor:

1. Is alternative therapy available? If not, what will happen if I don't have a hysterectomy? If so, is alternative therapy likely to cure the problem or will relief be only temporary?
2. If alternative therapy includes conservative surgery short of hysterectomy, what are my chances of needing hysterectomy later?
3. What are the risks of alternative therapy and of hysterectomy?
4. If I want to become pregnant, is it possible or safe to get pregnant?
5. Is this condition likely to improve on its own or get worse?
6. Is hysterectomy *medically necessary* or is it *recommended* to relieve my symptoms?

Here are some questions to ask yourself and to discuss with your husband or partner before you decide on elective hysterectomy:

1. Do I want to become pregnant in the future?
2. What are my feelings about my no longer having a uterus?
3. How will my job and life style be affected by a major operation at this time?
4. What is my husband's or partner's attitude about this surgery?

Risks of Hysterectomy

Although hysterectomy is one of the safest operations, no major surgery is without some risk. Fever and infection, the most frequent of the complications of hysterectomy, occur more often with vaginal hysterectomies. Infection usually involves the bladder or upper vagina and almost always responds promptly to antibiotic therapy. Serious complications such as blood clots or severe bleeding occur less than one percent of the time. Damage to other organs such as the intestines or bladder also occurs infrequently and is usually repaired at surgery. Such injuries may prolong your stay in the hospital, however. Mortality from hysterectomy is related to general condition and the reason for having surgery. Overall, approximately one death occurs for every two thousand hysterectomy operations. This frequency is considerably lower for women without chronic health problems such as heart disease or high blood pressure.

Recovering from Hysterectomy

Following hysterectomy, most women stay in the hospital four to six days. Complete recovery usually takes six to eight weeks. During the first two weeks at home, get plenty of rest and do only the simplest tasks which require little or no lifting. You will probably feel tired, perhaps more so than you expected. It is generally safe to climb stairs, shower, and wash your hair. In the third and fourth weeks following surgery, you can gradually increase your activities, including light chores and driving; and if you work outside the home you may consider returning to your job part-time as long as heavy lifting is avoided. In the fifth and sixth postoperative weeks, you may gradually return to your preoperative activities, except for vigorous exercise. By the sixth week, and sometimes before, you may take tub baths and resume sexual activity.

The time required to recover from surgery varies from individual to individual. Because of this fact and the difficulty in forecasting how you will feel, schedule your postoperative checkup no later than four weeks after surgery. If you have any questions about your activity limitations, call your physician before this checkup. Most women can return to work by the sixth week after surgery. You may, however, want initially to resume work half-time, especially if heavy lifting or strenuous activity is part of your job.

Long-term Effects of Hysterectomy

Many misconceptions and unnecessary fears surround the subject of hysterectomy and its possible effects—hormonal, sexual, and emotional. Following hysterectomy, a woman will not go through the menopause any sooner than nature intended unless both ovaries are removed, because hysterectomy alone causes no change in hormone levels. Surgical removal of both ovaries in women who have not reached menopause usually causes hot flashes, which can be prevented with estrogen replacement therapy (see Chapter 27). You will not need hormone replacement if one ovary is preserved, because one ovary functions well enough for two. Removal of the ovaries in women already past menopause will not cause hot flashes or other menopause symptoms.

For the great majority of women hysterectomy, with or without removal of the ovaries, has not been associated with loss of sexual desire, responsiveness, or satisfaction. Nevertheless, this subject has not been thoroughly studied and more research is needed. For many women relief from fear of pregnancy results in heightened sexual enjoyment following hysterectomy. Vaginal dryness, which may occur following removal of the ovaries, can be relieved by estrogen pills or creams or by using a water-soluble lubricant like K-Y lubricating jelly. Occasionally, hysterectomy shortens vaginal length and results in slight discomfort during intercourse.

The emotional impact of hysterectomy, like that of other major operations, depends on the woman's preparation, the nature of the problem requiring surgery, and the support of friends and family. As with the surgical removal of any organ, it is normal to go through an adjustment period and to experience feelings of loss. The adjustment to hysterectomy, however, is often more difficult. It is encouraging to note that in a recent carefully designed study by Coppen and others, sixty women who underwent hysterectomy experienced an improvement of mood and a general sense of well-being following this surgery (see reference list at the end of this section). However, most older studies show that twice as many individuals are likely to experience serious depression following hysterectomy as compared to other forms of surgery. Such depression is more likely when the woman is younger than forty or if the condition requiring hysterectomy interfered with desired childbearing (for example, pelvic infection leading to sterility). Depression is also more common when the operation is performed for a serious disease (such as cancer) or if a woman feels she had little choice in making this decision (in an emergency, for instance). Don't hesitate to seek help from friends, other women who have undergone hysterectomy, your clinician, or a counselor

if depression seems prolonged. Even the woman who is well prepared for hysterectomy and accepts the necessity for the surgery may experience some mental stress. However, women who have reacted to previous stress with positive efforts—recognition that feelings of loss are temporary, discussion of feelings with friends, realization of worthwhile results from surgery—may expect to respond similarly to hysterectomy.

References for Section Nine

Chapter 40—Deciding About Surgery

Burchell, R. C. Obtaining truly informed consent for surgery. *Contemporary OB/GYN* 13:163–168, Apr 1979.

Gizynski, M. N. Psychic trauma of gynecologic surgery. *The Female Patient* 37–39, Feb 1978.

Nierenberg, J., and Janovic, F. *The Hospital Experience.* Indianapolis: Bobbs-Merrill, 1978.

Chapter 42—Sterilization Options

Moses, V. I., et al. Tubal sterilization among women of reproductive age, United States, update for 1979-1980. *Urban Health* 38-42, Jan 1984.

Destefano, F., et al. Complications of interval laparoscopic tubal sterilization. *Obstetrics and Gynecology* 61(2):153-158, 1983.

Fortney, J. A., et al. A new approach to measuring menstrual pattern change after sterilization. *American Journal of Obstetrics and Gynecology* 147:830-836, 1983.

Corner, G. W., Jr., and Harris, B. A., Jr. Sterilization by mini-laparotomy. *The Female Patient* 51–53, Feb 1979.

Phillips, J. M. (ed.) *Laparoscopy.* Baltimore: Williams and Wilkins Co., 1977.

Center for Disease Control: Surgical Sterilization Surveillance. HEW Publication No. (CDC) 79–8378, 1979.

Letchworth, A. T., et al. Laparoscopy or minilaparotomy for sterilization of women. *Obstetrics and Gynecology* 56(1):119–121, 1980.

Chapter 43—Terminating Pregnancy

Stubblefield, P. G. Current technology for abortion. *Current Problems in Obstetrics and Gynecology* 2(4):3–44, 1978.

Centers for Disease Control: Abortion Surveillance 1983. Department of Health and Human Services, Atlanta, Georgia.

Maine, D. Does abortion affect later pregnancies? *Family Planning Perspectives* 11(2):98–101, 1979.

Cates, W., and Tietze, C. Standardized mortality rates associated with legal abortion: United States 1972–1975. *Family Planning Perspectives* 10(2):109–112, 1978.

Cates, W., Schulz, K. F., et al. The effect of delay and method of choice on the risk of abortion morbidity. *Family Planning Perspectives* 9(6):266–273, 1977.

Harlap, S., et al. A prospective study of spontaneous fetal losses after induced abortions. *New England Journal of Medicine* 301(13):677–81, 1979.

Cates, W., Jr. D & E after 12 weeks: safe or hazardous? *Contemporary OB/GYN* 13:23–29, Jan 1979.

Committee on Technical Bulletins of the American College of Obstetricians and Gynecologists: Methods of Midtrimester Abortion. Technical Bulletin #56, 1979, American College of Obstetricians and Gynecologists, Washington, D.C.

Harman, C. R., et al. Factors influencing morbidity in termination of pregnancy. *American Journal of Obstetrics and Gynecology* 139(3):333–337, Feb 1981.

Chapter 44—Hysterectomy and Its Alternatives

Mattingly, R. F. (ed.) *TeLinde's Operative Gynecology*, ed. 5. Philadelphia: Lippincott, 1977.

Roeske, N. C. Evaluating hysterectomy's psychosocial impact. *Contemporary OB/GYN* 12:95–102, Dec 1978.

Dennerstein, L., Wood, C., et al. Sexual response following hysterectomy and oophorectomy. *Obstetrics and Gynecology* 49(1):92–96, 1977.

Ananth, J. Hysterectomy and depression. *Obstetrics and Gynecology* 52(6):724–730, 1978.

Pratt, J. H. Deciding for hysterectomy. *Contemporary OB/GYN* 13:151–158, Apr 1979.

Wales, E. Sexual rehabilitation after gynecologic surgery. *The Female Patient* 61–67, Jul 1980.

Coppen, A., et al. Hysterectomy, hormones and behavior. *Lancet* 126–128, Jan 17, 1981.

Ten

A Healthy Life Style

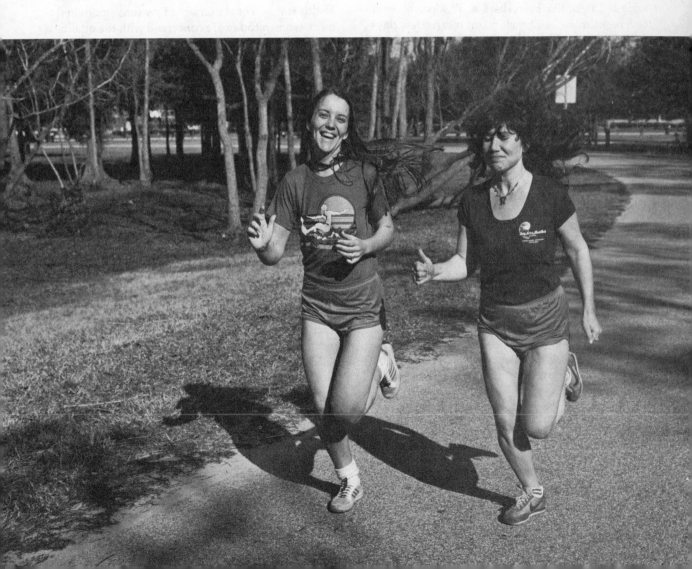

45

Staying Healthy

Just what is good health? It can mean different things to different people, often depending upon their history of previous illness. People who have not lived with a chronic health problem might view good health as the absence of acute illness, such as colds and flu. Older persons might say that good health consists of having the energy and the physical capability to accomplish what they want to do without the restrictions imposed by serious illness, like heart disease. To a person with severe arthritis, being well might mean a few days without pain in the joints. In general, we can say that good health is a condition of physical and mental well-being, free from disease, pain, or defect, that enables us to live our lives with choices and with vitality.

Whatever our definition of good health, one thing is for sure: it's easy to take good health for granted as long as we have it. Sometimes it is only after we become ill or unexpectedly disabled that our health becomes more of a concern; we may then concentrate on getting "well" or getting "back to good health."

The question now comes up: How much of good health results from chance, determined purely by luck, and how much results from our own decisions, our own responsibility? Certainly a genetic predisposition to, say, heart disease, diabetes, or obesity is real. Disablement that results from an accident is an unfortunate happening. But to what extent can chronic illness and degenerative diseases associated with aging be prevented or delayed? Studies have shown that there *are* certain actions we can all take to promote a state of good health and consequently live longer, more productive lives with greater freedom from disease. Although the experts don't always agree, there is a good deal of consensus in three areas: there is value in getting adequate, regular exercise, in eating a nutritious diet regularly, and in avoiding smoking.

In addition to good dietary and exercise habits and no smoking, we want to mention a few other basics crucial to good health. Recent research indicates the following factors also increase your life expectancy: seven to eight hours of sleep a night, regular meal taking, daily breakfast, maintenance of normal weight, and no more than moderate alcohol intake. Evidence suggests that people who adhere to these habits as well as maintain regular exercise and avoid smoking live about ten years longer than those who cultivate three or fewer of these practices.

Certainly in terms of longevity, the health status of women in the 1980s has improved over former times. Females born in the 1980s have a life expectancy of 81 years—33 years longer than their grandmothers. The age-adjusted death rate for women is now 4.6 per 1,000, half the level of 40 years ago.

But mortality statistics are only one indicator of health status. For a number of reasons, more and more women today are concerned with the quality of their level of wellness. This change in interest is due partly to increasing health consciousness on the part of our society generally.

In addition, women are aware of a variety of new social and work-related pressures which expose them to increased risks for stress-related illness, such as heart attacks. Today more women are employed outside the home than ever before and often must assume multiple roles in society as workers, homemakers, wives, and mothers. The impact of stress on the health status of women is uncertain and difficult to measure. Many professionals, including health educators, believe that women will soon catch up to men in many stress-related illnesses, such as heart disease and ulcers. With the tremendous changes in life style and work-related activities that have occurred in recent years, American women need, perhaps more than ever before, to use their resources for preserving wellness.

Most of the diseases we suffer from now are those related to body deterioration for which there are limited treatments—for example, heart disease or cancer. It is far easier to limit your risks for getting ill than to suffer through the pain and expense of hospitalization and treatment. It is far easier to maintain good health than to allow disease processes or an unhealthy condition to take over.

Just what *should* you do to bring about and maintain good health? We discuss, either below or in separate chapters that follow, several topics relevant to the maintenance of good health. In all of these areas you can take much of the responsibility for your own continued wellness.

Good Nutrition

Eating a well-balanced diet on a regular basis and staying at your ideal weight are critical factors in maintaining your emotional and physical well-being. Chapter 46 tells you some of the things you need to know about good nutrition. Maintaining your ideal weight is very important; the obese person is much more likely to develop certain chronic conditions such as diabetes, high blood pressure, and heart disease. Chapter 87, Weight Gain and Weight Loss, discusses the subject in some detail and tells you how to determine your ideal weight based on your height and body frame.

Regular, Adequate Exercise

Benefits of a consistent exercise program, an essential part of health maintenance, usually include some loss of weight (especially in overweight individuals) and a lowered blood pressure in persons with high blood pressure. Chapter 47 discusses the subject of physical exercise in some detail.

No Smoking

The best way to avoid smoking is never to start; but, unfortunately, studies show that smoking by women is on the rise. The numbers of teen-age smokers, as well as older women smokers, are increasing.

Cigarettes contain nicotine, a drug that exerts a dependency action on the body, creating a habit that is hard to break. Just one cigarette upsets the flow of blood and air in your body by temporarily constricting blood vessels and paralyzing the little filaments (cilia) in the lung that normally move back and forth continuously to rid air passages of tiny dirt particles from the air we breathe. Clear-cut evidence from numerous studies indicates that smokers, both men and women, have a much greater risk of getting lung cancer, emphysema, bronchitis, and coronary heart disease. Pregnant women who smoke have a greater chance of pregnancy complications and low birth weight babies. It has also been found that smokers significantly affect the health of the nonsmokers around them, including their families and co-workers. It is especially important that babies and young children not be subjected to cigarette smoke; if you or anyone who takes care of your children smokes, it is a good idea not to smoke when the children are present.

Further discussion about the hazards of smoking is presented in Chapters 31 and 59.

Avoidance of Drug Abuse

A drug is any substance that can alter the chemical functioning of the body or mind and includes over-the-counter medications and, of course, alcohol. Section Seven (Chapters 29, 30, and 31) discusses the subject of women and the use of drugs.

Enough Rest, Relaxation, and Stimulation

The competitive pulls and stresses of our society make it difficult to preserve the necessary balance of work and rest and relaxation that is so necessary for maintaining good mental and physical health. Stresses arise within our family life, schools, jobs, and even our retirement. It is important to evaluate your life style and your goals from time to time: are you trying to do too much? So often women feel that they must be successful in everything they do—from sex to work to play to motherhood. No one can do everything perfectly! But the belief that perfection is or *should* be possible is one of the main causes of depression and other forms of emotional distress in our society today. For this reason it may be helpful to appraise your goals periodically and make certain to plan for enough rest and relaxation.

Avoidance of Environmental Hazards

Environmental hazards are present everywhere. Because almost three of every five women seventeen and older are in the labor force today, hazards in the work world are an important consideration in women's health maintenance. Safety hazards, air as well as noise pollution, hazards from vibrations, frequent temperature changes, and the daily effect of working among smokers have all been shown to have potential health risks. We need to make ourselves aware of the possible specific hazards in our own environment, and we need to learn how to deal with them sensibly and safely.

Another environmental hazard that dermatologists have been warning us about for years is the sun. Excessive sun exposure can cause wrinkling, spotting, drying, and aging of the skin, to say nothing of the potential for skin cancer. To minimize these effects, women who want to have a suntan should be sure to use a suntan lotion that contains PABA (para-aminobenzoic acid), which is the ingredient that will protect you from sunburn. The amount of sunscreen protection provided by some of the so-called tanning lotions on the market now is indicated on the label by means of a numbering system. Numbers range from 1 to 15 and indicate the degree to which a particular product may help reduce such things as wrinkling of the skin and skin cancer due to sun overexposure. A number 1 rating means the product provides the least amount of sunscreen protection, and a number 15 rating, the most. You should choose the rating that is most beneficial for your type of skin; if you burn easily, choose a product with a higher number rating.

Good Body Hygiene

Hygiene habits are established early in childhood; bad ones can be either eliminated or changed in adult life. Because women sometimes base their self-esteem on their appearance, they are often easy prey to the many pressures to buy numerous products—to keep "young looking," to be attractive, to have more energy, to be more "feminine," to look tan and "healthy," and so on and on.

The best rule for maintaining a healthy, clean body is to use common sense. Cleanliness with the use of a neutral soap and water and a moisturizer if you have dry skin are all that is usually necessary. (Studies haven't clearly shown one type of cosmetic to be more helpful than the rest—or everyone would be using it!) Take a long, hot bath if it relaxes you. Taking regular care of your nails, hair, and feet represents good hygiene and promotes a sense of well-being as well.

Regular douching is not an element of good hygiene and may at times be harmful. Concentrations of douche ingredients may not be listed on the package because some products are considered cosmetics instead of drugs. Among the ingredients in most douches are agents which act as local anesthetics (phenol, menthol), perfumes (eucalyptol), or substances which increase or decrease vaginal acidity. Many such ingredients may cause local allergic reactions or, by their local anesthetic effects, mask symptoms of infection, possibly delaying effective treatment. One of the most effective over-the-counter products for vaginal infections is Betadine douche. When used daily for one to two weeks, Betadine may clear up some types of vaginal infections, especially trichomonas and bacterial types. However, most douches and similar feminine hygiene products cannot be generally recommended since they have not been proven to be effective for either treatment or prevention of vaginal infections (see Chapter 85).

If you do douche, here are some precautions:

1. If you have symptoms of a vaginal infection which does not clear up after using Betadine douche for one week, get medical attention.
2. If you douche for hygiene purposes, do not douche more than twice a week.
3. If you are pregnant, avoid douching, especially in late pregnancy when your bag of waters could possibly be ruptured by use of the douche.
4. Do not use a douche as a contraceptive; it is a very ineffective method.
5. Do not douche within six hours of using a contraceptive cream or jelly since contraceptive effectiveness may be diminished.
6. Do not douche after intercourse if you are trying to get pregnant since some douche ingredients may destroy sperm.
7. Do not douche within twenty-four hours before a visit to your doctor for a routine pelvic exam, a Pap smear, an exam for a vaginal infection, etc.

Good Oral Hygiene

Oral hygiene, or regular care of your teeth and gums, is very important. We are mentioning it here because of the prevalence of periodontal disease. Periodontal disease affects three out of four adults. Surveys show that most people brush their teeth regularly but still get periodontal disease. The reason for this is that brushing alone does not necessarily get rid of plaque (the microorganisms that grow on the teeth). Plaque tends to accumulate at the gumline near the base of the teeth, areas that often are not well cleaned through typical toothbrushing. It usually is necessary to use an additional cleansing mechanism, such as dental floss, to remove the plaque.

Periodontal disease usually shows itself initially as an inflammation of the gums (gingivitis); and, if it progresses, it destroys the alveolar bone and periodontal tissues supporting the teeth. With severe periodontal disease, loss of a tooth or teeth follows. Early signs of gingivitis include redness, swelling, and bleeding of the gums. Fortunately, this condition is reversible. It can be eliminated with proper home oral hygiene. It is best to discuss this condition with your dentist or dental hygienist *before* you have evidence of a problem.

Currently dentists recommend a soft toothbrush with two to three rows of bristles that are rounded at the tips. Brushes should be replaced frequently. Since plaque requires twenty-four hours to build up in order to exert its harmful effects, at least one thorough plaque removal per day is needed. Your dentist or dental hygienist can help you appraise the efficiency of your toothbrushing, through the use of a special coloring substance, and teach you how to properly use dental floss, the two best techniques for plaque removal. Daily use of floss is advisable, as it is the most effective way to remove the plaque from between the teeth. As a person ages, the gums often recede as a result of gradual damage from improper brushing and/or periodontal disease. This alters the normal structure of the gum, allowing more food and plaque to accumulate between the teeth. This condition may necessitate flossing and brushing more often.

Resources

The following resources can be helpful in providing information about general health:

American Dental Association
Bureau of Health Education and Audiovisual
    Services
211 East Chicago Avenue
Chicago, Illinois 60611

American Public Health Association
1015 Fifteenth Street, N.W.
Washington, D.C. 20005

Council on Family Health
633 Third Avenue
New York, N.Y. 10017

National Mental Health Association
1800 North Kent St.
Arlington, Virginia 22209

Nutrition

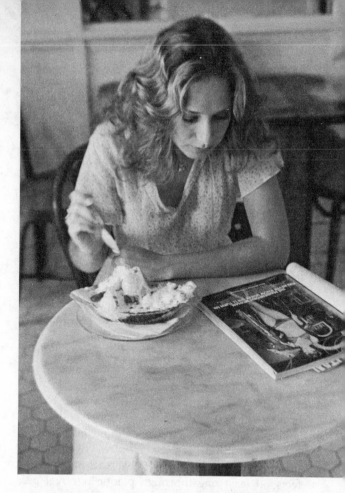

Nutrition plays a key role in maintaining health and in the prevention of many diseases. Dietary factors have been related to six of our leading causes of death: stroke, diabetes, heart disease, some cancers, hardening of the arteries, and cirrhosis of the liver. Today's American woman is concerned with a variety of issues relating to nutrition, from the proper use of vitamins to the health risks of food additives. She is bombarded daily with new books and magazine articles about various diets some of which promise easy answers to weight control or offer the prospect of controlling certain conditions, such as arthritis and heart disease. This chapter, because it discusses basic information we think most American women should know about nutrition, should help you to better evaluate what you read on the subject.

Nutrients

Nutrients are chemical substances derived from food during the process of digestion. The major nutrients—proteins, carbohydrates, and fats—are needed by the body for growth, repair, maintenance, and energy. The amount of energy supplied by a nutrient is measured in calories, but the nutritive values of different foods cannot be measured by calories alone. Good nutrition requires a balance of the right nutrients, that is, getting the proper amount, or proportion, of each one. Nutrients can be classified as follows:

Proteins

Proteins are an essential part of every cell in your body. Proteins help to repair worn-out or diseased tissue and to build new tissue. Protein is used, for example, in the formulation of hormones, enzymes, red blood cells, and antibodies and in the formation of milk for breast-feeding. When di-

gested, protein breaks down into smaller units called amino acids, some of which (the so-called essential ones) must be obtained from food. Proteins derived from animal foods, such as fish, meat, eggs, and dairy products, are "complete" proteins because they each contain all the amino acids, including the essential amino acids, in sufficient quantities and in proportion to one another. Vegetable proteins are "incomplete" because each one lacks one or more essential amino acids, or those that are there are not in good proportions to one another. However, when vegetable proteins and proteins in whole grains are used in certain combinations of foods (such as dried beans and rice, or cereal and milk), they supply all the required amino acids.

Carbohydrates

Carbohydrates function primarily to provide energy, supplying about two-thirds of an individual's total energy needs. When insufficient carbohydrates are eaten, body fat and proteins are then broken down to meet the body's energy demands. Foods high in carbohydrates include grains, vegetables, fruits, and seeds. Carbohydrates also include simple sugars found in sweets, candy, and pastries. Sugar is a "low-density" source of calories which are rapidly used up, thus promptly leading to a renewed desire for food. When used in moderate quantities, sugar isn't harmful as long as it doesn't replace other foods that have needed nutrients. Excess dietary sugar may lead to obesity, low blood sugar, and dental caries (tooth decay) and also has been linked to a possible increased risk of developing diabetes in later adult life.

Fats

The most concentrated source of food energy is found in fats, or lipids. They are necessary for the absorption and utilization of certain vitamins (A, E, D, and K). Fat deposits surround and protect body organs, such as the heart and liver, and help to maintain body temperature against outside environmental influences. Excess fat is stored in the body tissues and leads to weight gain.

High amounts of fat in the American diet have been linked to an increased risk for cancer and heart disease. The American Cancer Society recently announced results of a twelve-year study which found that excessive consumption of both saturated and unsaturated fats was linked to the development of breast and colon cancer. The American Heart Association (A.H.A.) also suggests that Americans consume fewer dietary fats (no more than 30-35% of total calories). Two specific types of fat—saturated fats and cholesterol—are the most important to restrict because they tend to raise the level of cholesterol in the blood and a high cholesterol contributes to hardening of the arteries and heart disease. Saturated fats are found in animal meats, butter, cream, and whole milk. Cholesterol-rich foods include eggs, liver, shellfish, red meats, and milk. You should replace cholesterol and saturated fats with heart-healthy foods such as fish, chicken, fresh fruit, and vegetables. In addition, the A.H.A. encourages every adult to have a blood test to measure her level of cholesterol. Some individuals inherit a tendency toward high cholesterol, but for most Americans the reason for high cholesterol is dietary.

Fiber

Although, strictly speaking, fiber is not a nutrient, fiber plays a vital role in the digestive process by softening bile waste and speeding up the process of elimination of undigested food. Some research suggests (but has not been proven) that increased amounts of dietary fiber may help protect against the development of colon cancer. In older women especially, foods high in fiber, such as raw fruits and vegetables, may help prevent constipation and certain colon conditions such as diverticulitis (see glossary). In some individuals excessive fiber intake can be a problem, too, causing bloating, gas, and diarrhea.

Vitamins and Minerals

Vitamins are organic substances which have no caloric or energy value but which contribute to nutrition by allowing chemical reactions to occur normally throughout the body. These reactions, known collectively as metabolism, are responsible for numerous functions, such as converting fats and carbohydrates into energy and utilizing proteins to repair injured tissue. Vitamins act as essential catalysts in these processes.

Table 70 U.S. RECOMMENDED DAILY ALLOWANCES OF VITAMINS

Vitamin	U.S. Recommended Daily Allowance (U.S. RDA) (in I.U.* or mg**)	
	For Adult Women	For Pregnant or Breast-feeding Women
Vitamin A	5,000 I.U.	8,000 I.U.
Vitamin D	400 I.U.	400 I.U.
Vitamin E	30 I.U.	30 I.U.
Vitamin C	60 mg	60 mg
Folic acid	0.4 mg	0.8 mg
Thiamine	1.5 mg	1.7 mg
Riboflavin	1.7 mg	2.0 mg
Niacin	20.0 mg	20.0 mg
Vitamin B$_6$	2.0 mg	2.5 mg
Vitamin B$_{12}$	6.0 mg	8.0 mg
Biotin	0.3 mg	0.3 mg
Pantothenic acid	10.0 mg	10.0 mg

* International Units

** milligrams

Minerals are chemical substances, such as calcium, sodium, iron, and potassium, which participate in many chemical reactions essential in human nutrition. Minerals are similar to vitamins in that they don't directly provide energy; but, unlike vitamins, minerals do act as components of major body structures, including bones, teeth, blood, and soft tissue.

Except during pregnancy and breast-feeding, supplemental vitamins and minerals are usually unnecessary in healthy women who eat well-balanced diets. Table 70 shows the recommended daily allowances (RDAs) of vitamins for women. The slightly increased needs for certain vitamins in pregnant or breast-feeding women are also shown. Women who are on restricted diets, who are dieting, or who have certain chronic illnesses may require supplementation of vitamins or certain minerals. In women, by far the most common mineral likely to be deficient in the diet is iron.

Table 71 SYMPTOMS OF VITAMIN DEFICIENCY

Vitamin	Early Symptoms of Deficiency	Food Containing Vitamin	Comment
A (Retinol)	night blindness, dry skin	liver, eggs, butter, whole milk, vegetables	deficiency rare
B_1 (Thiamine)	numbness, tingling, loss of sensation or shooting pains in the extremities, especially the legs	bran, whole grains, cereals, fruits, nuts, vegetables, fish	deficiency associated with excessive use of alcohol
B_2 (Riboflavin)	ulcer of mouth, cracking of lips, dimness of vision	liver, milk, eggs, vegetables	deficiency rare
B_3 (Niacin or Nicotinic acid)	weight loss, rough skin, mouth sores, burning of tongue, weakness, diarrhea	fish, meat, whole grains, cereals, vegetables	deficiency rare
B_6 (Pyridoxine)	depression, mouth soreness, dizziness, nausea	meat, vegetables, bran	deficiency rare but occasional depression is seen in women taking birth control pills
B_{12} (Cyanoco-balamine)	weakness, shortness of breath, numbness and tingling in fingers and toes	meat, fish, milk	deficiency rare; however, strict vegetarians should supplement their diets with this vitamin
C (Ascorbic acid)	gum bleeding, swelling, or infection; bleeding into the skin causing bruising	citrus fruits, fresh vegetables	deficiency very uncommon
D (Calciferol)	bowed legs, deformed spine	fish, egg yolks, vitamin-D-fortified milk	deficiency rare; vitamin D is also formed in the skin from the sun's rays
E	none	vegetables, whole grains, cereals, fruits	no deficiency state known
Folic acid	weakness, numbness and tingling of fingers and toes, mouth ulcers, sore tongue	liver, vegetables, nuts, whole wheat	deficiency rare; supplementation needed in pregnancy and in women taking some anticonvulsant drugs
K	bleeding	vegetables	deficiency rare
Pantothenic acid	headache, fatigue, loss of coordination	liver, eggs, potatoes, vegetables	deficiency rare

Table 72   QUESTIONS COMMONLY ASKED ABOUT TAKING VITAMINS

Question	Yes	No	Comment
Are "natural" vitamins better than synthetic ones?		X	There is no evidence that they are.
Does vitamin E have any proven therapeutic value?		X	And vitamin E deficiency is virtually unknown. (See Chapter 57.)
Do I need to take vitamins while on the birth control pill?		X	Blood levels of folic acid and vitamin B_6 may be slightly but not significantly lowered.
Does vitamin A prevent or control acne?		X	The dosage required to prevent acne produces toxic side effects.
Is excessive alcohol intake associated with vitamin deficiency?	X		Especially thiamine.
Is B_{12} an appetite stimulant?		X	Injectable B_{12} has been used to improve mood and provide a sense of well-being—the effect is entirely placebo.
Does B_6 help to control nausea and vomiting in early pregnancy?	X		B_6 sometimes helps but no studies have been done to document its effectiveness.
Do vitamins provide energy?		X	They are organic compounds necessary for changing food into energy.
Do so-called average or normal eaters usually need supplemental vitamins?		X	Except perhaps during pregnancy.
Are cracked nails a common sign of vitamin deficiency?		X	Much more common causes are trauma to the nail base or a fungal infection of the nail.

Iron-deficiency anemia associated with heavy menstrual periods, for example, may necessitate the use of supplemental iron from time to time.

A few words should be said here about the absorption of iron by the body. Certain substances in some of the foods we eat, like the tannic acid in tea, for example, inhibit the body's absorption of the kind of iron that is in plant foods. Certain other substances work in an opposite way and increase the amount of iron absorbed by the body from the foods we eat. These substances include high quality protein, like that provided by soybeans, and ascorbic acid (vitamin C), as found in orange juice. Not only do these substances increase the absorption of iron, they also reverse the inhibiting effects of substances like tannic acid. But in order for this reversal effect to take place, the foods must be eaten at the same meal. So if you drink tea, for example, with a meal, try to include some food high in vitamin C at the same meal.

The presumed beneficial effects of vitamins and minerals have been widely promoted by drug manufacturers. The consumer cannot easily evaluate the variety of claims being made for these products, and many of these claims are misleading. Vitamins do not, for example, provide energy or produce a sense of well-being. According to the FDA, vitamins are indicated only for the treatment or the prevention of deficiency states (see Table 71). Similarly, iron is indicated only when iron-deficiency anemia is present, but iron supplementation does not prevent listlessness or fatigue in individuals who are not anemic.

Vitamin preparations

There are numerous vitamin preparations available, some containing iron. If what you need is iron, you are just as well off and can save money by selecting an iron preparation with vitamin C (which helps the body to absorb the iron) rather than an iron and multiple vitamin combination. Vitamin products vary widely from expensive name brands which contain minerals rarely needed, such as manganese, to simple vitamin C. Over-the-counter products are almost always just as good as prescription vitamins. Neither are necessary in most healthy, nonpregnant women eating well-balanced diets.

Prescription vitamins, as distinguished from over-the-counter preparations, usually contain a larger dose of folic acid than is available in over-the-counter preparations. However, significant folic acid deficiency is uncommon except in women with certain chronic digestive diseases or who take anticonvulsants such as Dilantin. Women who are pregnant or who are taking birth control pills have a slightly increased need for folic acid, which can be met by a diet plentiful in fresh, green vegetables. It is questionable whether folic acid makes any significant contribution to the nutritional status of the vast majority of women, even in pregnancy.

The whole practice of vitamin supplementation in pregnancy is more of an expected tradition than a medical necessity in most healthy women. But because many vitamin preparations also contain the one mineral supplement that may be needed in pregnancy—iron—vitamins and iron tend to be prescribed and taken together in one pill, the so-called prenatal vitamins.

Table 72 answers some questions commonly asked about taking vitamins.

Megavitamins

Vitamins with a dose of more than ten times the Recommended Daily Allowance (RDA) (see below under Planning for Good Nutrition) are considered megavitamins. The megavitamin concept rests largely on the speculation that the vitamin needs of many people cannot be met from ordinary diets and on the belief that human nutrient needs vary over a range greater than ten times the RDA. However, both human and animal studies have shown that maintenance of a satisfactory state of health seldom requires nutrient supplementation beyond the requirements of the RDA. Despite the many possible harmful effects of megavitamin dosages (see Table 73), these dosages continue to be popular perhaps because of a placebo effect; that is, if both patient and doctor believe something will relieve a symptom, it often will. The National Nutrition Consortium, made up of a number of professional societies, has gone on record as recommending against large amounts of

vitamins. Vitamin C megadose supplementation during pregnancy can lead to serious problems in the newborn. After having been exposed to large dosages of this vitamin before birth, the newborn may develop a relative deficiency state after birth, resulting in scurvy and possible life-threatening bleeding. Very high doses of vitamin A and vitamin D have been associated with birth defects in the newborn.

Table 73   POSSIBLE SIDE EFFECTS OF MEGAVITAMINS

Megavitamin*	Possible Side Effects
Vitamin C	diarrhea, kidney stones and kidney damage, increased susceptibility to gout, increased susceptibility to sickle-cell crisis in women with sickle-cell anemia
Nicotinic acid	flushing, itching rash, vomiting, jaundice, liver damage, peptic ulcer
Vitamin E	headache, nausea, dizziness, blurred vision
Folic acid	increased seizures in women with epilepsy
Vitamin A	headaches, diarrhea, blurred vision, nervous system damage, liver damage, bone damage
Vitamin D	headaches, weakness, nausea, blurred vision, nervous system or kidney damage
Vitamin K	decreases the effectiveness of blood thinners, such as Coumadin
Pyridoxine (vitamin B₆)	seizures

* 10 times Recommended Daily Allowance or more

Iron preparations

You are much more likely to need and benefit from iron than from vitamins. Iron may be sold generically as ferrous sulfate, ferrous fumarate, or ferrous gluconate. These are the most economical forms of iron. The common side effects of iron are stomach irritation and constipation. Women who have a history of stomach ulcers should use iron

Table 74   COMPARISON OF IRON-CONTAINING DRUGS

Type of Iron	Common Brand Names	Comment
Simple iron, usually ferrous sulfate or ferrous fumarate	many brands	Many generics available and may be less costly. Liquid form generally costs more than capsule or tablet.
Timed-release iron products	Fero-Gradumet Fergon many other brands	Many generics available and may be less costly. Intended to prevent stomach irritation.
Iron plus a stool softener	Ferrosequels several other brands	Useful after surgery or childbirth.
Iron plus vitamin C	many brands	Vitamin C intended to promote absorption (slight effect) and decrease stomach irritation.
Iron plus multiple vitamins	many brands	Not needed in simple iron-deficiency anemia.

preparations cautiously since such use sometimes brings on ulcerlike symptoms. Stomach irritation may occur as nausea, gas, or indigestion. Some iron products contain timed- or sustained-release forms of iron which are less irritating to the stomach. The addition of vitamin C in the product may also decrease stomach irritation as well as increase iron absorption. For this reason, some iron preparations are sold in combination with this vitamin alone. Another way iron is prepared is in combination with a stool softener (sulfosuccinate). This combination may be helpful after surgery or childbirth when constipation is more likely to be a problem. All iron preparations may cause the formation of black-colored stool. See Table 74 for information on various types of iron preparations available and Table 75 for answers to questions commonly asked about taking iron.

Table 75   QUESTIONS COMMONLY ASKED ABOUT TAKING IRON

Question	Yes	No	Comment
Do iron tablets usually require a prescription?		X	Almost never necessary.
Can iron overdose occur?	X		One of the more common fatal accidental poisonings in children.
Can iron interfere with absorption of tetracycline?	X		Avoid taking these products within two hours of each other.
Can I get enough iron during pregnancy by eating a well-balanced diet?		X	Iron is needed during pregnancy to double the amount of blood in your body and for the fetus. The amount of iron absorbed from food is limited.
Is iron deficiency the commonest cause of anemia in women, both pregnant and nonpregnant?	X		
Is one form of iron less likely to cause stomach irritation than another?		X	Stomach irritation is related to the total amount of iron rather than the specific type of iron taken.
Should iron be taken between meals to allow maximum absorption?	X		However, it may be taken just after meals if stomach irritation occurs.

Planning for Good Nutrition

The four basic food groups

A report from the Food and Nutrition Board of the National Academy of Sciences in May, 1980, noted that eating a variety of foods is still the most important way to maintain good nutrition. Table 76 shows the recommended daily consumption from the four basic food groups for both pregnant and

---

Table 76   RECOMMENDED DAILY CONSUMPTION FROM THE FOUR BASIC FOOD GROUPS FOR PREGNANT AND NONPREGNANT WOMEN*

Note: Foods listed are meant only as examples for each group. Many more foods, of course, are available in each group.

I.   The Milk and Dairy Group supplies calcium, high-quality protein, riboflavin (a B vitamin), and vitamins A and D.
    Pregnant: 6 servings   Nonpregnant: 4 or more servings

Food	Amount	Calories	Food	Amount	Calories
Whole milk	1 cup	160	Ice milk	1 cup	285
Buttermilk	1 cup	90	Dry milk powder	¼ cup	63
Skim milk	1 cup	90	(nonfat instant)		
Cheddar cheese	1 oz.	105	Creamed cottage cheese	1 cup	240
Ice cream	1⅔ cup	492			

II.   The Meat and Egg Group provides protein, iron, and some B vitamins.
    Pregnant: 3 servings   Nonpregnant: 2 or more servings

Food	Amount	Calories	Food	Amount	Calories
Lean ground beef (broiled)	3 oz.	245	Peanut butter	4 tbsp.	380
			Dried beans (red)	1 cup	230
Chicken (broiled)	3 oz.	115	Egg (scrambled with milk and fat)	1	110
Lamb (baked)	3 oz.	211			
Liver (fried)	3 oz.	195	Fish (broiled)	3 oz.	135

III.   The Fruit and Vegetables Group supplies roughage, carbohydrates, vitamins (especially A and C), and minerals.
    Pregnant: 4 to 5 servings   Nonpregnant: 4 servings

Food	Amount	Calories	Food	Amount	Calories
Potato (baked)	1 med.	90	Apple (raw)	1	70
Broccoli	1 cup	40	Banana (raw)	1	85
Coleslaw	1 cup	120	Orange (raw)	1	60
Peas	1 cup	115	Orange juice	1 cup	110

IV.   The Bread and Cereal Group provides carbohydrates, B vitamins, and iron and other minerals.
    Pregnant: 4 to 5 servings   Nonpregnant: 4 servings

Food	Amount	Calories	Food	Amount	Calories
White bread	1 slice	65	Rye bread	1 slice	55
Whole wheat bread	1 slice	56	Spaghetti (cooked)	½ cup	78
Muffin (plain)	1 average	118	Oatmeal (cooked)	½ cup	65
Macaroni (cooked)	½ cup	85	Corn flakes	1 oz.	110
Rice (cooked)	½ cup	93	Granola cereal	½ cup	195

---

* Modified from patient education booklet, Women's Hospital, Tampa, Florida.

nonpregnant women. Together the four groups contain the essential nutrients needed by the human body every day. In order to evaluate your diet, write down everything, including snacks, that you ate during the past two or three days. How many daily servings from each group did you receive? Analysis of your daily menu should show you what kinds of nutrients your diet is both providing and lacking.

Optimum weight and energy balance

Your weight and energy balance are determined by three factors: the rate of your metabolism, the number of calories you eat, and the amount of exercise you get. The reasons for individual tendencies to gain weight are not always known. Individual variation with respect to metabolism is largely inherited so that some women never seem to have weight problems regardless of diet. Metabolism normally declines approximately 15% between the ages of twenty-five and seventy, representing a drop in calorie needs of about 1% every three years during this period. Metabolism is higher for males than for females at almost all ages. Obesity tends to start affecting women in their thirties whereas men are less likely to be affected until they reach their forties. During these times, a declining metabolic rate is likely to be paralleled by a decrease in activity. If the slowdown in metabolism and activity level in middle age is not accompanied by a decrease in calorie intake, weight gain occurs.

Obesity or excessive overweight is the number one nutrition problem in the United States today. Excessive weight gain is not good for your health because it places an additional strain on your heart and may contribute to certain diseases such as high blood pressure, gallstones, and diabetes. The risk of uterine, breast, gallbladder, kidney, stomach, and colon cancer is also increased. Insurance statistics show that the lowest mortality rates among women are associated with a weight of 15 to 20% below ideal weight for height. Chapter 87 on weight gain and weight loss provides information about weight-loss dieting as well as on losing and keeping off extra pounds. Table 104 (in Chapter 87) shows suggested weights for heights.

Food labeling

The U.S. Recommended Daily Allowances (RDAs) are the amounts of basic nutrients established by the Food and Nutrition Board of the National Research Council to meet the recognized needs of "practically all healthy people." These allowances are revised about every five years to reflect current research findings in nutritional science. U.S. RDAs are now used widely in nutrition labeling to indicate the percentage of RDA provided in each nutrient category of a given food. However, the nutrition label is legally required only if a manufacturer adds ingredients or advertises nutritional claims, such as on the label (for example, fortified or enriched foods). The number of servings in a container, the size of the serving, the number of calories per serving, and the amount of fat, protein, and carbohydrates per serving as well as the U.S. RDA per serving of protein, calcium, iron, and certain vitamins and minerals are included. The listing of other vitamins and minerals is optional.

Food additives

A food additive is any material other than the basic raw ingredients necessary for the production of a specific food. Additives are commonly used in most processed foods. Most additives are used for flavor, preservation of food, or color. Vitamin and mineral additives are used to enrich foods such as cereals, flour, and milk. Food additives are regulated by the FDA, which classifies them into two groups—newer additives and older ones which form the Generally Recognized As Safe list (GRAS). Sometimes older additives are reclassified by the FDA as possibly unsafe, as happened with saccharin. Ironically, saccharin was developed to avoid the presumed health risks of what is perhaps the most widely used additive—sugar. Although saccharin has not been found to cause cancer in humans, it has been linked to cancer in animals when very large doses were given. The risk of years of saccharin use in humans remains unclear.

Food additives may be a source of excess dietary salt. It is the sodium in salt that we need to be concerned with. Labeling on packages gives us the sodium content of the product, measured usually in mg (milligrams); 1000 mg is equal to 1 gram. Relatively large amounts of sodium are added as a preservative in most processed foods such as luncheon meats. More than sufficient sodium is obtained in the average American diet without adding salt at the table. The amount of sodium needed for healthy adults is 1 to 3 grams per day; the amount for you should depend on your physical activity and the amount of water you lose daily. Remember that the amount of sodium you consume will come from your total intake for the day, including those amounts "hidden" in foods (and some antacids) and not just what comes out of your salt shaker. The Dietary Goals for the United States recommends limiting total sodium consumption to 5 grams daily. A salt-restricted diet has one gram of sodium or less daily. It has been estimated that the average American consumes much more salt than is needed for good nutrition. A heavy salt intake may be a health risk for some women, especially those with a personal or family history of heart disease or high blood pressure. Even in normal individuals, excess dietary salt is suspected of playing a contributing role in the development of these conditions. (See the reference list at the end of this section.)

Food snacks

Eating habits of Americans have changed enormously during the last twenty years. More meals are eaten on the run and often consist of so-called fast foods. Overall, the nutritional value of meals provided by fast-food chains is short on essential vitamins and minerals, and these meals give you far more fats, salts, and sugar than you would get if you selected from the four basic food groups in the right proportions. Even if you "have it your way," it is almost impossible to get sufficient fruits and vegetables at the hamburger, chicken, fish, and pizza fast-food chains. Snacking is one of the features of the American eating habits which plays a significant role—often detrimental—in the determination of the quality of our diet. Even less nutritious than fast-food meals are snacks consisting of sugar-laden "junk foods," such as candy, pastries, and soda pop. On the other hand, snacks from the four basic food groups are ideal. Examples are:

Breads and cereals:	cheese wafers, graham crackers, sandwiches (use enriched or whole-grain bread)
Fruit and vegetables:	juices, dried fruits, fresh fruit and vegetables
Meat:	tacos, bean sandwiches, boiled eggs, meatballs, pizzas (with meat), peanut butter, nuts

Milk:	cheese, ice cream, yogurt, milkshakes, pudding, milk-containing dips, cottage cheese

Nutrition in the Later Years

As women get older, they need the same essential nutrients from the four basic food groups but fewer calories, as a result of decreasing metabolism and lessened physical exercise. In recent years, certain specific nutritional needs of older women have become recognized. Dietary surveys have revealed that women, starting in their forties and fifties, often have deficiencies in calcium and ascorbic acid related to inadequate consumption of milk, fruit, and vegetables. Older women may benefit from increased amounts of dietary fiber. Fiber, which forms much of the undigested roughage in food, helps to prevent certain intestinal problems that increase with age, including diverticulitis and constipation.

Osteoporosis (see Chapters 27 and 49) is a debilitating illness affecting women in middle and older age and accounts for approximately five million fractures in women each year. Among the factors making a woman more susceptible to bone loss and, therefore, osteoporosis are the nutritional stresses of childbearing accompanied by inadequate dietary calcium and sedentary life styles in later years. While the average nonpregnant woman needs at least 1000 milligrams of calcium daily before menopause and 1200 milligrams to 1500 milligrams a day after menopause, it is estimated that most American women over the age of fifty consume barely half this amount in their diets. Older women are likely to decrease their consumption of calcium-rich dairy products when going on weight-loss diets or because of digestive intolerance to dairy products (such intolerance may cause diarrhea or cramping) that sometimes occurs with age. Another factor opposing adequate calcium utilization is the high content of phosphorus in the American diet. This mineral competes with calcium for absorption, with the result that the more phosphorus-rich foods you eat (such as meat, carbonated beverages, and processed foods), the less calcium is absorbed. To acquire the recommended daily 800 to 1000 mg of calcium from her diet, an adult woman should consume a quart (four 8-oz. glasses) of milk each day, or the amount of other dairy products that will yield an equivalent amount of calcium. Vitamin D helps increase calcium absorption. However, supplementation with this vitamin is probably unnecessary if you drink vitamin-D-enriched milk or take a calcium supplement, such as calcium carbonate, available at most drugstores.

It is difficult to define the exact requirements of the essential nutrients for one's later years. Following the adult requirements (U.S. RDA) is probably adequate. The greatest protection lies in consuming a wide variety of foods with as little processing as possible. Chronic conditions may require a special diet—for example, salt restriction with high blood pressure or heart disease. Be certain to find out from your clinician if any medications you are taking will affect your nutritional needs.

Nutrition in Pregnancy and Breast-feeding

Adequate fetal growth and development depends upon a constant supply of nutrients from the mother. Inadequate nutrition, in fact, is considered a major risk factor in pregnancy and can lead to fetal malnutrition and low birth weight babies, which have more than their share of difficulties after birth. (See also Chapter 87 on weight gain and weight loss.)

During pregnancy, your diet should consist of a variety of foods selected from the four basic food groups shown in Table 76. Emphasize fresh fruits, vegetables, meat, and milk. Eat as few canned and processed foods as possible. The effects on the fetus of food additives such as monosodium glutamate (MSG) and nitrates are unknown.

The recommended vitamin requirements for pregnant and breast-feeding women are given in Table 70. Fresh fruits, vegetables, and whole grain products provide a dietary source for these vitamins although prenatal vitamins are often prescribed routinely, as noted earlier in this chapter.

The recommended daily amount of calcium during pregnancy and breast-feeding increases significantly from 800 to 1200 mg (an increase of approximately two 8-oz. glasses of milk). Eggs and fortified milk are nutritious sources of calcium and protein as well as vitamins A and D for pregnant and breast-feeding women. If you dislike drinking milk, try getting some of your calcium in creamed foods, yogurt, puddings, or cheese or ask your doctor for a calcium supplement.

Salt does not have to be restricted in pregnancy in healthy women. Research in recent years has shown that salt intake has little or no relationship to the development of toxemia (see Chapter 20).

When you are breast-feeding, you need to eat slightly more of most nutrients than you did during your pregnancy, especially as your baby grows. This is because your body requires more energy to produce the milk, and the milk itself requires substantial calories. In order to produce about one quart of milk per day when breast-feeding, you need to consume about 900 extra calories daily. This is not the time to start a weight-loss diet. There are no nourishing foods that need to be eliminated from your diet. Chocolate sometimes has been found to have a laxative effect on some babies; and broccoli, Brussels sprouts, cabbage, dried beans, and cauliflower sometimes create gas. Spicy foods may flavor the milk or cause gas pains in your baby. Moderation is a helpful rule, as most foods eaten by a breast-feeding mother in small amounts are well-tolerated by newborns.

If you don't breast-feed and you want to lose weight, you can begin a weight-loss diet at once after your baby is born. You may, however, want to wait several weeks before beginning any strenuous diet to lose weight because the process of childbirth is stressful and nutritionally demanding as are the first weeks at home. Refer to Chapter 87, on weight gain and weight loss, for healthy approaches to dieting and for a suggested diet plan to lose weight.

Resources

For more information on nutrition write to:

Community Nutrition Institute
1146 Nineteenth Street, N.W.
Washington, D.C. 20036

The American Dietetic Association
430 North Michigan Avenue
Chicago, Illinois 60611

Department of Foods and Nutrition
American Medical Association
535 North Dearborn Street
Chicago, Illinois 60610

Physical Fitness

Long ago in our society the physical demands of daily living were far greater than they are today. People then didn't have to be concerned with "creating" physical exercise to keep fit. Today, however, our jobs and daily lives, for most of us, place very few physical demands on us. As a result we must actively look for ways to keep in good physical condition.

Since the early 1960s, when President Kennedy recognized and promoted the need for increased physical fitness, Americans have shown a steadily increasing interest in maintaining good health through various forms of physical exercise. Women have become more and more involved in sports and fitness programs. With more women working than ever before and becoming, in some cases, the sole support of the family unit, women have come to realize that to get daily physical exercise, they have to plan for it.

How do you know what kind of physical shape you are in? You may notice the extra exertion required when an unexpected activity, such as running to catch a bus, leaves you feeling completely winded; or you may feel chronically tired and irritable after a day's work, with little energy left to enjoy your free time. *Hypokinesis* is the term used by physicians to indicate body deterioration or lack of proper physical fitness, which may be the cause of the symptoms just described.

When you decide that you do want to become more physically fit, where do you begin? Before you embark on any new physical exercise program, it is wise to have a physical examination and an EKG (electrocardiogram) to check for possible heart abnormalities. Most experts feel that if you are over the age of thirty-five, you should have a cardiovascular *stress test* (see glossary) before beginning a vigorous exercise program. If you have a family history of premature heart disease (that is, before age fifty) or are severely overweight, you should have a stress test, regardless of your age.

Physical Fitness and You

Physical fitness is often assessed by measuring heart rate after exercise. Fitness can also be measured in terms of muscular endurance or the strength of specific muscles required to perform a task such as lifting weights. Muscular flexibility is also a measure of fitness and refers to the range of motion of a particular joint. An example of this is how close you can come to touching your toes.

Your goal for physical fitness should be personal and should relate to your own needs (see Table 77). People may exercise for relaxation, to increase their muscular flexibility or strength, to improve their heart-lung functioning (see Aerobic Exercise below), to increase motor skills, to alter their body shape (lose inches), or for weight control or weight loss (see Table 78). People may do the same exercises for different reasons, as in adult ballet classes, where the goal may be to strengthen certain muscles, improve flexibility, or develop specific motor skills.

When you decide to begin a program of exercise, you should:

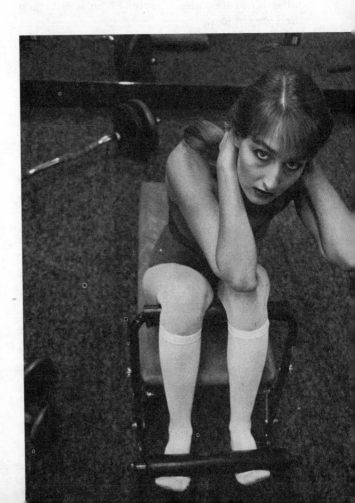

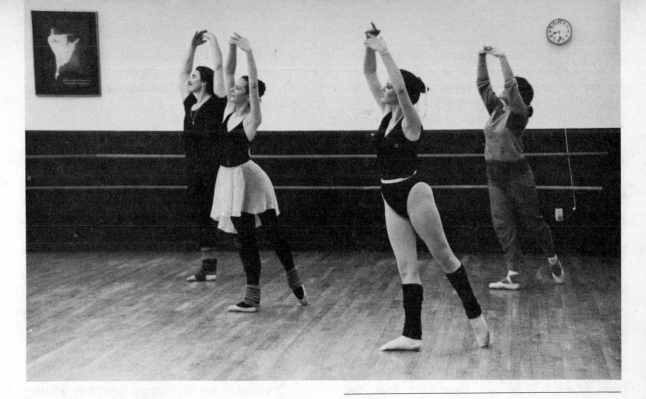

1. Be certain that your exercise plan will not aggravate any chronic physical condition you may have, such as arthritis. Check with your doctor first.
2. Pick an exercise that uses skills different from those you may use at work.
3. Consider choosing an activity you already enjoy or would like to try.
4. Begin exercising gradually and work up slowly to your desired level of fitness.
5. Use equipment that is the right size or weight for your level of skills and physical size.
6. Begin each exercise time with a gradual warm-up period (at least five minutes) and end your exercise with a cool-down period, gradually bringing your body back to rest.
7. Be certain to get enough daily rest.
8. Use common sense in your exercise program. Pay attention to your own body's signals when they tell you to slow down.
9. Never exercise after a heavy meal or after drinking alcohol. If you feel sick or dizzy, stop immediately.

After exercise, prevent dehydration by drinking water, orange juice, or perhaps one of the commercially available liquids, like Gatorade, which replace salt and other minerals lost in sweat.

If you live in a warm climate and you exercise outdoors, to avoid the possibility of heatstroke, exercise in the early morning or late evening when

Table 77   GOALS OF EXERCISING

Goal of Exercise	Exercise Program
improved motor skill	an exercise related to desired skill, e.g., backboard practice for tennis, pitching for softball, etc.
increased muscular strength	softball, weight lifting, tennis, karate, Royal Canadian Air Force Exercise Plan
increased muscular flexibility (range of motion in a joint)	stretching movements, such as those done in ballet, gymnastics, yoga, sailing, tennis
increased endurance	any aerobic exercise program, i.e., jogging, cycling, walking briskly, certain kinds of dancing, swimming, skiing
changed shape (lose inches)	gymnastics, modern dance, specific exercise program
weight control or weight loss	any exercise if done in combination with a reduction in calories (weight-loss diet) to lose weight
increased relaxation	isometric exercises, yoga, walking, bicycling, running, horseback riding; any exercise that can be done comfortably without great mental concern about a specific skill

it is cooler. When the humidity is high (over 80%), exercise cautiously or not at all as moisture in the air tends to slow sweat evaporation and puts an extra strain on the heart.

If you live in a cold climate and you exercise outdoors in the winter, take sensible safeguards: Cool down very gradually after you have worked up a sweat. Protect yourself against frostbite. If the air is very cold, you may want to put a loose-knit scarf over your mouth to help warm up the air you are breathing in. Or you may try to arrange to use a local school gym during off hours—say, in the early morning or evening hours.

Aerobic Exercise

Aerobic exercise refers to forms of exercise which are designed to strengthen your heart and lungs. Examples of aerobic exercises are jogging, swimming, cycling, and running. With proper conditioning aerobic exercises allow your heart and lungs to utilize oxygen more efficiently; in other words, for a given activity, your heart is able to deliver oxygen through your blood to your body doing less work, as evidenced by a lowered pulse rate. The concept of aerobic exercise was developed by Dr. Kenneth H. Cooper. A useful book, *Aerobics for Women*, by M. Cooper and K. Cooper, fully explains aerobic exercise programs for all age groups of women.

Women and Sports

Active participation by increasing numbers of women in many types of athletic competition is a relatively recent trend. Women have been encouraged to enter sporting activities by Title IX of the Federal Educational Assistance Act of 1972, which legalized equal Federal financial support for school programming of male and female sports. Sports opportunities for girls and women of all ages are blossoming, particularly in elementary and secondary schools. These new opportunities should enable a young girl to develop the kind of preconditioning necessary for participation in skilled athletics as an adult.

One area of special concern to women athletes is the effect of exercise on the menstrual cycle. It is now known that some women, especially professional athletes, develop menstrual irregularities or stop menstruating for several months or more after engaging in a program of strenuous exercise.

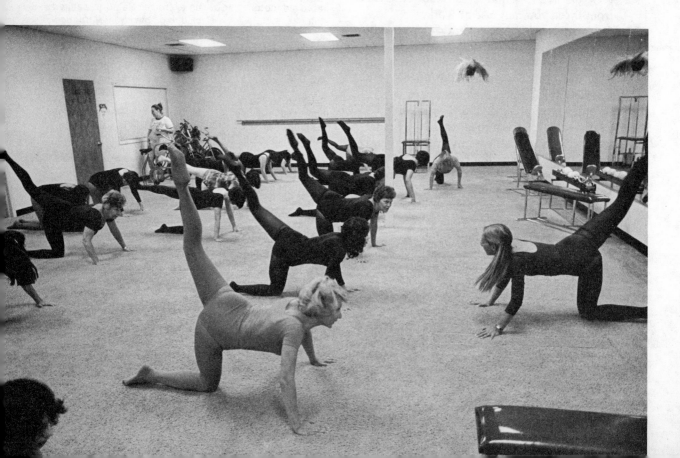

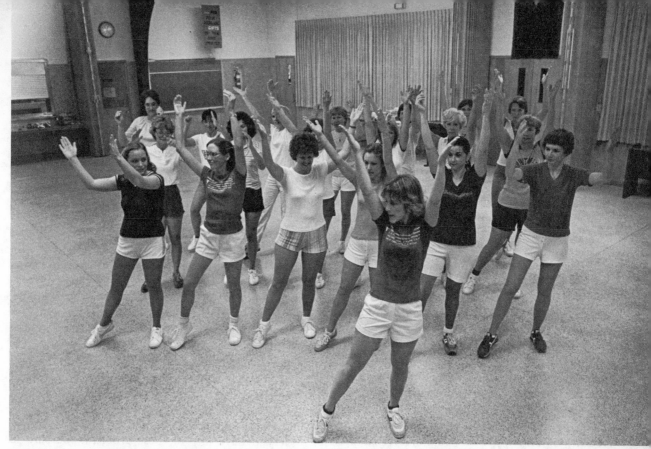

The reason for this is not clear. Possibly the stress involved—both physical and emotional—leads to hormone changes that disrupt normal menstrual cycles. When the woman stops or decreases the amount of exercise, her periods usually return to normal.

Sports are not only fun to take part in, they can also be an excellent part of a weight-control or weight-loss program. Table 78 will give you an idea of the number of calories you use up when you participate in certain sports activities.

Exercise During and After Pregnancy

Doctors now agree that certain forms of exercise are not only safe for pregnant women but highly recommended as well. Exercise helps prepare a woman's body for labor and delivery. If you experience pain or spotting when exercising, these are signals for you to stop. Unless you have a high-risk condition, most physicians don't restrict you from continuing, with some exceptions, exercises that you did prior to pregnancy as long as the exercises do not cause fatigue or discomfort. These exceptions might include the following: contact sports, such as basketball, where a severe blow to the abdomen could occur, and water skiing in

Table 78 **CALORIE EXPENDITURE FOR SOME COMMON SPORTS ACTIVITIES**

Activity	Estimated No. of Calories Used Up per Hour*
Bicycling (5.5 mph)	190 – 265
Bowling	225 – 335
Golf (foursome)	240 – 350
Gymnastics	200 – 270
Racquetball	620 – 850
Roller-skating	275 – 350
Running	400 – 550
Skiing	460 – 558
Swimming	400 – 550
Tennis	330 – 440
Walking or hiking	230 – 335

* Range is based on body weight of 110 lbs. to 150 lbs. The exact amount of calories you burn up per hour depends on how much you weigh (the more you weigh, the more calories you burn up per hour of exercise) and on how hard you work at your exercise. Going up a hill when you are bicycling, walking, or running, or carrying a backpack when you are hiking, will increase caloric expenditure.

which water could be forced into the vagina during a fall. These sports may be somewhat risky for the pregnant woman especially as pregnancy progresses beyond the first three months. Scuba diving also is not advisable because the effects of pressure changes on the developing fetus are unknown. If you are or could be pregnant, most physicians recommend limiting your diving to 33 feet. Helpful exercises for pregnancy and postpartum are listed in *Essential Exercises for the Childbearing Year*, written by a physical therapist, Elizabeth Noble, and published by Houghton Mifflin.

Preferably your fitness program will have started before you became pregnant. Pregnancy isn't the best time to take up a new exercise or sport, but you can get involved in something like taking walks, swimming, or doing certain floor exercises (stretching, bending, etc.). Swimming is a popular and very appropriate exercise during pregnancy, because this activity uses most muscles and your body is supported by water, which helps you to be more comfortable.

After you have your baby and your weight returns to normal, you may find that certain parts of your body appear heavier. This is due to stretching of tissues and sometimes increased fat deposits that accumulate in pregnancy. After your six-weeks checkup, set aside a regular time to exercise, and do exercises that tone your thighs, stomach, waist, and hips. There are no contraindications to exercise while you are breast-feeding, as long as you drink lots of fluids to remain well hydrated. Your general body conditioning and how you are feeling will determine how soon you can participate in active sports. Use your common sense and discuss exercise plans with your clinician.

Exercise and Certain Medical Problems

Exercise, in general, does much to improve your whole body functioning and, in particular, depending on the kind of exercise you do, improves your heart and lung functioning (that is, the oxygen and blood supply to all your tissues), increases your muscle tone and muscle strength, and decreases your body fat deposits. Because of these and other benefits, exercise can have a direct beneficial effect on many specific conditions and symptoms, among them the following: urinary stress incontinence, diabetes, insomnia, anxiety, nervousness, mild depression, some lung conditions, and some heart and blood vessel problems. If you have any of these problems, be sure to check first with your physician as to the appropriate beneficial exercises for you before you begin a vigorous exercise program.

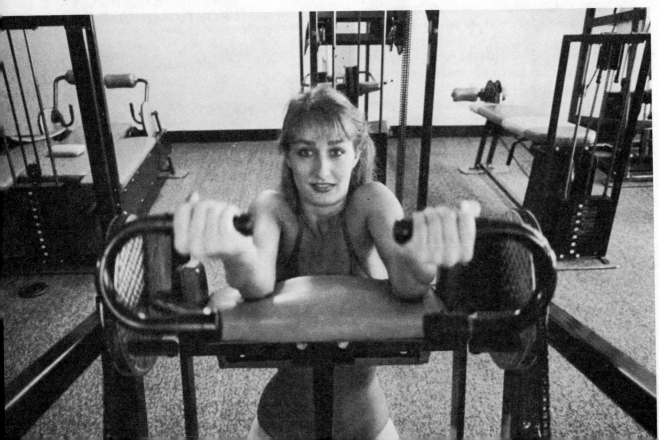

Resources

American Alliance for Health, Physical Education, Recreation and Dance
1900 Association Drive
Reston, Virginia 22070

Community recreation centers
Senior citizen centers

References for Section Ten

Chapter 45—Staying Healthy

Rosch, P. J. Effects of stress on women. *The Female Patient* 9(1):14–32, Jan 1984.

Ibrahim, M. A. The changing health state of women. *American Journal of Public Health* 70(2):120–121, Feb 1980.

Rice, D., and Cugliani, A. Health status of American women. *Women & Health* 5(1):5–22, spring 1980.

Martin, L. L. *Health Care of Women*. Philadelphia: J. B. Lippincott Co., 1978.

Suomi, J. D. Methods for the prevention of periodontal diseases. *Family and Community Health* 3(3):41–49, Nov 1980.

Schatzin, A. How long can we live? A more optimistic view of potential gains in life expectancy. *American Journal of Public Health* 70(11):1199–1200, 1980.

Iveson-Iveson, J. The general picture and diet. *Nursing-Mirror* p. 27, Sep 13, 1979.

Smoking and Health: A Report of the Surgeon General. DHEW Pub. No. (PHS) 79–50066, Government Printing Office, Washington, D.C., 1979.

Chapter 46—Nutrition

Williams, S. R. *Basic Nutrition and Diet Therapy*, 6th ed. St. Louis: C. V. Mosby Co., 1980.

Grundy, S. M., et al. Rationale of the diet-heart statement of the American Heart Association, Circulation 65, No. 4, 1982, American Heart Association, 7320 Greenville Avenue, Dallas, Texas.

Willard, M. D. *Nutrition for the Practicing Physician*. Menlo Park, Calif.: Addison-Wesley, 1982.

Weg, R. B. *Nutrition and the Later Years*. Los Angeles: Southern Calif. Press, 1978.

Beal, V. A. *Nutrition in the Life Span*. New York: John Wiley and Sons, 1980.

Recommended Dietary Allowances, Revised, 1980. Food and Nutritional Board, National Academy of Sciences – National Research Council, Washington, D.C.

Worthington-Roberts, B., and Taylor, L. *Nutrition During Pregnancy and Breast Feeding*. Chicago: Budlong Press Co., 1981.

Yen, P. What can you learn from labels? *Geriatric Nursing* 1:138–141, July, Aug 1980.

Hansen, R. Planning for the inevitable: snack foods in the diet. *Family and Community Health* 1:31–39, Feb 1979.

The Healthy Approach to Slimming (pamphlet). Monroe, WI: American Medical Association, 1978.

Appel, J., and King, J. Energy needs during pregnancy and lactation. *Family and Community Health* 1:7–18, Feb 1979.

Price, J. H., and Pritts, C. Overweight and obesity in the elderly. *Journal of Gerontological Nursing* 6(6):341–346, June 1980.

Dietary Goals for the United States, Second Ed. Report of U.S. Senate Select Committee on Nutrition and Human Needs, U.S. Government Printing Office, Dec 1977.

Heyn, D. The nutrition free-for-all. *Family Health* p. 24+, Jan 1981.

Harper, A. E. Meeting recommended dietary allowances. *Journal of the Florida Medical Association* 66(4):419–424, April 1979.

Harper, A. E. Vitamins and megavitamins: fact and fancy. *Urban Health* 22–26, Jul/Aug 1979.

Harper, A. E. Recommended dietary allowances - 1980. *Nutrition Reviews* 38(8):290–294, Aug 1980.

Albanese, A. A. Calcium nutrition in the elderly. *Postgraduate Medicine* 63(3):167–172, Mar 1978.

Chapter 47—Physical Fitness

Harris, R., and Frankel, L. (eds.) *Guide to Fitness After Fifty*. New York: Plenum Press, 1977.

Mirkin, G., and Hoffman, M. *The Sportsmedicine Book*. Boston: Little, Brown, 1978.

Wilmore, J. H. Medical aspects of exercise. *The Female Patient* 5(10):23–28, 1980.

Shangold, M. M. Do women's sports lead to menstrual problems? *Contemporary OB/GYN* 17(3):52–62, 1981.

Cooper, K. *The New Aerobics*. New York: Bantam Books, 1970.

Cooper, M., and Cooper, K. *Aerobics for Women*. New York: Bantam Books, 1972.

Hanson, D. *Health Related Fitness*. Belmont, Calif.: Wadsworth Publishing Co., 1970.

Hale, R. Women and sports: keeping up with female athletes' needs. *Contemporary OB/GYN* 13:85–95, Apr 1979.

eleven

What Your Symptoms Mean

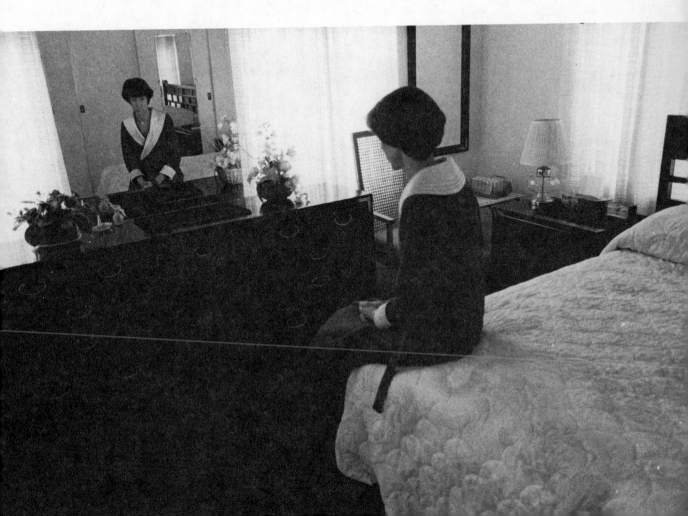

How To Use This Section

This section is about common symptoms—what they mean, what medical care can do, and what you can do to help yourself. Whether you see a general practitioner, a nurse practitioner, a family doctor, an internist, or a gynecologist, there are about one hundred symptoms or areas of concern that women commonly give as the reasons for visiting their clinicians. These problems are listed alphabetically below, along with a reference to the appropriate chapter or chapters in this section where each problem is discussed. Some symptoms, such as irregular menstrual periods and vaginal discharge, are directly related to conditions affecting the female reproductive system. We have included other symptoms (backaches, joint pains) because they bring about high disability in women.

Certain chapters in this section deal with conditions (hypertension, migraine headaches) affecting women more frequently than men.

Each chapter begins with basic information about a particular symptom and what the symptom can mean, as well as how pregnancy may be involved. Under the heading *What Medical Care Can Do*, the usual methods of diagnosis and treatment are explained. Finally, under *What You Can Do (Self Care)*, we suggest ways you can handle the problem yourself and suggest when you should seek medical care. Flow charts are provided in each chapter with references to appropriate chapters to help you decide when medical care or self-treatment is needed.

Health Concerns

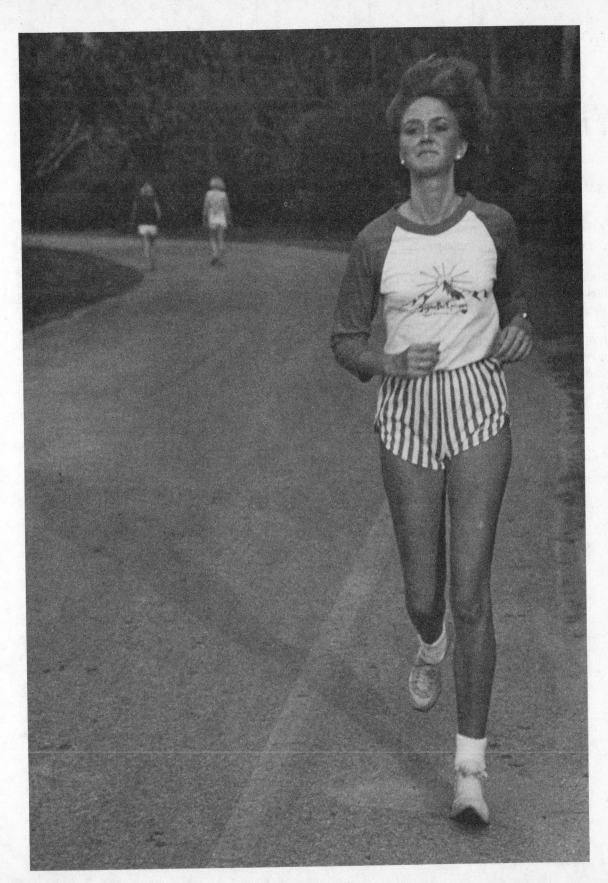

48

Acne

Acne, the most common skin problem in women, is a disorder of the hair follicle and oil (sebaceous) glands. It first occurs during puberty and affects about 75% of adolescent women. Certain hereditary predispositions to acne account for the persistence of this condition over many years in some women. Normally secretions from skin glands travel up the hair follicle to the surface. In acne, the hair follicle is blocked, resulting in a build-up of oil and bacteria which ultimately ruptures into the skin. Secondary infections from the skin bacteria then occur, causing pimples and other skin changes characteristic of acne. Pimples and blackheads are the most common finding in acne and may cause cosmetic problems when scarring occurs.

Acne is predominantly a response of the skin gland to androgens, weak male hormones produced in small amounts by the ovaries and adrenal glands in women. During puberty, there is a temporary hormone imbalance favoring a slight increase in the ratio of androgens to estrogens. Psychological factors may also affect the course of acne. In times of stress, our bodies release additional androgens. Among the factors that do not contribute to acne are failure to wash properly, sexual activity, and diets high in sweets.

Acne may be affected by different factors during the woman's life cycle. Some women characteristically have an increase in acne the week prior to menses. Some women who do not ovulate regularly and have irregular, infrequent periods have a disproportionate amount of acne as a result of the increased androgen production in their ovaries. Estrogens, such as found in birth control pills, sometimes alleviate acne by diminishing skin

ACNE

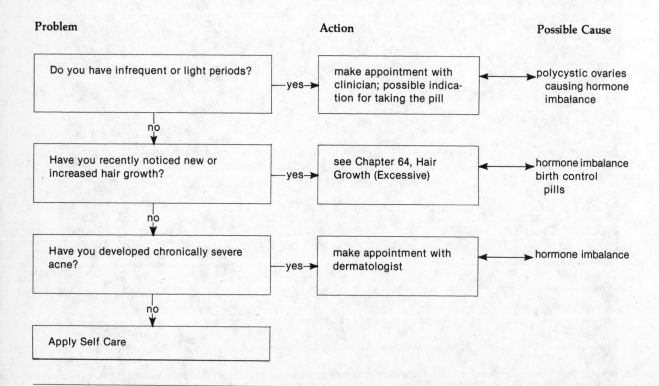

Problem

Do you have infrequent or light periods? —yes→

↓ no

Have you recently noticed new or increased hair growth? —yes→

↓ no

Have you developed chronically severe acne? —yes→

↓ no

Apply Self Care

Action

make appointment with clinician; possible indication for taking the pill

see Chapter 64, Hair Growth (Excessive)

make appointment with dermatologist

Possible Cause

polycystic ovaries causing hormone imbalance

hormone imbalance birth control pills

hormone imbalance

sensitivity to androgens. Withdrawal of birth control pills (oral contraceptives), known popularly as the pill, may produce a worsening of acne in some women.

Frequently in some women the skin improves during pregnancy as a result of the effects of high levels of estrogen. In other women, however, acne becomes worse in pregnancy for reasons not understood.

What Medical Care Can Do

In the nonpregnant woman, retinoic acid, benzoyl peroxide, and tetracycline antibiotics are the most effective prescription medicines used to treat moderately severe acne. Retinoic acid (Retin-A Cream) produces rapid cell turnover in the skin glands and should be used sparingly to determine the extent to which skin drying and peeling will occur. Retinoic acid, a potent derivative of vitamin A, may produce side effects of vitamin A overdose including cracked lips, dry skin, and headache. Vitamin A by itself, however, has no proven beneficial effect in the treatment of acne. Topical preparations (that is, preparations to be applied locally) containing benzoyl peroxide (Desquam, PanOxyl, Persa Gel, etc.) are peeling agents like Retin-A but also have antibiotic activity. Overexposure to sun, wind, and cold should be avoided when you use these preparations, because your skin is more sensitive.

When used to treat acne, tetracycline is taken twice a day for about six weeks. As improvement occurs, tetracycline is reduced to a daily dose and ultimately the drug is discontinued. When tetracycline therapy is ineffective, topical antibiotics may be tried but their use remains controversial.

For the woman who uses oral contraceptives as a birth control method or for some other valid medical reason, the pill may also be used for the treatment of acne. Because of the risks involved, however, the pill should not be used exclusively for the purpose of treating acne. An individual's skin response to taking birth control pills is highly variable and improvement may take as long as six months. Certain pills, such as Ovral, LoOvral, Norlestrin, and Loestrin, tend to increase acne although the acne condition may get better on its own after two or three months of pill use. There is no way to predict how a woman who has had severe acne as an adolescent will react to pregnancy or to taking the pill.

What You Can Do (Self Care)

Exposure to sunlight in small doses is sometimes helpful. Avoid oils, greasy cleansing creams, and other cosmetics. If you use makeup, be certain to wash your hands before applying it. Keep your makeup stored in the refrigerator to limit bacterial growth. Discard old makeup and buy new makeup frequently; unused portions of eye makeup should be discarded after three to four months' use. Don't use anyone else's makeup, only your own. Use an ordinary mild soap, such as Ivory, to keep your skin clean. Neutrogena acne soap may be helpful in preventing secondary bacterial infections. A number of over-the-counter products containing sulfur alone or in combination with resorcinol or salicylic acid (Fostex cream, Rezamid lotion) have proven helpful, but individual response to these products varies. X-ray treatments for acne are dangerous because they may lead to cancer. Remember that any chronic condition including anemia and poor nutrition may make acne worse. Eat plenty of fresh fruits and vegetables. Avoid a high-fat diet and such foods as chocolate and peanuts. To prevent disfigurement in severe cases, see a dermatologist promptly.

49

Backache

As many as 25% of women having a routine checkup by their gynecologist complain of backache. Low backache is the most common form of back pain in women; it has numerous causes, most of which are not serious. Some women experience back discomfort every month during menses. This pain is not usually a sign of disease since the uterus normally "refers" pain, or sends pain signals, to the back just as a toothache pain may be referred to the jaw. A popular misconception is that women with a "tilted" uterus are backache prone; pain occurs in this case only if the uterus is held back in this position as a result of disease such as endometriosis. Endometriosis produces severe low abdominal or back pain usually a day or two before as well as during menses. Certain conditions—uterine tumors such as fibroids, ovarian cysts, and pelvic infections of the tube or cervix—may cause low back discomfort at any time during the menstrual cycle. Table 79 tells you what symptoms are also present along with backache with certain conditions. Cancer of the pelvic organs almost never presents itself as backache alone. The backache of kidney infections is felt in the upper back toward the right or left side rather than in the low back and is usually associated with painful or bloody urination.

The terms *back strain* or *lumbosacral strain* usually refer to muscle spasm associated with trauma to the spinal column from your lifting objects that are too heavy or from a sudden spine-twisting turn. Even a bad mattress or poor posture can cause muscle spasms. Whatever the cause, the result is low back pain that is disabling. A much more serious problem that may result from straining your spine is a so-called slipped disc. In this painful condition, adjacent bones in the spine collapse upon each other as a result of rupture of the disc between them. This condition often irritates the spinal nerves, sending shooting pains down the backs of your legs.

Table 79 SYMPTOMS FOUND IN CERTAIN CONDITIONS THAT CAUSE BACKACHE

Condition Causing Backache	Associated Symptom(s)
Tube infection	Low abdominal pain, vaginal discharge, sometimes fever
Ovarian cyst	Low abdominal pain on one side
Endometriosis	Low abdominal pain occurring during and just before period
Cervical infection (cervicitis)	Chronic vaginal discharge
Uterine fibroid	Heavy or irregular menstrual bleeding
Kidney infection	Fever, painful urination, bloody urine

Older women are especially prone to two diseases of the spine: arthritis and osteoporosis. Osteoporosis affects about 30% of women over sixty years of age and is three to five times more common among women than men. This disease is characterized by gradual loss of bone from the spinal column, particularly after menopause, resulting in pain, a loss of height, and susceptibility to fractures. The condition of lower levels of estrogen following menopause has been suggested as a cause of osteoporosis (see Chapter 27). Arthritis of the spine is usually associated with chronic pain or stiffness in other joints, as well as in the spine.

Whatever the cause of backache, the role of stress must be evaluated. Most women have some minor back discomfort at one time or another for which no specific cause is found except tension. People under chronic stress tend to hold their muscles in an increased state of contraction, thereby contributing to back discomfort.

Most pregnant women suffer from at least minor degrees of back discomfort. This discomfort occurs predominantly in the second half of pregnancy as the enlarging uterus places more strain on the back muscles. Occasionally a shooting pain down the back of one or both legs may occur from pressure of the uterus on the pelvic nerves.

BACKACHE

Problem   **Action**   **Possible Cause**

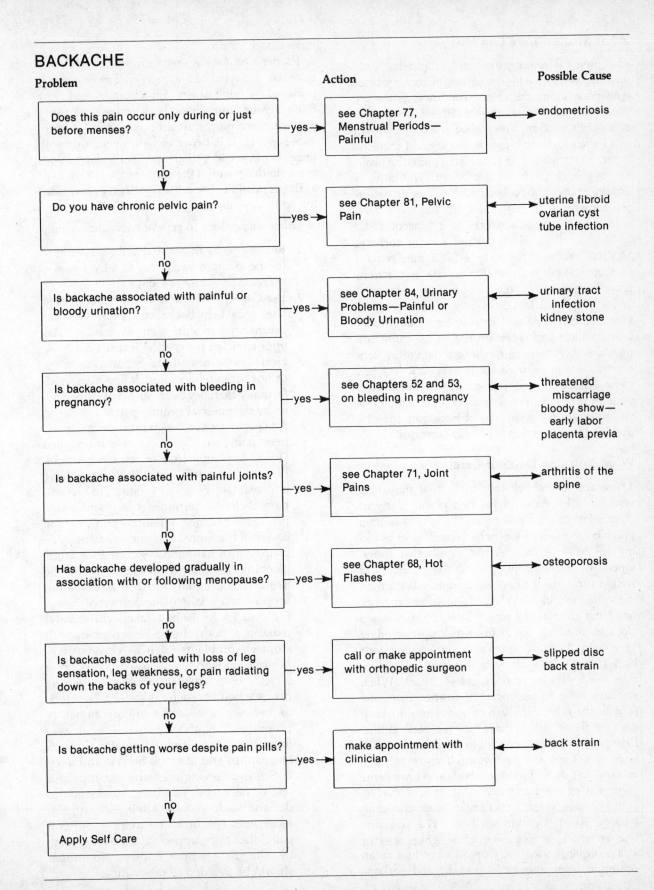

Does this pain occur only during or just before menses? —yes→ see Chapter 77, Menstrual Periods—Painful ←→ endometriosis

no ↓

Do you have chronic pelvic pain? —yes→ see Chapter 81, Pelvic Pain ←→ uterine fibroid ovarian cyst tube infection

no ↓

Is backache associated with painful or bloody urination? —yes→ see Chapter 84, Urinary Problems—Painful or Bloody Urination ←→ urinary tract infection kidney stone

no ↓

Is backache associated with bleeding in pregnancy? —yes→ see Chapters 52 and 53, on bleeding in pregnancy ←→ threatened miscarriage bloody show— early labor placenta previa

no ↓

Is backache associated with painful joints? —yes→ see Chapter 71, Joint Pains ←→ arthritis of the spine

no ↓

Has backache developed gradually in association with or following menopause? —yes→ see Chapter 68, Hot Flashes ←→ osteoporosis

no ↓

Is backache associated with loss of leg sensation, leg weakness, or pain radiating down the backs of your legs? —yes→ call or make appointment with orthopedic surgeon ←→ slipped disc back strain

no ↓

Is backache getting worse despite pain pills? —yes→ make appointment with clinician ←→ back strain

no ↓

Apply Self Care

What Medical Care Can Do

The physical examination will emphasize your posture, weight, and evaluation of any areas of tenderness along the spine. The lower limbs are usually checked for abnormal reflexes, weakness, or loss of sensation. You will be asked to lie down while the examiner lifts first one leg and then the other. If this maneuver elicits back pain, the problem is a back strain or disc injury. The latter is usually managed by a bone specialist or an orthopedic surgeon. If pelvic pain accompanies back pain, you may need a referral to a gynecologist.

Most back problems do not require surgery. Medical treatment for a slipped disc may require several weeks of bed rest with or without traction, prescription pain pills, or muscle relaxants. Sometimes local injections with anesthetics provide immediate pain relief. Newer modalities of therapy have had uncertain results. Acupuncture provides short-term pain relief but pain ultimately comes back in most cases. Biofeedback has had some limited success particularly in individuals with chronic tension and anxiety. A specific exercise program for your type of back pain may be obtained by referral to a physical therapist.

What You Can Do (Self Care)

There are several self-care tricks that may help you avoid backache in the first place. Many of them relate to good posture and body positioning. Wear comfortable shoes when standing or walking for long periods. Avoid high-heeled shoes, especially in pregnancy, since they shift your weight forward, thus placing additional strain on the spine and back. When lifting something, do not bend over at the waist. Instead squat down close to anything you plan to pick up, including your baby, bending your knees and keeping your back straight. Rise slowly from a bent-knees position, using your leg muscles, not your back. When standing for long periods, shift position from one foot to the other. The use of a footstool to keep one leg flexed at all times relieves back strain. Especially in pregnancy, roll to the side when you want to get up, and push yourself up using your arms. Don't do sit-ups unless both knees are bent. When caring for your baby, work at arm level to avoid bending over. For example, use a changing table or sit at your kitchen table. The pregnant woman who is gaining too much weight puts extra strain on her back, too. Control of weight to an optimum level also helps prevent and perhaps relieve back strain.

Proper positioning and sufficient rest are key essentials for relief of back strain. The best rest is achieved by lying down, not sitting. Avoid lying flat on your stomach or back unless you use a pillow under your pelvic area or low back to provide support. It is better to lie on your side with knees bent, keeping thighs perpendicular to your spine. In this position the curve of the back is kept as flat as possible. Use a firm mattress or bedboard for optimum support.

Other suggestions to relieve backache include:

1. Rest—slowing down your activity level even to the point of bed rest usually helps to decrease pain in a few days.
2. Exercise—"pelvic rock" and other back exercises may help backache especially during pregnancy or during menstruation. Ask your clinician for specific instructions.
3. Heat—moist heat through baths, showers, or hot packs relieves muscle spasm more effectively than dry heat, such as that provided by commercial heating pads.
4. Analgesics—over-the-counter drugs to relieve pain usually contain acetaminophen (Tylenol, Datril, etc.) or aspirin (Anacin, Bufferin, Excedrin, etc.). Both drugs have approximately equal ability to relieve pain. What determines the brand name product's potency depends mainly on the *dosage* of the ingredient or ingredients. Aspirin, which has been associated with fetal bleeding and birth defects, should be avoided in pregnancy. Also, aspirin's notorious potential to cause internal bleeding and ulcers (when taken chronically) make it a poor choice in a woman with stomach problems such as chronic indigestion. However, aspirin may be preferred over acetaminophen-containing drugs when backache is caused by arthritis because of aspirin's antiinflammatory properties. A third type of analgesic, ibuprofen, has antiinflammatory effects like aspirin and also has been found to be useful in relieving menstrual cramps and related backache. This drug, marketed under the trade names Advil and Nuprin, represents the first new nonprescription pain killer to be approved in twenty years by the FDA. Like aspirin, ibuprofen should be avoided in pregnancy.

50

Blackouts

The most common cause of blackouts is fainting, or *syncope*, the medical name for a temporary drop in pulse rate and blood pressure accompanied by a brief loss of consciousness. Pain, low blood sugar, sudden psychological stress, or fright can cause these blackouts. Accompanying symptoms may include blurred vision, sweating, nausea, and, when severe anxiety is present, numbness of mouth and hands from over-breathing (hyperventilation). Aggravating factors in fainting include prolonged sitting or standing, excessive coughing or straining, and collars or neck scarves that are too snug. You can faint during any procedure which stretches the cervix, such as insertion of an IUD, especially if you have never been pregnant.

The second major cause of blackouts in women is rapid blood loss from either external vaginal or rectal bleeding or internal abdominal bleeding as in the case of a ruptured cyst or tubal pregnancy. In women with peptic ulcer disease, tarry (black with the consistency of tar) stools may be the only sign of bleeding within the intestine. Internal bleeding is especially dangerous because it is less likely to be recognized early.

Other causes of blackouts, particularly in women over the age of forty, are heart problems, brain circulatory disorders, and, rarely, seizures. Heart disease is often accompanied by chest pain or shortness of breath. High blood pressure associated with small strokes may produce symptoms such as inability to move the arms or legs, loss of sensation, blurred vision, or difficulty with speech in addition to blackouts. These small strokes are usually temporary. Seizures are differentiated from blackouts by the rhythmic shaking movement that seizures often produce and by the accompanying loss of bowel or bladder control that frequently occurs.

An occasional cause of blackouts which may be overlooked is prescription drugs, such as those used to treat high blood pressure. These drugs may cause a person to faint when the person gets up suddenly from a reclining position. Tranquilizers, antidepressants, barbiturates, and antihistamines may also lead to blackouts if taken in excessive amounts.

In early pregnancy, fainting is common and frequently associated with low blood sugar or vomiting. Fainting in late pregnancy is due to changes in the circulation brought about by the weight of the uterus pressing on the major blood vessels to and from the heart.

What Medical Care Can Do

Your clinician will do a complete examination including taking your blood pressure and pulse rate, which usually varies from 60 to 100 beats per minute. Neurological examination is done if symptoms resemble a stroke or if you have a history of seizures; a referral to a neurologist may be made. In a woman with a suspected heart ailment, referral to a cardiologist may be made. An EKG (cardiogram) is ordered if the heartbeat is irregular or if chest pain is the presenting symptom. Medication to regulate heart rate or to control blood pressure may be needed. In addition to a complete examination, a blood count is done to rule out internal bleeding or chronic anemia. A history of stomach pain may require checking the stool for microscopic bleeding due to an ulcer.

What You Can Do (Self Care)

If you feel faint, lie down or sit down with your head between your knees. Use smelling salts or spirits of ammonia. If you faint easily, always rise from the reclining or sitting position slowly; and avoid sudden turning of your head or wearing tightfitting clothing around your neck, which may increase your susceptibility to fainting episodes. If you hyperventilate, breathe into a paper bag so that you rebreathe your own carbon dioxide and thereby prevent fainting. Take any medicines for blood pressure, heart problems, seizure disorders, or diabetes as directed, and avoid overuse of drugs that make you drowsy.

In pregnancy, fainting spells may be reduced by avoiding prolonged sitting and by getting up slowly after lying down. Eat frequent, small meals rather than three large meals a day to prevent rapid changes in blood sugar.

BLACKOUTS

Problem	Action	Possible Cause

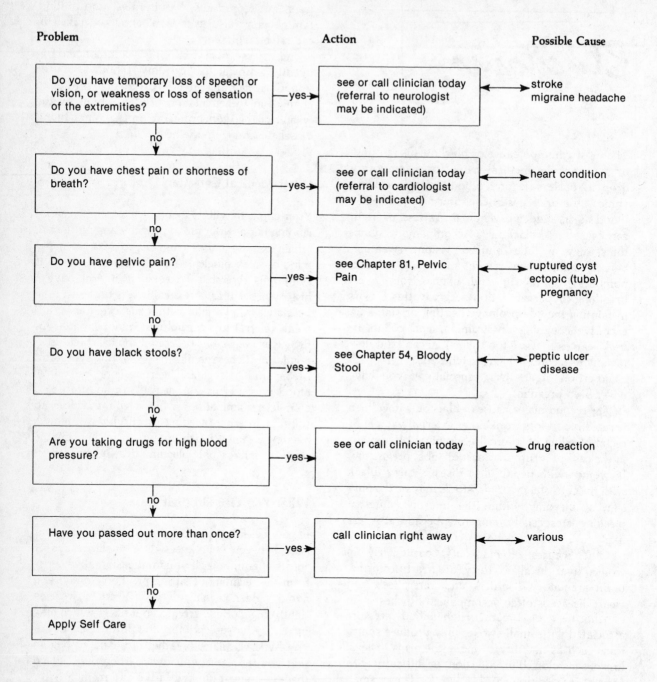

Problem

Do you have temporary loss of speech or vision, or weakness or loss of sensation of the extremities?
—yes→

no↓

Do you have chest pain or shortness of breath?
—yes→

no↓

Do you have pelvic pain?
—yes→

no↓

Do you have black stools?
—yes→

no↓

Are you taking drugs for high blood pressure?
—yes→

no↓

Have you passed out more than once?
—yes→

no↓

Apply Self Care

Action

see or call clinician today (referral to neurologist may be indicated)

see or call clinician today (referral to cardiologist may be indicated)

see Chapter 81, Pelvic Pain

see Chapter 54, Bloody Stool

see or call clinician today

call clinician right away

Possible Cause

stroke
migraine headache

heart condition

ruptured cyst
ectopic (tube) pregnancy

peptic ulcer disease

drug reaction

various

51

Bleeding After Intercourse

The most frequent cause of bleeding after intercourse is inflammation of the cervix, or *cervicitis*. This condition is usually a chronic one related to glandular changes in the cervix during pregnancy. Acute cervicitis is associated with symptoms of infection such as an irritating vaginal discharge. Bleeding is expected, and is normal, following initial intercourse because of stretching and small tears made in the hymen. Occasionally menses begins at the time of intercourse, so the appearance of blood is really coincidental. Tumors of the cervix, including polyps and cancer, are uncommon causes of spotting or bleeding after intercourse.

During pregnancy, bleeding after intercourse may occur as a result of the increased number of blood vessels and glands covering the cervix. This so-called pregnancy cervicitis is also accompanied by an expected increase in vaginal discharge. Sometimes it is impossible to differentiate between the bleeding caused by cervicitis and the bleeding caused by another disorder or by pregnancy. When bleeding persists, intercourse may need to be temporarily discontinued. Sexual activity does not cause miscarriage. However, in late pregnancy, bleeding due to intercourse may occur if the placenta lies directly over the cervix, a condition known as *placenta previa* (see Chapter 53). This condition necessitates abstinence through the remainder of

BLEEDING AFTER INTERCOURSE

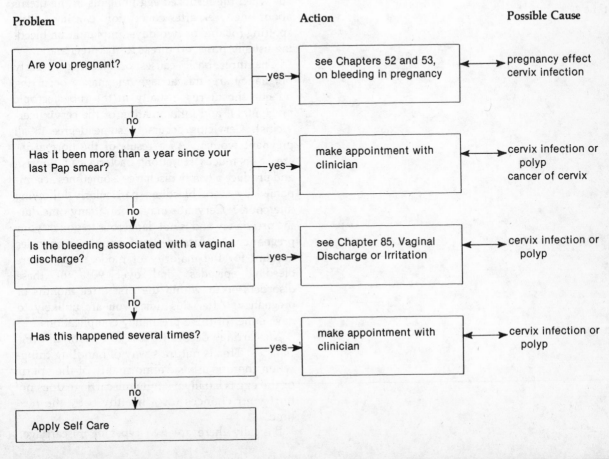

Problem	Action	Possible Cause
Are you pregnant?	—yes→ see Chapters 52 and 53, on bleeding in pregnancy	pregnancy effect, cervix infection
↓ no		
Has it been more than a year since your last Pap smear?	—yes→ make appointment with clinician	cervix infection or polyp, cancer of cervix
↓ no		
Is the bleeding associated with a vaginal discharge?	—yes→ see Chapter 85, Vaginal Discharge or Irritation	cervix infection or polyp
↓ no		
Has this happened several times?	—yes→ make appointment with clinician	cervix infection or polyp
↓ no		
Apply Self Care		

the pregnancy. Bleeding after intercourse which occurs in the second half of pregnancy should be evaluated promptly by a physician.

What Medical Care Can Do

A pelvic examination and Pap smear are done to diagnose the cause of bleeding. Usually cervicitis is found and a vaginal cream or suppository is prescribed. Cervical growths such as polyps are biopsied. Sometimes no cause for the bleeding can be determined. Persistent bleeding after intercourse may require further follow-up, often including cervical or endometrial biopsies (see Chapters 36 and 39).

What You Can Do (Self Care)

Betadine douches prepared by adding a tablespoon of Betadine douche (available in drugstores) to a quart of warm water may be used nightly for one week. This treatment will often clear up mild cervicitis. It is best to avoid intercourse during this time.

52

Bleeding in Early Pregnancy

It is possible to mistake what is really bleeding in early pregnancy for your regular menstrual period, especially if the pregnancy is unexpected or unaccompanied by the characteristic symptoms of breast tenderness and morning sickness. So it's smart to consider the possibility of pregnancy whenever your period is unusual for you: very heavy, very light, or delayed. Sometimes what is interpreted as a light period may actually represent implantation bleeding. This bleeding may occur when the fertilized egg implants in the uterus about one week after conception, causing a little spotting for one or two days; implantation bleeding usually poses no threat to the pregnancy.

The three basic causes of bleeding in early pregnancy are: miscarriage; pregnancy occurring outside the uterus, usually in the tube (ectopic pregnancy); and inflammation of the cervix (cervicitis). Cervicitis occurs to some degree in all pregnant women. As a result of the normal increase in mucus secretion, bacteria can flourish and produce a heavy discharge, sometimes accompanied by scant bleeding, particularly following intercourse. Cervicitis may occur at any time during pregnancy and is not dangerous to you or your pregnancy. Miscarriages and ectopic pregnancies account for the majority of moderate to severe bleeding episodes, and over 90% of these disorders occur within the first three months of pregnancy. After this time, you are unlikely to have either of these pregnancy complications.

Miscarriage occurs in 10% to 15% of all pregnancies. This is nature's way of handling things when there is a basic abnormality of the sperm or the egg. Usually a single miscarriage does not hurt your chances for a healthy baby the next time.

Basically there are two types of miscarriage.

The first and more usual type, *spontaneous abortion*, causes bleeding and cramping. Severe cramping is caused by strong uterine contractions which dilate the cervix and expel the fetus. Many women have what is called a *threatened miscarriage*; that is, they have some bleeding with little or no cramping. Bleeding is often in the form of light spotting which may go on for several days before it becomes known whether a miscarriage is going to occur or not.

The second and less common form of miscarriage is the *missed abortion*, in which the fetus, for reasons not well understood, fails to grow and develop normally. Consequently the uterus does not enlarge from one month to the next. The woman has little or no outward signs of problems, such as cramping or bleeding. In fact, her missed abortion may go undetected for several weeks unless pelvic exams are done in early pregnancy to confirm normal uterine growth. After the fourth month of pregnancy (16 weeks from the last menstrual period), failure to "show" or absence of fetal heart tones arouses suspicion of a missed abortion. The condition of missed abortion requires a D & C (see Chapter 41) to prevent infection and other complications.

Spotting may also indicate an ectopic pregnancy, that is, a pregnancy that occurs outside the uterus. The fetus cannot develop outside the uterus; and an ectopic pregnancy, which is uncommon, may be life-threatening for the mother.

Ectopic pregnancies are most commonly located in one of the Fallopian tubes and cause progressive pelvic pain and internal bleeding (see Figure 40). Tubal pregnancies leak most of the blood out the end of the tube into the abdomen; but some of the blood can trickle down into the uterus, accounting for the spotting characteristic of this condition. The apparent blood loss is deceiving since most of the bleeding occurs inside the body. Fainting commonly occurs. Pelvic inflammatory disease and IUDs are often associated with ectopic pregnancies.

Table 80 presents some of the findings associated with conditions causing bleeding in early pregnancy.

What Medical Care Can Do

The clinician approaches bleeding in early pregnancy by trying to answer three questions: 1) Is the woman in fact pregnant? 2) Is the pregnancy in the uterus? and 3) Is the woman miscarrying? He or she finds the answers through a combination of the pelvic exam, pregnancy testing, and sometimes a pelvic sonogram (see glossary).

The speculum exam may simply reveal a yellow discharge around the cervix, the hallmark of cervicitis or cervical inflammation (see Chapter 85). The clinician makes the diagnosis of miscarriage if tissue from the fetus or the placenta is seen coming

Figure 40   *An ectopic pregnancy is one that occurs outside the uterine cavity, usually in the Fallopian tube.*

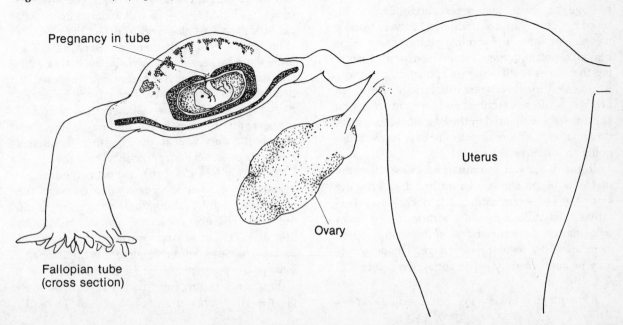

Pregnancy in tube

Uterus

Ovary

Fallopian tube
(cross section)

Table 80   FINDINGS ASSOCIATED WITH CONDITIONS CAUSING BLEEDING IN EARLY PREGNANCY (FIRST THREE MONTHS)

Condition	Medical Name	Typical Symptoms	Size of Uterus	Condition of Cervix
Threatening to miscarry	Threatened abortion	bleeding; mild cramping	enlarged	closed
Miscarriage (usual type)	Incomplete or spontaneous abortion	bleeding, often heavy; moderate to severe cramping; tissue may be passed	enlarged	open
Internal miscarriage (uncommon type)	Missed abortion	no bleeding or scant bleeding	normal size or enlarged less than expected	closed
Infection of cervix (mouth of uterus)	Cervicitis	vaginal discharge; bleeding after intercourse	enlarged	closed, discharge present
Pregnancy in tube	Ectopic pregnancy	bleeding, rarely heavy; moderate to severe pain, often on one side; fainting	enlarged minimally, if at all	closed
Hormone imbalance (not pregnant)	Dysfunctional bleeding	bleeding, variable	normal size	closed

through the dilated cervix. Usually, bleeding continues after a miscarriage, indicating that some tissue is still inside the uterus and will need to be removed by means of a D & C. In the absence of passage of tissue and severe abdominal pain, bleeding through an undilated cervix usually means you are "threatening" to miscarry. The bimanual examination is done next; and, assuming the uterus is still enlarged, no specific therapy is indicated for threatened miscarriage. Although bed rest is often prescribed and hormone pills and shots were widely used in the past, these measures do not alter the natural course of events if you are going to miscarry.

If the bimanual examination shows that the uterus is becoming smaller rather than growing since the last examination, the doctor may tentatively diagnose a missed abortion in a woman who has had prolonged spotting without the symptoms of a regular miscarriage. The diagnosis may be confirmed by pelvic sonogram before a D & C is done.

If the pregnant woman is spot bleeding and ex-

periences severe pain especially during the bimanual exam, then the clinician will suspect ectopic pregnancy. In the presence of a rapid pulse, low blood pressure, and a low blood count—signs of serious blood loss—she will undergo immediate culdocentesis (see glossary) to detect the presence of internal bleeding. If there is internal bleeding, immediate surgery is required. In less extreme circumstances, a pelvic sonogram may be used to determine the location of the pregnancy by as early as six weeks from the last menstrual period. If sonography is inconclusive or unavailable, surgery is the only way to distinguish a threatened miscarriage from a pregnancy in the tube. Laparoscopy (see glossary), a short procedure for visualizing the pelvic organs, may prevent the need for a regular abdominal incision by ruling out the existence of a pregnancy outside the uterus. When an ectopic pregnancy is confirmed by laparoscopy, definitive surgery is then done to remove the pregnancy in the affected tube.

Pregnancy testing (see Chapter 16) further complicates the evaluation of bleeding in early

Urine Pregnancy Test	Blood Pregnancy Test
positive	positive, hormone level variable
negative shortly after miscarriage occurs	positive, low hormone level
positive or negative	positive, low hormone level
positive	positive
positive or negative	positive, low hormone level
negative	negative

pregnancy. A positive pregnancy test does not necessarily mean, for example, that a woman is not going to miscarry. Most urine pregnancy tests will come out positive for a few days after a miscarriage. So, despite a positive pregnancy test, a miscarriage can occur and go unrecognized because only a minute amount of tissue is passed into the blood. In some instances, the only way for a physician to differentiate such completed miscarriages from a threatened miscarriage is to order a blood pregnancy test or to obtain a pelvic sonogram.

Negative pregnancy tests may also mislead the doctor in the presence of vaginal bleeding. Rather than being an ominous sign, a negative pregnancy test may merely mean the pregnancy is not far enough along for the test to turn positive. Again, the more sensitive blood pregnancy tests can accurately establish whether a woman is or recently has been pregnant. The blood pregnancy tests are also useful in detecting an early ectopic pregnancy. Routine urine tests are negative 50% of the time when pregnancy exists in the tube, but blood

pregnancy tests will always show some pregnancy hormone.

Pelvic sonograms, also known as *ultrasound*, are useful when ectopic pregnancy is suspected, because the developing fetus and amniotic fluid sac can be visualized as being either inside or outside the uterus by the sixth week of pregnancy. Since the diagnosis of tubal pregnancy indicates a need for immediate surgery, a sonogram is invaluable in such cases. In a woman with painless vaginal bleeding, indicating threatened miscarriage, this procedure may be less helpful, partly because it does not always provide information to help the doctor decide if a D & C needs to be done.

Table 81 shows the steps a doctor goes through to determine and treat the causes of bleeding in early pregnancy.

What You Can Do (Self Care)

If you are planning to become pregnant, keep a calendar record of your periods to help establish when you became pregnant. This information may help your clinician determine normal or abnormal uterine growth. If you develop severe pain, notify your physician. While many women have some form of low abdominal cramping in early pregnancy, this condition is rarely severe. You should also report to your health care provider any spotting or passing of tissue. Save any tissue that is passed for microscopic analysis later. Do not feel that activity, sexual or otherwise, contributes to bleeding; it doesn't. Most women who have bleeding in early pregnancy do not miscarry, and those who are going to miscarry will do so regardless of activity.

Table 81   HOW A DOCTOR EVALUATES BLEEDING IN EARLY PREGNANCY*

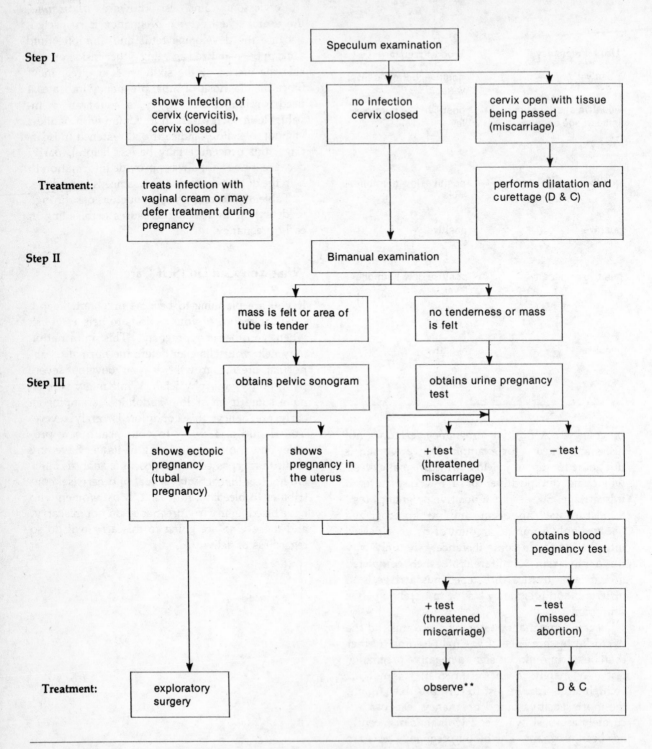

* Assume pregnancy has been established by examination (enlarged uterus) or by positive pregnancy test.

** Ectopic pregnancy precautions are given if sonogram has not been done; a repeat exam and pregnancy test in one week may be indicated.

BLEEDING IN EARLY PREGNANCY

Problem	Action	Possible Cause

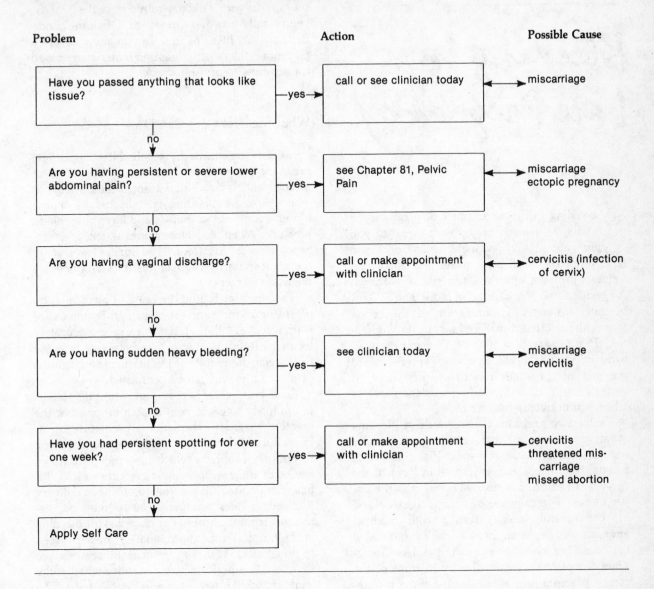

Problem		Action		Possible Cause
Have you passed anything that looks like tissue?	—yes→	call or see clinician today	←→	miscarriage
↓ no				
Are you having persistent or severe lower abdominal pain?	—yes→	see Chapter 81, Pelvic Pain	←→	miscarriage ectopic pregnancy
↓ no				
Are you having a vaginal discharge?	—yes→	call or make appointment with clinician	←→	cervicitis (infection of cervix)
↓ no				
Are you having sudden heavy bleeding?	—yes→	see clinician today	←→	miscarriage cervicitis
↓ no				
Have you had persistent spotting for over one week?	—yes→	call or make appointment with clinician	←→	cervicitis threatened mis- carriage missed abortion
↓ no				
Apply Self Care				

53

Bleeding in Late Pregnancy

Any bleeding in the second half of pregnancy is potentially serious and may pose a threat to you or your baby. Heavy vaginal bleeding occurs in fewer than 1% of all pregnancies and usually involves a problem with the afterbirth, or *placenta*. A specific cause is not found in more than 50% of bleeding instances. Inflammation of the cervix (cervicitis) is often considered a contributing factor. The passage of a blood-tinged mucus plug, sometimes called a "bloody show," occurs toward the end of the ninth month of pregnancy, is perfectly normal, and often heralds the onset of labor within twenty-four hours.

Of the two problems that often cause bleeding in late pregnancy, the more common and usually less serious is *placenta previa*. Placenta previa means that the placenta is located in front of the cervix instead of in its normal position in the upper uterus. Typically the bleeding occurs on and off for several weeks, starting with minimal amounts but becoming heavier during successive episodes. The bleeding is usually painless. Sometimes the placenta is not directly in front of the cervix (placenta previa) but lies just above it (low-lying placenta). Low-lying placenta is far more common but less likely to cause bleeding than placenta previa. Placenta previa is more likely to happen in women who become pregnant after the age of thirty, who are pregnant with twins, or who have had a previous cesarean birth.

Separation of the placenta from the uterus before labor begins is known as *abruptio placenta*. This condition occurs more often in women over thirty, especially where there is a history of high blood pressure. If the placenta detaches from the uterus, sudden bleeding may occur, accompanied by moderate to severe abdominal pain which feels like a strong, continuous contraction. With further separation, bleeding may be very heavy, and prompt delivery will be required since the fetal oxygen supply becomes threatened. Of all the conditions causing bleeding in late pregnancy, abruptio placenta is the most serious and may require blood transfusions to prevent shock.

What Medical Care Can Do

Immediate treatment of severe bleeding in late pregnancy depends on the overall condition of mother and fetus. Blood transfusions are given when excessive bleeding is indicated by a low blood count, rapid pulse, and dropping blood pressure. When blood loss causes shock, an emergency cesarean section will be done. However, in the great majority of instances, bleeding is not a medical emergency.

The best way to find the cause of bleeding is by means of a sonogram (see glossary). By the use of sound waves, the placenta can be accurately located within the uterus. If the placenta is found to lie over the mouth of the uterus, the diagnosis of placenta previa can be confirmed.

Since both placenta previa and abruptio placenta are likely to occur before the ninth month, the greatest hazard to the fetus is premature birth. Premature infants are likely to have many respiratory problems which may require days or weeks in the newborn intensive care unit. With placenta previa, it is possible to postpone delivery if bleeding does not persist. You may be discharged from the hospital or observed for bleeding in the hospital until approximately the 37th week of pregnancy. At that time, an amniocentesis (see Chapter 20) is performed to determine whether the fetal lungs will tolerate life outside the uterus. The doctor will postpone delivery until that time unless bleeding becomes heavy. A cesarean section is usually done since the fetus cannot be delivered in the normal manner when the placenta blocks the opening of the birth canal. In many instances of low-lying placenta, however, labor proceeds with little or no bleeding; and with the aid of a fetal monitor, vaginal delivery can be allowed.

With abruptio placenta, delivery cannot wait; fetal risks of delayed delivery outweigh the risks of prematurity. Bleeding is unlikely to stop by itself. Delivery is induced by rupturing the membranes and giving a drug (oxytocin) to stimulate

BLEEDING IN LATE PREGNANCY

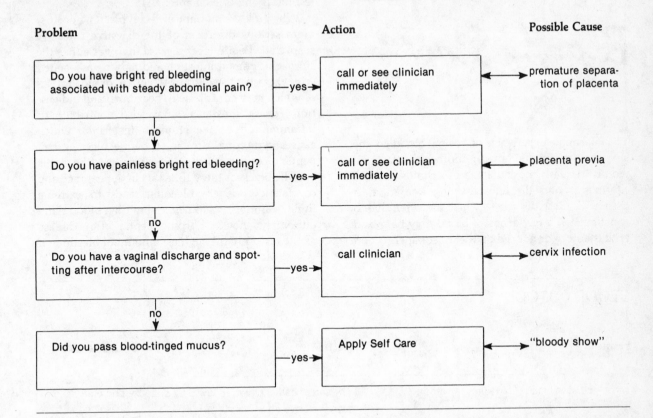

Problem	Action	Possible Cause
Do you have bright red bleeding associated with steady abdominal pain? —yes→	call or see clinician immediately ←→	premature separation of placenta
no ↓		
Do you have painless bright red bleeding? —yes→	call or see clinician immediately ←→	placenta previa
no ↓		
Do you have a vaginal discharge and spotting after intercourse? —yes→	call clinician ←→	cervix infection
no ↓		
Did you pass blood-tinged mucus? —yes→	Apply Self Care ←→	"bloody show"

contractions. Electronic monitoring is used to detect abnormalities in the fetal heart rate, and a cesarean section can be done if any problems occur.

What You Can Do (Self Care)

Bleeding in late pregnancy requires medical attention. In most instances, after a preliminary sonogram, you will be advised to rest in bed and to avoid intercourse, the use of tampons, and douching. Ask your doctor exactly what he or she thinks is going on and what the sonogram shows. If placenta previa or a low-lying placenta is excluded as the cause of the bleeding, there isn't any proven benefit to your lying in bed or otherwise reducing normal activity. If you have been given certain instructions during an office visit and the bleeding has not recurred, ask the physician on your follow-up visit if the same restrictions still apply. If bleeding, especially without pain, recurs from time to time, ask about having a sonogram to localize the placenta if this has not been done

before. If you have heavy bleeding, meet your doctor at the hospital rather than at the office. Usually spotting near your due date is from bloody show, sometimes brought about by a pelvic examination. However, if continuous abdominal pain occurs or if the baby's activity is markedly diminished, see your doctor at once.

54

Bloody Stool

The alarming experience of seeing blood in the stool occurs at some time or another to nearly all women. Usually the cause is hemorrhoids or an irritation around the anal opening known as a fissure. In these disorders, which are often due to constipation, a few drops of blood may be mixed with the stool or noticed on the toilet paper. Blood in the stool accompanies any cause of chronic diarrhea as a result of the irritation of the intestinal lining (see Chapter 61).

When a large amount of rectal bleeding occurs, more serious disorders of the digestive tract are suspected. Peptic ulcer disease involves either the stomach or small intestine and may be associated with excessive use of aspirin, coffee, or alcohol, all of which may contribute to heartburn and indigestion. These substances may also contribute to inflammation of the stomach (gastritis), which causes symptoms similar to peptic ulcer. When peptic ulcers or gastritis cause bleeding, the stools may be black or tarry (like tar) in appearance and consistency. Severe bleeding leads to extreme thirst, fainting, weakness, vomiting blood, and ultimately shock. Chronic peptic ulcer disease may cause only the slightest amount of bleeding; it

BLOODY STOOL

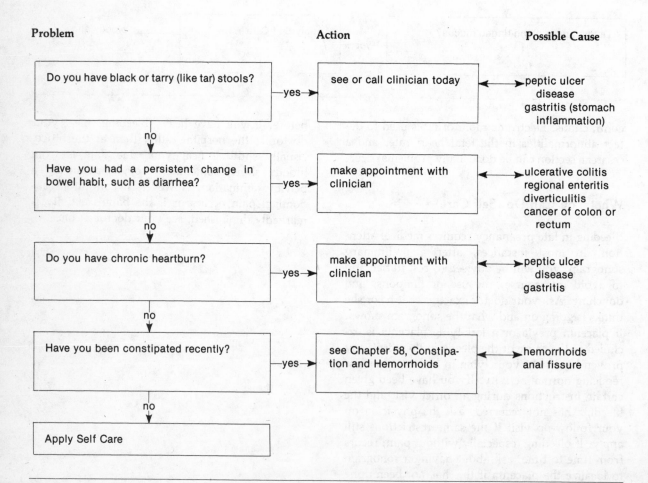

Problem	Action	Possible Cause
Do you have black or tarry (like tar) stools? —yes→	see or call clinician today	peptic ulcer disease / gastritis (stomach inflammation)
↓ no		
Have you had a persistent change in bowel habit, such as diarrhea? —yes→	make appointment with clinician	ulcerative colitis / regional enteritis / diverticulitis / cancer of colon or rectum
↓ no		
Do you have chronic heartburn? —yes→	make appointment with clinician	peptic ulcer disease / gastritis
↓ no		
Have you been constipated recently? —yes→	see Chapter 58, Constipation and Hemorrhoids	hemorrhoids / anal fissure
↓ no		
Apply Self Care		

may go unnoticed until a routine blood count shows you are anemic. Intestinal polyps, which may be hereditary, can cause bright red, painless bleeding and are usually benign. Because cancer of the colon and rectum is the second most frequent cancer in women, you should be aware that rectal bleeding is one of its symptoms. Fortunately, cancer is the least likely among the common causes of bloody stool mentioned here. Colon cancer occurs predominantly after the age of fifty and is usually associated with a persistent change in bowel habits, such as constipation or diarrhea.

What Medical Care Can Do

The evaluation of rectal bleeding depends on your overall condition. Heavy, bright red intestinal bleeding from an ulcer, for instance, is a medical emergency requiring blood transfusion and, sometimes, exploratory surgery. In the absence of acute bleeding, a very low blood count may be reason enough for hospitalization. Usually the basic X-rays—upper GI (gastrointestinal) series, lower GI series (i.e., barium enema), and sigmoidoscopy (see glossary for these tests)—can be done on an outpatient basis. Persistent rectal bleeding is sometimes evaluated by a subspecialist called a proctologist, who has had extra training in this branch of surgery.

What You Can Do (Self Care)

If you have hemorrhoids, you can treat occasional episodes of rectal bleeding at home (see Chapter 58). But you should see your doctor for repeated bouts of such bleeding. Use a mirror if there is any doubt as to whether the bleeding is from the rectum or the vagina. Remember that if you take iron, the color of the stool may be black, similar to the tarry stool seen with bleeding ulcers. Stopping the iron should be associated with return to the normal stool appearance within two to three days. Some physicians recommend that women over the age of forty have a stool specimen tested for microscopic bleeding as part of their routine annual examination.

55

Breast Discharge

A breast discharge may be noticed at many different times in a woman's life from adolescence to menopause (see Table 82). A clear or milky discharge from both breasts is known as *galactorrhea* and is associated with the brain's production of a hormone called prolactin. Galactorrhea is normal during pregnancy, in breast-feeding women, and in adolescents at puberty. Breast discharge may persist up to two years following pregnancy. The symptoms may also be provoked by manual stimulation during sexual activity. A variety of medications may produce galactorrhea, including antihypertensives, antidepressants, and tranquilizers. In addition, either taking or stopping birth control pills can bring on galactorrhea in some women. Chest wall disease such as shingles or chest surgery such as breast biopsy may also cause breast discharge. In women with galactorrhea, gynecologists are very concerned about the possibility of pituitary tumors, an uncommon but serious cause of breast discharge. Such tumors are usually associated with infrequent or absent menstrual periods and sometimes headaches or blurred vision.

In contrast to galactorrhea, conditions originating within the breast itself usually cause breast discharge from only one breast. The discharge may be bloody, green, brown, or yellow. Uncommonly, fibrocystic disease (see Chapter 33) may cause breast discharge. Breast tumors known as papillomas may occasionally produce a bloody discharge. Although a bloody discharge may be associated with cancer, a nonbloody discharge almost never is. Sometimes when it appears that a discharge is occurring from only one breast, manipulation of the opposite breast reveals that the discharge is actually coming from both breasts.

What Medical Care Can Do

Tell your physician about any accompanying

Table 82 POSSIBLE CAUSES OF BREAST DISCHARGE

Normal Causes	Comment
Pregnancy	usually in late pregnancy
Breast-feeding	may persist for up to two years after childbirth
Breast manipulation	may be associated with sexual stimulation

Localized Causes Due to Breast Conditions	Comment
Fibrocystic disease	usually clear or yellow discharge
Papilloma (benign tumor in breast duct)	sometimes bloody discharge
Breast cancer	almost always bloody discharge

Nonlocalized Causes	Comment
Pituitary (brain) tumors	uncommon; associated with lack of or infrequent periods; sometimes headaches
Chest wall surgery such as mastectomy on opposite side	sometimes any form of surgery can cause breast discharge as a result of hormonal changes associated with stress
Chest wall injury such as burns or disease such as shingles	
Birth control pills	also associated with going off the pill
Tranquilizers (such as Thorazine)	
Blood pressure pills (such as Aldomet or Reserpine)	
Antidepressants	
Hypothyroidism (low thyroid)	associated with fatigue, dry skin, cold intolerance, weight gain

symptoms you have such as headaches or blurred vision. You should also tell him or her about any medication you are taking and whether or not you have a history of cystic breast disease. The doctor will test the breast secretion to determine if it contains milk or another, nonmilky substance such as pus from an infection or fluid from a cyst.

During your physical, the doctor will examine your eyes to check for increased intracranial pressure which, if present, would implicate the rare pituitary tumor. Also, the thyroid is examined because certain thyroid conditions associated with diminished production of thyroid hormone may be associated with galactorrhea.

All women with abnormal galactorrhea should have a prolactin level taken, that is, a blood test of a hormone produced by the pituitary in the brain. If this test shows an increased level of prolactin, an X-ray of the skull is done to look for a pituitary tumor. Keep in mind that there are many harmless conditions that can also cause elevated prolactin levels. However, most women with a breast discharge have a normal prolactin level. When galactorrhea persists, prolactin levels are usually repeated in six months to a year.

If you have a discharge from only one breast, your doctor may recommend that you have a mammogram (see Chapter 33) to check for a cyst or tumor. Cytology, or cellular evaluation, of the breast discharge may be done, especially if the discharge is bloody. Table 83 describes the tests your doctor might use to diagnose abnormal breast discharge, when the tests are indicated, and the purpose of each.

A new drug is now available for treatment of breast discharge associated with irregular or absent periods. The drug, Bromergocryptine, is indicated only after skull X-rays and other appropriate steps are taken to rule out a pituitary tumor. Bromergocryptine has been very successful in establishing regular periods and in stopping breast discharge.

What You Can Do (Self Care)

Breast self-examination is essential and is unlikely to stimulate galactorrhea. Call your doctor if you have any type of breast discharge, especially if it is bloody or associated with cracking, scaling, or irritation around the nipples. Remember that most causes of breast discharge are benign, and even stress itself can be a factor accounting for this symptom.

Table 83 TESTS TO DIAGNOSE ABNORMAL BREAST DISCHARGE

Test	When Indicated	Purpose of Test
1. Sudan stain (microscopic smear of discharge for fat content)	Often useful except when discharge is bloody	To determine if discharge is milk (galactorrhea) or due to local breast disease (such as pus, cyst fluid)
2. Prolactin (blood test to measure a hormone produced in pituitary gland of the brain)	All cases of milky discharge (galactorrhea)	Screening test for pituitary tumor
3. Thyroid blood tests	Symptoms of low thyroid (weight gain, fatigue, dry skin, cold intolerance)	Detect low thyroid condition
4. Skull X-rays	Headaches or blurred vision or lack of or infrequent periods or abnormal prolactin test (elevated level)	Detect pituitary tumor
5. Mammogram (breast X-ray)	Breast lump felt or fibrocystic disease or discharge from only one breast	Detect breast abnormalities, including cancer
6. Cytology (microscopic smear of discharge to detect cellular abnormalities)	Same as test 5	Same as test 5

Table 84 QUESTIONS COMMONLY ASKED ABOUT BREAST DISCHARGE

Question	Yes	No	Comment
Is a green or yellow breast discharge a sign of infection?		X	These discharges usually accompany benign fibrocystic disease and represent blood pigments.
Is milk secretion from both breasts in a nonpregnant, non-breast-feeding woman a sign of breast disease?		X	Such secretions are due to hormonal changes from a variety of causes.
Can manual stimulation cause breast discharge?	X		
Is a bloody nipple discharge usually cancer?		X	The commonest cause is a benign tumor of the breast ducts called a papilloma.
Are tranquilizers a cause of breast discharge?	X		Especially the phenothiazine types, such as Thorazine.

During pregnancy, the presence of breast milk is no cause for alarm. Some women have very little; others have moderate amounts in the early portion of their pregnancy. Wash away any dried milk with soapy, warm water so your nipples will not become itchy, irritated, or sore.

Table 84 will answer some questions you may have about breast discharge.

56

Breast Lump

Breast lumps are among the most common complaints of women who visit gynecologists. Breast lumps may be associated with pain or breast discharge. Localized breast changes such as swelling, redness, skin dimpling, or recent nipple inversion (the nipple turns "inside out") should be investigated promptly by your doctor.

Three conditions must be distinguished in women with breast lumps: fibrocystic disease, fibroadenoma, and breast cancer (see Breast Diseases, Chapter 33). Women with fibrocystic disease may feel many tiny cysts when they examine their breasts, and a consistency of lumpiness or doughiness may be felt (see also Chapter 57). Fibroadenomas are solitary, firm, mobile, benign tumors commonly found in young women in their twenties. Breast cancer often presents itself as a hard, painless lump in one breast. Although breast cancer is rare under the age of thirty and very uncommon before age forty, the disease must be at least considered in any woman with a persistent breast lump. Risk factors include a family history of breast cancer in a close relative such as your sister or mother, first pregnancy after the age of thirty, and menopause after the age of fifty.

What Medical Care Can Do

Breast lumps can be evaluated initially by inserting a small needle, under local anesthesia, into the cavity of the mass and then withdrawing any fluid present into a syringe. This process of fluid removal is called *aspiration*. If the fluid obtained is clear and the lump disappears following aspiration of the fluid, no further treatment is needed except for routine examinations every six months.

Table 85   HOW A DOCTOR EVALUATES A LUMP IN THE BREAST

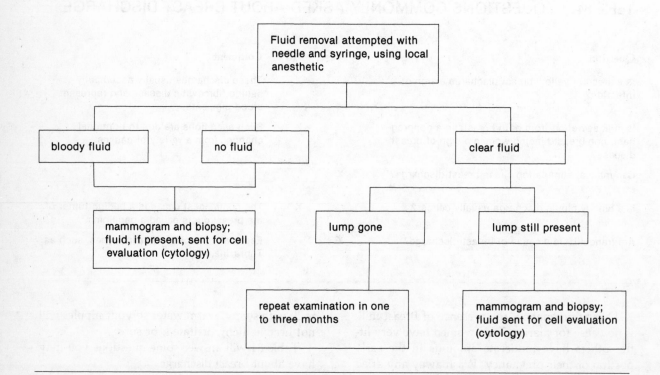

Such masses are usually due to fibrocystic disease. If the fluid is bloody or the mass is still present after the procedure, mammography (see Chapter 33) and biopsy are indicated. A frequent cause of bloody fluid in a breast lump is a benign tumor called a *papilloma*. But since a breast cancer could also be the cause, the fluid is sent to the lab for cytology (examination of the cell characteristics). Women who have recurrences of cysts previously drained by aspiration will usually need a biopsy to rule out the presence of cancer. Fortunately most biopsies are benign. The biopsies are done by general surgeons as opposed to gynecologists and may be done on an outpatient basis. This way, if the biopsy shows a malignancy, there is time to make a decision as to the type of further surgery or treatment indicated.

Table 85 summarizes how a doctor evaluates a lump in the breast.

What You Can Do (Self Care)

The hallmark of prevention of breast disease is the monthly breast self-examination (see Chapter 3) which is best done just after menses or, if you are past menopause, at a regular time every month. If you discover a lump in your breast, call your clinician. You should report any lump, regardless of how indefinite it may seem. If you are over forty, in addition to your self-exam, you should have your clinician examine your breasts approximately every twelve months. Mammography is indicated for women at risk for breast cancer (see Table 3, in Chapter 4, and Table 53, in Chapter 33).

57

Breast Tenderness

In nonpregnant women, cyclic breast tenderness before a period is common. At least 30% of women between the ages of thirty-five and fifty have tenderness associated with cystic breast changes sometimes known as *fibrocystic disease* (see Chapter 33). Fibrocystic disease means that there are multiple tiny cysts in one or both breasts. This condition, which may produce breast discharge, seems to be hormone dependent and tends to subside as menopause approaches. The use of oral contraceptives, while often diminishing breast pain associated with fibrocystic disease, is becoming increasingly controversial in women with this condition. Many studies indicate at least a twofold increased risk for breast cancer for women with fibrocystic disease regardless of pill use. For pill users it is possible that an already existent unrecognized cancer, stimulated by estrogen in the pill, might grow more rapidly than otherwise (see Chapter 9).

Injury to the breast, which can go unnoticed, also causes breast tenderness and bruising. Black and blue areas subside in about two weeks. The presence of a tender lump may arouse fear of cancer. However, breast cancer rarely causes pain unless it is far advanced. Estrogens also cause breast tenderness in some women on birth control pills as well as in women taking Premarin or other estrogens.

Breast tenderness is most commonly associated with pregnancy and breast-feeding. During pregnancy, the breasts may feel heavy or may tingle and may be especially tender during examination. Breast infections are most frequent during the postpartum period during breast-feeding when bacteria from the skin may be introduced into the breasts. Early symptoms of a breast infection are tenderness, redness, and fever.

What Medical Care Can Do

Nonpregnant women with cyclic breast tenderness may be treated with diuretics, although response to this treatment varies. The use of a birth control method other than the pill should be strongly considered since women who have fibrocystic disease may have an increased risk of breast cancer. Progesterone pills such as Provera may be tried for breast tenderness and are occasionally effective. Progesterone has not been associated with breast cancer or blood clots. Danazol, a new hormonal drug (see Chapter 35), shows promise in alleviating breast tenderness and has recently been approved by the FDA for this purpose.

Following delivery, the presence of redness around the breast accompanied by fever in breast-feeding women indicates infection. Antibiotics such as penicillin are usually prescribed.

What You Can Do (Self Care)

In nonpregnant women, mild cyclic breast tenderness does not require treatment. A low-salt diet may decrease engorgement of the breasts during the premenstrual period of your cycle. A supportive bra is advisable if you are prone to breast soreness, especially during physical activity such as jogging.

Recent reports indicate that fibrocystic breast disease may improve with the reduction or elimination of caffeine and caffeinelike foods from the diet. Several studies have shown that women who eliminated these substances, which include chocolate, tea, coffee, and cola, from their diet experienced a marked decrease in breast cysts and tenderness. In another recent study, vitamin E when taken for two months was reported to decrease symptoms of fibrocystic breast disease. Although further research is needed to confirm its effectiveness, taking vitamin E, 400 to 600 units daily, may help reduce your symptoms.

During pregnancy and lactation, the best way to prevent sore breasts is by the use of a supportive bra worn twenty-four hours a day if necessary. During pregnancy, after washing your breasts with soap and water, briskly dry the nipples with a stiff terry cloth towel to help "toughen" the nipples for lactation. If you decide to breast-feed, limit the time spent nursing to no more than ten to fifteen minutes on each breast. If necessary, use breast shields to protect your nipples from cracks, which can lead to breast infections. If breast infection does occur, hot compresses may reduce your symptoms; however, antibiotic treatment is generally necessary if fever occurs. Breast engorgement can be treated with ice packs and a supportive bra. Hormonal therapy to prevent breast engorgement in mothers who will not be breast-feeding their infants is not effective after seventy-two hours following delivery.

58

Constipation and Hemorrhoids

Constipation, a symptom reported twice as often by women as by men, exists when bowel evacuation is delayed several days or when the stool is unusually dry and hard or difficult to pass. The frequency of bowel movements varies greatly among healthy women; it is not necessary to have a bowel movement every day. The chief causes of constipation are improper diet, lack of exercise, certain drugs, excessive use of laxatives, and failure to establish a habit of regular defecation. Specific medical causes of constipation include certain digestive disorders such as irritable bowel syndrome and, less frequently, cancer of the colon, which is usually associated with a marked unexplained change in bowel habits. Low thyroid, or hypothyroidism, may cause constipation; but other symptoms such as fatigue, weight gain, or dry skin are also usually present. During pregnancy, hormone changes produce a relaxation of intestinal muscles, making constipation a frequent problem. Taking iron pills also contributes to constipation in pregnancy as does the pressure from an enlarging uterus.

Hemorrhoids may be a consequence of or contributor to constipation. Hemorrhoids, or piles, are varicose veins located at the anal opening (external hemorrhoids) or just within the anus (internal hemorrhoids). You can't see internal hemorrhoids. Both types may be brought on or aggravated by straining due to constipation. Failure to respond to the urge to defecate because of hemorrhoid pain may lead to further constipation and development of a vicious circle. Common symptoms of external hemorrhoids may include a soft tissue protrusion from the anus with or without itching, pain, or bleeding. Internal hemorrhoids show up as rectal bleeding, often without other symptoms. Hemorrhoids are common during pregnancy, which may help to explain the greater frequency of this condition among women as compared to men.

What Medical Care Can Do

An otherwise healthy woman can take care of common constipation at home. But if you are troubled with diarrhea, pelvic pain, or bloody stool (see these symptom chapters), you might need to consult your clinician. If conservative treatment of hemorrhoids (see below under What You Can Do) is unsatisfactory, there are a number of office procedures which may be tried. These include injecting chemicals into internal hemorrhoids and "freezing" the external hemorrhoids using cryosurgery (see glossary). These procedures may not cure the problem; hemorrhoids can recur. When a blood clot (thrombosis) forms in an external hemorrhoid, the hemorrhoid takes on a bluish appearance and becomes swollen and exquisitely tender. The pain is immediately relieved by surgical removal of the clot under local anesthesia. For severe cases or recurrences, complete external and internal hemorrhoidectomy (removal of hemorrhoids) by a general surgeon is indicated and curative. Sigmoidoscopy and a barium enema (see glossary) are done if the only symptom is rectal bleeding.

What You Can Do (Self Care)

You can take an occasional mild laxative, such as milk of magnesia or Metamucil, for simple constipation. Avoid chronic use of any laxative.

In general these guidelines are the safest approach to treating constipation:

1. Establish a pattern of regular evacuation by responding to the urge to defecate. Even in the absence of this urge, set aside a regular time after a meal for a bowel movement.
2. Drink six to eight glasses of fluid a day.
3. Increase the roughage (fiber) in your diet by eating plenty of fresh fruits, salads, and raw vegetables. Bran, another good source of roughage, can be sprinkled in fruit juice, mixed with another cereal, or eaten as a snack, such as granola bars. Prunes, dates, figs, raisins, and whole wheat bread also

add roughage to your diet. These high-fiber foods stimulate muscle activity in the lower bowel and rectum in contrast to dairy products which may be constipating.

4. Get some exercise each day.
5. Avoid or minimize the use of drugs that may cause constipation (see Table 86).
6. Following childbirth or pelvic surgery when elimination may be painful, the use of a stool softener helps and it is not habit-forming. This will help you maintain regular bowel habits and prevent constipation.

Most of the time you can treat hemorrhoids yourself. Take a warm bath to relieve local pain. Take mineral oil or stool softeners temporarily to facilitate elimination, but avoid harsh laxatives such as castor oil. Over-the-counter ointments and suppositories such as Anusol provide relief of local symptoms. Suppositories may be preferable since external hemorrhoids may be repositioned when the suppository is inserted. Ointments containing anesthetics may cause localized allergic reactions and are best avoided. For a severe bout with hemorrhoids, your doctor will call your drugstore and order a prescription drug; request drugs such as Anusol-HC, Wyanoids-HC, or Proctofoam-HC. The *HC* stands for hydrocortisone, a potent antiinflammatory ingredient not found in over-the-counter drugs. The HC-containing drugs have not been established as safe to use in pregnancy, however.

Table 87 lists common nonprescription laxatives that are presently considered safe to use during pregnancy. Table 88 lists the ones to avoid during pregnancy.

CONSTIPATION

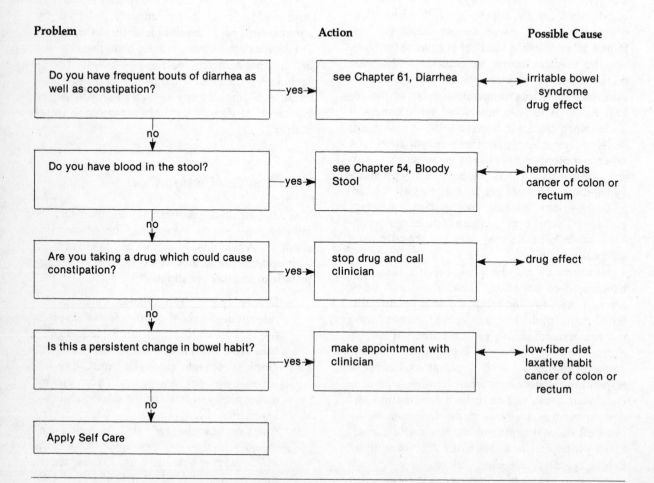

Problem	Action	Possible Cause
Do you have frequent bouts of diarrhea as well as constipation? —yes→	see Chapter 61, Diarrhea	←→ irritable bowel syndrome drug effect
↓ no		
Do you have blood in the stool? —yes→	see Chapter 54, Bloody Stool	←→ hemorrhoids cancer of colon or rectum
↓ no		
Are you taking a drug which could cause constipation? —yes→	stop drug and call clinician	←→ drug effect
↓ no		
Is this a persistent change in bowel habit? —yes→	make appointment with clinician	←→ low-fiber diet laxative habit cancer of colon or rectum
↓ no		
Apply Self Care		

Table 86   DRUGS THAT MAY CAUSE CONSTIPATION

Antacids

Iron preparations

Narcotics (includes any drug containing codeine)

Antihistamines

Water pills (diuretics)

Antidiarrhea drugs

Table 87   NONPRESCRIPTION LAXATIVES PRESENTLY CONSIDERED SAFE TO USE DURING PREGNANCY

Brand Name	Type
Colace	Stool softener
Dialose	Bulk laxative (mild) plus stool softener
Doxinate	Stool softener
Dulcolax	Mild stimulant
Kasof	Stool softener
Metamucil	Bulk laxative (mild)
Milk of magnesia (various brands)	Mild but rapid-acting (2–3 hrs) stimulant
Modane Bulk	Bulk laxative (mild)
Modane Soft	Stool softener
Senokot	Mild and slow-acting (8–10 hrs) stimulant
Senokot DSS	Mild stimulant plus stool softener
Surfak	Stool softener

Table 88   NONPRESCRIPTION LAXATIVES TO AVOID DURING PREGNANCY

Name	Comment
Castor oil	Strong stimulant, may start uterine contractions
Doxidan	Contains danthron—safety not established
Ex-Lax	Strong stimulant
Haley's M-O	Inhibits vitamin absorption since it contains mineral oil
Mineral oil	Inhibits vitamin absorption
Modane tablets	Contains danthron—safety not established
Pericolace	Strong stimulant

59

Cough

Cough is the most common symptom of respiratory disease. Coughing is a reflex by which the body tries to get rid of an irritating substance somewhere along the respiratory tract in the throat, breathing tubes (bronchi), or lungs. Cough may be unproductive (that is, nothing is coughed up) as in the dry cough of influenza or may be productive of sputum as in asthma, bronchitis, or pneumonia. Colds and flu, the most common cause of coughing, are discussed in Chapter 63.

More serious respiratory conditions associated with a cough, such as pneumonia, occur when environmental factors decrease natural resistance of the body to infection. Such factors may include viral respiratory tract infections, poor nutrition, chronic alcohol or drug use, chronic fatigue, and cigarette smoking. In addition, industrial exposure to hazardous chemicals such as asbestos may contribute to chronic lung disease.

Cough may be a prominent symptom in bronchitis, pneumonia, emphysema, or lung cancer, all of which may bear a direct relationship to cigarette smoking. Pneumonia, or infection of the lungs, is an acute debilitating illness associated with sudden onset of fever, chills, and yellow sputum production, sometimes accompanied by chest or shoulder pain which increases while the patient takes a breath. Bronchitis is invariably associated with a productive morning cough. Chronic bronchitis associated with cigarette smoking ultimately leads to emphysema, the most common form of chronic lung disease in women. Unlike bronchitis, emphysema involves actual destruction of lung tissue and may be accompanied by progressive shortness of breath. Along with cough, common symptoms of lung cancer are weight loss, bloody sputum, and chest pain. Historically this disease has been more common in men, but women smokers are catching up. The National Cancer Institute reports that the female death rate from lung cancer has more than doubled between 1965 and 1974. It is estimated that by 1985 lung cancer will overtake breast cancer as the leading cause of death from malignancy in women.

Occasionally cough may be due to conditions unrelated to the respiratory tract. In older women with heart disease, an enlarged heart may cause cough and shortness of breath at night or during exertion. In women taking hormones, including the pill, cough accompanied by bloody sputum, chest pain, and fever may be a sign of blood clots in the lung (pulmonary embolus). Associated findings may include calf pain in instances where a blood clot has traveled to the lungs from an inflamed vein in the leg.

Women who chronically cough may ultimately develop urinary stress incontinence, a condition in which the bladder muscles become weakened as a result of the continuous strain of coughing and allow urine leakage. In addition, coughing tends to place a strain on the ligaments that support the uterus and may contribute to a "dropped," or prolapsed, uterus.

Of major importance is the increased incidence of women who smoke. For the past fifteen years since the Surgeon General's report on smoking and health confirmed the link between cigarette smoking and serious respiratory disease, the percentage of women who smoke has been on the rise. Increased cigarette use has been striking among young women, especially adolescents. Smoking often starts as early as age thirteen. Several studies indicate that mothers who smoke set the same pattern for their children, especially their daughters, who tend to follow their mother's smoking behavior and disregard their father's if he is a nonsmoker. Approximately one in three women of reproductive age now smoke, and the total of all women who smoke is almost as much as that for men.

Various reasons are given for the increase in smoking among women. Changing life styles and pressures of work and home which were formerly linked to the male domain have been suggested as contributing factors. So have the cigarette companies which continue to direct much of their brassy and "newly liberated" pitches directly at women. Women's magazines got a bonanza shortly after cigarette commercials were banned from television. Shortly after the ban, cigarette ads quadrupled in *Cosmopolitan*, *Ladies' Home Journal*, and *Woman's Day* compared to an identical period in the previous year.

During pregnancy, smoking is hazardous to the

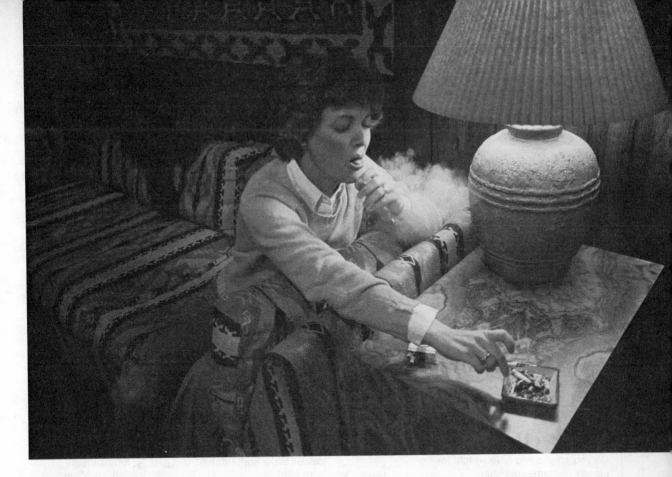

fetus for several reasons (see also Chapter 31). Many studies have indicated that smoking is associated, for reasons not completely understood, with lower birth weight babies as well as increased numbers of miscarriages, stillborns, and malformations of the newborn. Among conditions not related to smoking which cause cough, most do not become worse during pregnancy or have harmful effects on the fetus. Asthma, for instance, improves or remains unchanged in most women. Most colds and other respiratory infections are well tolerated in pregnancy by both mother and fetus.

What Medical Care Can Do

The physician initially will check your temperature and examine your throat, heart, and lungs. A chest X-ray and sputum tests may be obtained to diagnose infections such as pneumonia. Where tumor is suspected, the sputum is sent also for cytology, or cellular evaluation. Treatment of pneumonia will usually include penicillin antibiotics. During pregnancy, most medications used for treating pneumonia and asthma are not contraindicated with the exception of potassium iodide which may produce fetal goiter.

What You Can Do (Self Care)

All infections of the respiratory tract benefit from bed rest, an increase in fluids (especially hot tea or another hot drink) to loosen secretions, and steam inhalation by means of a vaporizer. Avoid cigarettes. When antibiotics are prescribed, take the full amount for the total number of days prescribed. If you have a tendency to chronic infections, bronchitis, or pneumonia, get early medical treatment when respiratory tract infections such as colds develop. When symptoms such as bloody sputum, chest pain, or shortness of breath occur, see your doctor. (See Chapter 63.)

Many programs have been developed to help people stop smoking. If you want to quit, contact your local branch of the American Lung Association, American Cancer Society, or American Heart Association, Smokenders, or the Seventh-Day Adventists. Look in your telephone directory, or see Appendix D for the addresses of the national headquarters. Write for information or to learn if there are clinics that you can attend.

Over-the-counter cough suppressants

Among the many ingredients in over-the-counter cough suppressants, the FDA has found very few

COUGH

Problem		Action		Possible Cause

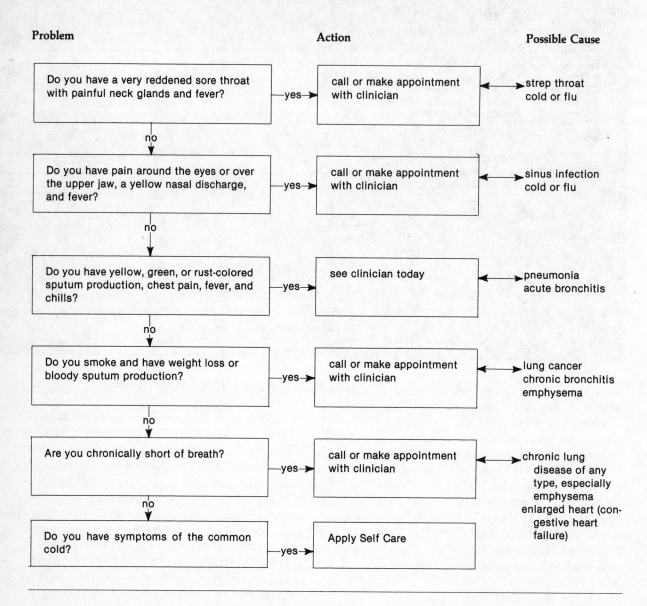

Do you have a very reddened sore throat with painful neck glands and fever? —yes→ call or make appointment with clinician ← strep throat / cold or flu

no ↓

Do you have pain around the eyes or over the upper jaw, a yellow nasal discharge, and fever? —yes→ call or make appointment with clinician ← sinus infection / cold or flu

no ↓

Do you have yellow, green, or rust-colored sputum production, chest pain, fever, and chills? —yes→ see clinician today ← pneumonia / acute bronchitis

no ↓

Do you smoke and have weight loss or bloody sputum production? —yes→ call or make appointment with clinician ← lung cancer / chronic bronchitis / emphysema

no ↓

Are you chronically short of breath? —yes→ call or make appointment with clinician ← chronic lung disease of any type, especially emphysema enlarged heart (congestive heart failure)

no ↓

Do you have symptoms of the common cold? —yes→ Apply Self Care

---

to be both safe and effective. They include dextromethorphan (found in Formula 44, Comtrex, and many other drugstore products) and codeine. Depending upon State law, codeine may be purchased in small doses without a prescription. Other ingredients of uncertain effectiveness include ethylmorphine, camphor, and cod liver oil. Medicated cough lozenges may contain various "medical" ingredients. Antibacterial ingredients contain doses too low to be effective. Local anesthetic ingredients may mask serious disease; hard candy can be just as effective to soothe an irritated throat. Chronic cough, cough with high fever or rash, or cough associated with asthma or bronchitis will normally require medical treatment.

Over-the-counter cough expectorants

Another group of over-the-counter products used in treating a cough, the expectorants, are intended to thin out phlegm to increase sputum production from the lungs. Two common ingredients used are glycerol guaiacolate (guaifenesin) and terpin hydrate. Although neither drug has proven effectiveness according to the FDA, they are included as ingredients in dozens of prescription as well as over-the-counter cough and cold remedies.

60

Depression

Depression, in one form or another, knows no age group. It is today the most common mental difficulty of both children and adults. Men and women both suffer depression, but women are more likely to seek relief from it.

Many women have a condition called premenstrual syndrome (PMS) in which depression and other symptoms such as fluid retention and irritability may occur regularly every month for several days up to two weeks before menses (see Chapter 82). This poorly understood but increasingly recognized syndrome seems to become more likely as women approach their late thirties and forties.

Specific health-related events in a woman's life, such as childbirth, a miscarriage, menopause, or a hysterectomy, may also trigger depression. Eighty-five percent of women become depressed, to some degree, at some time during the course of a normal pregnancy, and most experience the so-called postpartum blues.

Depression, along with the feelings and thoughts associated with it, ranges from the individual who occasionally feels blue to the individual who is so immobilized that the only alternatives he or she sees are either staying in bed or taking his or her life. In practice, people who experience depression usually fall into one large grouping we will call *mildly depressed* or another large grouping we will call *severely depressed*.

Mild depression among women is often experienced as a sad, blue, low-down feeling. A depressed woman may lose interest in almost everything, and nothing gives her joy. Some women can't sleep and others can only sleep. She has little energy and a lot of fatigue. There may be present an inability to concentrate, a poor self-image with low self-worth, and a hugely pessimistic attitude. The depressed woman sometimes experiences teary eyes, and occasionally she cries. Some mildly depressed women have thoughts of suicide and occasionally they attempt suicide.

Severe depression has the same symptoms as mild depression only more so. One of the most outstanding symptoms of severe depression is negativism, accompanied sometimes by irrational thinking. The person's appetite may be poor and there may be significant weight loss. The woman will complain of feeling hopeless and worthless. Some women may suffer memory loss. Suicidal thoughts and occasional gestures of suicide are usually present. Explosive anger that borders on rage is often reported. Sometimes the individual's moods will shift from anger to pessimism to a brooding, silent, dark sadness. The individual's moods may swing sometimes rapidly and sometimes slowly from agitated, anxious elation to the darkest depths of depression.

Elavil and Tofranil are two of the first antidepressants developed and two of the most prescribed antidepressants today. In recent years many new similar drugs have come on the market. These include Sinequan, Asendin, Ludiomil, Aventyl, Vivactyl, and certain combination drugs

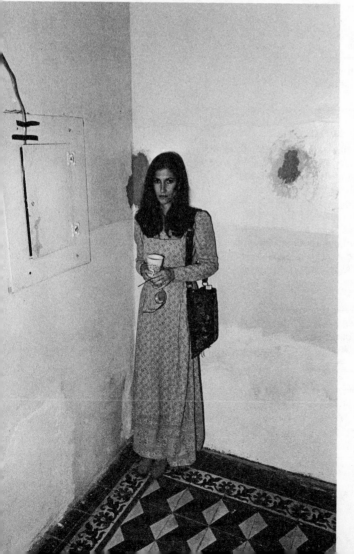

DEPRESSION

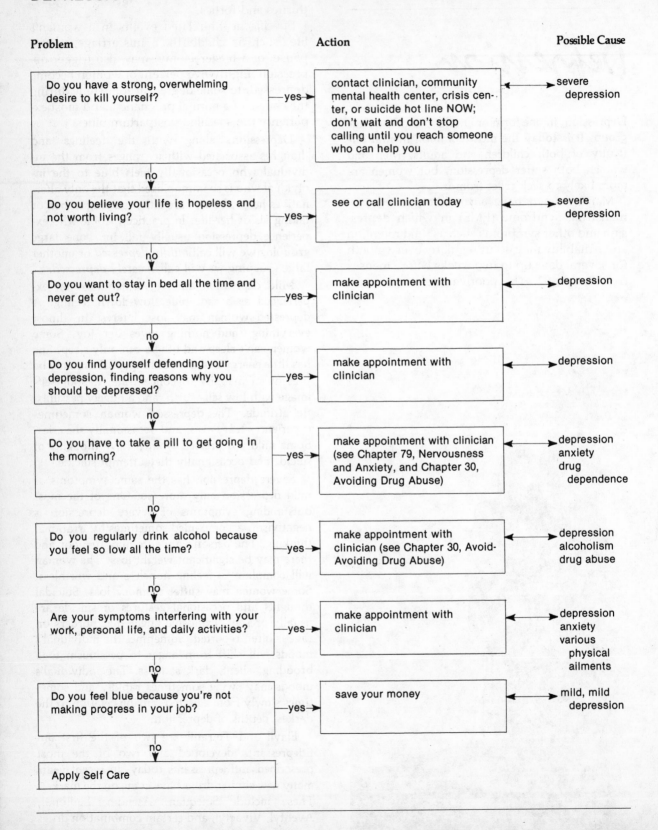

Problem	Action	Possible Cause
Do you have a strong, overwhelming desire to kill yourself? —yes→	contact clinician, community mental health center, crisis center, or suicide hot line NOW; don't wait and don't stop calling until you reach someone who can help you	severe depression
↓ no		
Do you believe your life is hopeless and not worth living? —yes→	see or call clinician today	severe depression
↓ no		
Do you want to stay in bed all the time and never get out? —yes→	make appointment with clinician	depression
↓ no		
Do you find yourself defending your depression, finding reasons why you should be depressed? —yes→	make appointment with clinician	depression
↓ no		
Do you have to take a pill to get going in the morning? —yes→	make appointment with clinician (see Chapter 79, Nervousness and Anxiety, and Chapter 30, Avoiding Drug Abuse)	depression anxiety drug dependence
↓ no		
Do you regularly drink alcohol because you feel so low all the time? —yes→	make appointment with clinician (see Chapter 30, Avoiding Drug Abuse)	depression alcoholism drug abuse
↓ no		
Are your symptoms interfering with your work, personal life, and daily activities? —yes→	make appointment with clinician	depression anxiety various physical ailments
↓ no		
Do you feel blue because you're not making progress in your job? —yes→	save your money	mild, mild depression
↓ no		
Apply Self Care		

such as Triavil, Limbitrol, and others. Most of these antidepressants share similar side effects, including drowsiness, blurred vision, and dryness of the mouth. Less frequent reactions to these drugs include dizziness, heart palpitations, and fainting.

Relief of depression through the use of antidepressant drugs usually takes between seven and thirty days and may require an increase or a decrease from the original dosage.

If an antidepressant or a tranquilizer has been prescribed for you, you should discuss the drug thoroughly with the physician who prescribed it, in order to learn about the medication. Alcohol in most cases must be avoided, and in some cases certain common foods must not be eaten. Antidepressants may interact with one another, with some tranquilizers, with other drugs, and sometimes with certain foods. They may also adversely affect a wide variety of existing medical conditions from thyroid problems to heart disease. Following prolonged use of an antidepressant or a tranquilizer, abrupt stopping of these drugs is to be avoided, because withdrawal symptoms (such as abdominal cramps, vomiting, and insomnia) may result.

Depression can accompany an illness, such as rheumatoid arthritis or hypoglycemia. Depression may also be drug-induced—for example, from blood-pressure-lowering drugs such as Reserpine, diet pills (amphetamines), tranquilizers like Valium, and alcohol. If you become depressed after starting to take a new drug, be certain to inform your doctor.

The probabilities are that if you have taken the time to read this chapter, you are either not depressed or only mildly depressed. But you may know someone close to you who is severely depressed. If so, she (or he) may need your help; she may not be able to help herself. Although depressed people need a great deal of social support, their extremely negative attitude often causes them to drive away the very people they need—their families and their friends.

The mental health professional never takes the suicidal threats of a severely depressed person lightly; neither should anyone else.

What Medical Care Can Do

The single most important function the physician can perform is to distinguish between mild and severe depression. If the depression is mild, your physician may recommend an antidepressant or may refer you for counseling. If the depression is severe, your physician may refer you to a specialist. The specialist may treat you with medication, counseling, and in some cases hospital treatment.

What You Can Do (Self Care)

1. Research has shown that one of the best treatments for depression is exercise. Try brisk walking, jogging, or swimming, and for detailed information on exercise see Chapter 47.
2. Keep up your daily routine; don't stop. Many people report feeling better during the times they work hardest.
3. If possible, join a women's counseling group. In many cities there is a women's center which has counseling groups for women who have undergone mastectomies, are going through a divorce, or are experiencing other traumatic events.
4. Talk to friends and relatives who will give you support. Remember that all people have limits in their ability to help others; a person may want to help you but is only able to go so far—you can and must help yourself.
5. Follow the directions and recommendations of your physician. Take the prescribed medication according to how it is prescribed.
6. If you have premenstrual syndrome, reduce your salt, caffeine, and sugar intake. Vitamin B_6 (50 to 100 mg per day) may help.
7. You can ask for help from any of the following, as appropriate:
   Community mental health center—these centers are required in most states to have service twenty-four hours a day, seven days a week.
   Crisis or suicide hotline—look up the telephone number and keep it near your telephone.
   Mental health association.
   Hospital—emergency room; psychiatric unit.
   Women's center.
   Your physician.

61

Diarrhea

Acute diarrhea, which lasts only a few days, is often due to simple intestinal infections or to drug side effects. The most common intestinal infection, gastroenteritis or stomach flu, typically begins with fever, vomiting, and stomach pains that may mimic appendicitis. In adults, intestinal infection is usually caused by a *virus*. However, if you have stomach flu following close contact with small children, the source may be *bacterial* gastroenteritis since this form is more prevalent in youngsters.

The most common prescription drugs causing diarrhea—antibiotics—include tetracycline, ampicillin, and cleocin, which are widely prescribed for female pelvic infections. Diarrhea accompanied by fever and abdominal cramping may develop during or several weeks following antibiotic treatment. Over-the-counter drugs which may produce diarrhea include iron, antacids (containing magnesium), and laxatives.

"Traveler's diarrhea" may occur when you are traveling from one country to another, especially when the change involves marked differences in climate, social conditions, or sanitation. This common ailment is usually due to alterations of intestinal bacteria but in some instances results from either bacterial or parasitic infection. Diarrhea from food poisoning, especially common among travelers, occurs from six to forty-eight hours after you have eaten contaminated food or liquid and is often accompanied by vomiting but usually not fever.

Chronic diarrhea, especially when associated with weight loss and weakness, may indicate a serious underlying disease. A "change in bowel habit" is one of cancer's seven warning signs and may indicate colon cancer, the second most frequent malignancy in women after breast cancer. However, ninety-nine percent of the time changes in bowel habits are due to benign causes, such as inflammatory diseases and what is called irritable bowel syndrome.

The principal inflammatory diseases causing chronic diarrhea are *diverticulitis*, *ulcerative colitis*, and *regional enteritis* (Crohn's disease). Symptoms of diverticulitis vary markedly from occasional mild diarrhea to acute episodes of severe diarrhea, which causes sharp pain in the left lower abdomen.

Ulcerative colitis, which involves the large intestine (colon), and regional enteritis, which involves the small intestine, afflict women more frequently than men. No one knows what causes these diseases, but physicians suspect that chronic stress triggers recurrences of the diseases. Both conditions may be associated with periods of bloody diarrhea, abdominal cramping, fever, and weight loss. Unpredictable periods of lessening and worsening of symptoms occur as well as long periods of freedom from symptoms. These conditions usually begin during the reproductive years but do not adversely affect menses or fertility. However, the effect of childbearing on these diseases may be serious if the disease becomes active or first develops at this time. The long-term effect of pregnancy may be to increase the severity of these two inflammatory conditions. Pregnancy should not be attempted during a flare-up of these conditions. However, unless symptoms are severe, these diseases do not require abortion or sterilization for medical reasons.

There are many names for irritable bowel syndrome, including *functional diarrhea*, *spastic colon*, and *nervous diarrhea*. Sometimes a set of symptoms for which no physical cause can be demonstrated by lab tests, X-rays, or surgery are lumped under one heading. This is the case with irritable bowel syndrome, which probably represents several separate disorders manifested differently in different women. Some individuals have recurrent bouts of watery diarrhea associated with anxiety or stressful situations and little, if any, abdominal pain. Other women have alternating episodes of diarrhea and constipation along with lower abdominal cramping. In pregnancy, the symptoms of irritable bowel syndrome often subside as a result of an increased tendency toward constipation.

What Medical Care Can Do

The doctor will prescribe antidiarrhea drugs for acute diarrhea unaccompanied by abdominal pain. Hospitalization is not necessary unless you have excessive fluid loss that requires immediate

DIARRHEA

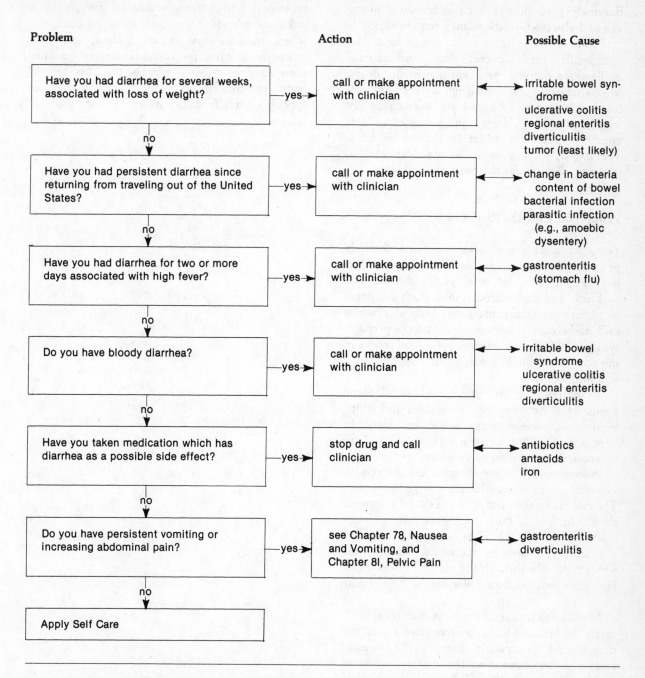

Problem	Action	Possible Cause
Have you had diarrhea for several weeks, associated with loss of weight? — yes →	call or make appointment with clinician	irritable bowel syndrome ulcerative colitis regional enteritis diverticulitis tumor (least likely)
no ↓		
Have you had persistent diarrhea since returning from traveling out of the United States? — yes →	call or make appointment with clinician	change in bacteria content of bowel bacterial infection parasitic infection (e.g., amoebic dysentery)
no ↓		
Have you had diarrhea for two or more days associated with high fever? — yes →	call or make appointment with clinician	gastroenteritis (stomach flu)
no ↓		
Do you have bloody diarrhea? — yes →	call or make appointment with clinician	irritable bowel syndrome ulcerative colitis regional enteritis diverticulitis
no ↓		
Have you taken medication which has diarrhea as a possible side effect? — yes →	stop drug and call clinician	antibiotics antacids iron
no ↓		
Do you have persistent vomiting or increasing abdominal pain? — yes →	see Chapter 78, Nausea and Vomiting, and Chapter 8l, Pelvic Pain	gastroenteritis diverticulitis
no ↓		
Apply Self Care		

intravenous fluid and mineral replacement. A stool specimen is examined for parasitic or bacterial infection if you recently traveled outside the United States or if you were recently exposed to a child with diarrhea. Bacterial infections respond well to prescribed antibiotics; viral infections do not.

When diarrhea is chronic, the clinician searches for the underlying cause. He or she can often diagnose cancer of the colon and the inflammatory conditions by an upper GI series and barium enema (see glossary), perhaps with the aid of sigmoidoscopy (see glossary). If these tests leave some doubt as to the diagnosis, further tests or surgery may be necessary. The physician treats flare-ups of ulcerative colitis and regional enteritis with powerful antiinflammatory drugs called corticosteroids, whose use in pregnancy is felt to be justified. Occasional complications of these inflammatory conditions, such as intestinal blockage and abscess formation, may require surgery.

Treatment of irritable bowel syndrome is also nonspecific although doctors often prescribe tranquilizers, sedatives, and antispasmodic drugs. Most studies suggest these drugs are minimally effective. It is best to avoid antidiarrhea or antispasmodic drugs during pregnancy since this condition poses no threat to mother or fetus. Therapy with a high-bulk diet and Metamucil is safe and effective for the pregnant woman.

What You Can Do (Self Care)

You can treat most forms of acute diarrhea yourself. Restrict solid foods during the first twenty-four hours, but drink plenty of fluids such as broth and carbonated drinks (such as ginger ale). Eliminate dairy products, especially whole milk and cream. Gatorade, a commercial preparation available in supermarkets, is a good source of mineral and fluid replacement, especially if vomiting occurs.

As diarrhea subsides, you can add small, bland meals while avoiding raw vegetables and fruits, fried foods, sweets, spices, coffee, and alcoholic beverages. Do not force yourself to eat if you have severe abdominal pain or vomiting.

Women with chronic diarrhea usually require vitamins, extra rest, and some change in the diet. The diet for women with irritable bowel syndrome should be free of milk, milk products, and raw fruits and vegetables. In addition, she may alleviate symptoms by increasing dietary bulk either naturally through the use of bran or other high-fiber foods or by supplementing the diet with Metamucil.

Most of the time an over-the-counter drug is safer, milder, and less expensive than a prescription drug for treatment of diarrhea. The strongest and most effective over-the-counter products, such as Donnagel PG and Parepectolin, contain small doses of paregoric which are not likely to be addictive if taken as directed. Milder over-the-counter drugs, such as Kaopectate, contain absorbent ingredients such as kaolin and pectin. Kaopectate is one of the safest drugs for diarrhea because the drug itself is not absorbed.

When traveling outside the United States, take Pepto-Bismol with you. Recent studies indicate that this over-the-counter drug effectively prevents and treats traveler's diarrhea. Take four tablespoons four times a day for the first two weeks of travel. If you are going to a country where medical services are limited, ask your physician to prescribe Lomotil, a common antidiarrhea drug. Also remember to drink bottled water, eat cooked foods, and avoid tap water or ice cubes made from tap water.

62

Dizziness and Vertigo

Dizziness means lightheadedness or giddiness. Vertigo refers to the sensation of objects spinning around you—that is, an object your eyes are focused on seems to move out of position. Lightheadedness commonly occurs when you suddenly stand up after sitting or lying down. This form of dizziness, known medically as *orthostatic hypotension*, is due to delayed adjustment of the circulatory system to changes in posture. The effect is more pronounced in pregnancy because the growing uterus compresses the blood vessels to and from the heart. Orthostatic hypotension may also occur in women taking blood pressure medication or having anemia.

More serious causes of dizziness in women include bleeding, high blood pressure, and low blood sugar. Chronic blood loss from an ulcer or heavy menstrual periods produces a low blood count which may be associated with weakness or dizziness. More rapid losses of blood also cause dizziness such as is found with ectopic pregnancy, in which the bleeding occurs internally and is not apparent immediately. Women with high blood pressure may have no symptoms or they may have occasional headaches or dizziness (see Chapter 67, High Blood Pressure). Hypoglycemia, or low blood sugar, may cause dizziness as well as headache, sweating, hunger, shakiness, and fatigue (see Chapter 73, Lethargy).

Vertigo, a more specific and disturbing symptom than dizziness, may be caused by an ear infection or by hardening of the arteries at the base of the brain, the latter usually occurring in elderly women. Other causes of dizziness and vertigo include drugs, particularly sedatives, tranquilizers, antihistamines, aspirin, and "water pills" (diuretics). The exact cause of dizziness is often not found; however, stress and emotional factors, particularly anxiety and depression, frequently play a role. Hyperventilation may occur when anxious individuals breathe rapidly, leading to dizziness and numbness in the hands and lips. Stress-related migraine headaches may also be associated with dizziness.

What Medical Care Can Do

Dizziness is usually diagnosed after a complete examination. A neurological examination is performed if there is evidence of neurological involvement from your history. The doctor will examine your eyes, which can reveal information about hardening of the arteries elsewhere in the body. A pelvic exam is done to check for uterine enlargement due to pregnancy or fibroid tumors which may cause heavy periods and anemia. Pertinent lab tests may include a blood count, examination of the stool for microscopic bleeding, and a pregnancy test. The clinician may refer you to a neurologist, an ear specialist, or an internist if he or she finds gross abnormalities in the examination of the nervous system, ear, or heart, respectively. In most cases the primary care clinician can deal with this symptom after excluding serious underlying disease.

What You Can Do (Self Care)

Drugs having the side effect of dizziness may need to be reduced in dosage or stopped altogether; consult with your doctor. However, if you are taking blood pressure medication, it may need to be increased. After the age of thirty, have your blood pressure checked annually. Get up slowly from the reclining position. In late pregnancy especially, this is best accomplished by turning to the side and slowly pushing yourself up with your arms. Avoid sweets in your diet because sweets may make you susceptible to hypoglycemia. Persistent dizziness associated with vertigo, suspected bleeding, or ear pain should be reported to your physician.

DIZZINESS AND VERTIGO

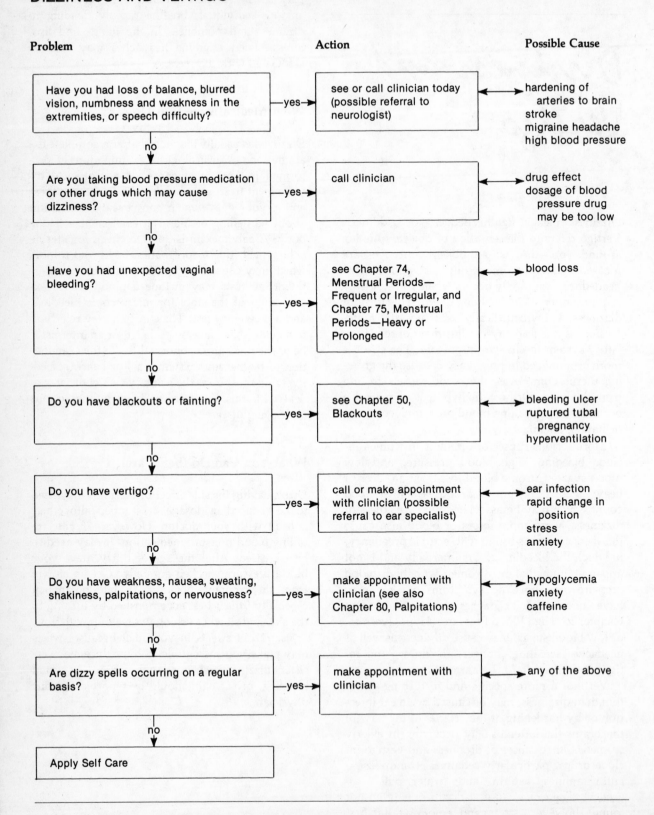

Problem	Action	Possible Cause
Have you had loss of balance, blurred vision, numbness and weakness in the extremities, or speech difficulty?	—yes→ see or call clinician today (possible referral to neurologist)	hardening of arteries to brain stroke migraine headache high blood pressure
↓no Are you taking blood pressure medication or other drugs which may cause dizziness?	—yes→ call clinician	drug effect dosage of blood pressure drug may be too low
↓no Have you had unexpected vaginal bleeding?	—yes→ see Chapter 74, Menstrual Periods—Frequent or Irregular, and Chapter 75, Menstrual Periods—Heavy or Prolonged	blood loss
↓no Do you have blackouts or fainting?	—yes→ see Chapter 50, Blackouts	bleeding ulcer ruptured tubal pregnancy hyperventilation
↓no Do you have vertigo?	—yes→ call or make appointment with clinician (possible referral to ear specialist)	ear infection rapid change in position stress anxiety
↓no Do you have weakness, nausea, sweating, shakiness, palpitations, or nervousness?	—yes→ make appointment with clinician (see also Chapter 80, Palpitations)	hypoglycemia anxiety caffeine
↓no Are dizzy spells occurring on a regular basis?	—yes→ make appointment with clinician	any of the above
↓no Apply Self Care		

63

Fever and Chills

Fever accompanies many illnesses, most of which are benign. Fever generally indicates infection somewhere in the body. Your temperature normally fluctuates on any given day up to as high as 100 degrees. The main significance of fever is not how high it is but what is causing it. This can usually be determined by the accompanying symptoms. Fever accompanied by chills usually means that an infection has spread to the bloodstream.

Common causes of fever which usually get better on their own are shown in Table 89. These include colds and stomach flu. You are probably all too familiar with the cold symptoms: headache, runny nose, sore throat, cough, hoarseness, and muscle aches. A low-grade fever is sometimes present. Influenza, or the flu, often occurs in epidemics and may be a more sudden and serious illness than the cold, producing extreme fatigue. The stomach flu (gastroenteritis) characteristically causes nausea, vomiting, or diarrhea in addition to the other symptoms.

Colds and stomach flu are caused by viruses and therefore do not respond to antibiotics. Although these ailments themselves are not serious, several of their complications are serious; and this is where medical treatment and sometimes antibiotics can help. The common complications of colds and flu in adult women are listed in Table 90. In addition to colds and flu, mononucleosis is a viral condition causing fever, sore throat, tender neck glands, and chronic fatigue. The condition is

Table 89 COMMON CAUSES OF FEVER

Cause	Possible Symptoms	Contact clinician if you have:
flu (influenza)	nausea, vomiting, diarrhea, muscle aches, headaches	vomiting of blood or severe abdominal pain lasting more than six hours
cold or upper respiratory infection	sore throat, runny nose, headache, cough	chest pain, shortness of breath, coughing up blood, or stiff neck
mono (mononucleosis)	sore throat and swollen neck glands, slight fever, chronic fatigue	yellow pigmentation of skin or eyes (jaundice) or any cold associated with fatigue that persists

Table 90 COMPLICATIONS OF THE COMMON COLD AND FLU

Complication	Diagnostic Test	Symptoms
pneumonia or bronchitis	chest X-ray	cough productive of green or yellow sputum fever and chills trouble breathing or you are wheezing chest pain especially when breathing
sinus infection	sinus X-ray	nasal discharge which is green or yellow sinus pain, especially around the eyes and over the upper jaw
strep throat	throat culture	very red throat often covered with a yellow or white drainage over tonsils tender neck glands

diagnosed by a blood test and generally runs an uncomplicated course.

Table 91 describes the more serious infections that require a visit to your clinician. These illnesses may become life-threatening if untreated. One of the most common infections in women is pyelonephritis, or kidney infection (see Chapters 83 and 84 on urinary problems). Another serious cause of fever in women is pelvic inflammatory disease (see Chapter 24, Sexually Transmitted Diseases).

During pregnancy, a high fever may be hazardous to the fetus by causing premature labor. Pregnancy does not significantly increase the susceptibility to illness. However, colds and flu, when complicated by bacterial pneumonia, may be particularly severe in pregnancy. Urinary tract infections are more frequent in pregnancy. However, pelvic inflammatory disease is less common during pregnancy because of the increased amount of cervical mucus, which acts as a barrier to bacteria. Despite the prevalence of varicose veins during pregnancy, the actual incidence of thrombophlebitis is not much different from that in nonpregnant women.

Among fever-causing conditions that are due to pregnancy itself, the most common is premature rupture of the membranes (see Chapter 20). The amniotic sac or fetal membranes may rupture prematurely, usually in the last third of pregnancy. Infection known as *amnionitis* may then occur, usually after twenty-four hours. This condition is associated with fever, a bad-smelling discharge, and abdominal pain and is potentially

---

Table 91   CAUSES OF FEVER REQUIRING MEDICAL TREATMENT

Cause	Typical Symptoms	How Diagnosed	Comment
pelvic infection (involving tube or ovary)	moderate to severe low abdominal pain persisting for several hours to days; vomiting may occur; vaginal discharge may be present	examination of abdomen and pelvis	diagnosis always presumptive; may be confirmed by laparoscopy or exploratory surgery
kidney infection	burning with urination; backache felt on one or both sides just above the waist; bloody or frequent urination may occur	urinalysis; urine culture	bladder infections cause the same symptoms without fever or backache
appendicitis	moderate to severe low abdominal pain persisting several hours and becoming worse on right side; vomiting usually occurs	examination of abdomen and pelvis	abscess of ovary or tube may cause same symptoms
pneumonia	cough with yellow or green sputum production; chest pain while taking a breath may occur; shortness of breath may occur	examination of the chest; chest X-ray confirms	in women over forty who smoke, these symptoms may be caused by lung cancer
meningitis	headache with stiff neck	spinal tap	relatively rare; flu may mimic these symptoms
thrombophlebitis	leg pain; swelling or redness particularly in area of the calf	examination of the lower extremities	associated with prolonged bed rest, use of birth control pills, recent surgery, or childbirth
connective tissue disease (such as lupus erythematosus)	joint pain; rash; chest pains	blood tests	although uncommon, may affect young women; multiple symptoms

Table 92 COMMON NONPRESCRIPTION COLD AND ALLERGY DRUGS*— WHAT THEY CONTAIN

Brand Name	Antihistamine	Decongestant	Pain Reliever	Expectorant	Cough Suppressant	Alcohol (at Least 3% by Volume)
Allerest	X	X				
Chlor-Trimeton	X					
Chlor-Trimeton Decongestant Tablets	X	X				
Chlor-Trimeton Expectorant	X	X		X		
Comtrex	X	X	X		X	X
Coricidin	X		X			
Coricidin Decongestant Nasal Mist		X				
Coricidin "D" Decongestant Tablets	X	X	X			
Coricidin Cough Syrup		X		X	X	
Neo-Synephrine Nasal Spray		X				
Novahistine	X	X				X
Novahistine Sinus Tablets	X	X	X			
Novahistine Cough Formula				X	X	X
Novahistine DMX		X		X	X	X
Robitussin				X		X
Robitussin-CF		X		X	X	X
Robitussin-DM				X	X	
Robitussin-PE		X		X		
Sinarest Tablets	X	X	X			
Sudafed		X				
Triaminic Syrup	X	X				
Triaminic Expectorant		X		X		X
Triaminic-DM Cough Formula		X			X	
Triaminicol Decongestant Cough Syrup	X	X		X	X	
Tussagesic	X	X	X	X	X	

* Not containing codeine or other narcotics.

very dangerous to the fetus. Except when the pregnancy is less than 34 weeks or so, labor is induced to prevent amnionitis. Childbirth fever sometimes occurs on the third or fourth postpartum day and is usually due to infection of the lining of the uterus (endometritis). This condition happens more commonly when delivery does not occur within twenty-four hours after rupture of the membranes. The symptoms are very similar to amnionitis. Other causes of fever following childbirth are urinary tract infections, breast engorgement or infection, and, much less commonly, thrombophlebitis.

What Medical Care Can Do

The symptoms and physical findings due to febrile conditions (that is, conditions in which fever is present) are numerous. Where the apparent cause seems to be an infection localized, for example, to the urinary tract or uterus, antibiotics are usually started immediately after appropriate cultures are obtained. Uncomplicated cases of colds and flu do not require antibiotics unless strep throat is confirmed by throat culture or there is a history of chronic lung disease.

When the cause of fever is unclear, screening tests may include a complete blood count (CBC), urinalysis, and chest X-ray. The CBC includes a white blood cell count which measures infection in the body. If you have severe abdominal pain or dehydration along with fever, you may be hospitalized. Occasionally surgery is indicated as in the case of pelvic abscess or appendicitis. Thrombophlebitis also requires hospitalization for initial medical treatment.

What You Can Do (Self Care)

In cases of fever due to colds and stomach flu, symptomatic treatment of such complaints as headache, diarrhea, or nausea is all that is indicated since the condition goes away by itself. (See individual chapters for these symptoms.) Getting plenty of rest will assist your body's natural defense mechanisms. Tylenol, or aspirin if you are not pregnant, may be used to lower fever, although temperatures between 100 and 101 degrees are not at all serious in otherwise healthy, nonpregnant individuals. Tepid baths may also bring down a fever without the use of drugs. Avoid smoking if

the problem is in the respiratory tract. Gargling with warm salt water is soothing to the throat and often helps decrease throat swelling. You need to replace the fluid lost through sweating when you have a fever. Try drinking a glass of tea, fruit juice, or other beverage at least every two hours. The increased water absorbed will also help to thin out and wash away mucous secretions. Cold steam through the use of a vaporizer is also effective for liquefying secretions and relieving cough. Good nutrition is as important as adequate hydration, because your need for calories increases from a fever, but eat and drink what you feel like. Don't force yourself to eat when you're nauseated. Resist the temptation to have antibiotics prescribed for the common cold or for influenza unless complications occur.

Common ingredients in many drugstore cold and flu remedies include pain relievers, expectorants (to help bring up secretions), and cough suppressants. Two other ingredients, antihistamines (see glossary) and decongestants (see glossary), are often included in cold remedies to reduce mucous secretions. Decongestants are far more effective in relieving symptoms of nasal and sinus congestion compared to antihistamines. In addition, antihistamines may cause unwanted drowsiness. Ingredients in some common over-the-counter drugs for treating cold and flu symptoms are listed in Table 92. Remember that these drugs treat symptoms but do not cure infection itself.

During pregnancy, avoid all drugs unless they are absolutely necessary (see Chapter 31, Drugs and the Pregnant Woman). Even cold remedies should be used cautiously (if at all) in pregnancy and only after consultation with your doctor. Drugs are necessary if you have a culture that indicates strep throat, a chest X-ray indicating pneumonia, or a sinus X-ray showing sinus infection.

64

Hair Growth (Excessive)

Excessive hair growth, called *hirsutism*, is a relatively common complaint among women partly because of our cultural stigma against the presence of hair on certain parts of the body. The quantity and distribution of hair depends on genetic, racial, and hormonal factors. Some families have an inherited tendency to more pronounced hair growth due to increased androgen. Androgen is the primary male sex hormone that is normally present in women in small quantities. Slight increases in androgen account for most cases of hirsutism in women. Often such an increase is a physiologic process during puberty or pregnancy when increased hair growth is temporary.

Another cause of hair growth in women of reproductive age is hormone imbalance. This condition is sometimes associated with irregular or absent periods, acne, obesity, and infertility. Some or all of these factors may be present, but in

HAIR GROWTH

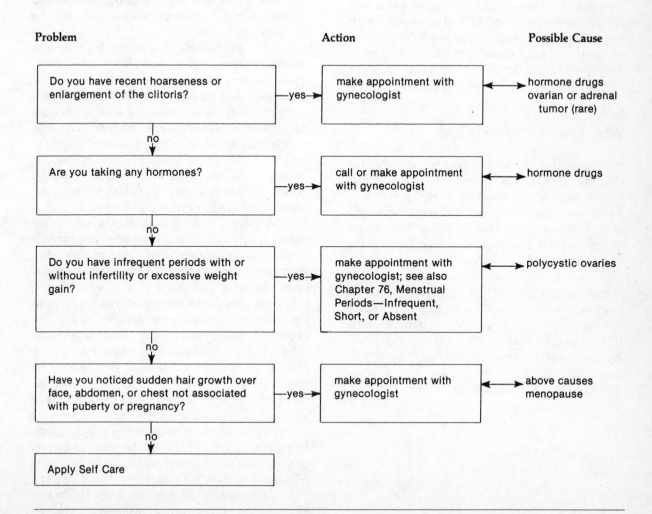

Problem	Action	Possible Cause
Do you have recent hoarseness or enlargement of the clitoris? —yes→	make appointment with gynecologist	hormone drugs ovarian or adrenal tumor (rare)
no ↓		
Are you taking any hormones? —yes→	call or make appointment with gynecologist	hormone drugs
no ↓		
Do you have infrequent periods with or without infertility or excessive weight gain? —yes→	make appointment with gynecologist; see also Chapter 76, Menstrual Periods—Infrequent, Short, or Absent	polycystic ovaries
no ↓		
Have you noticed sudden hair growth over face, abdomen, or chest not associated with puberty or pregnancy? —yes→	make appointment with gynecologist	above causes menopause
no ↓		
Apply Self Care		

any case, dark, coarse hair may appear on the face, abdomen, or chest.

During menopause, the drop in estrogen combined with a rise in androgen account for slightly increased hair growth. Drugs containing androgen, when taken near menopause, may also increase hair growth.

Rarely, an ovarian or adrenal tumor may account for excessive hair growth, sometimes associated with other symptoms such as hoarseness or clitoral enlargement.

What Medical Care Can Do

Since most causes of increased hair growth are due to inherited or physiologic processes, treatment is usually not indicated. Blood tests may be obtained to rule out the possibility of an ovarian or adrenal tumor. The physician may order birth control pills for treatment of hormonal imbalance when hair growth is extreme, especially if associated with acne. Some birth control pills work because the estrogen in them balances the androgen present. Keep in mind that removing the cause of hirsutism may not lead to loss of unwanted hair.

What You Can Do (Self Care)

Remember that hair growth patterns are inherited characteristics and that changing hair growth patterns normally accompany puberty, pregnancy, and menopause. Since these changes are mild and often temporary, the best treatment may be no treatment at all. Some women, however, try using bleaching solutions to lighten the hair color; this procedure is fine as long as the solution does not irritate your skin. Depilatory creams, such as Neet, and wax treatments may help temporarily but they may also cause skin irritations. Electrolysis by a certified technician is costly and may require several treatments to finally be effective. If you are taking any hormones, ask your doctor if this could be contributing to excessive hair growth.

65

Headache

Women seek care for headaches four times as often as men do. Although headache may be caused by head injury or infection, this symptom is due to stress, fatigue, or emotional distress over ninety percent of the time. A chronically suppressed desire to express anger is probably the most common psychological reason for headache. When the resulting inner tension and anger become self-directed, depression is produced and sometimes goes unrecognized as part of the headache symptoms.

Psychological stress can trigger both *tension headaches* and *migraine headaches*, the two basic types. *Tension headaches* are due to a tightening or contraction of the facial or neck muscles. Typical symptoms include a continuous ache or pressure that feels like a band around the head. The neck muscles may be tender, or pain may radiate to the neck or back. These headaches usually last for several hours and sometimes recur chronically. Tension headaches may be triggered by poor posture, eyestrain, or dental problems.

In *migraine headaches*, throbbing pain often starts on one side of the head and then spreads throughout the face and head. Some migraines are severe and may last for several days, accompanied by nausea, vomiting, diarrhea, or nasal stuffiness. Migraines affect some women only once a year or less often and other women twice daily. The average frequency is two or three times each month. Migraine headaches, which may be inherited, affect nearly 30% of all women at some time. Among factors that trigger migraines are changing hormone levels. During, before, and after a period, migraines may occur with increased frequency. Women on birth control pills frequently experience an increase in the severity of pre-existing migraine headaches. Use of birth control pills is not advisable if you suffer from migraines.

Certain foods may trigger migraine headaches: alcoholic beverages such as wine; aged cheeses;

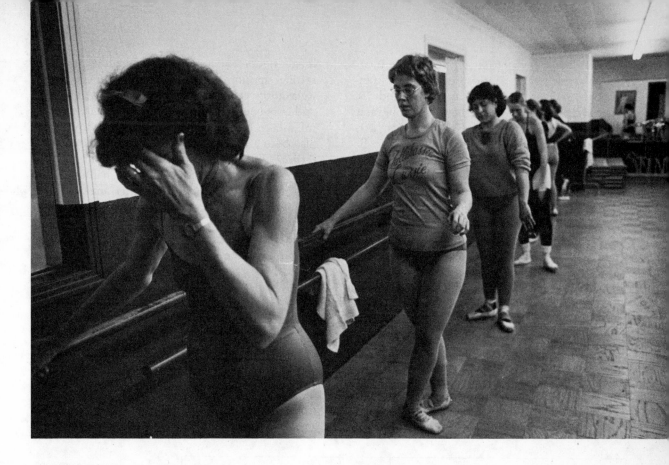

chocolate; citrus fruits; excessive caffeine; nitrate-containing foods such as cold cuts and hot dogs; and food with monosodium glutamate (MSG), which is often used in Chinese foods. In some women, not eating for several hours may set off a migraine as may any change in the pattern of sleep.

Some people experience warning symptoms just prior to a migraine attack. These symptoms frequently occur the same way each time. Such warning symptoms include some or all of the following: irritability, blurred vision, seeing multicolored or bright lights, or more alarming neurological symptoms such as temporary weakness or speech difficulty.

During pregnancy, particularly in the second half, migraine headaches are less common. Headaches experienced in the latter part of pregnancy may be associated with elevated blood pressure and other symptoms of toxemia (see Chapter 20), such as rapid weight gain and fluid retention.

During menopause, migraine headaches often disappear; however, because of irregular hormone levels during menopause, they may occur for the first time. In such cases, migraines usually subside completely in one to two years. Women near the menopause on continuous low doses of estrogen frequently experience a decrease in migraine frequency.

Table 93 shows you the extent to which several factors are involved in tension headaches and in migraine headaches.

What Medical Care Can Do

During the history-taking part of your visit, the clinician may ask questions concerning your family, job, and personal relationships since emotional factors play such an important role in headaches. A thorough head and neck and possibly neurological examination will be performed. X-rays of the skull, sinuses, and neck may be indicated. Occasionally an electroencephalogram (see glossary) is obtained. In general, more complex and costly procedures such as the CAT scan (see glossary) are reserved for atypical and very severe headaches.

Medical therapy for both tension and migraine headaches includes analgesics, antidepressants, tranquilizers, and antimigraine drugs. Over-the-counter analgesics usually contain aspirin or acetaminophen (Tylenol, Datril, etc.). Prescription pain pills for headache often contain multiple ingredients including a narcotic such as codeine or a narcoticlike ingredient like propoxyphene (Darvon, Wygesic, etc.). Antidepressants and tranquilizers are discussed in Chapters 60 and 79, respectively. If your headache is the migraine type, a specific antimigraine drug (which acts directly on the blood vessels in the head) may be the most effective remedy.

What You Can Do (Self Care)

Since emotional factors seem to be associated in most cases of tension and migraine headaches, you can do a lot by just evaluating the stress in your life. Talk about these stresses with your family and close friends. Identify problems and try to take some action. Be sure you are eating enough and as often as needed. Are you working longer hours than your health will allow? Are you setting up unrealistic expectations of yourself? Relaxation exercises, transcendental meditation, and brief counseling have been effective in treating migraines. Biofeedback and acupuncture have also been effective in the short run, but the long-term results are uncertain. Avoid the chronic use of tranquilizers and narcotics. See Chapter 49 for information about over-the-counter analgesics.

For immediate relief, a hot bath may be surprisingly effective. Avoid chronic use of over-the-counter analgesics because these may cause a rebound headache when they are discontinued.

To help prevent migraines, avoid the foods which seem to trigger the attack. If you find that MSG affects you badly and you like eating in Chinese restaurants, don't despair. You can ask that the MSG be withheld from the food you order.

HEADACHE

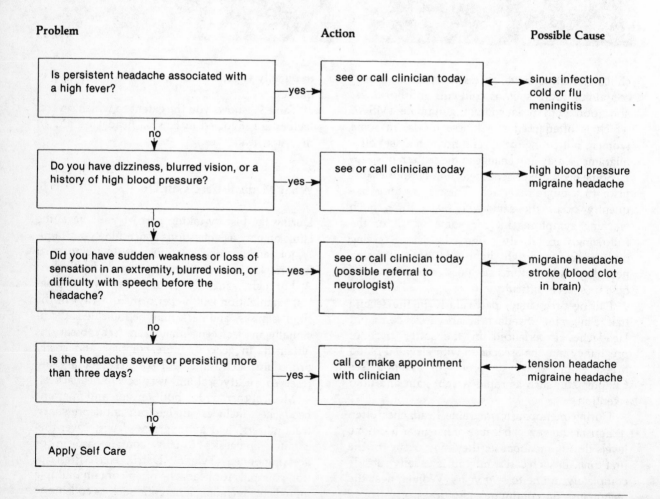

Problem	Action	Possible Cause
Is persistent headache associated with a high fever? —yes→	see or call clinician today	sinus infection, cold or flu, meningitis
↓ no		
Do you have dizziness, blurred vision, or a history of high blood pressure? —yes→	see or call clinician today	high blood pressure, migraine headache
↓ no		
Did you have sudden weakness or loss of sensation in an extremity, blurred vision, or difficulty with speech before the headache? —yes→	see or call clinician today (possible referral to neurologist)	migraine headache, stroke (blood clot in brain)
↓ no		
Is the headache severe or persisting more than three days? —yes→	call or make appointment with clinician	tension headache, migraine headache
↓ no		
Apply Self Care		

Table 93   COMPARISON OF TENSION AND MIGRAINE HEADACHES

Factor	In Tension Headache	In Migraine Headache
pain	continuous bandlike ache or pressure around head	throbbing pain, often limited to one side of the head
duration	lasts a few hours	may last many hours to a few days
accompanying symptoms	none	blurred vision, nausea, diarrhea
occurrence during sleep	rare	sometimes interrupts sleep
caused by psychological stress	often	often
caused by dietary factors	no	sometimes
caused by eyestrain	yes	no
associated with premenstrual tension	occasionally	sometimes
may be inherited	no	yes

66

Heartburn and Gas

Psychological stress plays an important role in causing heartburn and gas. Everyone swallows air to some degree when they eat. But anxiety can lead to excessive air swallowing while eating, thus causing belching and burping. Intestinal gas also comes from normal digestion of food, and the amount of intestinal gas varies from individual to individual and with different foods. In addition, spicy foods, excessive alcohol, and certain drugs

such as aspirin or antiarthritics are well-known causes of heartburn. What you may not know is that chronic dietary indiscretion (that is, continually eating foods that affect you badly, overeating, drinking alcohol to excess, taking too much aspirin, etc.) can eventually cause stomach inflammation called *gastritis*.

Two of the most common medical conditions associated with heartburn are peptic ulcer disease (erosion of the stomach lining) and gallbladder problems. Caused by excessive stomach acids, peptic ulcer disease is commonly associated with a recurrent burning pain felt in the upper middle abdomen under the breastbone; this burning sensation is often relieved by food, milk, or antacids. When a bleeding ulcer develops, the first symptom may be black tarry stools. Gallbladder disease, which is more common among women than men, particularly affects individuals who are over the age of forty and who have a fair complexion. Women who take birth control pills also have a slightly greater frequency of gallbladder disease. The gallbladder is located in the upper abdomen on the right side just beneath the rib cage. When

HEARTBURN AND GAS

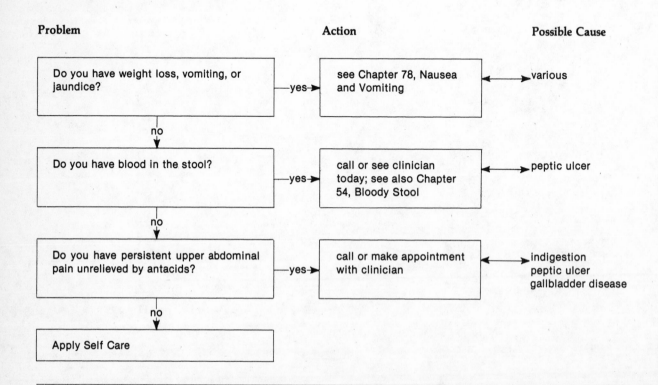

Problem	Action	Possible Cause
Do you have weight loss, vomiting, or jaundice? —yes→	see Chapter 78, Nausea and Vomiting ←→	various
↓ no		
Do you have blood in the stool? —yes→	call or see clinician today; see also Chapter 54, Bloody Stool ←→	peptic ulcer
↓ no		
Do you have persistent upper abdominal pain unrelieved by antacids? —yes→	call or make appointment with clinician ←→	indigestion peptic ulcer gallbladder disease
↓ no		
Apply Self Care		

the gallbladder is inflamed, cramping pain in this location, belching, and burping may occur, particularly after fatty or fried foods are eaten. If stones plug the gallbladder ducts, jaundice (see glossary) may develop and is sometimes associated with fever and severe pain. Heartburn affects 60% of pregnant women and usually starts about midway through pregnancy. This heartburn occurs primarily because the growing uterus impinges on the stomach. The increased frequency of gallstones in the pregnant woman is related to her changing hormones. Peptic ulcer disease, however, is rare in pregnancy because acid secretion in the stomach is actually decreased.

What Medical Care Can Do

The clinician will examine your abdomen and evaluate the pattern of your discomfort as well as your dietary habits. When severe or chronic abdominal pain occurs, an upper GI series (see glossary) or stomach X-ray may be obtained, as well as a gallbladder X-ray. These X-rays are contraindicated in pregnancy except in unusual circumstances. Stool may be tested for microscopic bleeding.

Treatment of many mild digestive disorders does not require prescription drugs. Peptic ulcer disease is commonly managed with antacids and antispasmodic drugs like Pro-Banthine which reduce hyperactivity of the digestive tract. A new drug called Tagamet (cimetidine) has proved useful in treating peptic ulcer. Gallbladder disease ultimately requires surgery for definitive treatment.

What You Can Do (Self Care)

To prevent heartburn, eliminate or reduce the intake or use of stomach irritants, such as coffee, cigarettes, aspirin, and alcohol. You may also want to try eliminating spicy foods for a while. Antacids may be used successfully to relieve heartburn. Antacids containing simethicone or products containing simethicone alone, such as Mylicon, may be used specifically for gas. This symptom can also be controlled by eating slowly and by avoiding gas-producing foods, like beans, cabbage, cucumbers, and any other foods you find cause gas for you. It is important to look for causes of chronic stress in your life which so often

precede the development of an ulcer in the form of recurrent heartburn.

During pregnancy, decrease the size and increase the frequency of meals; and eat a relatively bland diet. If indigestion persists at night, you may sleep with your head propped on pillows or elevate the head of the bed. Avoid drugs, such as tranquilizers, particularly during the first third of pregnancy (see Chapter 31).

67

High Blood Pressure

High blood pressure, called *hypertension*, is being diagnosed in women between the ages of twenty-five and fifty-five with increasing frequency. The condition is more common among women than men. Hypertension is sometimes called "the silent killer" because it has potentially lethal complications, although most people with high blood pressure feel no ill effects in the early stages. Hypertension that remains uncontrolled, however, may lead to severe headaches, blurred vision, damaged blood vessels, and other conditions.

In 85% of women with high blood pressure, no underlying cause for the high blood pressure is found. This situation is known as *essential* *hypertension*, a disease associated with hardening and narrowing of the walls of the blood vessels, a process that occurs with age. In the other 15% of women with high blood pressure, causes such as kidney disease or the use of certain drugs (e.g., estrogens, many diet pills) account for the high blood pressure. Factors associated with an increased risk of high blood pressure include obesity, a family history of high blood pressure, cigarette smoking, diabetes, elevated blood cholesterol, and psychological stress. High blood pressure is a major cause of stroke, heart disease, and kidney failure, especially when these risk factors are present.

During pregnancy, blood pressure is normally unchanged or temporarily decreased because of the hormones that relax blood vessels. Hypertension may develop by itself or represent continuation of previous high blood pressure. High blood pressure in pregnancy is rarely severe enough to warrant abortion. However, sterilization may be medically indicated when blood pressure elevation is especially high or when complications involving the heart or kidneys occur.

What Medical Care Can Do

The clinician will check your blood pressure

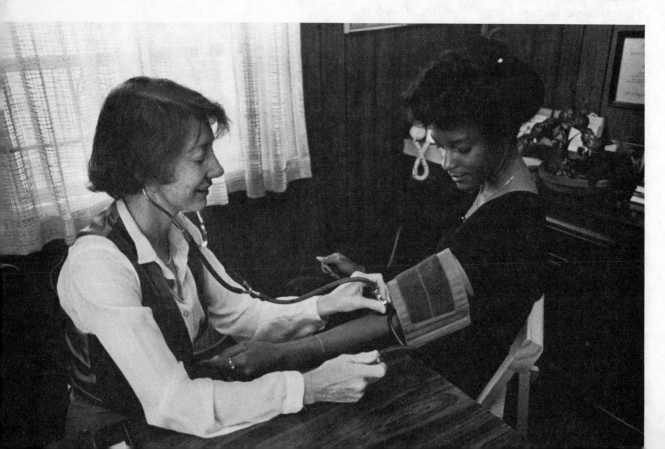

HIGH BLOOD PRESSURE

Problem	Action	Possible Cause

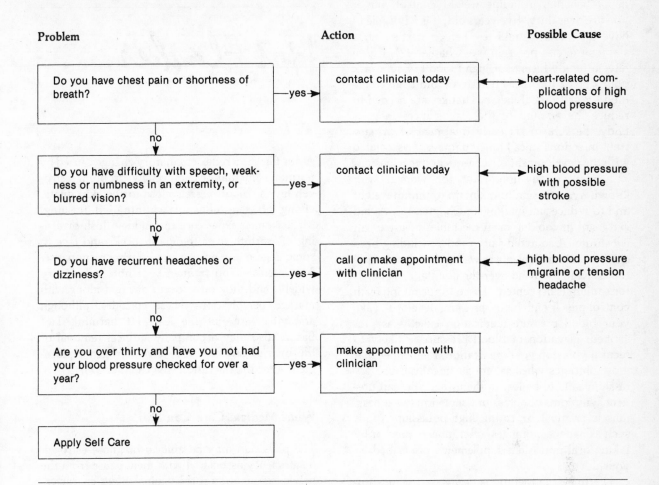

Problem	Action	Possible Cause
Do you have chest pain or shortness of breath?	—yes→ contact clinician today	←→ heart-related complications of high blood pressure
↓ no		
Do you have difficulty with speech, weakness or numbness in an extremity, or blurred vision?	—yes→ contact clinician today	←→ high blood pressure with possible stroke
↓ no		
Do you have recurrent headaches or dizziness?	—yes→ call or make appointment with clinician	←→ high blood pressure migraine or tension headache
↓ no		
Are you over thirty and have you not had your blood pressure checked for over a year?	—yes→ make appointment with clinician	
↓ no		
Apply Self Care		

several times, first in one arm and then in the other, while you are lying down and again while you are sitting. Since blood pressure varies with activity, emotions, and posture, it is important to evaluate blood pressure after you have been sitting or resting quietly for at least five minutes. Several elevated blood pressures are required to confirm a diagnosis of high blood pressure. In general, physicians consider a blood pressure of 120/80 or less normal; 140/90 causes suspicion of hypertension. And elevation to 160/95 or more, even intermittently in the office, almost certainly indicates the presence of at least mild hypertension.

During the physical exam, the clinician examines your eyes to look for blood vessel changes that occur with high blood pressure and evaluates your heart, lungs, and pulse. He may obtain an electrocardiogram (EKG) (see glossary), a chest X-ray, blood tests, and a urinalysis. These tests

are often completely normal unless complications of high blood pressure have begun to occur. Once the physician diagnoses hypertension, he or she prescribes diuretics (water pills) or other drugs that lower blood pressure. Drug therapy controls but usually does not cure high blood pressure unless a correctable underlying cause is found. In pregnancy, the treatment of hypertension consists of bed rest and may necessitate early delivery by induction of labor if high blood pressure becomes severe (see Chapters 20 and 21).

What You Can Do (Self Care)

Nearly half of the people who have high blood pressure don't know they have it, so you should have your blood pressure checked at least once a year after the age of thirty. Reduce as many risk factors as possible. Don't smoke and do keep your weight under control. Certainly, exercise has many benefits, including weight control, but if you are over thirty-five years old, it is advisable to have an exercise stress test before starting on a serious exercise program (see Chapter 47). If you have a family history of high blood pressure, ask your doctor to order cholesterol and triglyceride blood tests to see if dietary changes are needed to reduce the amount of these substances in your body. Be sure to get early treatment of urinary tract infections since kidney damage is associated with the development of subsequent hypertension.

It is especially important for women with known hypertension to maintain optimum weight and to reduce salt intake (see Chapter 46). Avoid extra salt in cooking or at the table, or use a salt substitute. Also avoid salty foods, including hard cheeses and lunch meats as well as other processed foods. Read food and over-the-counter drug labels for sodium (salt) content. Discontinue taking birth control pills if high blood pressure develops. Take your blood pressure medication exactly as prescribed; elevation of blood pressure is likely to recur if you stop your medication. Remember that most diuretics when taken chronically cause potassium salts to be lost in the urine. You can prevent symptoms of potassium depletion (weakness, muscle cramps) by eating high-potassium foods such as bananas, oranges, or cranberry juice or by taking oral potassium supplements prescribed by your doctor.

Lifetime drug therapy is necessary for most individuals with hypertension. The best way to prevent hypertension complications (such as heart disease) in the long run is to adopt a life style that minimizes as many risk factors as possible, especially in the areas of smoking, obesity, diet, and chronic stress (see Chapter 45). Consider purchasing a blood pressure cuff and learning from your doctor or a nurse how you or a family member can check your blood pressure at home.

For more information about high blood pressure, write to:

High Blood Pressure Information Center
120/80 National Institutes of Health
Bethesda, Maryland 20205

68

Hot Flashes

A *hot flash* is a reflex circulatory change caused by hormone fluctuations, especially dropping estrogen levels. Blood vessels close to the skin dilate, giving off sensations of warmth and flushing. Most women experience the sudden flush or feeling of warmth over the chest, neck, and face to some degree just prior to and during menopause. The intensity and frequency of hot flashes vary widely, and they often occur at night along with marked perspiration. These episodes, although annoying, are not the least bit harmful. Hot flashes also may accompany surgical removal of the ovaries unless you receive estrogen replacement after the operation (see Chapter 27).

What Medical Care Can Do

The physician may be able to diagnose estrogen insufficiency associated with menopause from the pelvic examination if the vagina shows characteristic thinning and paleness. The most reliable blood tests to diagnose the problem are the levels of certain brain hormones—FSH and LH (see glossary). These brain hormones reach a high level in the blood as menopause approaches (see Chapter 26).

The use of estrogen in treating symptoms of menopause is discussed in Chapter 27. The use of tranquilizers to treat hot flashes alone is not recommended.

What You Can Do (Self Care)

For ease and comfort, wear loose and layered clothing so you can take off outer layers during a hot flash. Some women find it helps to drink a glass of ice water immediately after a hot flash.

It helps to realize that menopausal symptoms do not represent anything wrong and that these

HOT FLASHES

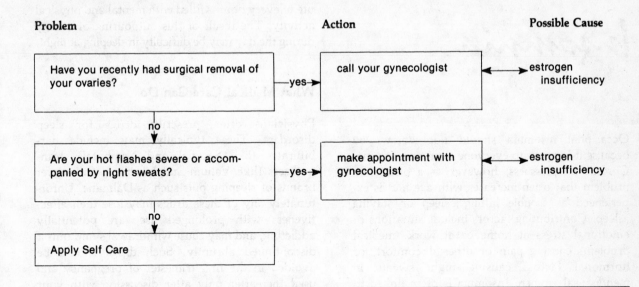

Problem	Action	Possible Cause
Have you recently had surgical removal of your ovaries?	—yes→ call your gynecologist	← → estrogen insufficiency
↓ no		
Are your hot flashes severe or accompanied by night sweats?	—yes→ make appointment with gynecologist	← → estrogen insufficiency
↓ no		
Apply Self Care		

temporary symptoms just mark one of the many natural changes which occur in the lifetime of all women. If you are taking hormone replacement, tell your clinician about the occurrence of any side effects of these pills, such as abnormal bleeding.

69

Insomnia

Occasional insomnia should not worry you because it happens to everyone from time to time. Chronic sleeplessness, however, is a distressing problem that often increases with age and is experienced as trouble falling asleep or staying asleep. Contributing factors include situations of emotional stress at home or at work, medical problems causing pain or other discomfort, or hormonal factors causing night sweats in menopausal women. Insomnia is often linked to common symptoms of depression such as daytime napping, inability to concentrate, loss of appetite, and loss of sexual desire. Some women by necessity or choice arrange their lives so that every minute of every hour is filled with mental and physical activity. The result of this outpouring of energy during the day may be difficulty in sleeping at night.

What Medical Care Can Do

Physicians often prescribe drugs for sleep disorders. These typically may include barbiturates (like Seconal and Nembutal), tranquilizers (like Valium and Librium), and newer brands of sleeping pills such as Dalmane. Unfortunately any of these drugs may lose their effectiveness with prolonged use, are potentially addicting, and may cause withdrawal symptoms if discontinued abruptly. Such drugs should be avoided in the first trimester of pregnancy and used thereafter only after discussion with your doctor. One of the safest sleeping pills to use in

INSOMNIA

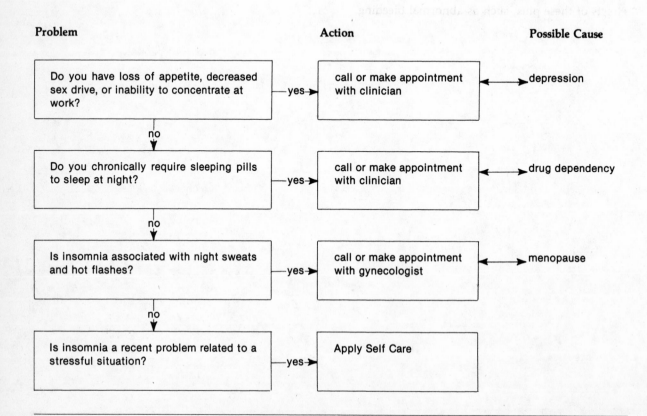

Problem	Action	Possible Cause
Do you have loss of appetite, decreased sex drive, or inability to concentrate at work? —yes→	call or make appointment with clinician ←→	depression
↓ no		
Do you chronically require sleeping pills to sleep at night? —yes→	call or make appointment with clinician ←→	drug dependency
↓ no		
Is insomnia associated with night sweats and hot flashes? —yes→	call or make appointment with gynecologist ←→	menopause
↓ no		
Is insomnia a recent problem related to a stressful situation? —yes→	Apply Self Care	

pregnancy is the antihistamine Benadryl, a less potent but more extensively studied drug than many other drugs currently used for this purpose. When depression causes insomnia, the doctor may prescribe antidepressant medication, preferably in combination with some form of counseling to help identify your underlying emotional conflicts. Like tranquilizers, antidepressant medication improves your symptoms only as long as you take the drug.

What You Can Do (Self Care)

Women vary in the amount of sleep needed, which may be more or less than eight hours a night. Some women are "day people" and prefer to go to bed early and rise early. Other women are "night people" who feel better if they sleep during the day and stay awake at night. The important thing is not when or how long, but how well you sleep. Here are some suggestions:

1. Avoid stimulants such as coffee, tea, cola, and amphetamine-type drugs two or three hours (or even longer) before going to bed. Also avoid large meals at this time since the digestive process can interfere with sleep. Some people find that a glass of warm milk is an effective sleep tonic. A hot bath each night before you go to bed may also help you relax.
2. Try to develop regular sleeping habits. Sleep at the same time and the same place every night in a comfortable bed. Plan to get to sleep within a half hour after lying down. Use your bedroom for sleeping and not for working activities.
3. Establish a quiet activity, such as reading, prior to going to bed. Avoid big decisions or family worries at this time. As you go to sleep, develop a habit of thinking of pleasurable plans or events which bring you happiness.
4. Avoid daytime napping.
5. Avoid chronic use of tranquilizers or alcohol to help with insomnia for the reasons mentioned above.
6. Plan for regular, daily exercise (see Chapter 47).

70

Itching, Rash, and Skin Pigmentation

Common Causes of Itching

One of the most common causes of itching is dry skin. As we grow older, our skin thins and decreases its capacity to retain moisture, causing dry skin. At other times itching may be localized, as in the case of rectal hemorrhoids. Emotional factors also play an important role in itching and, in some instances, may be the only identifiable cause. Other common causes of itching in women fall into three categories: allergy-related conditions, conditions causing vaginal itching, and drug reactions.

Allergy-related conditions

Allergy in the form of itching or rash is one way the body reacts to a foreign substance or an irritant. Hives and contact dermatitis are common skin conditions which may be allergic reactions. Women who acquire contact dermatitis or hives usually have a history of other allergic conditions such as asthma or hay fever.

Hives appear as pink, itchy skin swellings which represent a generalized reaction of the skin to a local irritant such as an insect bite, or to an ingested substance such as strawberries or a drug. Occasionally hives are induced by emotional tension or excitement.

Contact dermatitis is a common type of eczema or skin inflammation causing itching, burning, or stinging from contact with chemicals or other irritants such as poison oak. Skin blisters develop first; then they ooze and ultimately crust and flake in this process. There is always a potential for infection whenever the skin is broken. Your skin may be sensitive to any number of ordinary substances: soaps, detergents, metal, jewelry, creams, and so on. The affected area gives a clue to the cause of contact dermatitis. For instance, a scalp rash may be caused by a hair dye; a rash at the base of one finger could indicate sensitivity to the metal in a ring.

Conditions causing vaginal itching

This itching can be one of the most agonizing symptoms affecting women. The most common cause is a vaginal infection, especially yeast (see Chapter 85). Itching without discharge may represent an allergic reaction to a new soap, vaginal contraceptive foam, or a prescribed vaginal cream or suppository.

Infectious causes of itching without vaginal discharge include lice and scabies. These infestations are characterized by severe itching, often at night, of the pubic area. Although they are not life-threatening, lice and scabies are highly communicable and very much a nuisance. Both conditions are usually acquired through close personal contact though not necessarily through intercourse.

Pubic and scalp lice live on hair and skin; body lice are found in clothing. Lice infection is probably the only disease that is readily acquired from sitting on a contaminated toilet seat. The usual way of getting pubic lice, however, is through close physical contact, especially during intercourse.

Scabies produces itching in warm, moist areas of the body, particularly around the external genitalia. The organism, *Sarcoptes scabiei*, is about the size of a pinhead and burrows in the skin, making little tunnels that look like pencil dots.

In older women, a disorder called vulvar dystrophy is a major cause of intense itching of the external genitalia. Dystrophy causes thinning and shrinkage of the vulva, resulting in painful intercourse. A combination of infections and allergic factors, along with decreasing levels of estrogen, contribute to this condition.

Occasionally chronic vaginal itching may be the first symptom of cancer of the vulva. This disease should be suspected in a woman over the age of fifty when prolonged use of vaginal creams is unsuccessful in relieving her symptoms.

Table 94 summarizes the causes and method of diagnosis of vaginal itching.

Table 94 VAGINAL ITCHING— CAUSES AND DIAGNOSIS

Cause of Vaginal Itching	How Diagnosed
Vaginal infection (usually yeast)	microscopic examination of secretions
Skin disease (e.g., psoriasis)	characteristic skin changes not restricted to vulva
Diabetes	glucose tolerance test
Dystrophy of vulva	biopsy of suspected area of vulva
Infestation (scabies, lice)	finding an organism
Allergic reaction	history of use of vaginal hygiene or contraceptive product, new soap, or condom
Psychological stress	emotional factors predominate; other causes ruled out
Cancer of the vulva	biopsy of vulva

Drug reactions

Itching and rash are the most common forms of drug reaction. Almost any drug may produce nearly any type of rash. The rash may occur suddenly after the drug is taken and involve the entire body. Or the onset may be gradual with the rash beginning on, say, the abdomen. With repeated exposure to a drug, the chance of an allergic reaction is more likely. Sun exposure will increase the chance of a reaction to some drugs, such as diuretics (water pills), barbiturates, mood elevators, tetracycline, and sulfa. The tendency to develop a drug rash following sun exposure is known as photosensitivity.

Birth control pills may occasionally cause a rash, but the principal skin effect is increased pigmentation, that is, darkening of the skin, particularly over the face. This occurs in up to 30% of women on birth control pills. Pigmentation may persist even if the birth control pills are discontinued.

In pregnancy, itching is the most common complaint related to the skin. Itching, sometimes accompanied by a fine, red rash over the abdomen, is more common in the second half of pregnancy. The itching goes away after delivery but may come back with subsequent pregnancies or after birth control pills are started. These symptoms are probably due to increased levels of estrogen.

The most common skin change in pregnancy is an increase in pigmentation which occurs over the face (known as chloasma), nipples, and lower abdomen (*linea nigra*). Chloasma, or increased facial pigmentation similar to that produced by the pill, is known as the *mask of pregnancy* and affects over 50% of pregnant women, particularly brunettes. This type of pigmentation usually fades after pregnancy. Other common skin changes occurring in pregnancy include the formation of stretch marks, or striae, increased size and pigmentation of moles, and increased sweating. About 10% of women develop reddish skin spots

ITCHING AND RASH

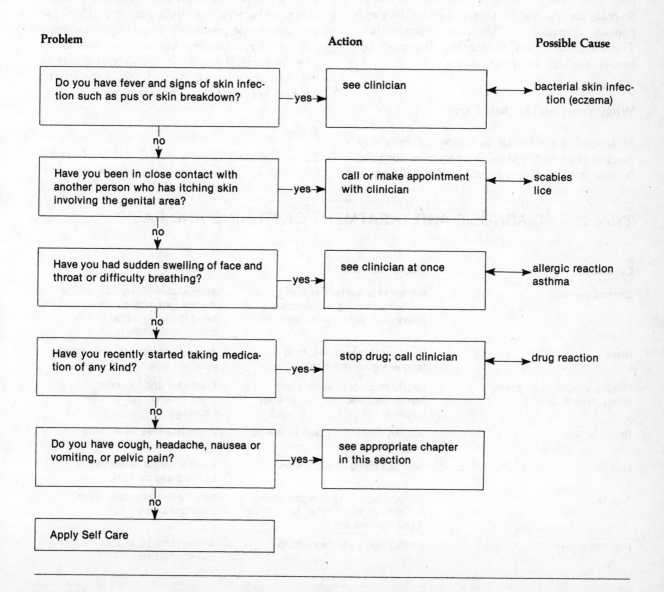

Problem	Action	Possible Cause
Do you have fever and signs of skin infection such as pus or skin breakdown? —yes→	see clinician	bacterial skin infection (eczema)
no ↓		
Have you been in close contact with another person who has itching skin involving the genital area? —yes→	call or make appointment with clinician	scabies lice
no ↓		
Have you had sudden swelling of face and throat or difficulty breathing? —yes→	see clinician at once	allergic reaction asthma
no ↓		
Have you recently started taking medication of any kind? —yes→	stop drug; call clinician	drug reaction
no ↓		
Do you have cough, headache, nausea or vomiting, or pelvic pain? —yes→	see appropriate chapter in this section	
no ↓		
Apply Self Care		

on the face, neck, and upper chest. These spots are dilated blood vessels which may have a spidery appearance. Most of these skin spots also disappear after delivery.

What Medical Care Can Do

The clinician will ask you about previous allergy to food or drugs, recent contacts with new chemicals or cosmetics, and a history of skin disease. The diagnosis is usually made from the characteristics and location of the skin lesion. Treatment is often nonspecific, involving antihistamines or sedatives to alleviate itching and antibiotics to prevent secondary bacterial infections. Steroids are reserved for severe cases of hives and contact dermatitis to decrease inflammation. Treatment of vulvar dystrophy, diagnosed by biopsy, includes hormone creams.

What You Can Do (Self Care)

In general, it's essential to follow carefully any medical regimen the physician prescribes for you. If you are treating yourself, start with small amounts of a cream or salve to be sure you are not allergic to it. Stop any drug that seems to produce a local irritation or an allergic response. Don't take a drug which previously caused a rash because subsequent reactions may be more serious. Taking over-the-counter antiinflammatory cream (hydrocortisone) or antihistamines on a short-term basis may help to control itching.

Some suggestions are given below for specific problems.

Contact dermatitis

Cooling baths to which two tablespoons of baking soda are added may be helpful. Minimize heat and keep the area clean. Avoid scratching irritated skin since bacterial infections can occur. Don't use substances that previously caused skin reactions. Use only hypoallergenic cosmetics or none at all when possible. If you think your detergent may be the cause, wash out your clothes with baking soda, to get rid of the detergent.

Hives

Take cornstarch or oatmeal baths (Aveeno Oatmeal works well and is available over-the-

---

Table 95   DIAGNOSIS AND TREATMENT OF ITCHING AND RASH

Condition	Diagnostic Features	Treatment
Contact dermatitis	Recent skin contact with an irritant or allergy-causing substance, e.g., poison oak, detergents, cosmetics	Antihistamines; various topical medications may be prescribed; avoid irritants; cornstarch or baking soda baths
Hives	History of insect bites; drug or food allergies; emotional stress	Antihistamines; cornstarch baths; calamine lotion
Fungus infections (of scalp, hands, feet, body)	Localized chronic scaling and itching patches over part of body involved	Keep skin dry; Tinactin; prescription drugs may be necessary
Drug reaction	Sudden generalized rash following drug use	Antihistamines; avoid drug
Lice	Intense itching of pubic area	Kwell lotion or cream; wash bedding and clothing
Scabies	Itching, especially at night, often involving genitals; other family members involved	Kwell lotion or cream; wash bedding and clothing
Pregnancy rash	Itching over abdomen with rash	Antihistamines; low-fat diet; cornstarch baths

counter with directions), and smooth on calamine lotion after bathing.

Lice and scabies

Be sure all family members and other possible contacts are treated and that all bedding and clothing are laundered or dry-cleaned. Kwell is the drug of choice and a prescription may be called in to your drugstore by a physician. If you use Kwell shampoo, repeat the shampoo in twenty-four hours. If you use Kwell cream or lotion, leave it on for twenty-four hours. Do not use Kwell during pregnancy without physician supervision as it may harm the fetus.

Dry skin

If you have dry skin, never use strong soaps or bubble baths. Small amounts of bath oil, such as Alpha Keri, may be helpful. Excessive bathing should be avoided and may itself cause itching if you have dry skin. Over-the-counter products for dry skin may contain many ingredients, including estrogen, which increases the water-holding capacity of skin. However, the FDA limits the amount of hormone that can be contained in these cosmetics, and they have no effect on the course of dry-skin conditions. Much of the effectiveness of estrogen-containing creams, and any decrease in wrinkles, are due to the cream's base, rather than to the hormone itself.

Pregnancy itching and rash

Oral or topical Benadryl relieves itching; your physician can call your drugstore and order a prescription. Cornstarch baths may also be helpful. A low-fat diet may help by putting less strain on the liver. If yellow pigmentation involving skin or eyes occurs (jaundice), contact your clinician.

Table 95 summarizes the diagnosis and treatment of itching and rash.

71

Joint Pains

Recurrent joint pains in women are usually due to one of the many forms of arthritis which afflict women. Arthritis is an inflammation in the area called the joint, where two bones meet. A capsule containing lubricating fluid encases all the body's joints. Swelling and inflammation within the joint capsule may cause stiffness, rigidity, and pain upon movement. Eventually a scar between the bones may develop, resulting in joint deformity. These processes occur regardless of the cause of the arthritis.

Rheumatoid arthritis, a chronic condition with some family predisposition, afflicts 75% of women, often beginning in a woman's reproductive years. The most painful and disabling form of arthritis in women, rheumatoid arthritis typically begins as a chronic nonfebrile (no fever) condition associated with fatigue, loss of appetite, and aching joints. Joint stiffness occurs in the morning but usually subsides during the day. Joints of the hands, feet, and ankles are commonly affected. Occasionally other organs are involved, causing anemia, rash, or diarrhea. This disease is usually progressive but controllable; early treatment may prevent deformities.

Osteoarthritis, a degenerative disease which occurs as a result of aging, is increasingly common after age fifty. The weight-bearing joints, such as the hip and back, are affected as are the joints in the ends of the fingers, which may become enlarged, stiff, and painful. Joint stiffness occurs at the end of the day with osteoarthritis, which is milder than rheumatoid arthritis and does not usually involve other parts of the body.

Infectious arthritis may result from a bacterial infection such as gonorrhea, causing an acute inflammation of one or more joints, sometimes associated with a rash. Joint deformity does not occur.

Systemic lupus erythematosus is the most common of several conditions known collectively as

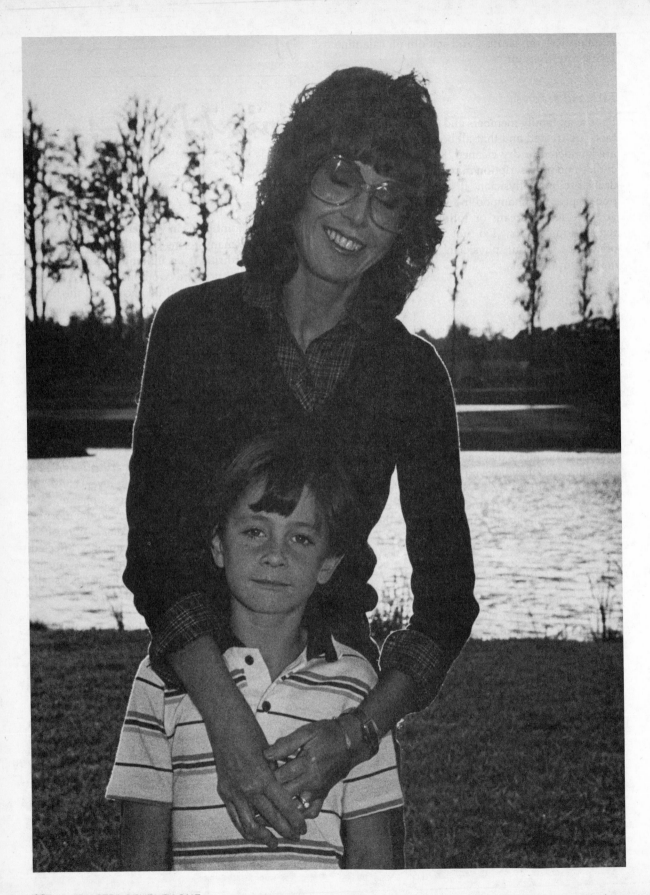

connective-tissue or *auto-immune disease*. Lupus, as it is sometimes called, affects women almost exclusively, often during the early childbearing years. The cause of lupus, which may affect varied areas of the body such as the skin, blood, and kidneys, is unknown.

Traumatic joint injury due to vigorous exercise or strenuous sports activity may damage the ligaments and tendons. The knees, elbows, and shoulders are most commonly affected. These conditions, as well as muscle strains, must be distinguished from arthritis.

Rheumatoid arthritis has no known deleterious effect on pregnancy, fertility, or the fetus. No one knows why rheumatoid arthritis often gets better during pregnancy and then worsens during the postpartum period. Systemic lupus erythematosus has a variable course during pregnancy but becomes worse during the postpartum period in

many women. The treatment of lupus requires powerful antiinflammatory drugs called steroids which may be necessary during pregnancy to control the disease. Unless severe, lupus is not a medical indication for termination of pregnancy or for sterilization.

What Medical Care Can Do

The physician will examine the affected joints for movement and localized swelling or tenderness. He or she may order specific lab tests to distinguish arthritis from other disorders or to differentiate among the types of arthritis. A cervix culture is obtained if gonorrhea is suspected. X-rays can determine the extent of disease and can follow the course of chronic arthritis.

Treatment of arthritis varies depending on the

JOINT PAIN

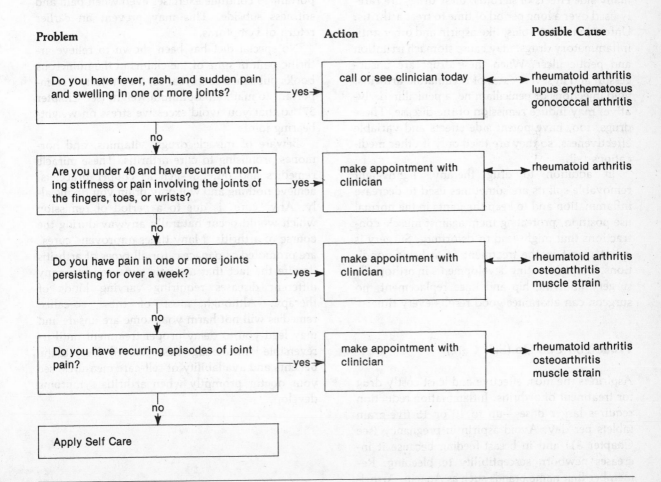

Problem	Action	Possible Cause
Do you have fever, rash, and sudden pain and swelling in one or more joints? —yes→	call or see clinician today	rheumatoid arthritis lupus erythematosus gonococcal arthritis
no ↓		
Are you under 40 and have recurrent morning stiffness or pain involving the joints of the fingers, toes, or wrists? —yes→	make appointment with clinician	rheumatoid arthritis
no ↓		
Do you have pain in one or more joints persisting for over a week? —yes→	make appointment with clinician	rheumatoid arthritis osteoarthritis muscle strain
no ↓		
Do you have recurring episodes of joint pain? —yes→	make appointment with clinician	rheumatoid arthritis osteoarthritis muscle strain
no ↓		
Apply Self Care		

cause, and in the case of severe forms a rheumatologist, or specialist in arthritis, may be consulted. The physician prescribes antibiotics for infectious forms of arthritis. In most other cases, treatment usually begins with aspirin because of its antiinflammatory properties. If aspirin is ineffective, the doctor may prescribe one of the antiinflammatory drugs for arthritis.

Recently many new drugs for treating arthritis have become available. These include Motrin, Tolectin, Naprosyn, Nalfon, and Clinoril. Presumably these newer antiinflammatory drugs have fewer side effects, like ulcer formation, intestinal bleeding, impairment of vision or hearing, and other reactions, compared to earlier drugs in this group such as Indocin. Nevertheless any antiinflammatory medication can be hazardous and requires close medical supervision for adverse side effects.

Steroids, the most potent of the antiinflammatory drugs, are used for treatment of the connective-tissue disorders, but because of the many side effects of steroids, these drugs are rarely used over a long period of time to treat arthritis. Unfortunately steroids, like aspirin and other antiinflammatory drugs, may cause stomach irritation and peptic ulcer. When these drugs are unsuccessful and in severe cases of rheumatoid arthritis, gold injections or penicillamine, a penicillin derivative, may induce remission of the disease. These drugs, too, have potent side effects and variable effectiveness, so they are tried only if other medications fail.

In addition to drug therapy, lightweight removable splints are sometimes used to decrease inflammation and to keep the joints in the normal use position, protecting them against muscle contractions that might lead to deformity. Surgery is a last resort in the treatment of arthritic conditions. Despite exciting developments in orthopedic surgery allowing hip and knee replacement, no surgeon can guarantee good results every time.

What You Can Do (Self Care)

Aspirin is the most effective and least costly drug for treatment of arthritis. Inflammation reduction requires larger doses—up to 10 or 15 five-grain tablets per day. Avoid aspirin in pregnancy (see Chapter 31) and in breast-feeding because it increases newborn susceptibility to bleeding. Remember that name brands such as Anacin, Arthri-

tis Pain Formula, and Arthritis Strength Bufferin cost more than generic aspirin. The chance of stomach irritation is reduced by taking aspirin-containing drugs with meals or with a glass of milk.

Heat in the form of hot baths, especially in the morning, is effective as are hot water bottles and heating pads.

A proper balance of rest and exercise is essential. Regular rest is particularly important with rheumatoid arthritis since flare-ups often occur during fatigue. When flare-ups do occur, bed rest is indicated. Exercise can be good or bad depending on the type of arthritis. Since arthritis affects each woman differently, there is no one program suitable for all. The most helpful exercise allows joints to move slowly through their full range of motion with no resistance. Swimming in a heated pool accomplishes this. Avoid exercises or activity which requires twisting, bending, jarring, or stooping. Jogging or other strenuous athletics may place strain on the ankle and knee joints. It is important to continue exercises even when pain and stiffness subside. This may prevent an earlier return of symptoms.

No special diet has been shown to relieve arthritic pain in spite of the claims in the numerous books published each year on the subject. It is important to maintain optimum weight (see Chapter 87) so that you avoid excessive stress on weight-bearing joints.

Beware of miracle drugs, vitamins, and hormones promising to cure arthritis. These miracle remedies and others, such as copper bracelets, achieve nothing and will only drain you financially. Any "cure" is due to a period of remission which would occur naturally anyway during the course of arthritis. Many times unproven "cures" are promoted as panaceas for all types of arthritis despite the fact that arthritis is caused by many different diseases requiring varying kinds of therapy. Although most of these so-called remedies will not harm you, some are unsafe and may lead you to delay proper treatment until irreversible joint damage has occurred. Despite the benefits and availability of self-care measures, see your doctor promptly when arthritis symptoms develop.

72

Leg Aches and Pains

In the nonpregnant woman, leg aches and pains are likely to be related to strenuous exercise, varicose veins, or low back problems. Daily exercise, such as jogging, may lead to aching in both calves as a result of muscle strain. When a person stands for a prolonged period of time, poor circulation in blood vessels returning blood to the heart from the lower extremities (a condition resulting from varicose veins) may cause leg aches or cramps. A tendency toward varicose veins is largely inherited. Varicose veins, which afflict women far more frequently than men, may predispose one to blood clots in the leg (thrombophlebitis) but, unless severe, are not usually considered a contraindication to the use of birth control pills. Low back pain may be associated with pain down the backs of both legs (see Chapter 49). In the postmenopausal woman early signs of diminished circulation to the lower legs may include calf pain brought on by walking and relieved by rest.

During pregnancy, leg cramps may result from varicose veins or from mineral problems—usually a deficiency of calcium or an excess of dietary phosphorus. Since high levels of phosphorus are found in meat, cheese, and milk, increasing the intake of these foods does not prevent and may even worsen this symptom. Leg cramps may occur while the woman is lying down and may awaken her from sleep, particularly after the first three months of pregnancy.

Varicose veins contribute to leg cramps during pregnancy because the growing uterus may affect blood circulation to and from the legs. Varicose veins tend to become worse as pregnancy progresses and may involve the vulva, producing an aching sensation. Severe varicosities afflict fewer than 20% of pregnant women and subside promptly following delivery. With subsequent pregnancies, varicose veins tend to become more severe and produce symptoms earlier.

What Medical Care Can Do

The clinician will examine your legs for signs of inflammation, range of motion, and the presence of varicose veins. X-rays may be necessary to rule out a fracture if trauma has occurred. Often the problem is one of muscle strain, and muscle relaxants or narcotic pain medication may be prescribed. They should be used sparingly and are best avoided completely in pregnancy. The treatment of severe varicose veins may require surgery in the nonpregnant woman.

What You Can Do (Self Care)

In nonpregnant women, acute muscle pains tend to be temporary, mild, and often related to muscle strain. These conditions are self-curing with time, rest, heat, and drugstore analgesics. Liniments containing methylsalicylate may provide some relief from muscle spasm.

Both pregnant and nonpregnant women with varicosities may benefit from the use of elastic stockings, frequent elevation of the legs, and avoidance of prolonged sitting or standing.

During pregnancy, the application of heat and massage and a diet which moderately restricts high-phosphorus foods may help leg cramps. Restrict meat to one or two servings a day and milk to one pint a day if symptoms are severe. If leg cramping persists, ask your doctor to prescribe calcium lactate, 600 milligrams, taken three times a day before meals. If necessary, you might ask your physician about the special support devised for pregnant women with severe vulvar varicosities.

LEG ACHES AND PAINS

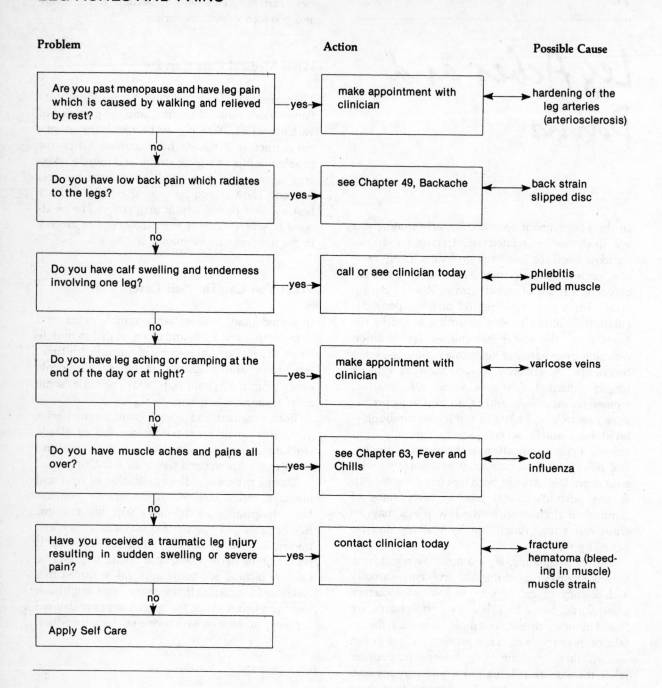

Problem	Action	Possible Cause
Are you past menopause and have leg pain which is caused by walking and relieved by rest?	—yes→ make appointment with clinician	hardening of the leg arteries (arteriosclerosis)
↓ no		
Do you have low back pain which radiates to the legs?	—yes→ see Chapter 49, Backache	back strain slipped disc
↓ no		
Do you have calf swelling and tenderness involving one leg?	—yes→ call or see clinician today	phlebitis pulled muscle
↓ no		
Do you have leg aching or cramping at the end of the day or at night?	—yes→ make appointment with clinician	varicose veins
↓ no		
Do you have muscle aches and pains all over?	—yes→ see Chapter 63, Fever and Chills	cold influenza
↓ no		
Have you received a traumatic leg injury resulting in sudden swelling or severe pain?	—yes→ contact clinician today	fracture hematoma (bleeding in muscle) muscle strain
↓ no		
Apply Self Care		

73

Lethargy

All of us feel lethargic now and then. Most of the time a little extra relaxation and sleep will clear up this fatigue. If it doesn't, you may want to consider other causes. Persistent lethargy without other apparent symptoms is often due, for example, to depression. Look for these symptoms that suggest depression: poor ability to concentrate, morning fatigue or headache, loss of appetite, decreased sex drive, and insomnia. Lethargy may also be a sign of one of numerous underlying conditions, from the common cold to cancer. You should see your doctor if lethargy is associated with a chronic cough, weight loss, persistent pelvic pain, or change in bowel habits. Sometimes low thyroid conditions (hypothyroidism) begin with lethargy associated with dry skin, brittle nails, and thinning of the hair. An occasional cause of persistent lethargy in young women is mononucleosis, which initially presents itself as a mild sore throat and fever.

In women, two major causes of lethargy are hypoglycemia and anemia. You are probably familiar with hypoglycemia, or low blood sugar, because this condition has been extensively covered in the press in recent years. Hypoglycemia is frequently confused with anxiety or depression since all of these conditions may produce fatigue, headache, mental sluggishness, and an inability to concentrate, as well as palpitations, sweating, hunger, and tremor. Often hypoglycemia afflicts women with premenstrual syndrome (see Chapter 82). In early pregnancy, many women tend to get hypoglycemia as a result of the frequency of nausea and vomiting and because the fetus selectively uses maternal carbohydrates for nutrition and growth at this time.

Anemia due to iron deficiency is probably the most frequent medical condition causing fatigue or lethargy in women. This is due usually either to heavy periods or to bleeding somewhere in the digestive tract. In women beyond the menopause, severe iron-deficiency anemia is likely to be due to stomach ulcers or an intestinal tumor. Iron-deficiency anemia may go unnoticed when it is mild or occurs gradually over several weeks or months. Chronic blood loss results in compensatory adjustments in the body's circulation as well as in increased production of blood cells so that symptoms of lethargy and weakness are minimal. For this reason, your blood count should be checked at least once a year, especially if you are over forty. A hemoglobin of less than 11 grams would be considered moderate anemia.

Iron-deficiency anemia affects well over half of all pregnancies. It is more common in women who have had more than one baby, especially when the pregnancies have been closely spaced. This deficiency happens because the build-up of maternal iron stores following childbirth takes several months. The amount of dietary iron which can be absorbed from the stomach is limited, averaging only about 20% of the ingested amount. During pregnancy, there are increased iron needs. The need for supplemental iron is greatest during the second half of pregnancy and continues through lactation in women who breast-feed.

The second most common form of anemia in pregnancy is folic-acid deficiency. In women eating a well-balanced diet, including green leafy vegetables, folic-acid deficiency is rare. Although folic acid is included in most prenatal vitamins, it is probably unnecessary for most women.

Sickle-cell anemia (see glossary) tends to become much more severe during pregnancy and predisposes the woman with sickle-cell disease to crisis as well as to increased rates of miscarriage, stillbirth, and premature labor.

What Medical Care Can Do

Low thyroid conditions and mononucleosis are diagnosed by simple blood tests. When you have the symptom of lethargy and no other symptoms, your doctor's evaluation will often concentrate on ruling out hypoglycemia and anemia. With hypoglycemia, a glucose tolerance test (see glossary) is needed for diagnosis. Anemia is initially evaluated by a complete blood count, including an evaluation of how the blood cells appear under the microscope. With iron-deficiency anemia, the cells are smaller and paler than normal. A blood test for the iron level is the most accurate method of diagnosing this form of anemia. If you have a very low blood count, further tests to evaluate causes of chronic blood loss may require a stool specimen, to test for internal bleeding, and X-rays of the upper and lower intestines (upper GI series and barium enema—see glossary). If the cause of anemia cannot be determined, you may be referred to a hematologist, a specialist in the blood. Usually the cause of anemia is iron deficiency, which is readily treated with iron over several weeks or months (see Chapter 46).

If elective surgery is planned, postpone it until your blood count rises to normal. Transfusions of blood for iron deficiency should not be done to "prepare" you for elective surgery because of the

LETHARGY

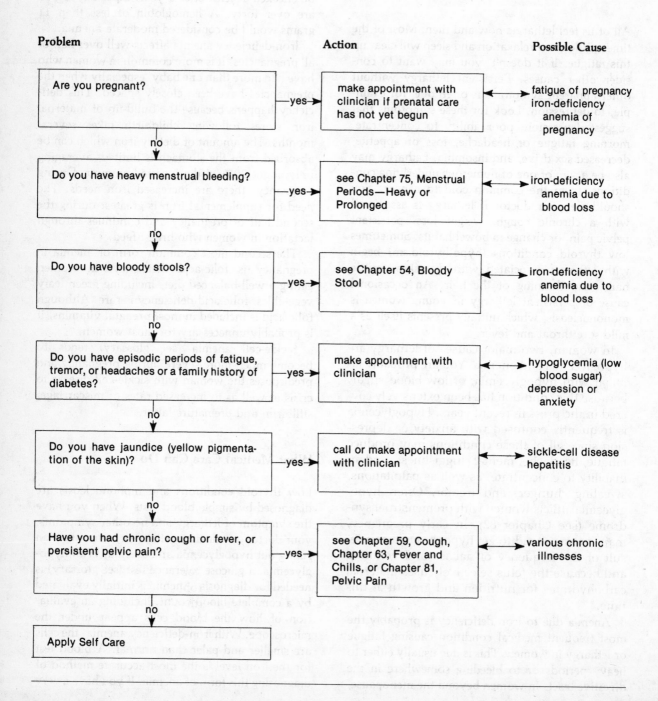

Problem	Action	Possible Cause
Are you pregnant?	—yes→ make appointment with clinician if prenatal care has not yet begun	fatigue of pregnancy iron-deficiency anemia of pregnancy
Do you have heavy menstrual bleeding?	—yes→ see Chapter 75, Menstrual Periods—Heavy or Prolonged	iron-deficiency anemia due to blood loss
Do you have bloody stools?	—yes→ see Chapter 54, Bloody Stool	iron-deficiency anemia due to blood loss
Do you have episodic periods of fatigue, tremor, or headaches or a family history of diabetes?	—yes→ make appointment with clinician	hypoglycemia (low blood sugar) depression or anxiety
Do you have jaundice (yellow pigmentation of the skin)?	—yes→ call or make appointment with clinician	sickle-cell disease hepatitis
Have you had chronic cough or fever, or persistent pelvic pain?	—yes→ see Chapter 59, Cough, Chapter 63, Fever and Chills, or Chapter 81, Pelvic Pain	various chronic illnesses
Apply Self Care		

risk of blood transfusions, including hepatitis and transfusion reactions.

What You Can Do (Self Care)

Since working long hours, lack of sleep, or emotional factors play a major part in causing lethargy, look into your own life style to see if you can reduce some of the stress (see Chapter 45). When possible, minimize the use of sedating drugs, particularly tranquilizers, sleeping pills, and alcohol, all of which are a potential cause of daytime drowsiness. When you have a checkup, make sure you know if your blood count is normal or low. If your hemoglobin (see glossary under complete blood count) is 11 grams or higher, it is most unlikely that your symptoms are due to anemia. If your hemoglobin is below 11 grams, iron-deficiency anemia is probably contributing to your symptoms. This condition can be corrected by simply taking over-the-counter iron preparations such as ferrous sulfate three times a day for three months or more.

Hypoglycemia is sometimes incorrectly diagnosed. If you have a family history of diabetes or if symptoms of hypoglycemia keep recurring, a glucose tolerance test would be advisable. Women with premenstrual syndrome may benefit by avoiding an excess dietary intake of sugar, since sweets may precipitate hypoglycemia, especially during the week before menses.

74
Menstrual Periods— Frequent or Irregular

Regular menstrual cycles depend on a delicate hormonal balance which may be affected by physical or emotional factors. It is important to understand that many patterns which do not conform to the five-day monthly period are nonetheless completely normal. In fact, frequent or irregular menses is the natural state of events at two times during a woman's life—during adolescence and for several years before menopause. During these times, production of the ovarian hormones, estrogen and progesterone, is slightly uneven; estrogen is produced in slightly greater amounts than progesterone. In the adolescent this condition exists because estrogen is the only hormone produced until the ovary matures and secretes progesterone. Menstrual periods may be very irregular and heavy for many months until this normal imbalance corrects itself. In the older woman approaching menopause, the opposite happens. The aging ovary stops producing progesterone first, which results in a relative excess of estrogen that may cause irregular bleeding. Many other temporarily abnormal patterns are associated with stressful events such as moving to an unfamiliar city, starting a new job, or experiencing serious personal or family problems.

Women taking birth control pills tend to have very regular cycles. Most other women will start their period on a different day of the month each cycle. Some women normally have a period every three weeks; for others, every five weeks is the rule.

Irregular menses may take many forms. Some women experience spotting for several days just before a period. Others notice scant bleeding midway between periods as a result of the normal hormonal changes associated with ovulation. Daily spotting which comes and goes is one of the most common bleeding patterns causing women to consult a gynecologist. Although physical causes such as tumors, infections, and pregnancy must be ruled out, the most common cause of this bleeding pattern is hormone imbalance.

What Medical Care Can Do

A blood pregnancy test may be ordered to diagnose an early pregnancy. A blood count is done to assess the severity of your bleeding. A hemoglobin (see glossary under complete blood count) of less than 11 grams often indicates anemia, possibly from recent blood loss. The pelvic examination may reveal the presence of uterine tumors such as polyps or fibroids (see Chapter 34). In addition to a Pap test, an endometrial biopsy (see Chapter 39) may be performed in women over the age of forty to diagnose tumors within the uterus that cannot be felt by examination. Special tests to measure hormone levels are rarely needed unless other problems such as hair growth, excessive weight gain, or breast discharge occur (see Chapters 64, 87, and 55, respectively).

The simplest treatment for irregular periods in a woman who needs contraception is birth control pills. For the adolescent not needing contraception or for the woman who wants to be fertile, a few days of progesterone pills (such as Provera) each month will usually regulate the cycle. Because of rare hazardous fetal effects these pills should not be used unless pregnancy has been ruled out. Progesterone therapy, which works best in women with minor degrees of hormone imbalance, is supposed to bring on a so-called withdrawal period starting two to seven days after the last progesterone pill—so don't be alarmed by this second period. When uncontrolled by hormone therapy,

Table 96   MENSTRUAL CYCLE IRREGULARITIES

Bleeding Pattern	Medical Name	Is Treatment Indicated?	Comment
periods start on different day each month	(normal)	no	some variation is normal
periods occur regularly every three weeks	polymenorrhea	no	unless this pattern is a change for you
spotting midway between periods for one day	ovulatory bleeding ("mittelschmerz" refers to the pain)	no	due to hormone changes during ovulation and sometimes accompanied by a sharp pain
light bleeding for several days before a period	premenstrual spotting	yes	initial treatment usually consists of progesterone (tablets) after ruling out tumors and pregnancy
continuous spotting for over a week (under age forty)	menometrorrhagia or "anovulatory bleeding"	yes	initial treatment usually consists of progesterone (tablets) after ruling out tumors and pregnancy
continuous spotting for over a week (over age forty)	menometrorrhagia or "anovulatory bleeding"	yes	treatment and diagnosis requires endometrial biopsy or D & C
bleeding after the menopause	postmenopausal bleeding	yes	treatment and diagnosis requires D & C

unscheduled bleeding lasting more than a few days or occurring in two or more cycles requires further investigation. The safest treatment for women over the age of forty is a D & C (see Chapter 41) to rule out the possibility of uterine cancer.[1]

Table 96 summarizes the types of irregular

bleeding problems that nonpregnant women have and tell which ones call for treatment.

What You Can Do (Self Care)

Lie down or decrease your activity as much as

[1]Sometimes a new procedure, hysteroscopy (see glossary), helps in evaluating difficult-to-diagnose bleeding problems. Hysteroscopy is as yet not widely used partly because for technical reasons it may be difficult to visualize the uterine cavity.

MENSTRUAL PERIODS—FREQUENT OR IRREGULAR

Problem	Action	Possible Cause

Are you pregnant? —yes→ see Chapter 52, Bleeding in Early Pregnancy ←→ miscarriage / tubal pregnancy

↓ no

Are you taking birth control pills? —yes→ see Chapter 9, Birth Control Pills (Oral Contraceptives) ←→ effect of pill

↓ no

Do you have pelvic pain? —yes→ see Chapter 81, Pelvic Pain ←→ tube infection / uterine infection associated with IUD / complication of unsuspected pregnancy

↓ no

Are you over 40 years of age? —yes→ make appointment with clinician ←→ hormone imbalance / cancer of the uterus or cervix

↓ no

Has it been over a year since your last Pap smear? —yes→ make appointment with clinician ←→ hormone imbalance / cancer of cervix

↓ no

Has the bleeding occurred during other cycles or lasted more than three days? —yes→ make appointment with clinician ←→ hormone imbalance

↓ no

Apply Self Care

possible. Reduce stress where feasible since this is a major cause of irregular bleeding. Take an over-the-counter iron preparation twice daily. A blood count by your clinician is the most accurate way to determine your need for iron supplements. If you are taking estrogen (e.g., Premarin), contact your physician. See Chapter 9, Birth Control Pills (Oral Contraceptives), if you have bleeding while taking the pill. If you have heavy bleeding, contact your physician.

75

Menstrual Periods—Heavy or Prolonged

This chapter deals with the problem of heavy or prolonged periods in women who have regular cycles. Normally a woman loses up to four table-spoons of blood during a menstrual period. Sometimes when menstrual flow is a little heavier than usual, the blood will clot. The fact that your blood clots does not necessarily mean that anything is wrong; in fact, it indicates your blood-clotting system is working as it should. Bleeding for more than seven days is considered excessive. Excessive menstrual bleeding is usually produced by conditions which interfere with the uterine mechanism for limiting menstrual blood loss. Benign uterine tumors located within the uterine wall (adenomyosis) or within the uterine cavity (fibroids or polyps) are among the most common causes of heavy periods. These conditions may also cause bleeding between periods. Intrauterine devices (coil, IUD) are another source of heavy or prolonged periods especially if associated with vaginal discharge, pelvic pain, and fever, all of which are signs of a uterine infection. Hormone imbalances, ovary infections, or cancer of the uterus rarely cause heavy periods and are more likely to show up as continuous or irregular on and off spotting.

What Medical Care Can Do

The clinician will do a pelvic exam to search for uterine infection, polyps, fibroids, or cancer. Infections are typically treated medically and usually do not require removal of the IUD if you have

MENSTRUAL PERIODS—HEAVY OR PROLONGED

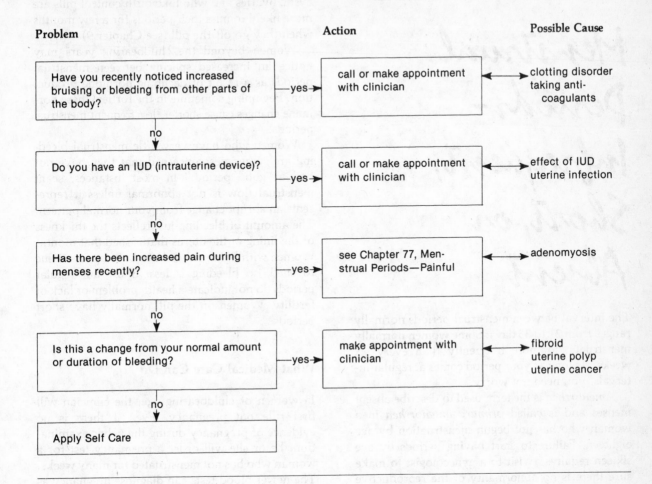

Problem	Action	Possible Cause

Have you recently noticed increased bruising or bleeding from other parts of the body? —yes→ call or make appointment with clinician → clotting disorder / taking anti-coagulants

↓ no

Do you have an IUD (intrauterine device)? —yes→ call or make appointment with clinician → effect of IUD / uterine infection

↓ no

Has there been increased pain during menses recently? —yes→ see Chapter 77, Menstrual Periods—Painful → adenomyosis

↓ no

Is this a change from your normal amount or duration of bleeding? —yes→ make appointment with clinician → fibroid / uterine polyp / uterine cancer

↓ no

Apply Self Care

---

one. If you are premenopausal and your uterus is enlarged, the doctor will order a pregnancy test, even when your periods are regular. If your blood count indicates anemia and your uterus is enlarged, an endometrial biopsy, a D & C, or a hysteroscopy (see glossary) may be done to establish a definite diagnosis. These procedures may also be therapeutic as in the case of a benign polyp. Conditions originating in the uterine wall, such as fibroids or adenomyosis, cannot be diagnosed by D & C since tissue cannot be readily biopsied. When such conditions are suspected and bleeding is heavy despite medication and a D & C, exploratory surgery with hysterectomy may be necessary as a last resort or even an emergency measure. Persistent heavy periods for which no apparent cause is found even after a D & C may cause severe anemia. Some women may elect to have a hysterectomy for this problem depending upon its

severity, their desire for future childbearing, and the degree of debilitation and inconvenience involved.

What You Can Do (Self Care)

Chronically heavy periods which do not represent a change from your normal pattern do not usually require surgery or other treatment aside from iron supplementation and periodic checkups.

Get as much rest as possible during your period. Inactivity tends to decrease menstrual bleeding. Have a blood count done every six months. It should be possible to obtain this blood count without having a complete examination. If you have fibroid tumors, avoid estrogen or birth control pills since these hormones stimulate the tumors to grow and may increase the amount of bleeding.

76

Menstrual Periods— Infrequent, Short, or Absent

The interval between menstrual periods normally ranges from 21 to 35 days. Some women normally menstruate no more frequently than every six weeks. As long as your period comes at regular intervals, you need not worry.

Amenorrhea is the term used to describe absent menses and is called *primary amenorrhea* in a woman who has not begun menstruation by age eighteen. Failure to start having periods by age sixteen requires a visit to a gynecologist to make sure there is no abnormality of the reproductive organs. Most women with primary amenorrhea are perfectly normal, the problem being just an inherited tendency to begin periods later in life.

The term *secondary amenorrhea* refers to menstrual periods that occur four months or more apart. This condition is much more common than primary amenorrhea. Such delays in menses may occur temporarily because of hormone imbalances related to stressful situations such as emotional problems, crash diets, or marked changes in weight or to the effects of a variety of drugs, including tranquilizers and antidepressants. Women with a condition known as cystic ovaries may have a chronic tendency to have their periods at intervals ranging from every six weeks to every six months. In this common condition, sometimes called the *polycystic ovary syndrome*, the ovaries are unable to regularly secrete the hormones that trigger menstruation. While infrequent ovulation is one cause of infertility, the use of fertility drugs,

like Clomid (see Chapter 13), can usually overcome these difficulties. Women who have polycystic ovaries and who take birth control pills are more likely to miss their periods for a few months when they go off the pill (see Chapter 9).

Women beyond the childbearing years may notice an increased spacing between menstrual periods as a result of declining hormone production. Beginning sometime in the forties, these hormone changes cause shorter, less frequent menstrual periods.

Women who have very little menstrual bleeding are sometimes concerned that they have not had a "good period." In most instances, scant menstrual flow is not abnormal unless it represents an abrupt change from your normal pattern. The amount of bleeding just reflects the thickness of the lining of the uterus that is shed that month. Women with light menses have built up less tissue to shed, so bleeding is less. Short but regular periods do not indicate a health problem or lack of fertility. Women on the pill normally have short periods.

What Medical Care Can Do

In women of childbearing age, the clinician will first rule out pregnancy. Even if there is no evidence of pregnancy during the pelvic examination, he or she will order a pregnancy test for a woman who has not menstruated for many weeks. The newer blood tests can diagnose pregnancy as early as one week after conception.

If the problem is hormone imbalance, progesterone may be given by injection or tablet to bring on, or induce, a period. The tablet form (synthetic progesterone) should never be taken if you could be pregnant since it may cause birth defects. The pure hormone used in injectable progesterone has not been associated with these defects. In either case, if you are already pregnant, the hormonal medication will not bring on a period. In most cases of hormone imbalance, progesterone will trigger a period within a week of the last progesterone pill taken. It may be a rather heavy period or just slight spotting, depending on your response. No further treatment is needed except that you should have a period induced at least every four months if you normally have only one or two periods each year. This treatment is recommended because markedly infrequent periods are associated with excessive stimulation of the uterus

MENSTRUAL PERIODS—INFREQUENT, SHORT, OR ABSENT

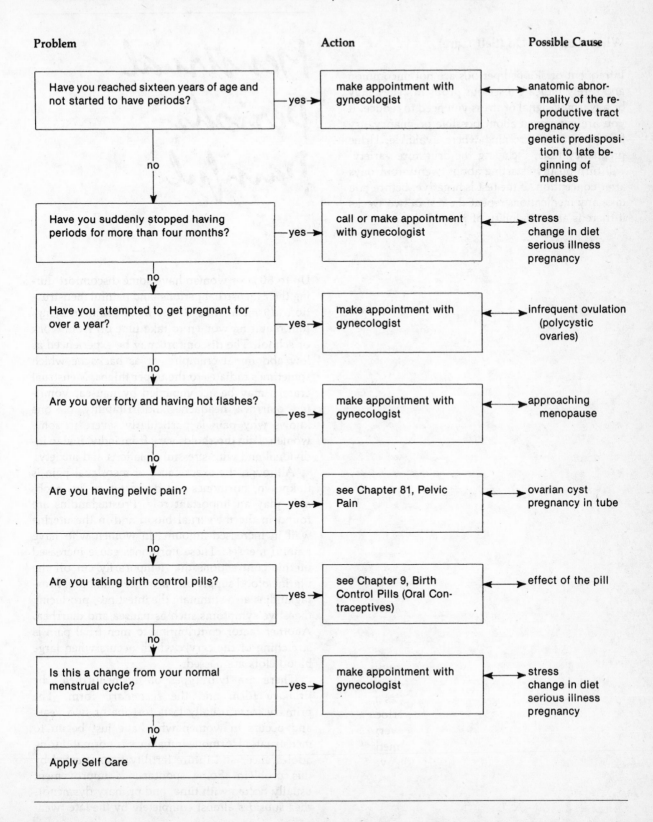

Problem | Action | Possible Cause

Have you reached sixteen years of age and not started to have periods? —yes→ make appointment with gynecologist ← anatomic abnormality of the reproductive tract / pregnancy / genetic predisposition to late beginning of menses

no ↓

Have you suddenly stopped having periods for more than four months? —yes→ call or make appointment with gynecologist ← stress / change in diet / serious illness / pregnancy

no ↓

Have you attempted to get pregnant for over a year? —yes→ make appointment with gynecologist ← infrequent ovulation (polycystic ovaries)

no ↓

Are you over forty and having hot flashes? —yes→ make appointment with gynecologist ← approaching menopause

no ↓

Are you having pelvic pain? —yes→ see Chapter 81, Pelvic Pain ← ovarian cyst / pregnancy in tube

no ↓

Are you taking birth control pills? —yes→ see Chapter 9, Birth Control Pills (Oral Contraceptives) ← effect of the pill

no ↓

Is this a change from your normal menstrual cycle? —yes→ make appointment with gynecologist ← stress / change in diet / serious illness / pregnancy

no ↓

Apply Self Care

by estrogen and a slightly greater risk of uterine cancer.

What You Can Do (Self Care)

Infrequent or skipped periods are not uncommon and rarely indicate a serious problem. They may be a warning signal of stress you need to reduce. If you are concerned about possible pregnancy, try free pregnancy screening where available. Urine pregnancy tests, including the drugstore variety, will turn positive starting about twenty-four days after conception. If the test is negative, before you take any medications repeat the test in two weeks if there is any possibility of pregnancy.

77

Menstrual Periods— Painful

Up to 80% of women have some discomfort during their menstrual periods, and painful menstruation (*dysmenorrhea*) is the most common symptom requiring women to take time off from work or school. The discomfort may be experienced as low abdominal cramping or as backache which sometimes radiates to the upper thighs. Menstrual cramps may be accompanied by nausea, vomiting, diarrhea, headache, and irritability. No one knows why pain is particularly severe in some women. Pain thresholds vary from individual to individual and with stressful situations and anxiety.

Although the exact cause of menstrual pain is unknown, hormones called *prostaglandins* probably play an important role. Prostaglandins are found in the menstrual blood and in the uterine wall in increased amounts in women who have painful menses. These hormones cause increased uterine contractions that temporarily cut off the uterine blood supply and produce cramping. Prostaglandins also stimulate the intestines, producing digestive symptoms such as nausea and diarrhea. Another factor contributing to menstrual pain is stretching of the cervix which occurs when large blood clots are passed.

There are two types of dysmenorrhea, the *primary* form and the *secondary* form. The primary form usually lasts for one or two years and occurs in women who have just begun to menstruate. Hormone imbalance is normal during adolescence, and future fertility is unaffected by this problem. Some spontaneous improvement usually occurs with time, and primary dysmenorrhea subsides almost completely by the late twen-

Table 97 QUESTIONS COMMONLY ASKED ABOUT PAINFUL PERIODS

Question	Yes	No	Comment
Does a tilted uterus cause painful menses?		X	A tilted uterus may cause painful menses only if the reason it is tilted is a result of disease, such as endometriosis.
Does hormone imbalance cause painful menses?		X	Painful menses is a sign of fertility and is associated with regular cycles and normal ovulation.
Is alcohol recommended to prevent painful cramps?		X	Alcohol relaxes the uterine muscles only slightly and is of limited benefit.
Is aspirin as good as most other painkillers except narcotics?	X		Because of its prostaglandin-inhibiting properties, aspirin is one of the most effective nonnarcotic analgesics for menstrual cramps.
Are painful periods normal in a woman with normal pelvic findings on examination?	X		Painful periods occur as a result of normal physiologic processes.
Do water pills help?	X		In some women who experience excessive fluid retention each month, cyclic weight gain and uterine cramping are reduced.
Do birth control pills usually relieve painful periods?	X		Failure of the pill to relieve painful periods indicates that a physical cause may be present.

ties. Childbirth dramatically relieves this form of dysmenorrhea, possibly from stretching of the cervix or from increasing uterine blood supply during pregnancy.

Secondary dysmenorrhea refers to menstrual pain that develops in women who previously had little or no cramping with their periods. This form of dysmenorrhea is much less common than the primary form. It is usually associated with some type of physical abnormality of the reproductive organs, such as benign uterine tumors (polyps, fibroids), pelvic infections, or endometriosis (see Chapter 35). Fibroids or polyps occur inside the uterine cavity and may stimulate forceful uterine contractions in an attempt to expel these tumors during menses. The pain of endometriosis occurs one or two days before the onset of menstrual bleeding. In contrast, pelvic infections often cause pain after menstrual bleeding has begun. Another common cause of painful periods is the intra-uterine device, especially in women who have never been pregnant. Cramps normally diminish a few cycles after IUD insertion, but if menstrual pain persists, removal of the IUD may be necessary.

Although pain anywhere in the body may have a psychological component, physicians have tend-ed to view dysmenorrhea as a psychosomatic ill-ness more often than other painful conditions. But it is now known that painful periods are most often not psychosomatic but are based on physical factors.

What Medical Care Can Do

The treatment of this condition depends on the findings during the pelvic exam. Usually the examination is normal and treatment depends on the severity of the woman's pain and her willingness to take birth control pills. Birth control pills decrease menstrual cramping both by blocking the action of prostaglandins and by decreasing the amount of tissue buildup within the uterus so that there is less stretching of the cervix. Among over-the-counter pills, aspirin is the best because of antiprostaglandin effects. None of the other nonnarcotic drugs have been found to be more effective than aspirin until recently. The newest group of drugs for menstrual cramps is the antiprostaglandin medications previously used to reduce arthritis inflammation. These include Ponstel and Anaprox, which the FDA has approved specifically for the treatment of painful periods (lower dose nonprescription brands of this type of drug are also available—see below). These drugs effectively decrease uterine contractions although side effects such as nausea and diarrhea sometimes occur.

In patients whose pain is unrelieved by medical measures, a procedure called laparoscopy (see glossary) may be performed to check for cysts or endometriosis. Surgery is much more likely to be necessary for the secondary form of dysmenorrhea since it is more commonly associated with physical abnormalities of the reproductive tract.

What You Can Do (Self Care)

The chapter on the female reproductive system (see Chapter 3) will help familiarize you with female anatomy and its functions during the menstrual cycle. Understanding where the pain comes from and how it is produced will help you deal with it. Among over-the-counter painkillers try aspirin or ibuprofen, an antiprostaglandin drug (see above) approved in 1984 by the FDA under the brand names Advil and Nuprin. Ibuprofen is indicated for minor aches and pains and especially menstrual cramps since it acts in part by reducing uterine contractions. Sexual activity may

MENSTRUAL PERIODS—PAINFUL

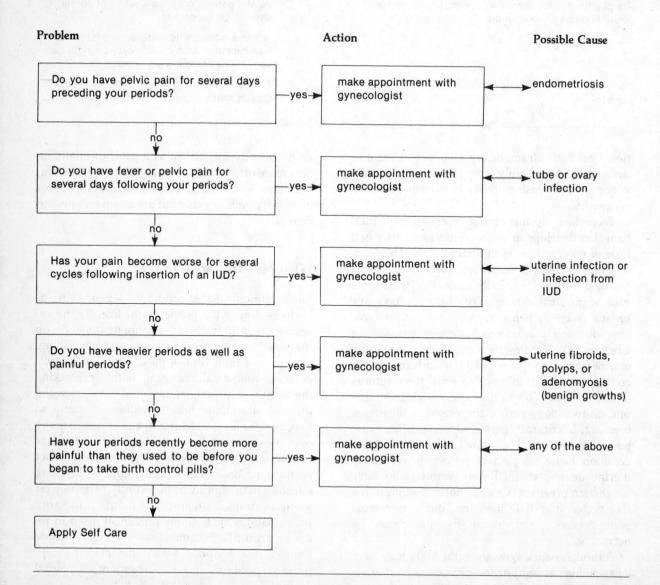

Problem	Action	Possible Cause
Do you have pelvic pain for several days preceding your periods? —yes→	make appointment with gynecologist ←	→ endometriosis
↓ no		
Do you have fever or pelvic pain for several days following your periods? —yes→	make appointment with gynecologist ←	→ tube or ovary infection
↓ no		
Has your pain become worse for several cycles following insertion of an IUD? —yes→	make appointment with gynecologist ←	→ uterine infection or infection from IUD
↓ no		
Do you have heavier periods as well as painful periods? —yes→	make appointment with gynecologist ←	→ uterine fibroids, polyps, or adenomyosis (benign growths)
↓ no		
Have your periods recently become more painful than they used to be before you began to take birth control pills? —yes→	make appointment with gynecologist ←	→ any of the above
↓ no		
Apply Self Care		

relieve some of the congestive symptoms that accompany menses. Masters and Johnson have shown that orgasm, achieved either alone or with a partner, shortly after the onset of menses may reduce pelvic cramping and backache. The use of heat (warm baths, heating pads) and exercise may improve blood flow and decrease pelvic pain. When lying down, keep your legs elevated with a pillow under your knees; or when lying on your side, bring your knees up to your chest. If none of these measures work, request one of the newer drugs, such as Ponstel, from your clinician rather than using narcotics.

In addition to taking physical measures, consider your own feelings toward menstruation. Cultural attitudes convey many negative messages about this natural process. Many women feel uncomfortable, mildly depressed, or unattractive at this time. You can guard against some of the cultural conditioning by simply being aware of it. Do you experience the same feelings with each period? Are there certain triggering factors aside from pain which produce these feelings? Use this opportunity to learn more about your emotional rhythms since this is a time when your level of inner perception and sensitivity is likely to be high.

Table 97 answers some questions you may have about painful periods.

78

Nausea and Vomiting

Although nausea and vomiting may accompany serious disease, these symptoms more often result from minor disorders. Intermittent nausea without vomiting almost never necessitates a visit to your doctor. Persistent vomiting, especially when accompanied by other symptoms such as abdominal pain, does require a physician consultation. Hospitalization may be necessary if vomiting causes excessive fluid loss.

Conditions Causing Nausea and Vomiting

Here is a brief guide to potentially serious conditions that cause nausea and vomiting.

Digestive disorders

Frequently accompanied by abdominal pain, digestive disorders often cause nausea and vomiting. Upper abdominal pain is associated with stomach or intestinal ulcers, gallbladder disorders (cholycystitis), inflammation of the pancreas (pancreatitis), and inflammation of the liver (hepatitis). Lower abdominal pain is associated with appendicitis and intestinal flu (gastroenteritis). Generalized abdominal pain and vomiting may be caused by a ruptured appendix, food poisoning, or blockage of the intestine (bowel obstruction). Among these conditions intestinal flu, a communicable disease spread by a virus, is by far the most frequent and least serious. For more information about digestive causes of nausea and vomiting, refer to Chapter 66, Heartburn and Gas, Chapter 61, Diarrhea, and Chapter 54, Bloody Stool.

Drug reactions

Vomiting is a common side effect of many drugs, particularly the tetracyclines, aspirin, narcotic pain pills, and estrogens, including birth control pills.

Stress

Emotional factors play a role in these symptoms.

In some illnesses, such as migraine headaches, it may be difficult to differentiate between physical, psychological, and stress-related factors causing nausea.

Vomiting as an avoidance of possible weight gain may result in a condition called bulimia, an emotional illness which has been recognized only recently. In this condition episodes of binge eating (eating large amounts of food at one time) are

NAUSEA AND VOMITING

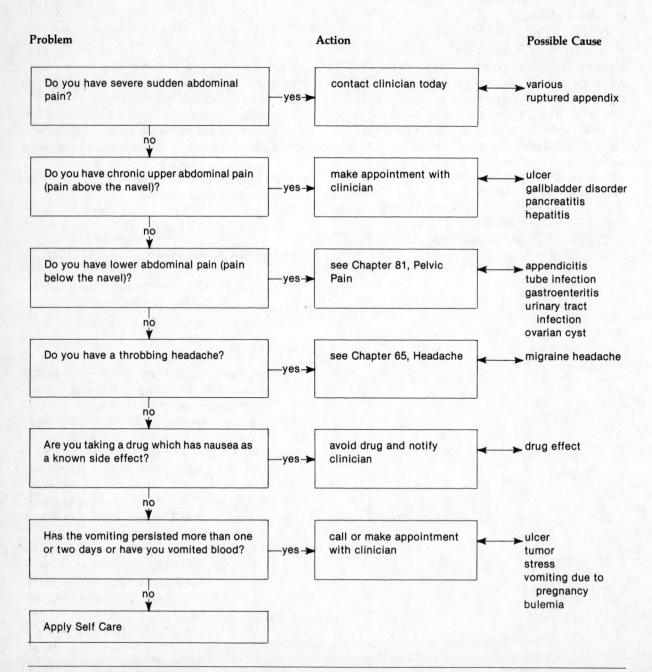

Problem	Action	Possible Cause
Do you have severe sudden abdominal pain? —yes→	contact clinician today	various ruptured appendix
Do you have chronic upper abdominal pain (pain above the navel)? —yes→	make appointment with clinician	ulcer gallbladder disorder pancreatitis hepatitis
Do you have lower abdominal pain (pain below the navel)? —yes→	see Chapter 81, Pelvic Pain	appendicitis tube infection gastroenteritis urinary tract infection ovarian cyst
Do you have a throbbing headache? —yes→	see Chapter 65, Headache	migraine headache
Are you taking a drug which has nausea as a known side effect? —yes→	avoid drug and notify clinician	drug effect
Has the vomiting persisted more than one or two days or have you vomited blood? —yes→	call or make appointment with clinician	ulcer tumor stress vomiting due to pregnancy bulemia
Apply Self Care		

followed by feelings of remorse or regret that are somewhat relieved by self-induced vomiting. This disorder is more common in adolescence or early adult life. People with bulimia are usually excessively concerned about their weight and try to control it by use of laxatives, dieting and vomiting.

Pregnancy

Sixty-five percent of pregnant women experience some degree of so-called morning sickness during the first three months of pregnancy. Emotional factors, hormone changes, and a sluggish digestive system may contribute to nausea and vomiting in pregnancy, though the specific cause remains unknown. Although feelings of nausea are most common in the morning, these symptoms may be experienced any time of day. If vomiting is prolonged, dehydration may occur and requires hospitalization.

What Medical Care Can Do

The physician will ask how long you've had nausea and vomiting and how your diet affects the symptoms. Eating fried foods, for example, often brings on a gallbladder attack which gives you pain, belching, and nausea. If vomiting is more prominent than abdominal pain, the doctor knows that pregnancy, a drug reaction, food poisoning, or intestinal flu is more likely. Vomiting of blood is an emergency requiring hospitalization and is often due to stomach ulcers (see Chapter 66, Heartburn and Gas).

Your doctor may prescribe antinausea drugs such as Compazine or Phenegran. These drugs come in rectal suppository form, which is preferable if vomiting accompanies nausea. But before taking any medication for morning sickness, especially in the first three months of pregnancy, discuss alternatives (for example, dietary measures) to drug treatment with your doctor.

Bulimia has been variously treated with antidepressant drug therapy, nutritional counseling, stress management, and psychotherapy. Women with this condition usually respond to a lower dose of antidepressant than is used in truly depressed patients.

What You Can Do (Self Care)

During pregnancy, nausea is sometimes relieved by your lying down immediately after meals. Meals should be frequent and small enough to keep your stomach from becoming completely empty or overly stretched out. If morning sickness occurs, try eating plain soda (saltine) crackers or dry toast before you get up. Get up slowly, avoiding sudden movements. Avoid greasy, fried, or spicy foods. Eat whatever appeals to you. It may help to eat only cold foods, or to eat solids and drink liquids an hour apart. Sometimes small amounts of apple juice, grape juice, or noncola carbonated beverages between meals helps to lessen nausea. You can take your vitamins and iron after you get through this period of your pregnancy since they may contribute to an upset stomach. Whenever possible, avoid taking drugs, especially in the first three months of pregnancy.

A woman afflicted with or with a tendency toward bulimia may find it helps to keep a diary recording when and what she eats, how often she vomits, and when she uses purgatives or laxatives. This information may help to make her aware that a problem exists or to set targets for gradual reduction in unwanted behavior. Professional counseling is usually recommended.

Nonpregnant women can apply the same dietary recommendations as for pregnant women. In recovering from illness, start nourishment with hot beverages (tea or clear broth) or cold beverages (iced tea, apple juice, cola, or ginger ale). Avoid drugs, such as aspirin, which may cause nausea. If vomiting persists for several days or you vomit blood, call your clinician.

79

Nervousness and Anxiety

Nervousness is another name for anxiety. Everyone experiences anxiety in one form or another during their daily lives. Anxiety may be good or bad.

Anxiety is good when it mobilizes the body for action. Controlled anxiety is the force which drives many people to accomplish their life's goals. Anxiety is often the fire behind the drive of creative, successful people. Without that driving force of controlled anxiety, the work of the world would not get done.

Sometimes anxiety may become a problem. When it does, there is usually a remedy readily available to bring it under control. Here are some forms anxiety may take.

Generalized anxiety is often experienced as trembling, jitteriness, or shakiness. Some women report a sensation like feeling their muscles jumping under their skin. Others experience anxiety as a tight band around the head or muscle tension in the limbs. Many people feel knots in their stomachs or backaches. Anxiety may be experienced as a fear or dread, which may be mistaken for depression. The anxious woman cannot relax; she feels tense and has trouble sleeping, eating, indulging in sex, working, and conducting her normal activities.

Some women experience anxiety as a reaction to a drug, such as diet pills (amphetamines) or Reserpine (a drug used to control blood pressure), to caffeine (in coffee, tea, cola, and chocolate), or to an alcoholic drink. Occasionally anxiety signals the onset of a disease, such as hyperthyroidism (overactive thyroid), in which the thyroid gland produces excessive amounts of thyroid hormone. And many women report anxiety as part of premenstrual syndrome (see Chapter

82). Often, when the situation causing the anxiety is corrected or settled, the anxiety will disappear.

Some women become anxious when they are in the presence of some specific object or animal—for example, a cat, a snake (often including objects made from a reptile), a doll, a door, etc.; almost anything can be a specific anxiety-producing thing.

Other women become anxious when they must perform a specific task or take part in a certain event—for example, take a test, fly in an airplane, give a speech, meet people on the street, etc.

Agoraphobia (a fear of being in open or public places) is a well-known form of anxiety. The woman becomes anxious and fearful when she is in a public place in which there are crowds of people—for example, shopping at a supermarket or a mall, going to a concert or a ballgame, or being in the lobby of a hotel. In some cases the effect of her anxiety may make the woman literally a prisoner in her own home.

To avoid anxiety some women develop repetitive, ritualistic behavior. The woman will go through a series of steps or procedures to avoid anxiety—for example, most simply, avoiding cracks in the sidewalk; more severely, explaining everything in minute detail, leaving nothing out.

Sometimes the woman may become obsessed by a thought that she knows is foolish but which she just can't get out of her mind—for example, thinking that if she is left alone she'll go crazy; or thinking she will hurt her newborn baby or hit someone while she is driving a car.

Some people become anxious merely anticipating an event—for example, an impending job interview. Other people may become anxious either directly after an event or several months later—for example, going calmly through a child's serious illness and then becoming anxious after all danger is past; or having an accident, recovering after a time, and then having an anxiety attack.

What Medical Care Can Do

If your physician cannot find a medical reason for your anxiety, then it is assumed to be psychological. Your physician and you after discussing your anxiety may discover that it is tied to and caused by a recent situation such as divorce, having to move, or sending a child off to school. Sometimes your physician may prescribe a tranquilizer to be taken over a short period of time and may recommend some short-term counseling. Counseling may involve a number of procedures such as hypnosis, biofeedback training, meditation, family or group counseling, and, if your physician feels you are physically able, jogging, swimming, or any of the aerobic type exercises (see Chapter 47).

Valium is the most prescribed tranquilizer in the United States. It is also considered by the FDA to be addictive with potential danger. For that

NERVOUSNESS AND ANXIETY

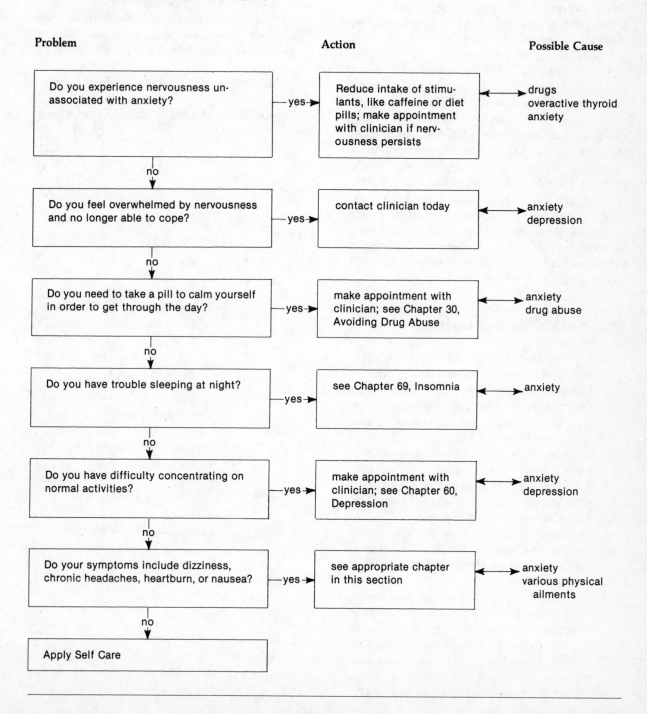

Problem / Action / Possible Cause

Do you experience nervousness un-associated with anxiety? — yes → Reduce intake of stimulants, like caffeine or diet pills; make appointment with clinician if nervousness persists ← → drugs, overactive thyroid, anxiety

no ↓

Do you feel overwhelmed by nervousness and no longer able to cope? — yes → contact clinician today ← → anxiety, depression

no ↓

Do you need to take a pill to calm yourself in order to get through the day? — yes → make appointment with clinician; see Chapter 30, Avoiding Drug Abuse ← → anxiety, drug abuse

no ↓

Do you have trouble sleeping at night? — yes → see Chapter 69, Insomnia ← → anxiety

no ↓

Do you have difficulty concentrating on normal activities? — yes → make appointment with clinician; see Chapter 60, Depression ← → anxiety, depression

no ↓

Do your symptoms include dizziness, chronic headaches, heartburn, or nausea? — yes → see appropriate chapter in this section ← → anxiety, various physical ailments

no ↓

Apply Self Care

reason it is a so-called controlled substance.

There are other tranquilizers used for anxiety besides Valium. The first tranquilizer on the market was Miltown, then Librium, and, following closely behind, Valium. Such drugs as Mellaril and Thorazine in low dosages may also be used.

If you are depressed, Valium and other tranquilizers alone may cause you to become more deeply depressed. Be certain your doctor understands your symptoms before he or she prescribes medication; depression and anxiety often have only a thin line separating them.

Tranquilizers may have pronounced additive effects causing marked sedation when taken at the same time as certain pain pills, alcohol, sleeping pills, or antidepressants. According to a recent study by the Institute of Medicine, some tranquilizers have additional hazards not previously recognized. Because of the long time required for the body's elimination of drugs like tranquilizers, chronic use may cause drug dependency (see Chapter 30). Also, unexpected toxic interactions with alcohol can occur when people take a drug like Valium for sleep and then drink alcoholic beverages the next day without realizing they still have high blood levels of the tranquilizer.

What You Can Do (Self Care)

1. Try to identify the situation which, when you think about it, makes you anxious.
2. Consider actions that would lessen the threat, and try them out (for example, attend childbirth preparation classes to deal with the stress of labor and delivery; eliminate or reduce caffeine intake if nervousness alone is the problem).
3. Avoid potentially dangerous ways of coping with anxiety—smoking, alcohol, drug dependence, overeating, undereating.
4. Express your feelings to someone you trust and can talk with comfortably. This unburdening of feelings often leads to a relief of anxious feelings.
5. Try relaxation techniques or meditation. Both or either often provides relief. Classes in yoga or stress reduction are often available through community programs.
6. If your doctor feels you are physically able to do so, try jogging, swimming, or any of the aerobic type exercises (see Chapter 47).

7. If nervousness regularly precedes menses, try reducing dietary salt to lessen this and other symptoms of premenstrual syndrome.
8. If your anxiety persists or becomes chronic, seek out a competent mental health professional.
9. You can ask for help from any of the following, as appropriate:

   Community mental health center—most are required to maintain service twenty-four hours a day, seven days a week.

   Mental health association—they can refer you.

   Health department—they can refer you.

80

Palpitations

Palpitations refer to fluttering sensations in the chest which occur when your heart skips a beat or beats rapidly. Palpitations are usually due to stress, fatigue, emotional factors, or drugs rather than to heart disease. Fear of heart disease may actually cause palpitations to become worse. Although palpitations alone are unlikely to indicate heart disease, you should see your doctor if you experience repeated episodes of palpitations associated with chest pain or shortness of breath. Among the most common causes of palpitations in women are excessive use of alcohol, cigarettes, or caffeine. Diet pills, water pills, decongestants containing ephedrine, and antidepressant drugs may cause these symptoms. An overactive thyroid (hyperthyroidism) can also cause palpitations along with weight loss, nervousness, shakiness, and heat intolerance. Palpitations are common in pregnancy and are especially noticeable when you lie down.

What Medical Care Can Do

The clinician will evaluate your pulse for rate and

PALPITATIONS

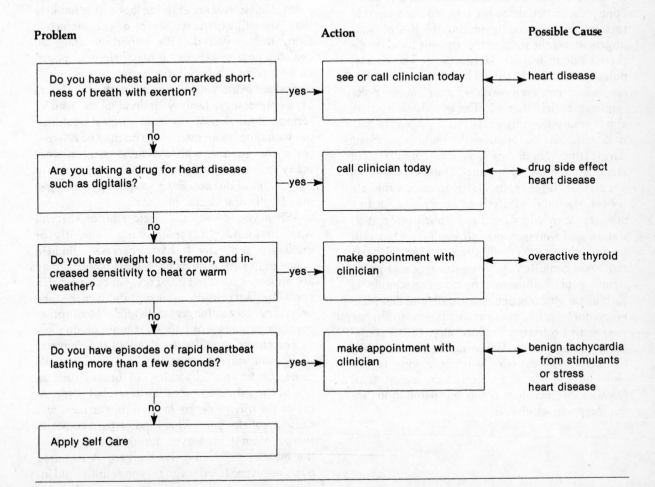

Problem	Action	Possible Cause
Do you have chest pain or marked shortness of breath with exertion? —yes→	see or call clinician today	heart disease
↓ no		
Are you taking a drug for heart disease such as digitalis? —yes→	call clinician today	drug side effect / heart disease
↓ no		
Do you have weight loss, tremor, and increased sensitivity to heat or warm weather? —yes→	make appointment with clinician	overactive thyroid
↓ no		
Do you have episodes of rapid heartbeat lasting more than a few seconds? —yes→	make appointment with clinician	benign tachycardia from stimulants or stress / heart disease
↓ no		
Apply Self Care		

regularity. He or she will examine your thyroid closely and may order thyroid blood tests. If you have chest pain or shortness of breath, the doctor will also obtain an electrocardiogram (EKG) (see glossary) and perhaps a twenty-four-hour Holter monitor, which records the workings of your heart as you participate in your normal daily activities. Or your doctor may choose to evaluate your heart by means of a stress test, which involves recording heart activity with an EKG as you go through increasingly strenuous exercises on a treadmill. The science of stress testing is far from exact, and many stress tests show heartbeat irregularities in perfectly healthy women. Only if palpitations are frequent and associated with symptoms of heart disease will the doctor prescribe drugs to control heart rhythm.

What You Can Do (Self Care)

If you have episodes of rapid heartbeat, try taking your pulse to determine the rate. You can learn to take your own pulse by placing the tips of your fingers across the wrist of the opposite hand on the thumb side to feel for the heartbeat. The normal pulse varies from 60 to 100 beats per minute during rest. If you exercise daily, your normal pulse rate may be less than 60. The two things to note about your pulse are its rate and rhythm. The rate is determined by counting the number of beats during one minute (or you can count for 15 seconds and multiply by four). The rhythm should feel regular. If the rhythm is irregular or if the rate is over one hundred after you have rested for five minutes, then you should call your doctor. You should also see your doctor if you take heart pills or are on antiarrhythmic drugs to control heart rate. You can often control uncomplicated palpitations yourself, however, by avoiding stimulants such as caffeine, cigarettes, alcohol, and diet pills. When these episodes occur, sit down or change your activity from something stressful to something you like to do. Get as much sleep as possible. Recurrent episodes warrant a visit to the physician's office if for no other reason than reassurance since most of the time palpitations are not due to heart disease.

81

Pelvic Pain

This chapter covers the complicated problem of severe or chronic pelvic pain. The subject is complicated because there are so many abdominal organs that can be the source of this pain. We're not talking about the pain related to your menstrual cycle or to the passing discomfort that accompanies, say, a bout with diarrhea. Rather, we want to discuss some possible causes of intense, unrelieved abdominal discomfort—pain that will definitely require a visit to your physician at some point. Unless you are entering labor, it is unlikely that you will experience severe or chronic pelvic pain. But if you do, it's important that you evaluate your own pain—it may help your physician pinpoint a difficult diagnosis.

Sudden acute pain lasting more than six hours in a previously healthy individual is usually serious. It may require prompt surgical treatment or evaluation by an internist. You may be referred for a consultation with a general surgeon since many causes of low abdominal pain are not due to gynecological disease. Even so, your gynecologist may be the first doctor you see.

When you do see the doctor, he or she will want to know *if the pain started abruptly or gradually* and how it has progressed. Sudden severe pain with little or no vaginal bleeding may accompany a ruptured tubal pregnancy or ovarian cyst. The pain subsides after rupture since the tube or ovary is no longer distended. Most other gynecologic causes of pain start more gradually.

The physician will also ask about *the character of the pain*, since the type of pain gives clues to its cause. Distention (stretching) of organs such as one of the Fallopian tubes (as in a tubal pregnancy) or the uterine cervix (as in a miscarriage) will cause a colicky pain. This kind of pain comes in sharp, intermittent waves during contractions of the muscles of the involved organ. A ruptured ovarian cyst or tubal pregnancy that spills fluid into the pelvic cavity can cause severe, steady pain.

Adhesions (see glossary) within or between organs may form after previous abdominal surgery, and they cause a dull ache or pulling pain.

Location of the pain, too, is important information for the clinician. It may not be easy for you to precisely locate your pelvic pain because the pelvic organs have fewer nerve endings than, say, the skin or muscles. The physician may help you more specifically locate the pain during the pelvic exam. Pain from the ovary or tube, for example, is usually well localized to an area two to three inches to the left or right of the midline (an imaginary line extending down from the navel; see Figure 38) and within an inch above the pubic hairline. Pain located above this region often is due to other organs, usually the large intestine or appendix. Ovarian pain commonly radiates to the inner part of the thigh. Uterine pain is located in the lower midline portion of the abdomen just above the pelvic bone. This pain may radiate to the buttocks or lower back, especially during menses. Bladder disease often causes pain similar to uterine pain but is usually accompanied by urinary symptoms, such as a burning sensation when you urinate. Vaginal disease rarely causes abdominal pain. Whether the pain is felt on both sides of the lower abdomen (bilateral) or only on one side (unilateral) is important. Pelvic inflammatory conditions involving the tube and ovary tend to be bilateral. Cysts and tubal pregnancies tend to cause unilateral pain.

Finally, the doctor will need to know *other symptoms that are associated with the pain*. It is helpful to your doctor if you can tell him or her the relationship of your pelvic pain to each of five specific physical events:

1. *Relationship to menses.* If you skipped your last period or you are having unscheduled vaginal bleeding, pregnancy disorders such as miscarriage or ectopic pregnancy (see Chapter 52) are more likely. Pain occurring just before and during menses suggests a common disorder called endometriosis (see Chapter 35). Pain beginning a few days after a period starts may be from an inflammatory process since your natural physiologic barrier to infection is temporarily removed at menses.

2. *Relationship to diet and digestion.* The absence of vomiting, diarrhea, or bloody stools tends to exclude the digestive tract as a cause of the pain.

3. *Relationship to bladder function.* The absence of painful urination, bloody urine, and frequent urination tends to exclude disease of the urinary tract and bladder.

4. *Relationship to fever and chills.* The absence of fever and chills rules against the likelihood of serious pelvic inflammatory conditions, such as acute tube infections or ruptured pelvic abscess, as well as other severe, nongynecologic infections.

5. *Relationship to intercourse.* Abdominal pain that increases with intercourse may indicate pelvic inflammatory disease or endometriosis.

Pain during early pregnancy may be associated with any of the causes of pelvic pain previously mentioned. After the first three months of pregnancy, pain is due mostly to pressure produced by the enlarging uterus. Pressure over the pelvic bones causes a variety of pains which may be sharp, dull, or stabbing and may radiate to the legs, hips, or vagina. A particularly common form of pelvic discomfort in late pregnancy is *round ligament pain*, due to stretching of these supporting ligaments found along both sides of the uterus. This type of pain may be more pronounced on one side, sometimes mimicking a kidney stone or appendicitis when severe. However, there are no accompanying symptoms such as fever, vomiting, or bleeding. One of the most serious causes of acute pain in late pregnancy is abruptio placenta (see Chapter 53).

Probably the most common pains in the second half of pregnancy occur as a result of uterine contractions. The differences between real and false labor, both of which may be quite painful, are summarized in Table 99. Knowledge of the signs of labor can be one of the most important aspects of childbirth education, since premature labor and delivery contribute, more than any other factor, to newborn respiratory distress and death during the first month of life. Premature labor (see Chapter 21) usually occurs spontaneously but may also occur following bleeding (abruptio placenta, placenta previa; see Chapter 53) or in association with high blood pressure (toxemia) or premature rupture of the membranes (see Chapter 20).

Acute Lower Abdominal Pain—What Medical Care Can Do

The cause of acute abdominal pain can often be identified from an evaluation of the pain as described above. Diseases of the urinary tract are usually excluded by a urinalysis in the office. The possibility of appendicitis requires hospitalization until the correct diagnosis can be confirmed. A surgical consultation is routine when nongynecologic disease is considered in the diagnosis of acute abdominal pain.

During the physical exam the doctor is concerned with deciding if you need surgery. The abdominal exam is all-important in the diagnosis of appendicitis but gives less information as to the exact source of gynecologic conditions causing pain. The speculum exam is essential in diagnosing miscarriage because tissue is visualized as it is passed through the dilating cervix. The presence of a uterine discharge seen during the speculum exam is consistent with pelvic inflammatory disease but does not prove the diagnosis. When a ruptured ectopic pregnancy is suspected, a culdocentesis (see glossary) is performed to rapidly detect the presence of internal bleeding, a potentially life-threatening situation. In ectopic pregnancy, the bimanual exam may provide little additional information to the gynecologist because severe pain makes relaxation of the abdominal wall impossible.

The common lab tests that evaluate low abdominal pain include: complete blood count (CBC), urinalysis, pregnancy test, cervical culture (transgrow), abdominal and kidney X-rays, and a sonogram.

The treatment of acute pelvic pain will often require surgery unless an infection, such as a tube or an intestinal inflammation, is suspected. In this case, antibiotics are given while your condition is observed in the hospital.

Among the surgical approaches in treating abdominal pain is dilatation and curettage (D & C) (see Chapter 41), which is the best treatment for a miscarriage. A laparoscopy (see glossary) is done when an ectopic pregnancy or ovarian cyst is suspected but has not shown signs of rupture. If the diagnosis is mistaken, a laparoscopy may

Table 98 FINDINGS ASSOCIATED WITH VARIOUS CAUSES OF ACUTE LOWER ABDOMINAL PAIN

	Cause of Acute Lower Abdominal Pain					
Finding	Infection of Tube or Ovary	Miscarriage	Rupture of Tubal Pregnancy or of Ovarian Cyst	Urinary Tract Infection	Appendicitis	Intestinal Inflammation (Colitis, Diverticulitis)
Pain location	Bilateral	Midline	Unilateral	Variable	Variable at first, shifts to lower right side	Variable
Fever	Yes	Sometimes	No	Yes	Yes	Yes
Missed periods	No	Yes	Sometimes	No	No	No
Bleeding	No	Yes	No	No	No	No
Foul vaginal discharge	Yes	No	No	No	No	No
Diarrhea	Sometimes	No	No	No	Sometimes	Yes
Urinary symptoms (burning) and urinalysis shows infection present	No	No	No	Yes	No	No

Table 99   SIGNS OF LABOR

Factor	Real Labor	False Labor
Intensity of discomfort	increases	remains the same
Time between contractions	gradually shortens	remains long
Regularity of contractions	regular	irregular
Location of discomfort	entire uterus and back	lower abdomen and groin
Effect of alcohol or other sedatives	unaffected	often relieved
Cervix opening	cervix dilated	cervix not dilated
Effect of previous childbirth	none	increases likelihood
Bloody show	often associated	not associated

CHRONIC PELVIC PAIN

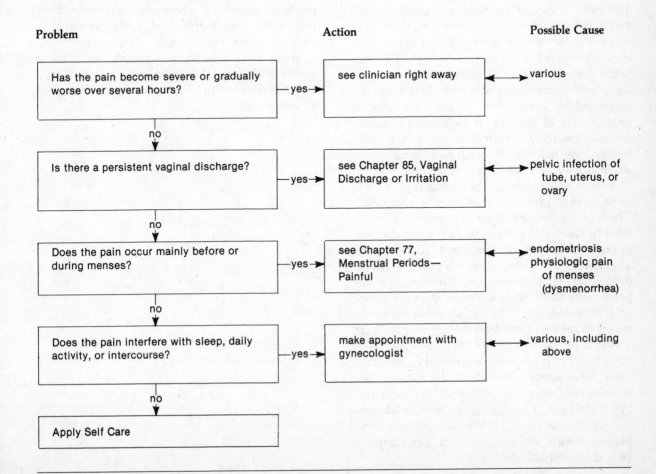

Problem	Action	Possible Cause
Has the pain become severe or gradually worse over several hours? →yes→	see clinician right away	various
↓no		
Is there a persistent vaginal discharge? →yes→	see Chapter 85, Vaginal Discharge or Irritation	pelvic infection of tube, uterus, or ovary
↓no		
Does the pain occur mainly before or during menses? →yes→	see Chapter 77, Menstrual Periods—Painful	endometriosis physiologic pain of menses (dysmenorrhea)
↓no		
Does the pain interfere with sleep, daily activity, or intercourse? →yes→	make appointment with gynecologist	various, including above
↓no		
Apply Self Care		

prevent an unnecessary incision and longer surgical recovery time. A laparotomy (see glossary) is indicated when the doctor diagnoses internal bleeding, a ruptured pelvic abscess, or some other condition requiring emergency surgery.

Table 98 summarizes the findings associated with various causes of acute lower abdominal pain.

Acute Lower Abdominal Pain—What You Can Do (Self Care)

If severe pain persists for several hours, get early medical attention. Do not eat or use an enema as long as the pain is severe. If you are pregnant, learn the signs of labor (see Table 99) and get prompt medical attention if pain is accompanied by bleeding or markedly decreased fetal movement.

Chronic Lower Abdominal Pain—What Medical Care Can Do

The same tests that are used to diagnose acute pelvic pain are used for chronic pelvic pain (that is, pain lasting several days or more) except that they are ordered on an outpatient basis. Chronic pelvic pain may be a frustrating problem for patients and doctors alike since no disease can be diagnosed by examination or lab tests approximately 50% of the time. If a diagnosis is made, medical treatment may include hormones, antibiotics, vaginal creams, and pain medication. Referral may be made to a urologist for urinary problems, to an internist for intestinal problems, or to an orthopedist for evaluation of your back. The role of emotional stress at home and at work must be taken into account because stress may aggravate pelvic pain. For this reason, it may be advisable for you to consult with a psychologist or other counseling professional. However, the apparent absence of physical disease does not imply an emotional basis for the pain. On the contrary, failure to respond to medical therapy may indicate a need to pursue the cause of the pain to rule out a malignancy. This is often accomplished by diagnostic laparoscopy which allows the doctor to see all the pelvic organs as well as the appendix and upper abdomen. Common gynecologic conditions causing chronic pelvic pain include pelvic inflammatory disease and endometriosis (see Chapters 24 and 35, respectively).

Chronic Lower Abdominal Pain—What You Can Do (Self Care)

Keep a record of your pain—when it occurs, its location, what makes it better or worse. Bring your record with you to the next office visit. Avoid whatever makes the pain recur. Many pains for which no cause is determined go away on their own. Pelvic inflammation responds to rest, warm Betadine douches, and temporary abstinence from sexual intercourse. Bladder infections also improve faster if intercourse is avoided and if you drink fluids during treatment. To help relieve the pain, try a heating pad over the abdomen or back. If an antibiotic or other medication has been prescribed, take the full amount even if symptoms begin to improve before you complete the prescription (see Chapter 29). Take Tylenol, or other analgesics containing only acetaminophen, in preference to aspirin-containing drugs; as a rule aspirin often causes stomach irritation. See also Chapter 49 for further discussion of over-the-counter analgesics (pain pills). Pain often produces emotional stress, and this stress then makes the pain worse; and a vicious circle is created. Make your health a high priority by allowing extra time for rest periods, including a good night's sleep. If the pain lasts for several days and interferes with your normal activities, see your doctor.

82

Swelling and Fluid Retention

In women the most common cause of generalized swelling (edema) is premenstrual fluid retention. Women in their thirties and forties are particularly affected. The addition of several pounds of water which gradually occurs during the two- to ten-day length of time before menses may cause a variety of symptoms including swollen legs, breast fullness, pelvic ache, headache, nervousness, irritability, insomnia, and loss of concentration. These symptoms peak in intensity just before menses and cease abruptly after the onset of bleeding. There is wide variation in the symptoms experienced among women. The condition is sometimes referred to as pre-menstrual syndrome (PMS).

Both the physical and emotional symptoms of premenstrual tension have some biochemical basis related to the high level of hormones in the second half of the menstrual cycle, when the estrogen level is higher. Recent research indicates that an important factor is the ability of estrogen to partially block salt and water excretion by the kidneys. As a result, the body retains fluid. Increased retention of fluid within the intestines helps to account for the frequency of diarrhea and cramping experienced by some women. Fluid retention involving the pelvic organs may have positive or negative effects. Some women experience congestion of the pelvic veins and feel this congestion as a dull, low abdominal aching pressure. Congestion around the vulva, on the other hand, may stimulate increased clitoral or vaginal awareness associated with greater sexual desire or responsiveness.

Women taking birth control pills (see Chapter 9) tend to have fewer and milder premenstrual symptoms compared to women using other contraceptive methods or none at all. This difference is due, perhaps, to the fact that the fixed ingredients of the pill prevent the slightest hormonal imbalance from occurring and because most birth control pills in current use contain relatively low dosages of estrogen. Premenstrual fluid retention and weight gain often subside after two or three months of birth control pill use.

Abdominal swelling unaccompanied by fluid retention elsewhere in the body is often due to a digestive problem. Gas, indigestion, and air swallowing cause temporary bloating and are likely to occur at times of psychological stress. A serious digestive disorder causing abdominal swelling is usually associated with abdominal pain, jaundice, vomiting, or bloody stool. In the gynecologic area pregnancy and ovarian tumors are the principal causes of abdominal swelling.

Pregnancy is associated with fluid retention of much greater magnitude than that of premenstrual tension, although the symptoms produced in each case may be strikingly similar. Characteristically, swelling, or *edema*, is worse at the end of pregnancy when the total amount of excess water retained may amount to 6½ quarts or more. About half of the water content is found in the fetus, bag of waters, and placenta. The rest is distributed to the mother's tissues, especially to the blood, breasts, and uterus. The mother's feet and legs usually swell the most because the growing uterus compresses the large veins that return blood from the lower extremities to the heart. When you lie down on your side, the uterus no longer blocks these vessels and swelling tends to go down. This is why at night more frequent urination occurs as fluid from the legs is available for excretion by the kidneys.

In pregnancy generalized edema involving the hands and face, as well as the legs, may be an abnormal finding signifying toxemia or high blood pressure, especially when the edema is accompanied by headaches, blurred vision, or dizziness. Rapid accumulation of water of more than five pounds in any given week may be the first sign of toxemia even before generalized swelling occurs.

What Medical Care Can Do

The treatment of premenstrual tension depends on the severity and type of symptoms experienced. The physician's medical management for premenstrual fluid retention consists of water pills (diuretics), hormones, and tranquilizers. For some women, the easiest way to get rid of weight and excess fluid is through water pills. When these drugs are taken chronically, potassium salts are lost in the urine and must be replaced with foods rich in potassium, such as bananas, oranges, or cranberry juice, or by potassium supplementation in the form of pills. Depletion of potassium may cause weakness and muscle cramps. Water pills are also used to control blood pressure. Because of the possibility of side effects, water pills, should be used sparingly when taken for relief of fluid retention or premenstrual tension.

A newer treatment for pre-menstrual syndrome (PMS) consists of progesterone vaginal suppositories. Some reports especially from England suggest the progesterone suppositories may represent a breakthrough in the treatment of PMS. However, since the suppositories are not yet FDA approved for this purpose, their availability in pharmacies and through physicians' offices is limited. Hormones in the form of birth control pills as well as progesterone in pill form may also relieve symptoms of PMS in some women.

If you are pregnant, you should avoid drug

SWELLING AND FLUID RETENTION

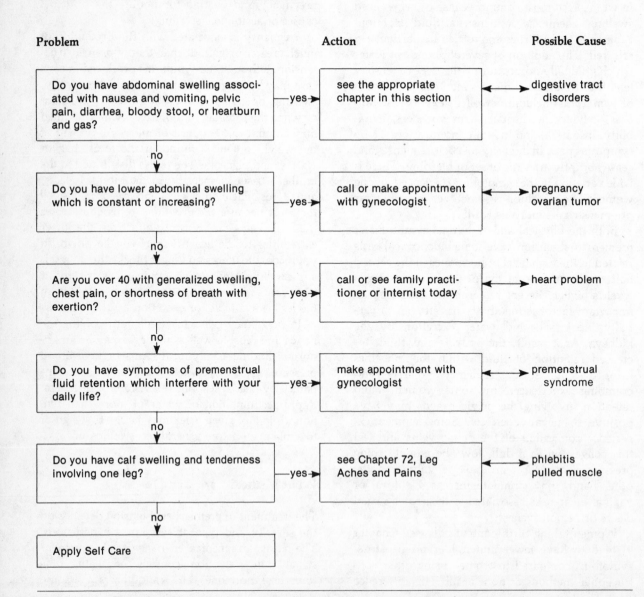

Problem	Action	Possible Cause
Do you have abdominal swelling associated with nausea and vomiting, pelvic pain, diarrhea, bloody stool, or heartburn and gas? —yes→	see the appropriate chapter in this section ←→	digestive tract disorders
no ↓		
Do you have lower abdominal swelling which is constant or increasing? —yes→	call or make appointment with gynecologist ←→	pregnancy ovarian tumor
no ↓		
Are you over 40 with generalized swelling, chest pain, or shortness of breath with exertion? —yes→	call or see family practitioner or internist today ←→	heart problem
no ↓		
Do you have symptoms of premenstrual fluid retention which interfere with your daily life? —yes→	make appointment with gynecologist ←→	premenstrual syndrome
no ↓		
Do you have calf swelling and tenderness involving one leg? —yes→	see Chapter 72, Leg Aches and Pains ←→	phlebitis pulled muscle
no ↓		
Apply Self Care		

therapy if possible. The use of water pills for treating uncomplicated leg swelling in pregnancy is not effective and is potentially hazardous to your unborn. The occasional use of diuretics for the pregnant woman with high blood pressure may be necessary.

What You Can Do (Self Care)

Your body retains water to dilute dietary salt, so restriction of salt is one of the most important steps in reducing fluid retention (see Chapter 46). The week before your period, avoid adding salt in cooking and don't eat salty foods, such as processed lunch meats, or highly seasoned foods. Drinking large amounts of water "to flush the kidneys and rid salt" from your body sounds like a good idea but has limited practical benefit in reducing symptoms of fluid retention. If you are on the pill, consider a change to a lower estrogen dose pill or to a mini-pill (see Chapter 9). In addition to rest and a nutritious diet (see Chapter 46), recreation and activity, especially sexual activity, relieves vascular congestion as well as emotional tension in many women.

During pregnancy, bed rest is the most effective way to reduce water retention. Elevate your legs whenever possible during the day. Fitted support hose may help. The restricted use of salt to control edema in pregnancy is controversial. Fluid retention and weekly weight gain are the result of many complex hormonal factors involving more than how much salt a woman takes in her diet. Although some women are particularly sensitive and respond to high salt intake with swelling, most do not and will not find symptomatic relief by restricting salt. Attempts to completely eliminate salt from your diet may, in fact, be hazardous to the fetus and is not recommended in normal pregnancies.

83

Urinary Problems— Frequent or Urgent Urination

If you experience frequent urination, called *urinary frequency*, or the sudden urge to urinate, called *urinary urgency*, you may have a urinary tract infection. Such infection usually involves some discomfort as well—either a burning sensation during urination or a dull pain in the lower abdomen toward the end of urination. A bladder infection (cystitis) may cause a constant desire to void (urinate) even when the bladder is nearly empty.

In the absence of painful or bloody urination, frequent or urgent urination is likely to result from other conditions, especially *urethral stenosis* and *cystocele*. Urethral stenosis, or stricture, refers to narrowing of the urethra. In women this condition occurs relatively frequently and from various causes. Urethral stenosis may be present from birth and first show up in adolescence or even earlier. At other times, this problem results from previous infection (such as gonorrhea—see Chapter 24), or it first develops after menopause from estrogen-deficiency related changes in the urethra (see Chapter 26). A cystocele (see Chapter 28) refers to a vaginal hernia or bulge that develops from a weakening of the vaginal muscles, especially in postmenopausal women. Cystoceles cause symptoms of urinary frequency and urgency because complete emptying of the bladder is prevented.

Frequent urination without urgency may be due

to excessive fluid intake, anxiety, alcohol, beverages containing caffeine, or diuretics (water pills), all of which increase urine formation. In addition, any pelvic mass, including a pregnancy, may press on the bladder, thereby producing more frequent urination.

Emotional stress can be a contributing cause, as well as an effect, of frequency and urgency and of *urgency incontinence*, the involuntary loss of urine. Such incontinence occurs from bladder spasms associated with severe urgency and clears up promptly once the underlying cause is treated. Urgency incontinence is quite different from another form of incontinence called *stress incontinence*, which is not associated with urinary frequency or urgency. With stress incontinence, the involuntary loss of urine occurs during physical (not emotional) stress, such as coughing, sneezing, laughing, or running. This form of incontinence results not from bladder spasms but from bladder muscle weakness or damage (for example, from childbirth) that prevents the bladder from containing the urine during strenuous physical activity. While stress incontinence is often relieved by surgery or special exercises, urgency incontinence is not.

URINARY PROBLEMS—FREQUENT OR URGENT URINATION

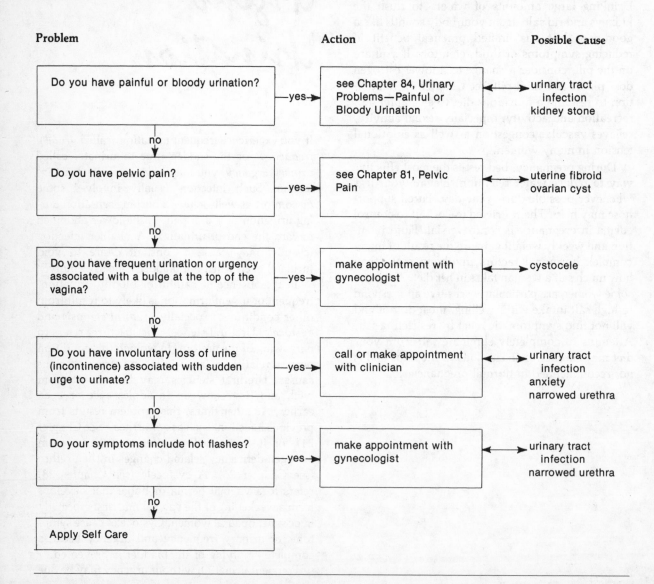

Problem	Action	Possible Cause
Do you have painful or bloody urination?	—yes→ see Chapter 84, Urinary Problems—Painful or Bloody Urination	urinary tract infection kidney stone
Do you have pelvic pain?	—yes→ see Chapter 81, Pelvic Pain	uterine fibroid ovarian cyst
Do you have frequent urination or urgency associated with a bulge at the top of the vagina?	—yes→ make appointment with gynecologist	cystocele
Do you have involuntary loss of urine (incontinence) associated with sudden urge to urinate?	—yes→ call or make appointment with clinician	urinary tract infection anxiety narrowed urethra
Do your symptoms include hot flashes?	—yes→ make appointment with gynecologist	urinary tract infection narrowed urethra
Apply Self Care		

What Medical Care Can Do

The physician does a pelvic exam to exclude pelvic tumors, pregnancy, or cystocele. He or she will also obtain a urinalysis or urine culture to check for bladder or kidney infection. In the absence of such infection, the doctor may prescribe antispasmodic drugs, such as Urispas, which relaxes the bladder muscle. If you have urgency or stress incontinence or urethral stenosis, you may need a referral to a urologist (bladder and kidney specialist).

What You Can Do (Self Care)

Urinary frequency and urinary urgency are usually temporary symptoms or are related to dietary or emotional factors which you may be able to minimize. Symptoms of stress incontinence may be reduced by a special exercise (called Kegel's exercise). (See Chapter 28, under Urinary Stress Incontinence, for instructions on how to do this exercise.) If incontinence becomes worse or persists or if you have bloody or painful urination, see your physician.

84

Urinary Problems— Painful or Bloody Urination

Painful or bloody urination is usually due to a urinary tract infection. Such infections affect women far more frequently than men because the urethra, which connects the bladder to the outside of the body, is located very close to the vagina and anus, both of which are sources of bacteria. Because of poor hygiene or during intercourse, childbirth, or gynecologic surgery, bacteria may enter the urethra and eventually cause infection of the lower or upper urinary tract (see Figure 41).

Lower urinary tract infections involving either the urethra (*urethritis*) or bladder (*cystitis*) are the most common. Cystitis will cause painful and sometimes bloody, frequent, or urgent urination. When the only symptom is a burning sensation on urination, urethritis is more likely to be the cause. Special kinds of urethritis may occur as a result of allergic reactions (to soaps, vaginal creams, etc.) or from venereal infection, especially gonorrhea (see Chapter 24). More often, urethritis and cystitis occur together as common symptoms of nonvenereal infections. No one knows why some women are more prone to urinary tract infections. Bladder infections often result from sexual activity and are sometimes known as *honeymoon cystitis* since they frequently occur among young women who have just become sexually active.

Figure 41
The female urinary system.

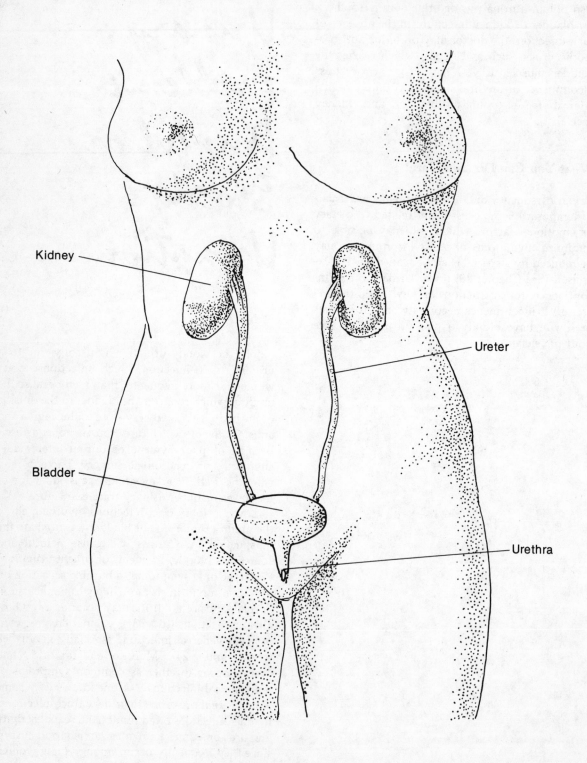

Kidney

Ureter

Bladder

Urethra

The urethra itself is especially susceptible to infection because of the number of pockets and crevices which line the wall of this complex tube. Several small pockets may form one large pouch, called a *diverticulum*, which may collect urinary debris. Swelling and inflammation of this diverticulum may prevent adequate drainage and result in chronic infection unresponsive to antibiotic therapy. In some women, the presence of a cystocele (see glossary) may make her susceptible to chronic infection because of the woman's inability to completely empty her bladder. Bacteria may grow rapidly in the urine which remains.

When cystitis spreads beyond the bladder, then upper urinary tract or kidney infection (*pyelonephritis*) occurs. Kidney infections, unlike bladder infections, are associated with symptoms such as weakness, nausea, backache, fever, and chills. Kidney infections, like bladder infections, usually respond rapidly to antibiotics. Occasionally kidney infections become chronic and result in kidney damage.

During pregnancy, hormonal changes cause a general relaxation in the muscle tone of the urinary system, resulting in retention of urine in the two ureters (the *ureter* is the tube carrying urine from each kidney to the bladder) and bladder. This urine retention makes the woman susceptible to symptomless bacterial growth. For this reason, physicians may routinely perform urine cultures during pregnancy, because kidney infections may be associated with premature labor.

Painful urination is not always associated with bacterial infection. Herpes infections, vaginal infections, intercourse, and chemical irritation from vaginal hygiene products may all cause urination discomfort. During menopause, lower estrogen levels increase susceptibility to bladder irritation, causing occasional burning with urination.

What Medical Care Can Do

The doctor will do a pelvic exam as well as a culture for gonorrhea if venereal infection is suspected. He or she diagnoses a urinary tract infection by urinalysis (see glossary) and urine culture. New screening methods have recently become available that use a paper strip (for example, N-Uristix) which changes color in less than a minute when the strip is dipped in infected urine.

But the most accurate diagnostic technique is the urine culture, which takes the laboratory twenty-four to seventy-two hours for the results. The culture tells which bacteria are causing the infection, and the doctor will know which antibiotic will destroy the bacteria. To collect a urine sample for a urine culture, here is what you do: first, you separate the lips of the vagina and clean the urinary opening with mild soap and water; next, you urinate a small amount into the toilet bowl; and then you urinate a portion of the urine into the sterile container. This process is known as a *clean-catch midstream* collection; and the specimen is much more reliable than a specimen collected from simply urinating into a cup, which may cause contamination of the urine specimen. When a urine culture reveals no bacterial growth, the physician rules out urinary tract infection and looks for other causes of the symptoms (see Chapter 83, Urinary Problems—Frequent or Urgent Urination).

The physician may refer you to a urologist if urinary tract infections occur chronically. An IVP (intravenous pyelogram—see glossary) is a kidney X-ray which may be ordered by a physician to check for signs of previous kidney infection, kidney stones, or slight anatomic variations in the urinary tract which sometimes make a person susceptible to infection. Cystoscopy is a procedure to examine the inside of the bladder. This may be done in the doctor's office or as an outpatient surgical procedure.

The treatment of urinary tract infection always involves taking antibiotics, usually for seven to fourteen days. Persistent infections may require a course of antibiotics lasting several months, even during pregnancy when changes in the urinary system make a woman susceptible to the growth of bacteria. If you have a long history of multiple bladder or kidney infections, your doctor may prescribe antibiotics as a preventative to be taken once before or immediately after intercourse. Hospitalization may be required for treating kidney infections that occur in pregnancy or for recurrent infections among nonpregnant women not responding to oral antibiotics.

What You Can Do (Self Care)

Drink plenty of fluids to help flush out the urinary tract. Drinking cranberry juice acidifies the urine, which helps prevent bacterial growth within the

Table 100   QUESTIONS COMMONLY ASKED ABOUT URINARY TRACT INFECTIONS

Question	Yes	No	Comment
Are kidney or bladder infections contagious?		X	They are not transmitted by intercourse, unlike venereal infection. However, gonorrhea may produce symptoms like a bladder infection such as burning with urination.
Is a kidney stone the commonest cause of bloody urination after urinary tract infection?	X		The stone may become lodged in the ureter (the tube between the kidney and bladder) and produce severe back or abdominal pain on one side.
Can chronic kidney damage cause high blood pressure?	X		High blood pressure may occur after multiple kidney infections.
Is kidney damage common?		X	Most urinary tract infections are limited to the bladder and urethra.
Should a previously prescribed antibiotic be taken for a urinary tract infection?		X	Although the symptoms may be the same, different infections may be caused by different bacteria and will require different antibiotic treatment.
Does wearing a tampon delay recovery from a urinary tract infection?		X	There is no effect on the course of the infection.
Are periods of increased sexual activity associated with an increased frequency of bladder infections?	X		Bacteria from the vagina may be mechanically introduced into the urethra (the tube through which urine passes from the bladder to the outside of the body).
Are bladder infections more common during and after menopause?	X		Estrogen loss during and after menopause makes the tissues more vulnerable to bacteria.
Is painful and frequent urination always a sign of a bladder or kidney infection?		X	Chemical irritation and vaginal herpes infections also cause these symptoms.

Table 101   CAUSES OF CHRONIC BLADDER AND URETHRAL INFECTIONS IN WOMEN

Cause	Source of Infection	Where Infection Occurs	Treatment
resistant bacteria	insufficient or wrong antibiotic	bladder or urethra	antibiotics for several weeks
cystocele (weakening or hernia of bladder wall)	incomplete bladder-emptying due to cystocele	bladder	surgery (in some cases)
diverticulum (pocket in urethra)	small amounts of bacteria chronically pocketed in diverticulum	bladder or urethra	surgery
venereal infection involving urethra (gonorrhea or chlamydia)	sexual intercourse with infected partner	urethra	antibiotics

urinary tract. Take antibiotics exactly as prescribed even though your symptoms subside in three or four days. It is a good idea to have a repeat urine culture two weeks after your treatment begins to make sure that the infection is cleared up. A consultation with a urologist is advisable when urinary tract infections persist despite antibiotic therapy.

Here are suggestions that will help you to prevent urinary tract infections:

1. Don't hold your urine for prolonged periods; respond to the urge to urinate.
2. Be sure to wash the external genitalia each time you bathe or shower.
3. Urinate soon after intercourse.
4. After a bowel movement, be sure to wipe from front to back to avoid contamination of the urinary tract.
5. Avoid the use of urethral irritants, such as vaginal perfumes and bubble baths. Continue to use vaginal contraceptive cream or foam (if this is your birth control method) since these products kill bacteria as well as sperm.

6. During pregnancy, have a urine culture ordered if you have a history of urinary tract infections. Many women do not realize that prenatal urine evaluations in the doctor's office, while checking for protein or sugar, may not include a test for infection.
7. If you have a history of frequent bladder or kidney infections, consider testing your urine for infection yourself on a periodic (for example, monthly) basis. This can be done by asking your pharmacist to order one of the new paper strip tests (such as N-Uristix) which detect urinary infection. These products, while mostly sold for use in doctors' offices, are available over-the-counter for home use as well.

Table 100 answers some specific questions about urinary tract infections.

Table 101 summarizes some information about the causes of chronic bladder and urethral infections in women.

URINARY PROBLEMS—PAINFUL OR BLOODY URINATION

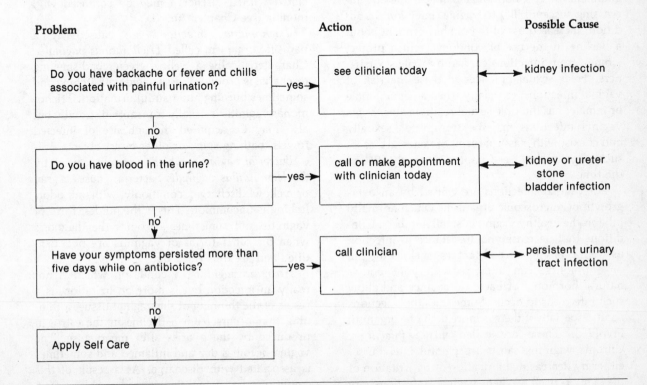

Problem	Action	Possible Cause
Do you have backache or fever and chills associated with painful urination? —yes→	see clinician today	←→ kidney infection
↓ no		
Do you have blood in the urine? —yes→	call or make appointment with clinician today	←→ kidney or ureter stone / bladder infection
↓ no		
Have your symptoms persisted more than five days while on antibiotics? —yes→	call clinician	←→ persistent urinary tract infection
↓ no		
Apply Self Care		

85

Vaginal Discharge or Irritation

Vaginitis is an inflammation of the vagina, often accompanied by pain, itching, discharge, and odor. It is most often due to an infection. Women who experience vaginitis are likely to describe it as "simply awful." The incidence of vaginal infections has been steadily increasing over the last decade, and this problem now accounts for more than five million clinician visits each year. Various explanations for the increase in vaginal infections include changing patterns of sexuality and contraceptive practices. Taking birth control pills alters the body's hormonal balance, thereby increasing susceptibility to vaginal infection. In addition, increased use of the pill has brought about a decline in the use of condoms, which protect women from infections carried by male sex partners. Freer sexual practices increase the risk of vaginal infections, especially when a person, male or female, has multiple sexual relationships. Some vaginal infections may be transmitted sexually and coexist with classical forms of venereal disease such as gonorrhea (see Chapter 24) nearly 10% of the time.

All vaginal infections are caused by an overgrowth of microscopic organisms which normally inhabit the healthy vagina in small numbers. Conditions that decrease your resistance to infection as well as environmental factors, such as the pill or antibiotics, can interfere with your body's natural hormonal or bacterial balance and allow such infections to occur. Sometimes the infections recur, especially if there is more than one organism involved. These are called *mixed infections*. Chronic vaginitis can cause painful intercourse, either by decreasing lubrication or by irritation of the vulva itself. When vaginal infections are chronic, there is usually inflammation of the cervix as well, the cervix often being secondarily infected. On the other hand, infection within the cervix, such as gonorrhea or a uterine infection associated with the use of an IUD, may be the primary cause of vaginal discharge.

The most common vaginal infections are discussed below.

Yeast infections, also known as *monilia* or *candidiasis*, are the most common type of vaginal infection. Yeast infections are caused by an overgrowth of a funguslike organism, *Candida albicans*. This organism is normally present in small amounts in the vagina as well as in the mouth and digestive tract. Monilia causes a white discharge which looks like cottage cheese. The most common symptom is intense itching of the external genitalia. Symptoms may vary from mild irritation to severe redness and swelling of the vulva. There may also be painful urination or pain during intercourse. Monilia is more common during pregnancy and in women taking hormones, including birth control pills. It is also more frequent when antibiotics are being taken because of the imbalance of normal bacteria that occurs. Chronic monilia may be the first sign of diabetes. Although monilia is the most common cause of vulvar itching, many other causes of itching or rash unassociated with a discharge may be confused with monilia (see Chapter 70).

Trichomonas infections are caused by a parasitic organism called *Trichomonas vaginalis*. Characteristically a yellow-green, bad-smelling discharge is produced, associated with itching and sometimes burning and painful urination. Trichomonas vaginitis is usually transmitted sexually but also may be acquired through use of infected towels, bathing suits, or other moist objects.

Bacterial vaginitis, which is usually caused by the *Hemophilus vaginalis* bacteria, causes a gray or yellow discharge, commonly with an odor. Itching is uncommon. This is the mildest form of vaginitis and sometimes becomes the diagnosis when the other forms of vaginitis are not identified and are thus ruled out.

Atrophic vaginitis, a condition which is not really an infection but is more an irritation, is a result of the thinning of the vaginal tissue, a thinning that occurs from a decline in the estrogen produced by the ovaries after menopause. The vagina becomes dry and inflamed and sometimes is associated with discharge. As a result of this condition, the vaginal tissues are less able to fend

Table 102 TREATMENT OF VAGINAL INFECTIONS (VAGINITIS)

Type of Infection	Typical Drugs to Treat This Infection	How Drug Is Taken	Comment
Monilia (yeast)	Gyne-Lotrimin (vaginal tablets or cream)	Insert tab or cream into vagina once daily for one week or insert two tabs once daily for three days.	Regardless of which medication is used, treatment may require two or more weeks when infection is severe.
	Monistat 3 (vaginal tablets)	Insert tab into vagina once daily for three days.	Mycolog cream often used in conjunction with one of the other medications.
	Monistat 7 (vaginal tablets or cream)	Insert tab or cream into vagina once daily for one week.	Allergic reactions (local burning or itching) are relatively common with Mycolog because of its multiple ingredients.
	Mycelex-G (vaginal tablets or cream)	Insert tab or cream into vagina once daily for one week, or insert two tabs once daily for three days.	
	Mycostatin (vaginal tablets, cream, ointment, or powder)	Insert into vagina twice daily for two weeks.	
	Mycolog (cream or ointment)	Apply to outer vagina (vulva) twice daily for one to two weeks.	
Trichomonas ("trich")	Flagyl (pills)* (relief of symptoms sometimes helped by certain vaginal preparations, especially Betadine, Vagisec, Triva Jel—see Table 103)	Take orally as directed.	Avoid alcohol—interacts with Flagyl to cause vomiting. Partner should also be treated. Avoid Flagyl in pregnancy.
Bacterial (Hemophilus)	Ampicillin (pills)	Take orally as directed.	Ampicillin rarely may cause severe allergic reactions if you are allergic to penicillin (see *anaphylaxis* in glossary).
	Flagyl (pills)*	Take orally as directed.	Flagyl—see comments above under trichomonas infections.
	Doxycycline (pills)	Take orally as directed.	Partner may need to be treated if infection persists after you have been treated.
	Sultrin (vaginal tablets or cream)	Insert tab or cream into vagina twice daily for one week.	
	Betadine douche	Douche daily for one week or as directed.	
Atrophic (estrogen-deficiency related)	AVC with Dienestrol (vaginal tablets or cream) Dienestrol (vaginal cream) Ogen (vaginal cream) Premarin (vaginal cream) (For information on oral estrogen therapy for atrophic vaginitis, see Chapter 27.)	Insert into vagina as directed.	All of these drugs contain estrogen and should be avoided if you might be pregnant or if you have had breast cancer or a history of blood clots. Less estrogen is absorbed with vaginal as opposed to oral products; however, the same precautions apply (see Chapter 27). Avoid using continuously—stop medication for one week every month. Discuss with your doctor the benefits and risks of taking these vaginal estrogen-containing drugs.

*Other equivalent brands include Metryl, Satric, and Protostat.

off bacteria. The tissues are also more susceptible to abrasion during intercourse, which, in turn, increases susceptibility to infection. Atrophic vaginitis may occur before menopause in women who have had surgical removal of the ovaries.

Noninfectious causes of vaginal discharge sometimes occur. The adolescent woman will probably experience a profuse watery discharge prior to or following the beginning of menstruation as a result of the hormonal surge that occurs at puberty. During the reproductive years, some vaginal discharge is considered physiologic, a normal consequence of ovulation especially in women who have had one or more pregnancies. Increased glandular secretions from the cervix may also occur normally as a result of taking birth control pills. Unlike vaginitis, physiologic discharges occur without odor and are perfectly harmless.

What Medical Care Can Do

Be sure to avoid douching for twenty-four to forty-eight hours prior to the office visit because the diagnosis of vaginal discharge is made on the basis of the pelvic examination and the results from a glass slide of vaginal secretions (*wet smear*). A culture for gonorrhea and a blood test for syphilis may be obtained if exposure to venereal disease is suspected. Mild physiologic discharge does not need any treatment at all. Excessive discharge without infection is sometimes treated by cautery of the cervix (see glossary), or by using a freeze technique, called cryosurgery (see glossary). If the discharge is due to a uterine or an ovarian infection, the physician will prescribe an appropriate antibiotic.

If a vaginal infection alone is diagnosed, specific antibiotic or local vaginal therapy is prescribed. Treatment of the main types of vaginitis is discussed in Table 102. When the exact cause of a vaginal infection cannot be found, the clinician then treats for *nonspecific vaginitis*. Table 103 outlines instructions and precautions for using some of the vaginal drugs commonly prescribed for nonspecific vaginitis. Treatment in

---

Table 103 COMMONLY USED PRESCRIPTION DRUGS FOR NONSPECIFIC VAGINITIS—INSTRUCTIONS AND PRECAUTIONS

Brand Name	How to Use	Precautions
Mycolog Cream	Apply to vulva as directed for relief of vulvar itching or burning. Often used along with a vaginal douche, suppository, or cream.	Avoid if you have active herpes vaginal infection.
AVC (cream or suppositories)	Apply cream or suppositories into vagina in morning and at bedtime; usually therapy requires 14 days.	Avoid if allergic to sulfa.
Vagitrol (cream or suppositories)	Apply cream or suppositories into vagina in morning and at bedtime; usually therapy requires 14 days.	Avoid if allergic to sulfa.
Vagisec (liquid douche and suppositories)	Use douche, followed by suppository in morning; use suppository at bedtime; continue therapy 14 days.	Avoid douche in pregnancy.
Triva Combination (gel and douche powder)	Use douche followed by gel at bedtime; continue therapy for 14 days.	Avoid douche in pregnancy.
Vagilia (cream or suppositories)	Apply cream or suppositories into vagina in morning and at bedtime; usually therapy requires at least 14 days.	Avoid if allergic to sulfa.
Trichotine (liquid, powder, or disposable douche)	Use as directed as additional therapy for vaginal infections.	Not sufficient treatment by itself for nonspecific vaginitis.
Aci-jel	One application intravaginally, in the morning and at bedtime	Not sufficient treatment by itself for nonspecific vaginitis.

this case is essentially based on a trial-and-error approach, which is less likely to be effective than when a specific cause of vaginitis is diagnosed from the wet smear.

VAGINAL DISCHARGE OR IRRITATION

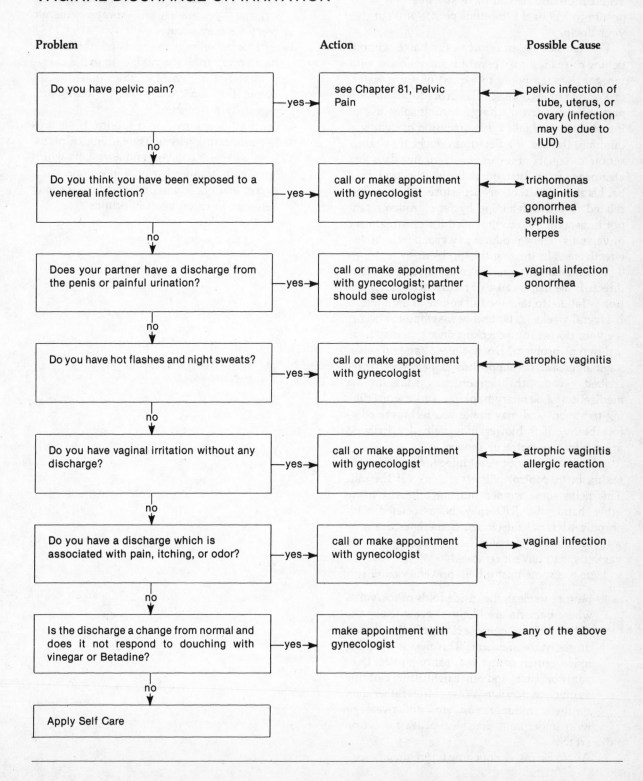

Problem	Action	Possible Cause
Do you have pelvic pain? —yes→	see Chapter 81, Pelvic Pain	pelvic infection of tube, uterus, or ovary (infection may be due to IUD)
no ↓		
Do you think you have been exposed to a venereal infection? —yes→	call or make appointment with gynecologist	trichomonas vaginitis gonorrhea syphilis herpes
no ↓		
Does your partner have a discharge from the penis or painful urination? —yes→	call or make appointment with gynecologist; partner should see urologist	vaginal infection gonorrhea
no ↓		
Do you have hot flashes and night sweats? —yes→	call or make appointment with gynecologist	atrophic vaginitis
no ↓		
Do you have vaginal irritation without any discharge? —yes→	call or make appointment with gynecologist	atrophic vaginitis allergic reaction
no ↓		
Do you have a discharge which is associated with pain, itching, or odor? —yes→	call or make appointment with gynecologist	vaginal infection
no ↓		
Is the discharge a change from normal and does it not respond to douching with vinegar or Betadine? —yes→	make appointment with gynecologist	any of the above
no ↓		
Apply Self Care		

What You Can Do (Self Care)

The sexually active woman should keep in mind that unusual vaginal discharge could represent a venereal disease. If you have any question of exposure to VD or if symptoms persist or recur, see your doctor.

Women having an odorless discharge without itching or redness may benefit from douching with vinegar (two teaspoons to a quart of warm water) one or two times a week. This procedure is helpful particularly when discharge accompanies use of the birth control pill. When irritation or itching is minimal, the use of a Betadine douche (one tablespoon to a quart of warm water) for five days and abstinence from intercourse during this time may be helpful. Most other drugstore douches and related so-called feminine hygiene products cannot in general be recommended for self-treatment of vaginitis. These products as a group lack proven effectiveness in treating this problem.

When medication has been prescribed, use it as directed; the major cause of recurrence of an infection is failure to take the full course of antibiotics. If several weeks go by and new symptoms occur, see your doctor for a checkup since you may have a different problem. Do not use a tampon when vaginal cream or suppositories have been prescribed because the tampon may soak up the medication. A sanitary napkin may be worn during treatment and may make you feel more comfortable. A hair blower may help dry irritated areas after you bathe or shower.

If you have chronic yeast infections and you are taking birth control pills, try going off the pill. This helps some women but not others. On the other hand, the IUD may be associated with chronic bacterial infections. Sometimes the only way to find out if your IUD is causing chronic vaginitis is to have it removed.

Here are some tips to help prevent vaginitis:

1. Be sure to clean the inside folds of the vulva where bacteria are likely to grow. Keep the vulva as dry as possible since infection thrives on moisture and heat. This means avoiding nylon-crotch pantyhose, panty girdles, tight pants or jeans, and other tightfitting clothing as much as possible. Wear cotton rather than synthetic (nylon, rayon, etc.) underwear, or wear underpants that have at least a cotton crotch.
2. Avoid excessive douching (more than twice a week), which may upset the normal chemical balance that helps ward off infection. Douching as a routine practice is probably never necessary.
3. Avoid strong detergent soaps and feminine hygiene deodorants and sprays. Allergic reactions may occur.
4. After a bowel movement, wipe toward the back, away from the vagina, to avoid carrying bacteria or yeast into the vagina.
5. Avoid the unnecessary use of antibiotics, especially for colds.
6. During intercourse use a lubricant, such as K-Y lubricating jelly or Transi-Lube, if necessary, to avoid irritation and abrasions which open pathways for bacterial infection.
7. A diet low in carbohydrates and sweets may help cut down on yeast infections.

86

Vaginal Lump

A lump in the vaginal area is a fairly common but upsetting finding, especially when the cause is unknown. Be assured that over 99% of vaginal lumps are benign. Most lumps are painless and are usually discovered inadvertently. Sometimes a woman or her sex partner feels the cervix for the first time and mistakes this part of the anatomy for a tumor.

Small, soft, nontender masses, usually no larger than a grape, are likely to be *retention cysts*. These fluid-filled solitary growths may occur anywhere within the vagina or vulva where glands are found; they are formed when gland ducts opening into the vagina or vulva are blocked. A vaginal cyst may also result from previous episiotomy repair (sewing up of the cut made at childbirth). Retention cysts must be distinguished from hair follicle infections, which are solitary tender areas that often drain intermittently and usually subside in a few days.

A larger type of cyst originating from one of the Bartholin's glands is found at the base of the vagina and typically measures 1 to 2 inches in diameter (see Figure 42). Like retention cysts, Bartholin's cysts are soft and nontender, but they have a much greater tendency to become infected and form an abscess.

Another cause of vaginal lumps is vaginal wall hernias called *cystoceles* and *rectoceles* (see Chapter 28). Cystoceles occur in the front vaginal wall whereas rectoceles are found in the back vaginal wall. These bulges are common in women who have given birth to several large babies; the result of such births is a stretching of the muscles supporting the vagina, bladder, and rectum. Associated symptoms may include vaginal pressure or ache, difficulty emptying the bladder, urinary stress incontinence, difficulty with elimination, or difficulty with penetration during intercourse.

Occasionally venereal warts, called *condylomata* (see Chapter 24), are responsible for the complaint of vaginal lumps. These lumps occur singularly or in groups as wartlike growths rarely larger than the tip of a pencil. Of all the vaginal lumps discussed here, condylomata are the only ones that increase in size and number during pregnancy.

In the postpartum period, the most common cause of vaginal lumps is painful complications of the episiotomy repair, including blood clot formation (hematoma) and infection.

What Medical Care Can Do

The pelvic examination readily distinguishes the causes of the vaginal lumps mentioned. Occasionally a biopsy is done under local anesthesia if

Figure 42
Blockage of the Bartholin's gland on either side of the vulva may result in the formation of a painless cyst. If the cyst becomes infected and forms an abscess, surgery may be required to drain the abscess.

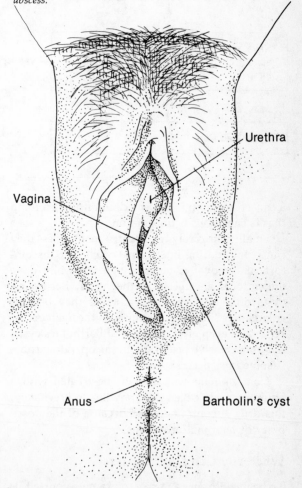

VAGINAL LUMP 379

VAGINAL LUMP

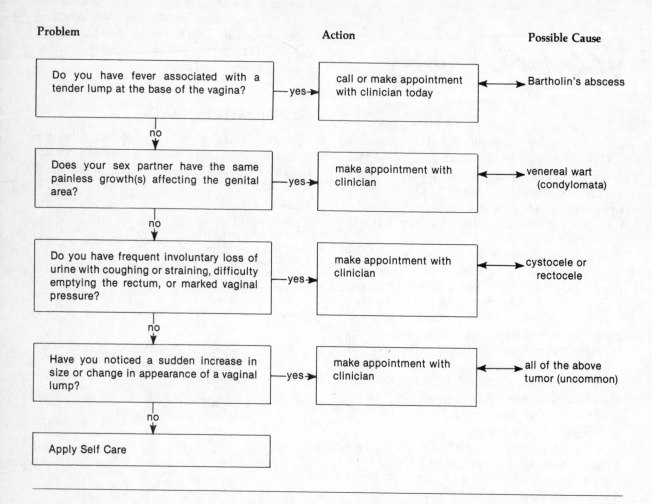

Problem	Action	Possible Cause
Do you have fever associated with a tender lump at the base of the vagina? —yes→	call or make appointment with clinician today	←→ Bartholin's abscess
↓ no		
Does your sex partner have the same painless growth(s) affecting the genital area? —yes→	make appointment with clinician	←→ venereal wart (condylomata)
↓ no		
Do you have frequent involuntary loss of urine with coughing or straining, difficulty emptying the rectum, or marked vaginal pressure? —yes→	make appointment with clinician	←→ cystocele or rectocele
↓ no		
Have you noticed a sudden increase in size or change in appearance of a vaginal lump? —yes→	make appointment with clinician	←→ all of the above tumor (uncommon)
↓ no		
Apply Self Care		

a cancerous lump is suspected, but finding a lump that is cancerous is uncommon.

Small cysts rarely require treatment unless they cause pain during intercourse or chronic discomfort. If removal is necessary, it is usually done under local anesthesia in the office. Bartholin's cysts often need to be drained if they become enlarged or infected. Because of the high recurrence rate even after drainage of Bartholin's cysts, a more extensive procedure in the operating room is sometimes necessary.

Condylomata will need to be treated with a liquid or paste called podophyllin. In pregnancy, this drug is contraindicated because of the possibility of fetal malformations.

What You Can Do (Self Care)

To begin with, use a mirror to examine yourself. Is the lump tender or leaking pus? Report any change or enlargement of a vaginal growth to your doctor. Painful inflammation of hair follicles, episiotomies, or Bartholin's glands responds to hot tub baths, which reduce pain and swelling. These infections may then drain on their own without need for medical treatment.

A cystocele and a rectocele appear as a swelling of the front and back vaginal wall, respectively, and become visibly enlarged when you strain down. These protrusions require surgery only when symptoms are severe. Cystoceles and rectoceles are less likely to develop or become worse if you maintain optimum weight, avoid strenuous lifting, and prevent chronic cough such as is associated with heavy cigarette smoking.

87

Weight Gain and Weight Loss

In a society which stigmatizes being overweight, some women take great risks to follow fashion's dictate to look thin by going on crash diets or participating in the latest fad diet. Many of these often unusual dieting techniques may be deceptively effective at first, because they get rid of body water rather than fat stores. The water rapidly reaccumulates, however, once you return to normal eating patterns. Some of the fad diets, such as the liquid protein diet, are harmful to your health. In fact, it is estimated that less than 6% of all weight-reduction techniques are both safe and effective. The reality is: to lose weight, you must eat less or exercise more, or both.

Excessive Weight Gain

Obesity, defined as being 20% over your ideal weight, is the number one nutrition problem in the United States. Women consistently outnumber men two to one in obesity and exceed men in amount of weight gained. It is estimated that 40% of American women in their forties are 20% above the ideal weight for their height and frame (see Table 104). To estimate your ideal weight you must take into account the comparative size of your body frame (wide or narrow shoulders and hips, large or small ankles and wrists). That is, if

Table 104   SUGGESTED WEIGHTS FOR HEIGHTS*

Height (without shoes)		Low		Average		High	
Feet & Inches	m**	lb	kg**	lb	kg**	lb	kg**
5′	1.52	100	45	109	50	118	54
5′1″	1.55	104	47	112	51	121	55
5′2″	1.57	107	49	115	52	125	57
5′3″	1.60	110	50	118	54	128	58
5′4″	1.63	113	51	122	55	132	60
5′5″	1.65	116	53	125	57	135	61
5′6″	1.67	120	55	129	59	139	63
5′7″	1.70	123	56	132	60	142	65
5′8″	1.73	126	57	136	62	146	66
5′9″	1.75	130	59	140	64	151	69
5′10″	1.78	133	60	144	65	156	71
5′11″	1.80	137	62	148	67	161	73
6′	1.83	141	64	152	69	166	75

Weight (without clothing)

* From *The Healthy Approach to Slimming*, American Medical Association, 1978.
** A meter (m) = 39.37 inches. A kilogram (kg) = 2.2 pounds (lb).

you have a large frame, your best weight is somewhere between the "average" and "high" figures in the table. For a small frame, you should probably weigh not less than the "low" figure and probably somewhere between "low" and "average." If you have a medium frame, your weight should probably be close to the "average" figure. Your ideal weight does not change as you grow older; what is ideal weight at age 25 remains ideal weight later in life.

Psychological factors often impede attempts at weight loss. Women who have dieted successfully and then regained the lost weight may experience an intense negative sense of their own worth or may feel hopelessly out of control in managing their weight. On the other hand, women who are depressed or under stress may resort to over-indulgence as a means of coping, even though this strategy is self-defeating. Although hypothyroidism (low thyroid) or other hormonal conditions occasionally account for obesity, most people gain weight simply because they take in more calories than they use up.

Excessive Weight Loss

The problem of weight loss is much less common than that of weight gain. Any unplanned weight loss amounting to 10% or more of your usual weight over three to six months could well be due to a medical problem. Although the clinician must rule out the possibility of serious illnesses, such as cancer or diabetes, more often sudden weight loss results from a change in eating habits that, in turn, results from nervousness, anxiety, or depression.

A condition known as *anorexia nervosa* is a disease marked by a chronic lack of appetite, accompanied by emotional distress, to the point where weight loss is very great (20% of original body weight). This condition is prevalent among teen-age girls and women and has afflicted more and more adult women as well. There are various theories for what causes anorexia nervosa; but no matter what the cause is, the important thing is to recognize the problem and seek professional help.

Normal Weight Gain During Pregnancy

Many scientific studies have shown the advantages of good nutrition before and during pregnancy. In general, fewer complications of pregnancy occur in women rated as having well-balanced diets consisting of foods from each of the four basic food groups (see Table 76 in Chapter 46). It is not so important to increase calories in pregnancy as it is to improve the quality of the diet. In the second half of pregnancy, however, caloric intake does need to be increased by approximately 10%, and this increase should continue through breast-feeding.

The subject of weight gain during pregnancy has been controversial for many years. Obstetricians now impose less severe restrictions on weight gain than in the past in an effort to decrease the number of babies with low birth weights. In general, bigger newborn babies are healthier babies. The National Research Council approves a weight gain of approximately twenty to thirty pounds during pregnancy. However, there may be considerable variation depending upon the woman's body size. In general, weight gain should not exceed 20% of ideal body weight.

There are several reasons for weight gain during pregnancy: the growing fetus and its surrounding amniotic fluid, the growth of specific organs such as the uterus and breasts, the increase in your blood volume, and fluid retention. The pattern of weight gain is more important than the total amount gained. You should gain weight gradually and primarily during the second two-thirds of your pregnancy. In the first third of pregnancy, weight gain averages three pounds but may be less if nausea and vomiting are severe.

Excessive Weight Gain During Pregnancy

A gain of more than 20% over ideal weight for height is excessive. Weight gain should not be equated with good nutrition. Obesity may result from eating calorically rich but nutritionally poor food such as pastries, potato chips, and sweet drinks. On the other hand, excessive weight gain sometimes occurs as a result of physiologic fluid retention in women eating well-balanced diets.

A weight gain of two to five or more pounds in one week is due largely to fluid. It takes an extra thousand calories a day to gain just two pounds a week from food overindulgence alone. Sudden fluid retention of more than five pounds in one week—a common finding in toxemia (high blood pressure during pregnancy)—warrants a call to your physician. Lesser amounts of weight increase are usually due mostly to an increased amount of normal fluid retention. Fluid is eliminated in the first week postpartum when an average weight loss of twenty pounds occurs. The remaining weight loss normally takes approximately three months.

Markedly excessive weight gain (that is, thirty-five to fifty pounds) increases the risk of developing high blood pressure or diabetes during pregnancy. Furthermore, in women who weigh close to two hundred pounds, the risk of the delivery itself, especially by cesarean section, is increased. In addition, postpartum bleeding, anesthesia complications, and vaginal tearing from childbirth are more likely to occur.

Too Little Weight Gain During Pregnancy

Some women delivering healthy babies gain only ten to twelve pounds each pregnancy. However, a gain of less than 15% of ideal weight for height often results from chronic illness, a nutritionally deficient diet, or severe vomiting during early pregnancy, all of which use up protein stores. During the last six months of pregnancy, weight loss or a gain of less than two pounds per month puts the fetus at risk for low birth weight. Toxemia is actually more common among women who gain too little weight than for those who gain too much. Subnormal weight gain is associated with closely spaced pregnancies and is more frequent among adolescents for whom prepregnancy nutrition is often inadequate.

What Medical Care Can Do

The treatment of overweight or obesity in the nonpregnant woman is basically up to the woman's own resourcefulness, although her physician should check her blood pressure and check her urine for sugar to screen for diabetes. Many physicians have difficulty dealing with obese patients, partly because nutrition has, until recently, received minimal attention in medical training. Some doctors prescribe diet pills rather than attempt to help women alter the basic behavioral patterns which led to overeating. Be wary of weight-loss clinics which promise quick results by severely restricting calories (500 to 1000 calories daily), by using hormone shots (HCG—human chorionic gonadotropin), or both. These approaches may prove to be unsafe and ineffective in the long run. Referrals to established weight control groups such as Weight Watchers or to a nutritionist may be helpful, however.

The clinician's evaluation of weight loss in the nonpregnant woman can involve numerous tests and X-rays unless there are accompanying symptoms which point to a specific cause, such as diabetes. If you have fever, anemia, or loss of appetite unassociated with nervousness or depression, hospitalization is sometimes necessary.

For weight loss that can be classified as anorexic, the woman must first be treated for possible medical problems, and then she may require one of various alternative psychological therapies.

The pregnant woman's weight is carefully monitored. During prenatal visits, the clinician determines fetal growth by measuring the height of the uterus (see Figure 15 in Chapter 16) and by assessing weight gain. Inadequate weight gain may be associated with abnormal fetal growth (see Chapter 16). If you have gained weight too quickly, the doctor will screen for toxemia by testing your urine for protein and checking your blood pressure. Toxemia (see Chapter 20) cannot be prevented or treated by restricting calories. Medical therapy consists of bed rest and occasionally drugs to control blood pressure. Again, in the area of weight gain, most of the treatment is up to you.

What You Can Do (Self Care)

If unplanned weight loss is associated with depression or nervousness, refer to Chapters 60 and 79 for suggestions for self care. Otherwise, consultation with your physician is advisable.

Self-treatment of overweight and obesity means recognizing that a tendency to be overweight will require lifetime changes in eating patterns. Your goal should be to establish a diet which you can stick to permanently. The best way to lose weight is to establish a life style in which you eat less and exercise more. Completely avoid the use, for the purpose of losing weight, of diet drugs, including amphetamines, thyroid, hormone shots (for example, HCG), and water pills. These drugs are unsafe when used to lose weight, and they interfere with a healthy change of dietary habits. Recently advertised "starch inhibitors" have not been carefully investigated to prove their effectiveness.

Concerning a weight-loss diet, the amount you eat is sometimes more important than the specific kinds of food you eat. You can get fat on a high-protein diet, for instance, if you eat too much, since excess calories can be converted to carbohydrates or fats. Most successful weight-loss diets are designed to have you eat smaller quantities of most of the foods you are presently eating. You need to retrain your appetite to be satisfied with less food in the interest of your future health. If you find yourself feeling starved on a diet, then suddenly binge eating (eating large amounts of food at one time) to relieve your feelings of hunger, then your diet may be too low in calories or carbohydrates. If you frequently feel the need to vomit after binge eating, contact your clinician as frequent vomiting can have harmful physiological effects. (See Chapter 78.)

For most women, it is unrealistic to expect a weight loss by dietary measures alone since a major part of overweight and obesity is due to low energy expenditure. Certain activities consume more calories than others. For example, running and swimming burn up about twice as many calories as walking or playing golf (see Table 78 in Chapter 47). Exercise should be regular and vigorous as opposed to occasional and strenuous. Duration of activity is more important than the exertion put into it. In tennis, for example, activity is intermittent, involving only a fraction of the total game-playing time. You will burn fewer calories in this instance as compared to a sport where activity is continuous. Women over thirty-five who are about to start an exercise program should first have a medical examination.

Nutrition research tells us that gradual weight loss is far more likely to be maintained than rapid weight loss. A realistic goal is to lose one or, at the most, two pounds per week. There are 3500 calories in each pound of stored fat; so you need to consume 500 fewer calories each day to lose one pound a week. Once you attain your ideal weight in pounds, multiplying this weight by 15 gives the number of calories you need each day to maintain this weight. The number 15 refers to the number of calories per pound of body weight needed by a woman who leads a moderately active life in order to keep her weight the same; this total will vary somewhat depending on the amount of exercise the woman engages in.

If on your present diet you are maintaining your weight (that is, not gaining or losing) and you want to determine how many calories a weight-loss diet for you should contain, do the following:

1. First estimate the number of calories present-

Table 105   1300-CALORIE DIET PLAN, BASED ON THE FOUR BASIC FOOD GROUPS

	Food Group*	Calories**
Breakfast	Fruit	80
	Bread-Cereal	70
	Milk	90
		240
Mid-Morning	Bread-Cereal	70
Lunch	Fruit	40
	Vegetable	50
	Bread-Cereal	70
	Meat	140
		300
Mid-Afternoon	Fruit	40
	Milk	90
		130
Dinner	Vegetable	80
	Bread-Cereal	70
	Meat	210
		360
Evening	Bread-Cereal	70
	Fruit-Vegetable	40
	Milk	90
		200
	Total Calories for Day	1300

* See Table 76 for examples of foods from each group.

** Calories from protein: 325 (25%)
Calories from carbohydrate: 728 (56%)
Calories from fat: 247 (19%)

ly in your diet. To do this, keep a record of everything you eat, including the amounts, over a period of several days or a week and, using a calorie counter, add up the calories. Divide the total by the number of days.

2. Then subtract 500 calories per day. This reduction in calories will allow for a weight loss of about one pound a week if you maintain your same physical activity level.

Your new diet should allow for a variety of foods from the four basic food groups (see Table 76 in Chapter 46). A 1300-calorie diet plan, using foods from the four basic food groups, is shown in Table 105. The number of calories shown are average amounts. You can vary the foods and servings as long as you make your choices in the right proportion from each food group and you do not exceed the total number of calories. For example: for breakfast you could have, for the "fruit" choice, about 6 oz. of orange juice or a small banana; for dinner, for the "bread-cereal" choice, you could have a slice of bread or a little less than half a cup of cooked spaghetti. In general, a diet of 1200 calories or more does not require vitamin supplementation in healthy women. Diets below 1000 calories per day may leave you tired or vulnerable to illness.

Eat regular meals, eat slowly, scale down portions, and avoid snacks. Learn the amount of calories in *everything* you eat. There are many books on the market that give the calorie content of hundreds of basic foods, and some books list the foods by brand name. Don't worry about small differences in calorie values among similar amounts of the same food. Remember, however, that processing often changes the total calorie count for some foods; for example, canned fruits packed in a heavy syrup have more calories than

WEIGHT GAIN

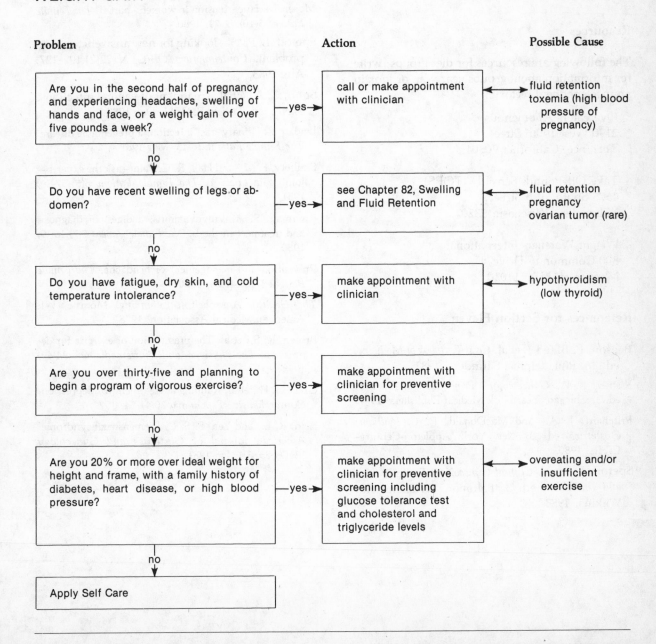

Problem	Action	Possible Cause
Are you in the second half of pregnancy and experiencing headaches, swelling of hands and face, or a weight gain of over five pounds a week? —yes→	call or make appointment with clinician	←→ fluid retention toxemia (high blood pressure of pregnancy)
Do you have recent swelling of legs or abdomen? —yes→	see Chapter 82, Swelling and Fluid Retention	←→ fluid retention pregnancy ovarian tumor (rare)
Do you have fatigue, dry skin, and cold temperature intolerance? —yes→	make appointment with clinician	←→ hypothyroidism (low thyroid)
Are you over thirty-five and planning to begin a program of vigorous exercise? —yes→	make appointment with clinician for preventive screening	
Are you 20% or more over ideal weight for height and frame, with a family history of diabetes, heart disease, or high blood pressure? —yes→	make appointment with clinician for preventive screening including glucose tolerance test and cholesterol and triglyceride levels	←→ overeating and/or insufficient exercise
Apply Self Care		

either juice-packed fruits, with no sugar added, or the same fresh fruits. (See Chapter 46 for more information about nutrition.)

Pregnancy is not a time to diet, especially during the last half, which is a critical time for fetal brain development. During this time, inadequate protein or carbohydrate intake may be harmful to the intellectual development of the fetus. Although crash dieting is harmful, some restriction in calories may be recommended in overweight women during the first half of pregnancy. Diet restrictions to limit weight gain throughout the entire pregnancy is seldom, if ever, advisable.

Resources

The following are resources for diet groups; write for information about groups near you, or look in your telephone directory.

Overeaters Anonymous
2190 West 190th Street
Torrance, California 90504

Take Off Pounds Sensibly (TOPS)
4575 South Fifth Street
Milwaukee, Wisconsin 53207

Weight Watchers International
800 Community Drive
Manhasset, N.Y. 11030

References for Section Eleven

Beeson, P. B. (ed.), et al. *Cecil Textbook of Medicine*, ed. 16. Philadelphia: Saunders, 1982.

Kistner, R. W. *Gynecology - Principles and Practice*, ed. 3. Chicago: Year Book Medical Publishers, 1979.

Pritchard, J. A., and MacDonald, P. C. *Williams Obstetrics*, ed. 16. New York: Appleton-Century-Crofts, 1980.

Speroff, L., et al. *Clinical Gynecologic Endocrinology and Infertility*, ed. 3. Baltimore: Williams and Wilkins, 1983.

Rakel, R. E. (ed.) *Current Therapy*. Philadelphia: Saunders, 1984.

Wolman, B. B. (ed.) *Psychological Aspects of Gynecology and Obstetrics*. Oradell, N.J.: Medical Economics, 1978.

Favazza, A. R. The primary care physician's approach to anxiety. *The Female Patient* 6(3):62-71, 1981.

Stellman, S. D., and Stellman, J. M. Women's occupations, smoking, and cancer and other diseases. *Ca-A Cancer Journal for Clinicians* 31(1):29-43, 1981.

Moser, M. Hypertension in women - part I. *The Female Patient* 5(9):27-34, 1980.

Moser, M. Hypertension in women - part II. *The Female Patient* 5(10):72-79, 1980.

Speroff, L. PMS—looking for new answers to an old problem. *Contemporary OB/GYN* 22(2):102-127, Aug 1983.

Sohn, C. A., et al. Treatment of vaginal infections. *The Female Patient* 8:33-44, Dec 1983.

Lindan, R. Urinary tract infection: a preventable disease. *The Female Patient* 36-43, Mar 1981.

Skultety, F. M., and Hall, R. C. Pain—ask the experts—joint pain—part 1. *The Female Patient* 6(5):57-59, 1981.

Kaufman, S. A. Vulvovaginitis: a digest of diagnosis and treatment methods. *The Female Patient* 5(7):16-19, 1980.

Prevention and management of headache. *The Female Patient* 5(10):46-54, 1980.

The Healthy Approach to Slimming. Monroe, WI: American Medical Association, 1978.

Brown, R. S., et al. The prescription of exercise for depression. *The Physician and Sportsmedicine* 6:34-49, 1978.

Greist, J. H., et al. Running as treatment for depression. *Comprehensive Psychiatry* 20:41-54, 1979.

Reid, R. L., and Yen, S. S. C. Premenstrual syndrome. *American Journal of Obstetrics and Gynecology* 139(1):85-104, Jan 1981.

Appendices

APPENDIX A

The Health History Profile is explained more fully in Chapter 4. Be certain to mark those items that apply to you and, when you see your clinician, be sure to mention them.

Health History Profile

1. **Current Problems**—be sure to mention if you have noticed any of the following recently:

   pelvic pain
   irregular bleeding
   vaginal discharge or itching
   breast pain, lump, or discharge
   hot flashes or night sweats
   loss of urine with coughing or sneezing
   fatigue, weakness, or fainting
   frequent or severe headaches
   chronic cough
   chest pain or palpitations

   shortness of breath
   swelling of hands, feet, or ankles
   frequent, painful, or bloody urination
   painful intercourse
   loss of sexual desire
   inability to reach orgasm or difficulty in reaching orgasm
   indigestion, stomach trouble, or ulcers
   nausea, vomiting, or bloating
   diarrhea or constipation
   hemorrhoids, rectal itching, or bleeding

2. **Menstrual History**

   Started at age _____ Length of cycle _____ days (from start of one period to start of next period)

   Number of days period usually lasts _____ Date last normal menstrual period started _____

   Periods regular? yes _____ no _____

   Have you started menopause? yes _____ no _____

   Pain or cramps? yes _____ no _____ sometimes _____

   Do you ever bleed between periods? yes _____ no _____

   Flow: light _____ medium _____ heavy _____ excessive _____

3. **Contraceptive History**

   Current method (type and dose of birth control pill, if applicable) _____

   _____

   Previous method(s) _____

   _____

4. **Pregnancy History**—include miscarriages and abortions

Year	Length of Pregnancy	Baby's Weight at Birth	Girl or Boy	Hours of Labor	Hospital (name & city)	Was anesthesia used?

Mention any of these complications:

1) prenatal hospitalizations such as for toxemia (high blood pressure in pregnancy)
2) special prenatal tests such as oxytocin stress test
3) premature births or stillbirths
4) prolonged labors or cesarean sections
5) newborn complications including congenital abnormalities or need for newborn intensive care
6) postpartum complications requiring antibiotics, blood transfusions, or prolonged hospital stay

5. **Previous Conditions**—mention if you have ever had any of the following:

high blood pressure	anemia	asthma, bronchitis, or pneumonia
heart disease	epilepsy	abnormal Pap smear
stroke	migraine headache	infection of female organ
phlebitis or blood clot	hepatitis	ovarian cyst
diabetes	gallbladder disease	fibroid (uterine tumor)
cancer	breast disease	kidney or bladder infection
thyroid disease	German measles (rubella)	

6. **Previous Hospitalizations**—give a review of your previous serious illnesses

	1	2	3
Type of operation or illness			
Date hospitalized			
Name and location (city) of hospital			
Doctor(s)			

7. **Family History**—it is important to mention any family history of the following:

heart disease	breast or uterine cancer	stroke
high blood pressure	twins	diabetes
bleeding disorder	kidney disease	birth defects, including mental retardation and Down's syndrome (formerly called Mongolism)
epilepsy	thyroid problems	

8. **Medication History**

Drug allergies _____

Current medications and dosages _____

APPENDIX B

Glossary

adhesion(s): bands of fibrous tissue that abnormally bind together two body structures. Adhesions within the abdomen may result from previous abdominal surgery or from prior infection, especially involving the pelvic organs.

afterbirth: the placenta and fetal membranes expelled from the uterus after childbirth (see *placenta*).

amniocentesis: a procedure for removing a small amount of amniotic fluid from the uterus during pregnancy. After the skin is numbed with a local anesthetic, a small needle attached to a syringe is inserted into the uterus through the abdomen to obtain the fluid. The fluid may be tested for chromosomal or other genetic abnormalities (usually between sixteen and eighteen weeks) or may be used to assess the fetal condition and gestational age (in late pregnancy). (See Chapters 11 and 20.)

anaphylaxis (or *anaphylactic reaction*): an allergic reaction usually caused by a drug (for example, penicillin), with symptoms ranging from itching and hives to more severe manifestations such as difficult breathing, throat swelling, or loss of consciousness (*anaphylactic shock*). Such reactions characteristically occur within minutes of taking the drug, regardless of dose, and may require immediate medical treatment.

antibody (pl. *antibodies*): a substance formed in the blood in an attempt to counteract or neutralize a foreign body such as a virus. For example, a woman who has had rubella (German measles) develops antibodies which protect her from getting the disease a second time. In other viral infections, such as herpes, antibodies lessen but do not prevent subsequent infections. Rh negative women may develop antibodies after a pregnancy in which the baby is Rh positive. In this case the production of antibodies may be harmful in a subsequent pregnancy (see Chapter 20).

antihistamine(s): a family of drugs found in many prescription and nonprescription cold and hay fever remedies.

atherosclerosis (or *arteriosclerosis*) ("hardening of the arteries"): the aging process within blood vessels, making a person susceptible to heart disease, stroke, and other circulatory disorders.

atypical cells: cells which appear slightly abnormal when studied under a microscope. Such cells may be associated with infection in the cervix (*cervicitis*) or with early precancerous changes in the cervix (*dysplasia*).

barium enema (or *lower GI series*): a procedure for examining the large intestine (colon) by means of X-rays, often obtained to evaluate chronic pelvic pain or bowel problems. An enema and/or laxative is given the night before the X-rays are taken to prepare the colon and make the X-ray picture more distinct. In this procedure the X-ray dye (barium) is introduced by means

of a small tube inserted into the rectum. After the procedure, the barium is expelled and usually a laxative is given to help get rid of remaining barium. (See also *GI* and *upper GI series*.)

biopsy: removal of tissue for microscopic diagnosis. Biopsy of the vulva, vagina, cervix, or endometrium can readily be done as an office procedure, usually with minimal discomfort. Breast biopsy, a more extensive procedure than the others mentioned, is usually performed in a hospital, often as an outpatient procedure.

birth canal: the passageway formed during labor by the dilated cervix and the vagina.

Braxton-Hicks contractions: slight uterine cramping or contractions that come and go throughout pregnancy, particularly during the last trimester.

breakthrough bleeding: bleeding, at a time other than a menstrual period, that sometimes results from taking estrogen-containing drugs, including birth control pills.

breast biopsy: see *biopsy*.

carcinoma-in-situ: a cancer which involves only the surface cells and which does not invade the underlying tissue.

catheterization of bladder: placement of a small rubber tube through the urethra and into the bladder to drain urine from the bladder. Catheterization is sometimes necessary during labor or in the first few days after childbirth when bladder emptying may temporarily become difficult. After abdominal or vaginal surgery the catheter, attached to a collection bag, may need to be left in for up to several days (see Chapter 40).

CAT scan (computerized axial tomography): a highly sophisticated, painless procedure that uses a computer to produce three-dimensional X-rays of the body, especially the brain. The test helps to diagnose a variety of conditions, especially tumors.

cauterization: see *cautery of cervix*.

cautery of cervix (cauterization): superficial burning of the lower end of the cervix by means of heat (*electrocautery*) or by freezing (*cryosurgery*). Usually done as treatment for mild to moderate dysplasia or for mild inflammation of the cervix accompanied by vaginal discharge.

CBC: see *complete blood count*.

cervicitis: inflammation or infection of the cervix, sometimes associated with a chronic discharge.

chemotherapy: treatment of cancer or other conditions by the use of special drugs.

chlamydia: a type of bacterialike microorganism responsible for certain sexually transmitted infections including some cases of nongonococcal urethritis (see Chapter 24).

cholesterol: a fatty substance present in the blood and in certain fatty foods. A high cholesterol level in the blood may make a person susceptible to heart disease. Cholesterol level in the blood may be influenced by heredity and is usually controllable by diet.

chromosomes: structures within cells that contain the genetic material (genes) which determine inherited characteristics (see Chapter 11).

climacteric: the several years preceding menopause when certain physical, emotional, and hormonal changes may occur (see Chapter 26).

colostrum: a thin, white breast discharge that normally precedes the production of breast milk and is secreted from the breast during the last few weeks of pregnancy.

colposcopy: a procedure for looking at and diagnosing abnormalities of the cervix through a special magnifying instrument called a colposcope. In a woman with an abnormal Pap smear this procedure, done in the doctor's office, allows the gynecologist to take a biopsy of the cervix from the most abnormal-appearing area.

complete blood count (CBC): a blood test for evaluation of the blood elements (red blood cells, white blood cells, and platelets). The parts of the CBC known as the hemoglobin and hematocrit are each a measure of the number of red blood cells. An elevated white blood count is often a sign of infection somewhere in the body, while a low red blood count indicates anemia. A CBC is ordered routinely before major surgery and during most hospital admissions.

condylomata (venereal warts): wartlike growths found on the external genitalia and caused by a sexually transmitted virus (see Chapter 24).

cone biopsy: an operation to remove a cone-shaped segment of tissue from the lower part of the cervix to diagnose the extent of cancerous or precancerous changes (dysplasia) (see Chapter 36).

cryosurgery: see cautery of cervix.

culdocentesis: a procedure to diagnose the presence of internal bleeding such as from a tubal (ectopic) pregnancy which has ruptured. In this emergency procedure, a needle attached to a syringe is inserted through the upper vagina into the abdominal cavity. The diagnosis is confirmed if blood is withdrawn into the syringe. (See Chapter 52.)

cystitis: bladder infection. Cystitis may cause painful or bloody urination as well as a frequent and urgent need to urinate (see Chapters 83 and 84).

cystocele: a vaginal hernia which causes a bulge in the upper vaginal wall and which becomes more pronounced during any activity involving straining (see Chapters 28 and 83).

cystoscopy: a procedure for looking at the inside of the bladder through a telescopelike instrument called a cystoscope. Cystoscopy is performed by a urologist (doctor specializing in diseases of the urinary system).

D & C (dilatation and curettage): a minor operation involving widening (dilatation) of the cervix opening and curettage (scraping and removing tissue) inside the uterus with a surgical instrument called a curette (see Chapter 41).

decensus: see prolapse.

decongestants: a family of drugs intended for relief of congestion of the nose, throat, and sinuses due to upper respiratory infections (colds and flu) and certain allergic conditions.

DES (diethylstilbestrol): the term DES refers both to a group of synthetic estrogen-containing drugs and to one of those drugs called diethylstilbestrol (see Chapter 37).

diabetes: a chronic hormone disorder associated with high blood sugar and sometimes inherited.

dilatation and curettage: see D & C.

diuretics: see water pills.

diverticulitis: inflammation of the small pockets (diverticula) in the wall of the colon. This condition produces cramping, abdominal pain, and diarrhea (see Chapter 61).

doptone: a device that uses sound waves to allow the clinician to hear the fetal heartbeat. The doptone can reliably pick up the fetal heart sounds by the fifth month of pregnancy and sometimes earlier.

dysplasia: abnormal microscopic appearance of cells obtained by taking a biopsy of the cervix. Although dysplasia may go away by itself in some instances, it can slowly progress over several years, from mild dysplasia to more severe forms of dysplasia or even to cervical cancer if left untreated (see Chapter 36).

ECG: see electrocardiogram.

ectopic pregnancy (or tubal pregnancy): pregnancy which occurs and develops outside the uterus, usually within one of the Fallopian tubes. Ectopic pregnancies often cause abnormal bleeding or pelvic pain (see Chapters 52 and 81).

edema: fluid retention within tissues, often producing swelling. Sometimes edema is normal as in pregnancy-related leg edema.

EEG: see electroencephalogram.

EKG: see electrocardiogram.

electrocardiogram (ECG, EKG): a graphic tracing of the electric current associated with contractions of the heart muscle. The ECG is used to diagnose various heart ailments.

electrocautery: see cautery of cervix.

electrocoagulation: burning of tissue using an electric current (see tubal ligation) (see Chapter 42).

electroencephalogram (EEG): recording of the brain's electrical signals (brain waves). The EEG is used to diagnose various conditions of the nervous system, including brain tumors.

endometrial aspiration: a procedure for removing cells lining the uterus (see endometrium) for diagnostic purposes (see Chapter 39).

endometrial biopsy: a procedure, done in the doctor's office, in which tissue lining the uterus (see endometrium) is removed for diagnosis (see Chapter 39).

endometrium: the inner lining of the uterus.

episiotomy: the small cut in the perineum which may be made at the time of childbirth to widen the birth canal (see Chapter 19).

estriol: an estrogen hormone produced in pregnancy and excreted in the urine. The amount of estriol measured in the urine may be used as a rough indication of fetal condition (see Chapter 20).

estrogen: principal hormone produced by the ovary. Estrogens play an important part in regulating the menstrual cycle and in the growth, development, and maintenance of the entire female reproductive system (see Chapter 3). Synthetic estrogen is used in most birth control pills and in drugs to treat certain symptoms associated with menopause (see Chapter 27).

fetal distress: a sign that the fetal oxygen supply may be less than optimal. Fetal distress in labor indicates the baby could be in danger (although it is often not in danger despite these signs) and may need prompt delivery if the distress is severe (see Chapter 21).

fibroadenoma: a relatively common, painless, benign breast tumor (noncancerous).

fibroids (leiomyomata): muscle tumors of the uterus which are almost always benign (see Chapter 34).

FSH (follicle stimulating hormone): a hormone secreted by the pituitary gland in the brain. By its interactions with hormones made in the ovary, FSH plays an important role in regulating the menstrual cycle (see Chapter 3).

galactorrhea: secretion of milky fluid from the breasts that is unassociated with pregnancy or the postpartum period (see Chapter 55).

gastroenterologist: an internist that subspecializes in diseases of the digestive system.

genes: components of chromosomes containing the genetic material determining inherited characteristics (see Chapter 11).

gestational age: the number of weeks of fetal growth or duration of pregnancy calculated from the last menstrual period. Term pregnancy is approximately 40 weeks. (See Chapter 16.)

GI: gastrointestinal (of the stomach and the intestines). See *barium enema* (lower GI series) and *upper GI series.*

glucose tolerance test (GTT): a series of blood tests obtained over three (or sometimes five) hours to diagnose diabetes or hypoglycemia (low blood sugar) (see Chapter 73).

goiter: a chronic enlargement of the thyroid gland not due to a tumor. Sometimes goiter is associated with excess thyroid hormone production (see *hyperthyroidism*) (see Chapters 79 and 80).

HCG (human chorionic gonadotropin): the hormone produced by the placenta in early pregnancy. All pregnancy tests are based upon the detection of this hormone in the urine or blood (see Chapter 16).

hematocrit: see *complete blood count.*

hemoglobin: see *complete blood count.*

high-risk pregnancy: a pregnancy in which one or more conditions exist prior to the pregnancy, or develop during the pregnancy, that place the fetus (and sometimes the mother) at increased risk for complications (see Chapter 20).

hyperthyroidism (overactive thyroid): a condition with various causes in which abnormally high amounts of thyroid hormone are produced. Symptoms include nervousness, loss of weight, palpitations, rapid pulse, trembling, and intolerance to heat. (See Chapters 79 and 80.)

hyperventilation: very rapid or deep breathing which may cause tingling of the face and fingers, dizziness, and fainting.

hypoglycemia: low blood sugar (see Chapter 73). Symptoms include headache, weakness, dizziness, nausea, and nervousness.

hypothyroidism (underactive thyroid): a condition with various causes in which abnormally low amounts of thyroid hormone are produced. Symptoms include dry skin, weight gain, and sluggishness (see Chapter 73).

hysterectomy (total, partial, or radical): surgical removal of the uterus including the cervix. The word *total* before hysterectomy is usually dropped since subtotal hysterectomy, in which the surgeon removes the upper uterus but not the cervix, is rarely performed. When hysterectomy is done without removal of the tubes and ovaries (a separate operation), the procedure is sometimes called *partial hysterectomy. Radical hysterectomy* is a more extensive operation performed for cancer of the uterus (endometrium) or cervix in which the upper vagina and nearby pelvic lymph nodes are removed as well as the uterus and cervix.

hysterosalpingogram (HSG): an X-ray of the uterus and tubes showing their inside appearance, including any blockages within these structures (see Chapter 13).

hysteroscopy: a new procedure using a thin, telescopelike instrument similar to the laparoscope for examining the inside of the uterus. Performed in the physician's office or in an outpatient setting, hysteroscopy can be used for evaluation of bleeding problems (sometimes combined with D & C), for infertility evaluation, or for removal of an IUD or of small uterine growths such as polyps and small fibroids.

intravenous pyelogram (IVP): X-rays of the urinary system (kidneys, ureters, and bladder) often obtained to help evaluate pelvic or back pain, bloody urine, chronic kidney infection, or high blood pressure. Shortly before the procedure a dye visible in X-rays is injected into the vein and becomes concentrated in the urinary system minutes later.

jaundice: a yellow coloration of the skin or of the white part of the eyes, usually due to liver damage and the resulting buildup of bile pigments in the blood. Jaundice is usually caused by liver disease but sometimes represents a reaction to drugs.

lactation: the production of breast milk which occurs a few days after childbirth.

laparoscopy: an operation performed through a small incision in the navel. The surgery can be done for diagnosis (for example, to evaluate the cause of pelvic pain) or for tubal sterilization (see Chapter 42).

laparotomy: an operation performed through an incision in the abdomen. The incision is usually four to five inches long except for the mini-laparotomy (see Chapter 42), which involves an incision of less than two inches.

leukorrhea: a white, not necessarily infectious, discharge from the vagina. Some leukorrhea is normally present and usually becomes increased around the time of ovulation.

LH: see *luteinizing hormone.*

linea nigra ("black line"): a line of increased skin pigmentation that develops during pregnancy and extends from the navel to the pubic hairline.

lower GI series: see *barium enema.*

low thyroid: see *hypothyroidism.*

luteinizing hormone (LH): a hormone, produced by the pituitary gland, which helps to regulate the menstrual cycle.

mammogram: breast X-ray used mainly to help diagnose and screen for breast cancer (see Chapter 33).

mastectomy: one of several types of breast removal operation usually performed for cancer of the breast (see Chapter 33).

meconium: brown coloration of the amniotic fluid (bag of waters) seen during labor and caused by a fetal bowel movement (stool). The presence of meconium in some instances indicates fetal distress (see Chapter 21).

menarche: the first menstrual period of a girl in puberty.

menopause: the time in a woman's life when the ovaries produce decreasing levels of hormones and menstrual periods have ceased for at least one year (see Chapter 26).

mini-laparotomy (or *mini-lap*): a type of sterilization operation performed through a small incision (less than two inches) in the lower abdomen (see Chapter 42).

miscarriage: the expulsion of a fetus from the womb before the fetus is developed enough to survive, usually accompanied by cramping and bleeding (see Chapter 52).

myomectomy: an operation on the uterus to remove one or more benign muscle tumors (fibroids) (see Chapter 34).

oophorectomy: an operation to remove one or both ovaries.

osteoporosis: a chronic condition especially common in postmenopausal women in which the calcium in bones gradually becomes depleted and makes the woman susceptible to fractures (see Chapters 27 and 49).

overactive thyroid: see *hyperthyroidism*.

partial hysterectomy: see *hysterectomy*.

perineum: the area between the vulva and rectum (see Chapter 3). An episiotomy (a cut which may be made to widen the birth canal during childbirth) involves a small incision in the perineum (see Chapter 19).

pessary: a device made of rubber or plastic or other synthetic material to lift up and support the uterus. A pessary may be used as an alternative to hysterectomy or other surgery to treat prolapse of the uterus (see Chapter 44).

photon absorptiometry: a test used to screen for osteoporosis by measuring bone density. A light beam is passed through bone (often the radius bone in the forearm) and a detector on the other side measures the beam's intensity as it emerges. A computer converts the photon absorption data and gives bone mineral content in grams per centimeter.

pigmentation: skin coloration. Darkening of the skin (increased pigmentation) in pregnancy often involves the face, nipples, and navel.

placebo: a pill with no active ingredients, given for its suggestive effects. The effects of a placebo, if any, are due to the expectations of the person taking it.

placenta: the organ which supplies oxygen and other nutrients to the fetus. One side of the placenta is attached to the uterus and remains in contact with the mother's circulation while the other side maintains contact with the fetal circulation through the umbilical cord. (See *afterbirth*.)

postpartum: the six-week time period following childbirth.

procto exam: see *sigmoidoscopy*.

progesterone: a major sex hormone produced by the ovary. This hormone plays an important role in regulating the menstrual cycle and in preparing the uterine lining (endometrium) each month for implantation of a fertilized egg. Progesterone is found in all birth control pills and in some intrauterine devices (IUDs). Progesterone is sometimes given to regulate the menstrual cycle or to treat certain conditions such as endometriosis. In pregnancy, the placenta produces large amounts of progesterone, which plays an important role in maintaining pregnancy.

prognosis: the predicted or expected probable course (outcome) of a disease.

prolapse (of the uterus): a condition in which the uterus has dropped down slightly, compared to its usual position, as a result of weakening of the surrounding muscles. Sometimes as a result of childbirth injuries and especially after menopause, some degree of symptomless uterine prolapse occurs (see Chapter 28).

pyelonephritis: a kidney infection. Unlike a bladder infection (see *cystitis*), kidney infections usually cause fever, chills, and backache (see Chapter 49).

quickening: perception of movement of the fetus beginning around the fifth month of pregnancy.

radical hysterectomy: see *hysterectomy*.

rectocele: a vaginal hernia which causes a bulge in the lower (back) vaginal wall and which becomes more pronounced during any activity involving straining (see Chapters 28 and 83).

regional enteritis: a chronic condition in which the small intestine becomes inflamed. This disease is associated with intermittent bouts of diarrhea and abdominal cramping (see Chapter 61).

rooming-in: a hospital procedure allowing for the newborn and mother to share the same room for all or part of the day. This arrangement provides for feeding on demand and gives the mother a chance to care for her baby. Fathers are usually allowed to visit both mother and baby often as well.

salpingectomy: surgical removal of the Fallopian tube. If both tubes are removed, the operation is known as bilateral salpingectomy (unilateral salpingectomy if only one tube is removed).

sedative: a drug that reduces nervousness and anxiety and often produces some drowsiness. Tranquilizers are typical sedatives, but many other types of drugs such as antihistamines found in many cold remedies may have sedative properties (see Chapter 30).

sickle-cell anemia: an inherited type of anemia, mostly affecting black people, in which the blood cells take on a sickle shape and become destroyed more rapidly than normal. Symptoms include episodes of joint and leg pains. A blood test can detect individuals who have or are carriers of this disease.

sigmoidoscopy (or *procto exam*, *proctological exam*): a procedure for looking at the lining of the lower colon (sigmoid) by means of an instrument with a built-in lens and light source (sigmoidoscope) which is inserted into the rectum.

sonogram: see *sonography*.

sonography (ultrasound): a painless technique using sound waves (as opposed to X-rays) for visualizing internal organs.

The resulting picture is called a sonogram. Sonography may be used to diagnose various gynecologic conditions such as ovarian cysts. In the pregnant woman sonography can be very useful in determining gestational age, assessing fetal growth, and diagnosing certain birth defects (see Chapter 16).

spina bifida: a birth defect involving the spinal column, in which part of the spinal cord or the membranes which cover it may protrude through the spinal column. Spina bifida may be crippling or fatal depending upon the extent and location of the defect in the spinal column. This birth defect may be diagnosed prenatally (see Chapter 11).

stillbirth: the birth of a fetus that is dead prior to delivery, after the twentieth week of pregnancy.

stress test (cardiovascular): a test to assess a person's overall fitness, especially the condition of the heart. The test involves a series of graduated exercises (running in place, etc.) during which the heart's rate and rhythm are measured.

stress test (oxytocin challenge test (OCT)): a test to assess the overall condition of the fetus during pregnancy (see Chapter 20).

Tay-Sachs disease: a hereditary disease, usually fatal in early childhood, found almost exclusively among Jews of central eastern Europe or their descendants. Carriers of this disease, which may cause mental retardation and blindness, may be identified by genetic screening (see Chapter 11).

total hysterectomy: see *hysterectomy*.

toxemia: high blood pressure during pregnancy (see Chapter 20).

tubal ligation (or *tubal sterilization*): any operation involving the Fallopian tubes which results in permanent contraception. The tubes may be tied with suture or thread ("ligated"), burned (electrocoagulated), or mechanically blocked with clips or bands (see Chapter 42).

ulcerative colitis: a chronic condition of the large intestine causing symptoms of cramping pain and bouts of bloody diarrhea (see Chapter 61).

underactive thyroid: see *hypothyroidism*.

upper GI series: a procedure for examining the esophagus, stomach, and small intestine by means of a series of X-rays. Flavored barium is drunk just before the X-rays are taken. The barium (an X-ray dye) shows up on the X-ray, outlining the upper digestive tract. This series is often done to evaluate upper abdominal pain or chronic indigestion that may be due to an ulcer.

ureter: one of the two tubes that carry urine from the kidneys to the bladder (see Figure 41).

urethritis: inflammation of the urethra, a condition associated with painful and frequent urination (see Chapters 83 and 84).

urgency incontinence: involuntary loss of urine associated with symptoms of a urinary tract infection, especially the sudden and frequent urge to urinate (see Chapter 28).

urinalysis: analysis of the urine to detect blood, sugar, protein, or other abnormalities. Microscopic examination of the urine to look for white cells (pus) may not be done routinely as part of the urinalysis in routine office checkups unless it is requested.

urinary stress incontinence: involuntary loss of urine when the bladder muscles are stressed as during coughing, sneezing, laughing, running, or other strenuous activity (see Chapter 28).

varicose veins: prominent, sometimes swollen veins usually occurring in the lower extremities. Such veins tend to have weak or improperly functioning valves so that circulation is impaired. Varicose veins may temporarily arise in pregnancy and become worse as a result of pressure from the enlarging uterus against the major veins that return blood from the legs and lower abdomen to the heart (see Chapter 72).

water pills: a class of prescription drugs, known as *diuretics*, which are used to treat high blood pressure, certain heart and kidney ailments, and sometimes simple fluid retention (see Chapter 82).

wet smear (vaginal smear): microscopic evaluation of vaginal secretions. This procedure is usually done to diagnose types of vaginitis (see Chapter 85).

APPENDIX C

Further Reading

General

Our Bodies, Ourselves: A Book by and for Women. The Boston Women's Health Book Collective. Simon and Schuster, 1976. The first and best-known comprehensive discussion of women's health issues written for the consumer.

Better Homes and Garden's Woman's Health and Medical Guide. P. J. Cooper. Meredith Corp., 1981. This comprehensive resource guide includes chapters on stress, relaxation, and death and dying, as well as common medical problems.

Talk Back to Your Doctor: How to Demand (and Recognize) High Quality Health Care. A. Levin. Doubleday, 1975. How to shop for and demand high-quality health care.

The Hospital Experience. J. Nierenberg and F. Janovic. Bobbs-Merrill, 1978. What the consumer should know about hospitals—from admission to discharge. Various operations discussed.

Symptoms: The Complete Home Medical Encyclopedia. S. Miller (Ed.). Thomas Crowell, 1976. Over 650 symptoms are discussed in easy-to-understand language, providing much usable information for men as well as women.

Medical Self-Care: Access to Health Tools. T. Ferguson (Ed.). Summit Books, 1980. Easy-to-understand discussion of many aspects of self-care. Includes references and resources for developing your own self-care program.

Ms. Guide to a Woman's Health. C. Cooke and S. Dworkin. Doubleday, 1979. Easy-to-read discussion of gynecological and health care problems.

EveryWoman's Health: The Complete Guide to Body and Mind. D. Thompson (Consulting Ed.). Doubleday & Co., 1980. Seventeen women physicians discuss all aspects of women's health, both mental and physical, in a scholarly fashion.

Pregnancy

First Nine Months of Life. G. Flanagan. Simon and Schuster, 1982. Beautiful pictures of fetal development with easy-to-understand explanations of what happens each month.

A Child Is Born. L. Nilson. Dell Publishing Co., 1979. Another look at fetal development, beautifully photographed.

The following pamphlets are available free from the American College of Obstetricians and Gynecologists:

Pregnancy and Daily Living
Food, Pregnancy, and Health
Travel During Pregnancy

Write to: Resource Center
The American College of Obstetricians and
Gynecologists
600 Maryland Ave., S.W.
Washington, D.C. 20024

Pregnancy, the Psychological Experience. A. Colman and L. Colman. Harper Magazine Press, 1975. The many emotional aspects of pregnancy are discussed.

Essential Exercises for the Childbearing Years. E. Noble. Houghton Mifflin, 1982. Exercises during pregnancy and postpartum with emphasis on prevention. Includes chapter on exercises after a cesarean birth.

A New Life: Pregnancy, Birth and Your Child's First Year. J. Queenan, Van Nostrand Reinhold Co., 1979. A beautifully illustrated, thorough discussion of pregnancy, childbirth, and the first year of life.

Making Love During Pregnancy. E. Bing and L. Colman. Bantam Books, 1982. Deals with common sexual feelings and fears that occur during pregnancy.

Having A Baby After Thirty. E. Bing and L. Colman. Bantam Books, 1980. This book and the following one provide sound information for the woman over thirty.

Parents After Thirty. M. Kappelmann and P. Ackerman. Rawson Wade Publishers, 1980.

Childbirth

Methods of Childbirth. C. Bean. Doubleday and Co., 1982. A good introduction to alternatives within the childbirth experience and education for childbirth.

Husband-Coached Childbirth. R. Bradley, Harper & Row, 1981. The main reference to the Bradley method of childbirth. Stresses the father's participation.

Childbirth Without Fear. Grantly Dick-Read. Harper & Row, 1979. Original description of the Dick-Read method. A pioneering work on the subject of prepared childbirth.

Thank You, Dr. Lamaze. M. Karmel. Harper and Row, 1983. One woman's account of the search for "natural" childbirth and an explanation of the Lamaze method.

The Experience of Childbirth. S. Kitzinger. Penguin, 1978. Emphasis on the author's touch relaxation method for use during labor and delivery.

Six Practical Lessons for Easier Childbirth. E. Bing. Bantam Books, 1981. Based on her modification of Lamaze techniques, this is a practical book in preparing for labor and delivery.

Birth Without Violence F. Leboyer. Knopf, 1975. Description of "nonviolent" birth or "gentle" birth, beautifully photographed and described.

What Every Husband Should Know About Having A Baby. J. Sasmor. Nelson-Hall, 1972. Excellent discussion of prepared childbirth emphasizing the father's role and feelings.

Have It Your Way. V. Walton. Henry Phillips, 1978. Discusses birthing alternatives within the hospital setting.

"Siblings at Birth: A Survey and Study," S. Anderson. *Birth and the Family Journal* 6:80-7, 1979. Presents guidelines for siblings attending childbirth.

Maternal-Infant Bonding. M. Klaus and J. Kennell. C. V. Mosby Co., 1976. Original work describing the importance of early mother-infant contact.

Bonding: The Beginnings of Parent-Infant Attachment. M. Klaus and J. Kennell. New American Library, 1983. A furthur discussion of the bonding process.

The Cesarean Birth Experience. B. Donovan. Beacon Press, 1978.

Having A Cesarean Baby. R. Hausknecht and J. Heilman. E. P. Dutton, 1983.

Cesarean Childbirth: A Handbook for Parents. C. Wilson and W. Hovey. Doubleday, 1980.

The Breastfeeding Book. M. Messenger. Van Nostrand Reinhold, 1982.

You Can Breastfeed Your Baby . . . Even In Special Situations. D. Brewster. Rodale Press, 1979. Hints for successful breastfeeding in all situations, from cesarean section mothers to cleft palate babies.

Nursing Your Baby. K. Pryor. Simon and Schuster, 1973.

Womanly Art of Breast Feeding. La Leche League International, 1981.

Growth and Development of Mothers. A. McBride. Harper & Row, 1981. This book and the following one deal with the realities of motherhood and what to expect.

The Mother Person. V. Barber and M. Skaggs. Schocken Books, 1977.

Premature Babies—A Handbook for Parents. S. Nance. Arbor House Publishing Co., 1983.

The Premature Baby Book. H. Harrison and A. Kositsky. Berkley Books, 1982.

Coping with a Miscarriage. H. Pizer and C. Palinski. New American Library, 1981.

The following articles from *American Baby* magazine may be available from your local library or may be obtained from:
American Baby, Inc.
575 Lexington Ave.
New York, N.Y. 10022

"The Bonding Experience," T. Munson. *American Baby* 42:204, April 1980.

"New Options in Childbirth, Part 1: Family-Centered Maternity Care." M. Montrose. *American Baby* 40:50-54+, May 1978.

"New Options in Childbirth, Part 2: Family-Centered Cesarean Births," M. Montrose. *American Baby* 40:52-53+, June 1978.

"New Options in Childbirth, Part 3: Having a Baby At Home," M. Montrose. *American Baby* 40:58-61+, July 1978.

"Photographing Your Baby's Birth," J. Beaderstadt. *American Baby* 41:48-49, March 1979.

"How to Enjoy Bottle Feeding and Not Feel Guilty," A. Whetsell. *American Baby* 40:14+, September 1978.

"Guilt and the Working Mother," S. Rad. *American Baby* 42:54+, January 1980.

"Common Myths about Motherhood," K. Woodworth. *American Baby* 41:12+, November 1979.

"Sex and the New Parent," J. Gochros. *American Baby* 39:16+, May 1977.

"Keeping in Touch," B. Nash. *American Baby* 40:56+, July 1978. (Leboyer birth experience)

"Good Nutrition for Oral Health," A. B. Natow et al. *American Baby* 42:54+, September 1980.

"Nutrition Needs In Pregnancy," R. Gause. *American Baby* 42:36, February 1980.

"Pregnancy and Weight Control," S. Jimenez. *American Baby* 42:50+, April 1980.

"Nutrition for the Nursing Mother," A. Natow. *American Baby* 41:18+, July 1979.

"Are You Nutritionally Ready for Pregnancy?" W. McGanity. *American Baby* 41:28+, March 1979.

"Running: How it Affects Pregnancy," M. Shangold. *American Baby* 41:42+, July 1979.

Gynecology

It's Your Body - A Woman's Guide to Gynecology. N. Lauersen and S. Witney. Berkley Pub., 1980. Comprehensive book with interesting discussion of historical as well as futuristic aspects of birth control, infertility, and female surgery.

My Body, My Health: The Concerned Woman's Guide to Gynecology. F. Stewart et al. Bantam Books, 1981. Sensitively written with especially thorough discussions of birth control, sterilization, and abortion.

The Birth Control Book. H. I. Shapiro. Avon Books, 1982. Detailed, well-explained information on birth control methods and all aspects of abortion.

Women and the Crisis in Sex Hormones. B. Seaman and G. Seaman. Bantam Books, 1978. Stimulating discussion of the use of estrogen and birth control pills.

Infertility: A Guide for the Childless Couple. B. E. Menning. Prentice-Hall, 1977. Helpful, comprehensive book dealing with the emotional as well as physical aspects of infertility.

Every Woman's Guide to Hysterectomy: Taking Charge of Your Own Body. D. Jameson and R. Schwalb. Prentice-Hall, 1978. Excellent resource for any woman considering having this operation.

Second Opinion. I Rosenfeld. Bantam Books, 1981. Tells you why, when, and sometimes where to ask for a second medical opinion about such subject areas as hysterectomy, cancer, and sexually transmitted diseases.

Sexuality

For Yourself: The Fulfillment of Female Sexuality. L. Barbach. Doubleday, 1975. A basic approach to understanding and experiencing your sexuality.

The Hite Report: A Nationwide Study of Female Sexuality. S. Hite. Dell, 1978. Summarizes the responses of 3,019 women who answered questions about sex and sexuality.

Our Right to Love. G. Vida (Ed.). Prentice-Hall, 1978. A good resource book about female homosexuality.

The Joy of Sex: A Cordon Bleu Guide to Lovemaking. A. Comfort. Simon and Schuster, 1974. Enjoyable reading about the variety possible in sexual behavior.

Sex After Sixty: A Guide for Men and Women for Their Later Years. R. N. Butler and M. I. Lewis. Harper & Row, 1976.

Rape

Fighting Back: How to Cope with the Medical, Emotional and Legal Consequences of Rape. J. Bode. Macmillan, 1978. Comprehensive discussion of the issues surrounding rape and how different communities handle them.

Drugs

The People's Pharmacy Two: A Guide to Prescription Drugs, Home Remedies and Over-the-Counter Medications. J. Graedon. Avon, 1980.

The Essential Guide to Prescription Drugs. J. W. Long. Harper & Row, 1982. This book and the preceding one are excellent consumer guidebooks providing information on the uses, risks, and side effects of common drugs. Information on drug use during pregnancy as well as possible effects on the fetus is included.

Physician's Desk Reference, ed. 38. Medical Economics Co., 1984. Known as the *PDR,* this best seller is annually updated to include the latest manufacturers' information about nearly all prescription drugs.

Physicians' Desk Reference for Nonprescription Drugs, ed. 5. Medical Economics Co., 1984. Information about nonprescription drugs, organized like the PDR above.

DATA: Drug, Alcohol, Tobacco Abuse During Pregnancy. Provides information on the effects of drug use and smoking during pregnancy.
Write to: March of Dimes Birth Defects Foundation
　　　　　Box 2000
　　　　　White Plains, N.Y. 10602

"Drugs and Pregnancy," P. Postotnik. *FDA Consumer,* October 1978. Gives information on the use of drugs during pregnancy.
Write: HFI 20, Food and Drug Administration
　　　　　5600 Fishers Lane, Room 15B-32
　　　　　Rockville, MD 20857

Physical Fitness

Especially for Women. E. Darden. Leisure Press, 1977.

Physical Fitness: A Way of Life. B. Getchell. John Wiley & Sons, Inc., 1976.

The Female Athlete. C. Klafs and J. Lyon. C. V. Mosby Co., 1978.

Total Woman's Fitness Guide. G. Shierman and C. Haycock. Anderson World Inc., 1979.

Running for Health and Beauty: A Complete Guide for Women. K. Lance. Bantam Books, 1978. Discussion of benefits of running on personal appearance and well-being as well as on physical conditioning.

Women's Running. J. Ullyst. Anderson World, 1976. Pertinent information for the beginner as well as the experienced runner. Areas such as running while pregnant and while breast-feeding are discussed.

Introduction to Yoga. R. Hitteman. Bantam Books, 1979. Easy-to-read presentation of yoga and its benefits for physical conditioning.

Slendercises. B. Pearlman. Doubleday & Co., 1980. An exercise program and discussion for body toning.

The New Aerobics. K. Cooper. Bantam Books, 1970. A thorough discussion and program of all exercises and their benefits for physical conditioning.

Aerobics for Women. M. Cooper and K. Cooper. Bantam Books, 1972. Discussion of benefits of aerobics for women and suggestions and exercise schedules.

Royal Canadian Air Force Exercise Plans For Physical Fitness. Pocket Books, 1976. Two excellent physical fitness plans, one for men and one for women, devised by the Royal Canadian Air Force.

Fit or Fat? C. Bailey. Houghton Mifflin Co., 1978. A helpful discussion of exercise and nutrition.

The Middle Years and After

Mid-Life: Developmental and Clinical Issues. W. H. Norman and T. J. Scarmella. Brunner/Mazel Publishers, 1980. Provides further detailed reading on such phases of adult life as changing roles of women at midlife, divorce, sexual problems.

Issues and Crises During Middlescence. J. Stevenson. Appleton-Century-Crofts, 1977. (paperback) General reading about the midlife crises, concerning role changes as well as other social, cultural, and emotional factors.

Marital Separation. R. S. Weiss. Basic Books, 1975. Deals with the decision to separate, effects of separation on friends and relatives, and starting over.

Using Your Medicines Wisely: A Guide for the Elderly. National Institute on Drug Abuse, Rockville, MD, 1979. Discussion of special concerns for older adults, particularly those with chronic conditions, in taking drugs and the possible combination or additive effects.

The Menopause Book. L. Rose (Ed.). Hawthorn Books, 1980. This easy-to-read book discusses social, physical, and emotional concerns of menopause.

Breaking Out of the Middle-Age Trap. L. Westoff. New American Library, Inc., 1980. Discusses midlife crises and other problems faced by the working woman and homemaker.

Nutrition

Eating for Two: The Complete Pregnancy Nutrition Cookbook. I. Cronin and G. Brewer. Bantam Books, 1983. Includes recent information about alcohol, caffeine, smoking, etc. and effects on pregnancy and breast-feeding.

Nutrition and the Later Years. R. B. Weg. Southern California Press, 1978. Comprehensive discussion of the nutritional needs of the older adult.

The Supermarket Handbook. N. Goldbeck and D. Goldbeck. The New American Library, Inc., 1976. Helpful hints in selecting your foods and information about their packaging and processing.

The Little Book of Baby Foods. K. Applegate. The Lightning Tree, 1978. A Spanish-English text full of practical and economical tips on feeding your baby.

The New Nuts Among the Berries. R. Deutsch. Bull Publishing, 1977. This informative book traces the history of food quackery in the U.S.

Realities of Nutrition. R. Deutsch. Bull Publishing, 1976. This fun book provides a comprehensive way to learn about nutrition.

Jane Brody's Nutrition Book. J. Brody. W. W. Norton Co., 1981. Written by a New York *Times* reporter, this is a comprehensive, well-researched look at the current issues in nutrition.

Diet for a Small Planet. F. M. Lappé. Ballantine Books, 1982. This is an excellent book that explains "protein complementarity"—the combining in the proper proportions of nonmeat foods to produce high-grade protein nutrition.

Recipes for a Small Planet. E. B. Ewald. Ballantine Books, 1975. A companion book to the book above, following the principle of good nutrition through the right combinations of foods.

The following pamphlets are available:

Food and Pregnancy. March of Dimes Birth Defects Foundation, Box 2000, White Plains, N.Y. 10602. (free)

The Healthy Approach to Slimming. The American Medical Association, Order Department, P.O. Box 821, Monroe, WI 53566. ($1.00)

Calories and Weight. USDA Information Bulletin No. 364; U.S. Government Printing Office, Washington, D.C. 20402. ($1.00)

Nutritive Value of Foods. USDA Home and Garden Bulletin No. 72; U.S. Government Printing Office, Washington, D.C. 20402. ($1.05)

Basic Bodywork for Fitness and Health. Order No. OP428; The American Medical Association, Order Department, P.O. Box 821, Monroe, WI 53566. ($.60)

Recommended Dietary Allowances, Revised, 1980. Food and Nutrition Board, National Academy of Sciences—National Research Council, Washington, D.C.

Dietary Goals for the United States, 2nd ed., December 1977. Available from: Superintendent of Documents, U.S. Government Printing Office, Washington, D.C. 20402.

APPENDIX D
Resource Groups

For information about —	Contact —	Chapter
health services; selecting a doctor, etc.	(See Table 1, Resources for Finding Health Care Alternatives.)	2
cervical caps (enclose $5.00 for information and a list of cap distributors)	National Women's Health Network 224 7th Street, S.E. Washington, D.C. 20003	7
birth control	Planned Parenthood Federation of America, Inc. 810 Seventh Avenue New York, N.Y. 10019 (212) 541-7800	10
birth control	Zero Population Growth, Inc. 1346 Connecticut Avenue, N.W. Washington, D.C. 20036	10
birth defects; inherited diseases	March of Dimes Birth Defects Foundation Box 2000 White Plains, N.Y. 10602	11, 31
birth defects; inherited diseases	National Clearinghouse for Human Genetic Diseases 805 Fifteenth Street, N.W., Suite 500 Washington, D.C. 20005	11
infertility	RESOLVE, Inc. P.O. Box 474 Belmont, MA 02178	13
infertility	The American Fertility Society 1608 13th Avenue South, Suite 101 Birmingham, AL 35256	13
infertility	Barren Foundation 6 East Monroe Street, Room 1407 Chicago, IL 60603	13
childbirth education	(See Table 25, Childbirth Education Organizations.)	14
alternative birth settings	National Association of Parents and Professionals for Safe Alternatives in Childbirth (NAPSAC) P.O. Box 267 Marble Hill, Missouri 63764	15
family-centered maternity care	The Cybele Society Suite 414, Peyton Building Spokane, Washington 99201	15
home birth	Home Oriented Maternity Experience (HOME) 511 New York Avenue Tacoma Park, MD 20912	15
home birth	Midwives' Alliance of North America 30 S. Main Street Concord, NH 03301	15
birth centers	National Association of Childbearing Centers R.D. 1, Box 1 Perkiomenville, PA 18074	15

For information about --	Contact --	Chapter
pregnancy	Resource Center American College of Obstetricians and Gynecologists 600 Maryland Ave., S.W. Washington, D.C. 20024	16
pregnancy	Office of Maternal and Child Health U.S. Dept. of Health and Human Services 5600 Fishers Lane, Room 7-39 Rockville, MD 20857	16
local baby care and parenting classes	American Red Cross 2025 E Street, N.W. Washington, D.C. 20006	14, 18
support groups for the pregnancy/ parenting experience	COPE 37 Clarendon Street Boston, MA 02216	18
breast-feeding	La Leche League International 9616 Minneapolis Avenue Franklin Park, Illinois 60134	19
cesarean birth	C/SEC, Inc. 66 Christopher Road Waltham, MA 02154 (617) 965-2781	21
cesarean birth	Cesarean Birth Council International P.O. Box 6081 San Jose, CA 95150	21
sexuality and sex counseling	American Association of Sex Educators, Counselors, and Therapists 600 Maryland Avenue, S.W. Washington, D.C. 20024	22
sexuality and sex counseling	Sex Information and Education Council of the U.S. 80 Fifth Avenue, Suite 801 New York, N.Y. 10011	22
sexually transmitted diseases	Technical Information Services Center for Prevention Services Centers for Disease Control Atlanta, GA 30333	24
sexually transmitted diseases	VD P.O. Box 100 Palo Alto, CA 94302	24
genital herpes	Herpes Resource Center P.O. Box 100 Palo Alto, CA 94302	24
rape	National Center for the Prevention and Control of Rape 5600 Fishers Lane, Room 15-99 Rockville, MD 20857	25
drug abuse prevention	National Institute on Drug Abuse Prevention Branch 5600 Fishers Lane, Room 10A-30 Rockville, MD 20857	30
women's drug abuse treatment programs	National Clearinghouse on Drug Abuse P.O. Box 416 Kensington, MD 20795	30
alcohol (including use and abuse in pregnancy)	National Clearinghouse for Alcohol Information P.O. Box 2345 Rockville, MD 20852	30, 31

For information about --	Contact --	Chapter
alcohol abuse	Alcoholics Anonymous P.O. Box 459 Grand Central Station New York, N.Y. 10163	30
alcohol abuse in relative or friend	Al-Anon Family Group Headquarters, Inc. P.O. Box 182 Madison Square Station New York, N.Y. 10159	30
breast cancer rehabilitation	Reach to Recovery 19 W. 56th Street New York, N.Y. 10019 (212) 586-8700	33
cancer	Cancer Information Service National toll-free telephone number: 800-638-6694	33
cancer	Office of Cancer Communications National Cancer Institute Bldg. 31, Room 10A-18 9000 Rockville Pike Bethesda, MD 20205	33
cancer	American Cancer Society, Inc. 777 Third Avenue New York, N.Y. 10017 (212) 371-2900	33
DES	Office of Cancer Communications National Cancer Institute Bldg. 31, Room 10A-18 9000 Rockville Pike Bethesda, MD 20205	37

nearest referral center for names of
  second surgical opinion physicians
	HEW:
	National toll-free telephone number (except Maryland):
	  800-638-6833; in Maryland: 800-492-6603
		40

sterilization	Association for Voluntary Sterilization, Inc. 122 E. 42nd Street, 18th Floor New York, N.Y. 10168 (212) 573-8350	42
sterilization	Planned Parenthood Federation of America, Inc. 810 Seventh Avenue New York, N.Y. 10019 (212) 541-7800	42
abortion	National Abortion Federation 110 E. 59th Street New York, N.Y. 10022 National toll-free telephone number (except in the State of New York): 800-223-0618; in New York call collect (212) 688-8516.	43
abortion	Planned Parenthood Federation of America, Inc. 810 Seventh Avenue New York, N.Y. 10019 (212) 541-7800	43
dental care	American Dental Association Bureau of Health Education and Audiovisual Services 211 East Chicago Avenue Chicago, Illinois 60611	45
general health	American Public Health Association 1015 Fifteenth Street, N.W. Washington, D.C. 20005	45

For information about --	Contact --	Chapter
general health	Council on Family Health 633 Third Avenue New York, N.Y. 10017	45
mental health and counseling services	National Mental Health Association 1800 North Kent Street Arlington, VA 22209	45
nutrition	Community Nutrition Institute 1146 Nineteenth Street, N.W. Washington, D.C. 20036	46
nutrition	The American Dietetic Association 430 North Michigan Avenue Chicago, Illinois 60611	46
nutrition	Department of Foods and Nutrition American Medical Association 535 North Dearborn Street Chicago, Illinois 60610	46
exercise	American Alliance for Health, Physical Education, Recreation and Dance 1900 Association Drive Reston, VA 22070	47
lung conditions and smoking (Write for information or enclose $5.00 for the two manuals on the "Freedom from Smoking" program.)	American Lung Association 1740 Broadway New York, N.Y. 10019 (212) 245-8000	59
quitting smoking	American Cancer Society, Inc. 777 Third Avenue New York, N.Y. 10017 (212) 371-2900	59
quitting smoking	American Heart Association 7320 Greenville Avenue Dallas, Texas 72531 (214) 750-5334	59
quitting smoking	General Conference of Seventh-Day Adventists Health Services Dept. 6840 Eastern Ave., N.W. Washington, D.C. 20012 (202) 723-0800	59
quitting smoking	Smokenders 3708 Mt. Diablo Blvd., Suite 100 Lafayette, California 94549	59
high blood pressure	High Blood Pressure Information Center 120/80 National Institutes of Health Bethesda, MD 20205	67
weight loss	Overeaters Anonymous 2190 West 190th Street Torrance, California 90504	87
weight loss	Take Off Pounds Sensibly (TOPS) 4575 South Fifth Street Milwaukee, Wisconsin 53207	87
weight loss	Weight Watchers International 800 Community Drive Manhasset, N.Y. 10030	87

APPENDIX E

A woman should perform a breast self-examination regularly as most breast cancers are first detected by the woman herself. The earlier cancer is detected, the better the results of treatment. According to the American Cancer Society every woman should perform this examination once a month.

The best time to do this examination is about a week after your menstrual period. During this time of your cycle you are less likely to have breast tenderness. Also, the week after menstruation you are less likely to experience cystic breast changes that some women regularly get before a period. After menopause or hysterectomy you should perform the breast self-examination at a convenient time each month. If you do find a breast lump, do contact your doctor so a definite diagnosis can be made. Fortunately the great majority of breast lumps evaluated turn out to be benign.

Breast Self-Examination

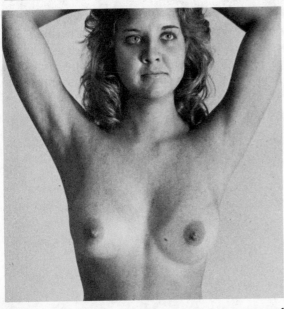

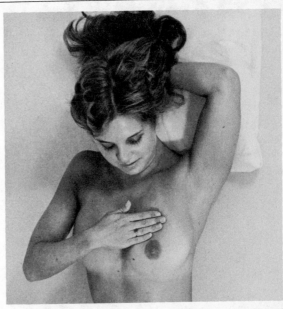

Step 1. Start by standing in front of a mirror and inspect both breasts for anything unusual such as dimpling of the skin or a distinct change in breast size or shape since your last examination. Do this first with your arms at your sides and then with your arms raised above your head.

Step 2. While lying down with your left hand underneath your head, examine your left breast using your right hand. Use the flat of your fingers (not the tips) to feel one area of your breast at a time. Move your fingers back and forth in a circular motion as you examine each area, pressing firmly enough so that the breast tissue moves back and forth under the skin. You will be feeling for a lump or thickening in your breast.

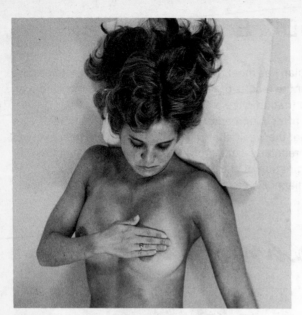

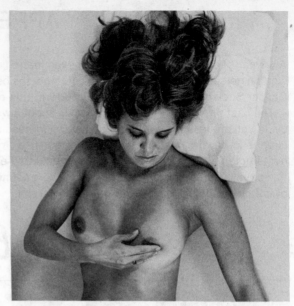

Step 3. Now repeat step 2 but keep your left hand at your side.

Step 4. With your arm still down examine and gently squeeze the nipple and the area around the nipple and note whether there is any discharge. Repeat steps 1–4 as you examine your right breast.

Index

bottle feeding, 123-124
Bradley husband-coached natural childbirth. *See* childbirth education.
breast. *See also* breast-feeding.
  anatomy of, 11-12
  cancer of, 197-200
  discharge from, 295-297
  diseases, noncancerous, of, 197
  examination of, 12, 19
  fibroadenoma of, 197
  fibrocystic disease of, 197, 198, 295, 298, 299-300
  infection of, 299
  lump within, 197, 198, 298-299
  mammograms, 198-199
  risk factors for cancer, 198
  screening of high risk women for cancer, 197-198
  self-examination, 12
  symptoms to report to your doctor, 198
  tenderness of, 299-300
  X-rays of, 198-199
breast-feeding, 122-123
  diet and, 265
  drugs and, 191-192
  sexuality and, 155
breast mass. *See* breast.
breech birth, 137-138
bronchitis. *See* cough.
bulimia, 354
caffeine,
  breast cysts and, 300
  frequent urination and, 368
  nervousness and, 356
  palpitations and, 359
calcium, 264, 265
cancer,
  of the breast, 48, 49, 174, 197-200, 210, 217, 257, 263, 296, 298, 299, 300
  of the cervix, 49, 207-208, 209, 217
  of the colon or rectum, 20, 257, 263, 295, 302
  of the lung, 304, 306
  of the ovary, 49, 212-213, 217
  of the uterus, 48, 49, 174, 213-215, 217
  of the vagina, 208
  of the vulva, 332
carcinoma-in-situ (of cervix), 204, 205, 207, 217
cervical cap, 35, 37
cervical mucus,
  infertility and, 70
cervical mucus method of birth control. *See* natural family planning.

cervical stenosis, 70
cervix, 10, 19-21. *See also* Pap smear.
  anatomy of, 10
  biopsy of, 205, 210
  cancer of, 207-208
  cone biopsy of, 206-207
  DES and changes in. *See* DES.
  infection of, 285, 286, 288, 289, 290, 291, 374
cesarean birth, 138-142
  breech position and, 141
  father-attended, 117-118, 142
  increasing rate of, 140-142
  vaginal delivery after, 140-141
childbirth. *See* labor and delivery.
childbirth education, 76-81
  Bradley husband-coached natural childbirth, 78
  Dick-Read method, 77-78
  hypnosis, 78
  Lamaze method, 78
  organizations, 81
  parenting classes, 79
  yoga, 78
childbirth settings, 81-87
  birthing centers, 85
  birthing rooms, 83-84
  home delivery, 85, 87
  hospital delivery, 83, 85
chills. *See* fever.
cholesterol, 42, 44, 46, 257, 328
chorion biopsy, 60
chromosome disorders, 57, 59-60, 61, 62
chromosomes, 56
circumcision, 125
climacteric, 16
clitoris, 10, 19
colds, 304, 315, 317, 318
colposcopy, 205, 210
conception. *See* fertilization.
condom, 74, 75-76
condylomata. *See* venereal warts.
constipation, 301-303
  dietary fiber and, 257
contact dermatitis, 331-332
contraception. *See* birth control.
contraceptive creams, foams, jellies, and suppositories, 36-37, 49-52
corpus luteum, 13
cough, 304-306
  lung diseases and, 304
  pregnancy and, 305
  remedies, 305-306

℗   Ⓜ

Reference Books from PLUME and MERIDIAN

More Healthy Eating Ideas from PLUME

Eating Well with PLUME